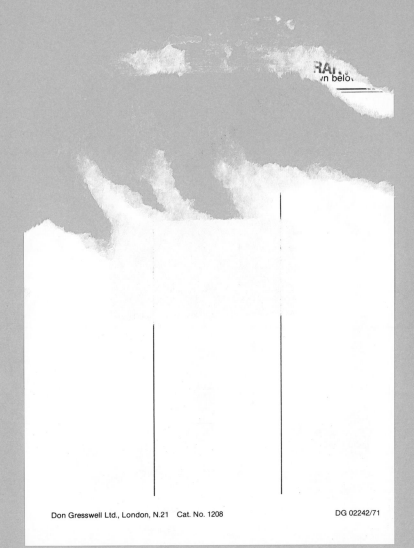

Dana-Farber Cancer Institute

Atlas of
DIAGNOSTIC ONCOLOGY

THIRD EDITION

MULTIMEDIA CD-ROM Single User License Agreement

1. NOTICE. WE ARE WILLING TO LICENSE THE MULTI-MEDIA PROGRAM PRODUCT TITLED **Atlas of Diagnostic Oncology 3e** ("MULTIMEDIA PROGRAM") TO YOU ONLY ON THE CONDITION THAT YOU ACCEPT ALL OF THE TERMS CONTAINED IN THIS LICENSE AGREEMENT. PLEASE READ THIS LICENSE AGREEMENT CAREFULLY BEFORE OPENING THE SEALED DISK PACKAGE. BY OPENING THAT PACKAGE YOU AGREE TO BE BOUND BY THE TERMS OF THIS AGREEMENT. IF YOU DO NOT AGREE TO THESE TERMS WE ARE UNWILLING TO LICENSE THE MULTI-MEDIA PROGRAME TO YOU, AND YOU SHOULD NOT OPEN THE DISK PACKAGE. IN SUCH CASE, PROMPTLY RETURN THE UNOPENED DISK PACKAGE AND ALL OTHER MATERIAL IN THIS PACKAGE, ALONG WITH PROOF OF PAYMENT, TO THE ATHORISED DEALER FROM WHOM YOU OBTAINED IT FOR A FULL REFUND OF THE PRICE YOU PAID.

2. **Ownership and License.** This is a license agreement and NOT an agreement for sale. It permits you to use one copy of the MULTIMEDIA PROGRAM on a single computer. The MULTIMEDIA PROGRAM and its contents are owned by us or our licensors, and are protected by U.S. and international copyright laws. Your rights to use the MULTIMEDIA PROGRAM are specified in this Agreement, and we retain all rights not expressly granted to you in this Agreement.

- You may use one copy of the MULTIMEDIA PROGRAM on a single computer
- After you have installed the MULTIMEDIA PROGRAM on your computer, you may use the MULTIMEDIA PROGRAM on a different computer only if you first delete the files installed by the installation program from the first computer.
- You may not copy any portion of the MULTIMEDIA PROGRAM to your computer hard disk or any other media other than printing out or downloading non- substantial portions of the text and images in the MULITMEDIA PROGRAM for your own internal informational use.
- Your may not copy any of the documentation or other printed materials accompanying the MULTIMEDIA PROGRAM.

Neither concurrent use on two or more computers nor use in a local area network or other network is permitted without separate authorisation and the payment of additional license fees.

3. **Transfer and Other Restrictions.** You may not rent, lend, or lease this MULTIMEDIA PROGRAM. Save as permitted by law, you may not and you may not permit others to (a) disassemble, decompile, or otherwise derive source code from the software included in the MULTIMEDIA PROGRAM (the "Software"), (b) reverse engineer the Software, (c) modify or prepare derivative works of the MULTIMEDIA PROGRAM (d) use the Software in an on-line system, or (e) use the MULTIMEDIA PROGRAM in any manner that infringes on the intellectual property or other rights of another party.
 However, you may transfer this license to use the MULTIMEDIA PROGRAM to another party on a permanent basis by transferring this copy of the License Agreement, the MULTIMEDIA PROGRAM, and all documentation. Such transfer of possession terminates your license from us. Such other party shall be licensed under the terms of this Agreement upon its acceptance of this Agreement by its initial use of the MULTIMEDIA

PROGRAM. If you transfer the MULTIMEDIA PROGRAM, you must remove the installation files from your hard disk and you may not retain any copies of those files for your own use.

4. **Limited Warranty and Limitation of Liability.** For a period of sixty (60) days from the date your acquired the MULTIMEDIA PROGRAM from us or our authorised dealer, we warrant that the media containing the MULTIMEDIA PROGRAM will be free from defects that prevent you from installing the MULTIMEDIA PROGRAM on your computer. If the disk fails to conform to this warranty you may as your sole and exclusive remedy, obtain a replacement free of charge if you return the defective disk to us with a dated proof of purchase. Otherwise the MULTIMEDIA PROGRAM is licensed to you on an "AS IS" basis without any warranty of any nature.

WE DO NOT WARRANT THAT THE MULTIMEDIA PROGRAM WILL MEET YOUR REQUIRMENTS OR THAT ITS OPERATION WILL BE UNINTERRUPTED OR ERROR-FREE. THE EXPRESS TERMS OF THIS AGREEMENT ARE IN LIEU OF ALL WARRANTIES, CONDITIONS, UNDERTAKINGS, TERMS AND OBLIGATIONS IMPLIED BY STATUTE, COMMON LAW, TRADE USAGE, COURSE OF DEALING OR OTHERWISE ALL OF WHICH ARE HEREBY EXCLUDED TO THE FULLEST EXTENT PERMITTED BY LAW, INCLUDING THE IMPLIED WARRANTIES OF SATISFACTORY QUALITY AND FITNESS FOR A PARTICULAR PURPOSE.

 WE SHALL NOT BE LIABLE FOR ANY DAMAGE OR LOSS OF ANY KIND (EXCEPT PERSONAL INJURY OR DEATH RESULTING FROM OUR NEGLIGENCE) ARISING OUT OF OR RESULTING FROM YOUR POSSESSION OR USE OF THE MULTIMEDIA PROGRAM (INCLUDING DATA LOSS OR CORRUPTION), REGARDLESS OF WHETHER SUCH LIABILITY IS BASED IN TORT, CONTRACT OR OTHERWISE AND INCLUDING, BUT NOT LIMITED TO, ACUTAL, SPECIAL, INDIRECT, INCIDENTIAL OR CONSEQUENTIAL DAMAGES. IF THE FOREGOING LIMITATION IS HELD TO BE UNENFORCEABLE OUR MAXIMUM LIABILITY TO YOU SHALL NOT EXCEED THE AMOUNT OF THE LICENSE FEE PAID BY YOU FOR THE MULTIMEDIA PROGRAM. THE REMEDIES AVAILABLE TO YOU AGAINST US AND THE LICENSORS OF MATERIALS INCLUDED IN THE MULTIMEDIA PROGRAM ARE EXCLUSIVE.

5. **Termination.** This license and your right to use this MULTIMEDIA PROGRAM automatically terminate if you fail to comply with any provisions of this Agreement, destroy the copy of the MULTIMEDIA PROGRAM in your possession, or voluntarily return the MULTIMEDIA PROGRAM to us. Upon termination you will destroy all copies of the MULTIMEDIA PROGRAM and documentation.

6. **Miscellaneous Provisions.** This Agreement will be governed by and construed in accordance with English law and you hereby submit to the non-exclusive jurisdiction of the English Courts. This is the entire agreement between us relating to the MULTMEDIA PROGRAM, and supersedes any prior purchase order, communications, advertising or representations concerning the contents of this package, No change or modification of this Agreement will be valid unless it is in writing and is signed by us

Dana-Farber Cancer Institute

Atlas of
DIAGNOSTIC ONCOLOGY

THIRD EDITION

Edited by

Arthur T Skarin

Associate Professor of Medicine
Harvard Medical School
Senior Attending Physician
Medical Director, Lowe Center for Thoracic Oncology
Dana-Farber Cancer Institute
Department of Medicine, Brigham and Women's Hospital

Associate Editors

Kitt Shaffer

Radiology Department
Harvard Medical School
Dana-Farber Cancer Institute
Brigham and Women's Hospital

Tad Wieczorek

Pathology Department
Harvard Medical School
Brigham and Women's Hospital

Foreword by

George P Canellos

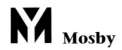 Mosby

*To my wife, for her patience, encouragement, and devotion
during the preparation of this atlas;*

To William C. Moloney, M.D., and Emil Frei III, M.D., who stimulated my interest in hematology and oncology

and

To all our patients who have contributed so much to medical education

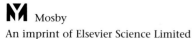 Mosby

An imprint of Elsevier Science Limited

© 2003, Elsevier Science Limited. All rights reserved.

The right of Arthur T Skarin to be identified as an editor of this work has been asserted by him in accordance with the Copyright, Designs and Patents Act 1988

Second edition 1996
Third edition 2003

ISBN 0 7234 3206 6

British Library Cataloguing in Publication Data
A catalogue record for this book is available from the British Library

Library of Congress Cataloging in Publication Data
A catalog record for this book is available from the Library of Congress

Note
Medical knowledge is constantly changing. As new information becomes available, changes in treatment, procedures, equipment and the use of drugs become necessary. The contributors and the publishers have taken care to ensure that the information given in this text is accurate and up to date. However, readers are strongly advised to confirm that the information, especially with regard to drug usage, complies with the latest legislation and standards of practice.

Commissioning Editor: Dolores Meloni
Project Development Manager: Louise Cook
Project Manager: Cheryl Brant
Design: Andy Chapman
Illustration Manager: Mick Ruddy
Illustrator: Robin Dean

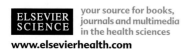 your source for books, journals and multimedia in the health sciences

www.elsevierhealth.com

Typeset by Marie McNestry
Printed in Spain by Grafos SA

The Publisher's policy is to use **paper manufactured from sustainable forests**

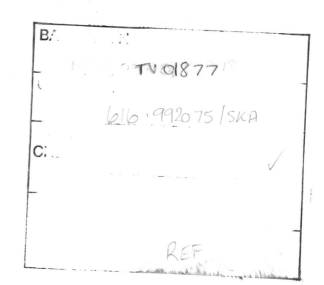

Contents

Foreword

This edition of the *Atlas of Diagnostic Oncology* represents the best of the three editions thus far. The editor and his associates in radiology and pathology have produced not only an excellent visual volume, but by upgrading the summary text that deals with the histology, staging, and clinical manifestations of these tumors the book has been brought up-to-date in all instances. There have been considerable advances in the radiographic and molecular diagnosis of disease. Many of these advances are incorporated in this issue. This atlas has become a classic and will serve as an excellent addition to the knowledge base of a practicing oncologist or fellow in training.

All of the contributors to this issue are members of the Harvard Medical School faculty and the Dana-Farber Cancer Institute. Eminent in their areas of expertise, they have been brought together by Dr Arthur Skarin who, in his own right, is a distinguished clinician in medical oncology. Dr Skarin is also a skilled medical photographer.

The *Atlas of Diagnostic Oncology* 3rd Edition will complement any knowledge base, whether it is textbook, CD-Rom or internet-based. The reader now has the opportunity of having a CD-Rom instead of the previously offered 35mm slide sets. This will enhance the ability of the clinician to search for the relevant areas. The new chapters on molecular biology and the revised chapters in other areas bring this volume as up-to-date as possible. It further emphasizes the important role of the cancer clinician as the lynchpin in the multi-disciplinary team that evaluates and recommends therapy for patients. It is an honor for me to write the Foreword for Dr Skarin who has been a close colleague for many years. I am further proud of the fact that 17 of the 38 contributors to this third volume were former fellows in medical oncology at the Dana-Farber Cancer Institute. Sometimes the most useful product is the people we train, and this volume is a testimony to that fact.

George P. Canellos, MD, DSc(Hons)
William Rosenberg Professor of Medicine
Harvard Medical School Senior Physician,
Dana-Farber Cancer Institute Boston, MA

Preface

Considerable progress has occurred in the field of oncology during the past ten years since the first edition of the *Atlas of Diagnostic Oncology*. As a result, three new chapters were added to the second edition, in addition to expansion of the original 14 chapters. The new chapters were Chapter 1, "The Role of Molecular Probes and Other Markers in the Diagnosis of Malignancy", Chapter 2, "Radiographic Evaluation of Cancer", and Chapter 17, "Aids Associated Malignancies". Additional cancer specialists assisted in the preparation and revision of the second edition. Because of further progress in cancer research, diagnosis, staging and management, a third edition was necessary. This required extensive revision plus the addition of Chapter 18, "Systemic and Mucocutaneous Reactions to Chemotherapy". Another 15 cancer specialists were selected as co-authors for the update of the third edition. They all have academic positions at the Harvard Medical School, Dana-Farber Cancer Institute, Brigham and Women's Hospital and/or the Massachusetts General Hospital, Boston, MA.

The chapter formats have remained the same: a general review of the cancer including incidence, epidemiology, etiology and histopathology with molecular biology when relevant and clinical features, which is followed by diagnostic studies and current clinical and pathologic staging. Detailed charts are used for histopathological classification, diagnostic studies, and prognostic factors when important. Generous illustrations with detailed figure legends are utilized for examples of histopathology, staging, radiographs, CT, MRI and PET images and differential diagnosis, along with examples of various clinical manifestations. As with previous editions, treatment recommendations are not included since these are outside the goals of this cancer this book. The reader is referred to standard oncology textbooks and current review articles for details concerning management of cancer patients.

Of note, previous editions of this Atlas had optional 35 mm slide sets available for teaching purposes. Advances in computer technology have made it possible to provide a CD-Rom with each copy of this edition. The disc contains all the illustrations and charts. We feel the CD-Rom will greatly improve the scope of this atlas and allow for a broader use in lectures and other teaching functions. This fulfills our original goals of preparing a unique and illustrative, educational *Atlas of Diagnostic Oncology*.

Arthur T. Skarin, MD
September 2002

Contributors

Annick Van Den Abbeele, MD
Associate Professor of Radiology, Harvard Medical School
Director, Division of Nuclear Medicine
Dana-Farber Cancer Institute
Department of Nuclear Medicine
Brigham and Women's Hospital
Boston, MA, USA

Kenneth C. Anderson, MD
Professor of Medicine, Harvard Medical School
Director, Jerome Lipper Multiple Myeloma Center
Adult Oncology Division
Dana-Farber Cancer Institute
Department of Medicine
Brigham and Women's Hospital
Boston, MA, USA

Karen H. Antman, MD
Associate Professor of Medicine
Harvard Medical School Director, Solid Tumor
Autologous Marrow Program
Dana-Farber Cancer Institute
Boston, MA
Present Position: Professor of Medicine &
Pharmacology
Director of Herbert Irving Comprehensive Cancer
Center
Chief, Division of Medical Oncology
Columbia University Medical Center
New York, NY, USA

Ramon Blanco, MD
Fellow in Surgical Pathology
Department of Pathology
Brigham and Women's Hospital
Boston, MA, USA
Present Position: Department of Pathology
Falmouth Hospital
Falmouth, MA, USA

Susana Campos, MD
Instructor in Medicine, Harvard Medical School
Gillette Center for Women's Cancer
Adult Oncology Division
Dana-Farber Cancer Institute
Department of Medicine
Brigham and Women's Hospital
Boston, MA, USA

John R. Clark, MD
Instructor in Medicine, Harvard Medical School
Attending Physician, Head and Neck Tumor Clinic
Adult Oncology Division
Dana-Farber Cancer Institute
Department of Medicine
Brigham and Women's Hospital
Boston, MA, USA
Present Position:
Oral and Maxillofacial Surgery Division
Massachusetts General Hospital
Boston, MA, USA

A. Dimitrios Colevas, MD
Instructor in Medicine, Harvard Medical School
Attending Physician, Head and Neck Tumor Center
Adult Oncology Division
Dana-Farber Cancer Institute
Brigham and Women's Hospital
Boston, MA, USA
Present Position: Senior Investigator
Investigational Drug Branch
National Cancer Institute, CTEP
Rockville, MD, USA

Christopher L. Corless, MD, PhD
Instructor of Pathology, Harvard Medical School
Department of Pathology
Brigham and Women's Hospital
Boston, MA, USA
Present Position: Assistant Professor of Pathology
Oregon Health and Sciences University
Portland, Oregon
USA

Faith Davies, MBBCh, MRCP, MD
Blood Component Laboratory
Adult Oncology Division
Dana-Farber Cancer Institute
Department of Medicine
Brigham and Women's Hospital
Boston, MA, USA
Present Position: Department of Health Clinician
Scientist and Academic Specialist Registrar
University of Leeds and Leeds General Infirmary
Leeds, UK

George Demetri, MD
Associate Professor of Medicine, Harvard Medical School
Director, Sarcoma Program
Adult Oncology Division
Dana-Farber Cancer Institute
Department of Medicine
Brigham and Women's Hospital
Boston, MA, USA

David Dorfman, MD, PhD
Associate Professor of Pathology, Harvard Medical School
Associate Pathologist
Department of Pathology
Brigham and Women's Hospital
Boston, MA, USA

Joseph Paul Eder, MD
Assistant Professor of Medicine, Harvard Medical School
Phase I Group
Adult Oncology Division
Dana-Farber Cancer Institute
Department of Medicine
Brigham and Women's Hospital
Boston, MA,USA

Marc B. Garnick, MD
Associate Professor of Medicine, Harvard Medical School
Associate in Medicine and Genitourinary Oncology
Adult Oncology Division
Dana-Farber Cancer Institute
Present Position: Clinical Professor of Medicine,
Harvard Medical School
Associate in Medicine and Genitourinary Oncology
Department of Hematology/Oncology
Beth Israel-Deaconess Medical Center
Boston, MA, USA

David R. Genest, MD
Associate Professor of Pathology, Harvard Medical School
Staff Pathologist
Department of Pathology
Brigham and Women's Hospital
Boston, MA, USA

Holcombe Grier, MD
Associate Professor of Pediatrics, Harvard Medical School
Associate Chief, Pediatric Clinical Oncology
Dana-Farber Cancer Institute
Children's Hospital
Boston, MA, USA

Daniel Hayes, MD
Assistant Professor of Medicine, Harvard Medical School
Gillette Center for Women's Cancers
Adult Oncology Division
Dana-Farber Cancer Institute
Boston, MA, USA
Present Position: Assistant Professor of Medicine,
University of Michigan School
Clinical Director, Breast Cancer Program
University of Michigan Cancer Center
Ann Arbor, Michigan, USA

F. Stephen Hodi, MD
Instructor in Medicine, Harvard Medical School
Cutaneous Oncology Program
Adult Oncology Division
Dana-Farber Cancer Institute
Department of Medicine
Brigham and Women's Hospital
Boston, MA, USA

Frederic A. Hoffer, MD
Associate Professor of Radiology, Harvard Medical School
Radiologist
Children's Hospital
Boston, MA, USA

Nancy E. Joste, MD
Instructor of Pathology, Harvard Medical School
Department of Pathology
Brigham and Women's Hospital
Boston, MA, USA

Present Position: Assistant Professor of Pathology
Department of Pathology
University of New Mexico School of Medicine
Albuquerque, New Mexico

Philip W. Kantoff, MD
Associate Professor of Medicine, Harvard Medical
School
Director, Lank Center for Genitourinary Oncology
Adult Oncology Division
Dana-Farber Cancer Institute
Department of Medicine
Brigham and Women's Hospital
Boston, MA, USA

Karen J. Krag, MD
Clinical Instructor in Medicine, Harvard Medical
School
Adult Oncology Division
Dana-Farber Cancer Institute
Department of Medicine
Brigham and Women's Hospital
Boston, MA, USA
Present Position: North Shore Cancer Center
Peabody, MA, USA

Matthew Kulke, MD
Assistant Professor of Medicine, Harvard Medcial
School
Gastrointestinal Cancer Program
Adult Oncology Division
Dana-Farber Cancer Institute
Department of Medicine
Brigham and Women's Hospital
Boston, MA, USA

Janina Longtine, MD
Assistant Professor of Pathology, Harvard Medical
School
Clinical Director Molecular Biology Laboratory
Department of Pathology
Brigham and Women's Hospital
Boston, MA, USA

Elizabeth A. Maher, MD, PhD
Instructor in Medicine, Harvard Medical School
Neuro-Oncology Program
Adult Oncology Division
Dana-Farber Cancer Institute
Department of Medicine
Brigham and Women's Hospital
Boston, MA, USA

Ursula Matulonis, MD
Assistant Professor of Medicine, Harvard Medical
School
Gillette Center for Women's Cancers
Adult Oncology Division
Dana-Farber Cancer Institute
Department of Medicine
Brigham and Women's Hospital
Boston, MA, USA

Ann C. McKee, MD
Instructor in Pathology, Harvard Medical School
Division of Neuropathology
Massachusetts General Hospital
Boston, MA, USA
Present Position: Associate Professor of Neurology
and Pathology
Boston University School of Medicine
Bedford, MA, USA

Francis D. Moore, Jr, MD
Associate Professor of Medicine, Harvard Medical
School
Chief, Division of General and Gastrointestinal
Surgery
Brigham and Women's Hospital
Boston, MA, USA

William Oh, MD
Assistant Professor of Medicine, Harvard Medical
School
Lank Center for Genitourinary Oncology
Adult Oncology Division
Dana-Farber Cancer Institute
Department of Medicine
Boston, MA, USA

Antonio Perez-Atayde, MD
Associate Professor of Pathology, Harvard Medical
School
Department of Pathology
Children's Hospital
Boston, MA, USA

Marshall Posner, MD
Associate Professor of Medicine, Harvard Medical
School
Head and Neck Cancer Program
Adult Oncology Division
Dana-Farber Cancer Institute
Department of Medicine
Brigham and Women's Hospital
Boston, MA, USA

Ravi Salgia, MD, PhD
Assistant Professor of Medicine, Harvard Medical
Schhool
Lowe Center for Thoracic Oncology
Adult Oncology Division
Dana-Farber Cancer Institute
Department of Medicine
Brigham and Women's Hospital
Boston, MA, USA

David Scadden, MD
Associate Professor of Medicine, Harvard Medical
School
Director, AIDS Hematology Oncology Research Unit
Deaconess Hospital
Boston,MA, USA
Present Position: Associate Professor of Medicine,
Harvard Medical School
Director of Experimental Hematology AIDS Research
Massachusetts General Hospital
Boston, MA, USA

Kitt Shaffer, MD, PhD
Associate Professor of Medicine, Harvard Medical
School
Clinical Director of Oncology Radiology
Dana-Farber Cancer Institute
Department of Radiology
Brigham and Women's Hospital
Boston, MA, USA

Mark A. Socinski, MD
Medical Oncology Fellow, Harvard Medical Schoool
Adult Oncology Division
Dana-Farber Cancer Institute
Department of Medicine
Brigham and Women's Hospital
Boston, MA, USA
Present Position: Assistant Professor of Medicine
Division of Medical Oncology
University of North Carolina
Chapel Hill, NC, USA

James N. Suojanen, MD
Instructor of Radiology, Harvard Medical School
Director of Neuroradiology
Deaconess Hospital
Boston, MA, USA
Present Position: Clinical Instructor of Radiology,
Harvard Medical School
Department of Radiology
South Shore Hospital
South Weymouth, MA, USA

Jerold R. Turner, MD, PhD
Instructor in Pathology, Harvard Medical School
Staff Pathologist, Department of Pathology
Brigham and Women's Hospital
Boston, MA, USA
Present Position: Department of Pathology
Harper Hospital
Detroit, MI 48201

Michael M. Wick, MD, PhD
Associate Professor of Dermatology, Harvard
Medical School
Laboratory of Molecular Dermatologic Oncology
Dana-Farber Cancer Institute
Department of Medicine
Brigham and Women's Hospital
Boston, MA, USA
Present Position: Vice President
CV Therapeutics Inc.
Palo Alto, CA, USA

Tad Wieczorek, MD
Clinical Fellow in Pathology, Harvard Medical School
Department of Pathology
Brigham and Women's Hospital
Boston, MA, USA

Acknowledgments

I would like to acknowledge the associate editors of the first edition, Dr Maxine Jochelson (currently Director of Oncologic Radiology and Women's Imaging, Cedars-Sinai Medical Center, Los Angeles, CA) and Dr Robert Penny (currently Director of Hematopathology, Community and St. Vincent's Hospital of Indianapolis, IN). Their immense help in organizing and evaluating the radiographic and pathology material for the chapters contributed significantly to the success of the Atlas. In the extensive revision and update of the third edition, I deeply appreciate the work of the current associate editors, Dr Kitt Shaffer, Clinical Director of Radiology at Dana-Farber Cancer Institute and Dr Tad Wieczorek, Clinical Fellow in Pathology at Brigham and Women's Hospital. Their expertise was invaluable in emphasizing the illustrative and teaching aspects of this edition. I also appreciate the work of the editorial staff at Elsevier Science in preparing the revised layouts and keeping everything on schedule.

Introduction

The increasing impact of cancer on patient populations and economics is well known. In the US about one in three people will be diagnosed with cancer during their lifetime, and every minute another person dies from cancer (Calabresi et al, 1995). Furthermore, about 1.3 million new cases will add to the more than 8 million individuals alive today who have already been diagnosed with cancer. The lifetime risk of being diagnosed with cancer is noted in Figure 1 (Stat Bite, 2001). Men have a 43% lifetime risk while women have a 38% chance of being diagnosed with any type of cancer. The incidence rates for selected childhood cancers are noted in Figure 2 (Stat Bite, 2001).

Detailed statistics concerning incidence and deaths in the US have been published annually by the American Cancer Society (ACS). The data on 2002 estimated new cases and deaths related to organ sites are summarized in Figures 3 and 4 (Jemal et al, 2002).

Of note, however, a continued decrease in cancer incidence and death rates has been reported by collaborative work from several groups including the NCI (National Cancer Institute) and ACS (Howe et al, 2001). Data reveals that from 1992 through 1998, the total cancer death rates declined in both men and women. Among specific tumor sites, breast cancer incidence rates in women increased slightly because of higher rates in some older age groups. Lung cancer mortality rates, a major cause of death in women, continued to increase but more slowly than in earlier years.

The increased incidence of many cancers is explained by known epidemiologic factors such as an improved detection of early prostate and breast cancers, cigarette smoking among women, HIV infection in young and middle-aged men, and sunlight exposure patterns (Devesa et al, 1995). A full understanding of cancer trends will require further research into the changing exposures to various carcinogens as well as progress in molecular epidemiology.

An important research database for the evaluation and study of cancer trends is the Surveillance, Epidemiology, and End Results (SEER) Program. A recent supplement to the journal *Cancer* presents data based on more than 1 million microscopically proven invasive cancers and 98 000 *in situ* cancers diagnosed during the period 1973-1987 (Percy et al, 1995). The special supplement entitled "Histology of Cancer" covers major anatomic sites or organ systems with important data regarding

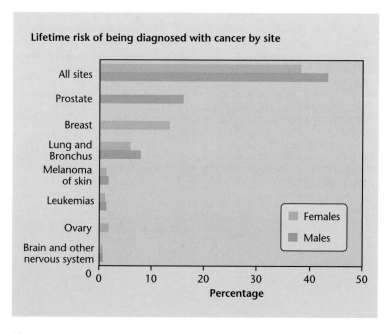

Fig. 1 Lifetime Risk of being diagnosed with cancer, by site. Used with permission, JNCI, V. 93, No. 10, May 16, 2001, p. 742.

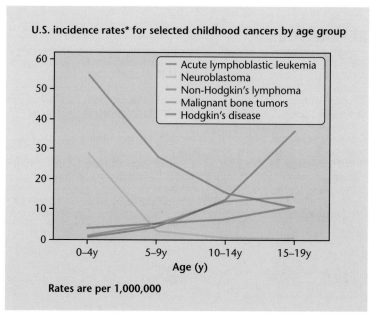

Fig. 2 U.S. Incidence notes for selected childhood cancers. Used with permission, JNCI, V. 93, No. 16, August 15, 2001, p. 1201.

frequency and histology rates, as well as 5-year survival rates. It is a useful complement to this *Atlas of Diagnostic Oncology*.

Two other ancillary references useful to those concerned with the care of cancer patients are a review of prognostic factors for various cancers (Burke et al, 1993), prepared by the American Joint Committee on Cancer (AJCC) and the AJCC Cancer Staging Manual (6th edition, Greene et al, 2002). All of the TNM staging information is now uniform between the AJCC and the UICC (International Union Against Cancer). However, major new changes in staging have only occurred in breast cancer and melanoma.

Discoveries of cancer susceptibility genes (see Chapter 1) are creating new opportunities for translational cancer control research. For example, carriers of the breast cancer gene (*BRCA1*) are at high risk for hereditary breast and ovarian cancers. While these carriers are potential candidates for early detection and chemoprevention studies, cancer pre-disposition testing poses important questions not only about ethical, legal and social issues, but also about technologic, logistic and economic challenges (Li, 1995).

Also, of great interest is the availability of new technology to perform DNA microarrays on tumor samples (Ramaswamy, 2002). Among many applications, this technique will allow for more accurate cancer diagnosis as well as for predicting prognosis.

Finally, continuing research in the area of environmental carcinogenic agents including logical measures in reducing the cancer epidemic, such as the elimination of cigarette smoking, cannot be underestimated.

Arthur T. Skarin, MD

Table 1 Estimated cancer statistics in US men, 2002

	New cancer cases*	Cancer deaths
Total number, all sites	637,500	288,200
Distribution by site (%)		
Prostate	30	10
Lung	14	33
Colon and rectum	11	10
Urinary	10	6
Leukemia and lymphoma	8	9
Melanoma of skin	4	2
Oral	3	3
Pancreas	2	5
Stomach	2	3
All other	16	19

*Excluding basal and squamous cell skin cncers and in situ carcinomas except bladder. (From Jemal *et al*, 2002)

Table 2 Estimated cancer statistics in US women, 2002

	New cancer cases*	Cancer deaths
Total number, all sites	647,400	267,300
Distribution by site (%)		
Breast	31	15
Lung	13	25
Colon and rectum	12	11
Uterus	8	4
Leukemia and lymphomas	7	8
Ovary	4	5
Urinary	4	4
Melanoma and skin	4	1
Oral	2	1
Pancreas	2	6
All other	13	20

*Excluding basal and squamous cell skin cancers and in situ carcinomas except bladder. (From Jemal et al, 2002). JNCI, V. 93, No. 10, May 16, 2001, p. 742

REFERENCES

Burke HB, Henson DE: Criteria for prognostic factors and for an enhanced prognostic system. Cancer 1993; 72: 3131-3135.

Calabresi P (Chairman), Antman K, Bettinghaus E, et al: Cancer at a crossroads: A report to Congress for the Nation. Cancer 1995; 76:135-148.

Devesa SD, Blot WJ, Stone BJ, et al: Recent cancer trends in the United States. JNCI 1995: 87:175-182.

Greene FL, Page DL, Fleming ID, et al: AJCC Cancer Staging Manual, 6th Ed. Springer-Verlag, New York, 2002.

Howe HL, Wingo PA, Thun MJ, et al: Annual report to the nation on the status of cancer (1973 through 1998), featuring cancers with recent increasing trends. JNCI 2001; 93:824-842.

Jemal A, Thomas A, Murray T, et al: Cancer statistics, 2002. CA Cancer J Clin 2002;52:23-47.

Li FP: Translational research on hereditary colon, breast, and ovarian caners. Monogr Natl Cancer Inst 1995;17:1-4.

Percy C, Young, Jr., JL, Muir C, et al: Histology of cancer incidence and prognosis: SEER population-based data, 1973-1987. Cancer 1995; 75:140-421.

Ramaswamy S, Golub TR: DNA Microarrays in clinical oncology. J Clin Oncol 2002;20:1932-1941.

Stat Bite: Lifetime risk of being diagnosed with cancer. JNCI 2001; 93: 742.

Stat Bite: US Incidence Rates for Selected Childhood Cancers. JNCI 2001; 93: 1201.

The role of molecular probes and other markers in the diagnosis of malignancy

Tad Wieczorek, Janina A. Longtine

Histopathologic assessment is a cornerstone in the diagnosis, classification and grading of malignancies. Light microscopic evaluation augmented by histochemical stains is sufficient in the majority of cases to provide adequate information for diagnosis and prognostication. However, it is limited by subjectivity and imprecision in the evaluation of poorly differentiated malignancies, tumors of unknown primary origin and unusual neoplasms. In an era of increasingly sophisticated therapeutic protocols and improved cancer survival as well as the ability to obtain samples by core biopsy or fine-needle aspiration (FNA), ancillary techniques have been developed to increase accuracy and reproducibility. They rely on cell-specific ultrastructural features, antigen expression or tumor-specific genetic changes.

Electron microscopy (EM) may assist in the diagnosis of poorly differentiated malignancies by revealing specific ultrastructural characteristics such as melanosomes in melanoma, neurosecretory granules in neuroendocrine carcinoma or desmosomes in carcinomas. It is limited by requirements for special fixation in glutaldehyde, by high labor and expense in processing and by sampling errors. In most instances, the advent of monoclonal antibodies directed against cellular proteins, coupled with the immunoperoxidase technique, has superseded EM in allowing more accurate designation of epithelial, mesenchymal, hematolymphoid, neuroendocrine or glial origin of neoplasms. One example is immunolocalization of cytoskeletal intermediate filaments which are differentially expressed in different cell types. Table 1.1 lists the intermediate filaments most useful in determining the cell lineage of tumors. The cytokeratins are a complex family of polypeptides that are expressed in various combinations in different epithelial cell types. Antibodies to cytokeratin subtypes can sometimes be utilized to identify the epithelial origin of metastatic carcinomas of unknown primaries. For example, the pattern of reactivity for cytokeratin 7 (54 kDa), which is expressed in most glandular and ductal epithelium and transitional epithelium of the urinary tract, and for cytokeratin 20 (46 kDa), which is more restricted in its expression, has been helpful in this regard.

In addition to the intermediate filaments, other monoclonal antibodies to cellular or tumor antigens are available. In the past decade, advances in the technique of immunohistochemistry have allowed consistent reliable application in routinely processed surgical pathology specimens. Antigen retrieval techniques, including proteolytic digestion and heat-induced antigen retrieval, sensitive detection systems, automation and a broad range of antibodies have all contributed to this advance. As a result, immunohistochemistry plays an important role in tumor diagnosis. Table 1.2 lists a panel of antibodies that can be utilized in routine formalin-fixed paraffin-embedded tissue to diagnose poorly differentiated neoplasms. (Specific markers in the immunophenotyping of leukemia and lymphoma are discussed in Chapters 13 and 14.) A differential diagnosis is generated by clinical and morphologic features which can then be further refined by the use of immunohistochemistry. It is important to realize that the majority of antibodies are not entirely specific in lineage determination and 'aberrant' staining patterns are observed. In addition, there is biologic variation in poorly differentiated neoplasms resulting in variation in protein expression. Therefore, accuracy is enhanced by using a panel of antisera to determine lineage or primary site. One application of this principle is distinguishing between poorly differentiated adenocarcinoma and mesothelioma in pleural tumors. Table 1.3 demonstrates the differential immunoprofile.

While a panel of monoclonal markers greatly aids in the diagnosis of a particular cancer, three malignancies can be confirmed solely by demonstrating the presence of a highly specific protein. Papillary and follicular thyroid carcinomas are characterized by immunoreactivity to thyroglobulin, prostate carcinoma by detection of prostate-specific antigen and breast carcinoma by a positive reaction for gross cystic duct fluid protein, which is present in approximately 50–70% of cases. It is noteworthy that the latter protein is also present in the rare apocrine gland carcinoma. Other antibodies which are not tissue-specific markers but useful in antibody panels include CD99 (cell surface glycoprotein p30/32 encoded by MIC2 gene) for Ewing's/peripheral neuroectodermal tumor, CD117 (c-kit) for gastrointestinal stromal tumors and CD31 (platelet endothelial cell adhesion molecule) for vascular endothelial neoplasms.

Somatic mutations, i.e. mutations that occur in the genes of non-germline tissues, are central to the development of cancer. A series of different mutations in critical genes is probably necessary for malignant transformation to occur. The mutations may be deletions, duplications, point mutations and/or chromosomal translocations in the DNA of the tumor precursor cell. The mutations affect regulation of the cell cycle, differentiation, apoptosis or cell–cell and cell–matrix interactions. Different neoplasms have different combinations of genetic alterations, which lead to clonal proliferations of cells. The genetic alterations can be used as diagnostic markers for malignancies. This is best characterized in lymphomas and leukemias where specific genetic translocations result in the production of chimeric mRNA and novel proteins. These translocations are the *sine qua non* for the classification of some leukemias, such as the Philadelphia chromosome [t(9;22)(q34;q11)] for chronic myelogenous leukemia and t(15;17)(q22;q11–21) for acute promyelocytic leukemia. (See Chapters 13 and 14 for further examples.) Chromosomal translocations also commonly occur in soft tissue tumors. Table 1.4 lists the soft tissue tumor translocations which are diagnostically useful.

Complete cytogenetic analysis requires fresh, viable tumor. Fluorescence *in situ* hybridization (FISH) can be performed on interphase nuclei obtained from frozen or fixed paraffin-embedded tissue and can identify characteristic cytogenetic abnormalities as an adjunct to tumor diagnosis. For example, FISH probes which flank the EWS gene region show a 'split apart' signal when an EWS rearrangement is present, as in Ewing's sarcoma (*see* Fig. 1.1). Many of the characteristic cytogenetic abnormalities of neoplasms have been cloned, allowing for the utilization of molecular biology techniques such as Southern blot hybridization or the polymerase chain reaction (PCR) in diagnoses. These techniques can utilize frozen tumor or even fixed, embedded tissue (in PCR) and improve diagnoses by identifying the characteristic chromosomal translocations of malignancies at the molecular level. A specific translocation can be detected in as little as 1 in 100 000 or 1 in 1 000 000 cells. Southern blot hybridization or PCR can also identify clonal rearrangements of the immunoglobulin or T-cell receptor genes as an adjunct to the diagnosis of lymphoma or lymphoid leukemias.

Genetic analysis of neoplasms may also provide prognostic information, such as identifying the bcr-abl rearrangement in Philadelphia chromosome-positive acute lymphocy leukemia (ALL) or N-myc amplification in neuroblastoma. The genetics of cancer also extends to inherited predisposition to neoplasms described in a number of families. These syndromes include germline mutations of tumor suppressor genes, such as familial retinoblastoma, and mutations of DNA repair genes as in ataxia-telangiectasia or hereditary non-polyposis colon cancer. Some of these are listed in Table 1.5.

Table 1.1 Cytoskeletal intermediate filaments

Cell Type	Intermediate Filaments	Molecular Weight or Subtype	Presence in Tumor
Epithelial	Cytokeratins	40–67	Keratinizing and non-keratinizing epithelial carcinomas
Mesenchymal	Vimentin	58	Wide distribution: sarcomas, melanomas, many lymphomas, some carcinomas
Muscle	Desmin	53	Leiomyosarcoma, rhabdomyosarcoma
Glial astrocytes	Glial fibrillary acidic protein	51	Gliomas, ependymoma
Neurons	Neural filament	68, 160, 200	Neural tumors, neuroblastoma

Table 1.2 Immunocytochemistry in the differential diagnosis of malignancies

Malignancy	Chromogranin/ Synaptophysin	EMA	HMB-45	Keratin	LCA	PLAP	SMA/ Desmin	S100
Carcinoma	–	+	–/+	+	–	–/+	–	–/+
Germ cell	–	–	–	+/–*	–	+	–	–
Lymphoma	–	–	–	–	+	–	–	–
Melanoma	–	–	+	–	–	–	–	+
Neuroendocrine	+	–	–	+/–	–	–	–	–
Sarcoma	–	–/+	–/+	–/+	–	–	+/–	–/+

+ positive   +/– mainly positive, occasionally negative
– negative   –/+ mainly negative, occasionally positive

*Keratin is usually negative in seminomas, but positive in non-seminomatous germ cell tumors

EMA, Epithelial membrane antigen   LCA, Leukocyte common antigen
PLAP, Placental alkaline phosphatase   SMA, Smooth muscle actin

Table 1.3 Antibody panel in the differential diagnosis of adenocarcinoma and mesothelioma

Malignancy	Keratin*	Calretinin	CD15 (Leu-M1)	CEA
Adenocarcinoma	+	−	+	+
Mesothelioma	+	+	−	−

*Keratin positivity in the appropriate clinicopathologic setting limits the differential diagnosis to adenocarcinoma and mesothelioma

+ positive, − negative

Table 1.4 Examples of cytogenetic translocations in soft tissue tumors*

Malignancy	Characteristic Cytogenetic Abnormality	Genes
Alveolar soft part sarcoma	t(X;17)(p11;q25)	Unknown
Chondrosarcoma, myxoid	t(9;22)(q22;q12)	TEC/EWS
Clear cell sarcoma (MMSP)	t(12;22)(q13;q12)	ATF1/EWS
Dermatofibrosarcoma protuberans	t(17;22)(q22;q13)	PDGFB/COL1A1
DSRCT	t(11;22)(p13;q12)	WT1/EWS
Ewing's sarcoma/PNET	t(11;22)(q24;q12)	FLI1/EWS
	t(21;22)(q22;q12)	ERG/EWS
	t(7;22)(p22;q12)	ETV1/EWS
	t(17;22)(q12;q12)	EIAF/EWS
	t(2;22)(q33;q12)	FEV/EWS
Infantile fibrosarcoma	t(12;15)(p13;q25)	ETV6/NTRK3
Liposarcoma, myxoid	t(12;16)(q13;p11)	CHOP/TLS
	t(12;22)(q13;q11–12)	CHOP/?
Rhabdomyosarcoma, alveolar	t(2;13)(q35–37;q14)	PAX3/FKHR
	t(1;13)(p36;q14)	PAX7/FKHR
Synovial sarcoma	t(X;18)(p11,q11)	SSX1/SYT
		SSX2/SYT

*PNET, Peripheral neuroectodermal tumor
DSRCT, Desmoplastic small round cell tumor
MMSP, Malignant melanoma of the soft parts

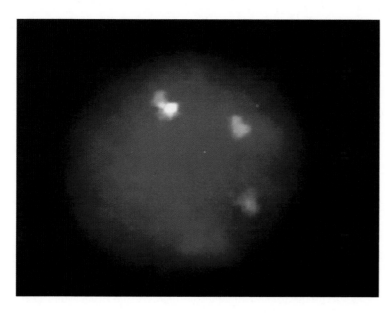

Fig. 1.1 Fluorescence *in situ* hybridization (FISH) on an interphase nucleus with red and green probes flanking the EWS gene demonstrate one fused and one split signal, the latter indicating rearrangement of the EWS gene region. (Courtesy of Dr Paola Dal Cin, Cytogenetics Laboratory, Brigham and Women's Hospital.)

Table 1.5 Examples of inherited syndromes predisposing to cancer

Syndrome	Chromosome Locus	Gene
Ataxia-telangiactasia	11q22	ATM
Hereditary breast/ovarian cancer	17q21	BRCA-1
Familial adenomatous polyposis	5q21	APC
Familial retinoblastoma	13q14	RB1
Hereditary non-polyposis Colorectal cancer (Lynch syndrome)	2p2 3p21–22	hMSH2 hMLH1
Li-Fraumeni	17p13	p53
Multiple endocrine neoplasia, Type 1	11q13	MEN1
Multiple endocrine neoplasia, Type 2	10q11.2	RET
Neurofibromatosis, Type 1	17q11	NF1
Neurofibromatosis, Type 2	22q12	NF2
von Hippel–Lindau disease	3p25	VHL

REFERENCES

Chan JKC: Advances in immunohistochemistry: impact on surgical pathology practice. Semin Diagn Pathol 2000; 17 : 170–177.

Chu P, Wu E, Weiss LM: Cytokeratin 7 and cytokeratin 20 expression in epithelial neoplasms: a survey of 435 cases. Mod Pathol 2000; 13(9):962–971.

Graadt van Roggen JF, Bovee JV, Morreau J, Hogendoorn PC: Diagnostic and prognostic implications of the unfolding molecular biology of bone and soft tissue tumors. J Clin Pathol 1999; 52 : 481–489.

Jones D, Fletcher CDM: How shall we apply the new biology to diagnostics in surgical pathology? J Pathol 1999; 187 : 147–154.

Lasko D, Cavenee W: Loss of constitutional heterozygosity in human cancer. Ann Rev Genet 1991; 25 : 281–314.

Moran CA, Wick MR, Shuster S: The role of immunohistochemistry in the diagnosis of malignant mesothelioma. Semin Diagn Pathol 2000; 17 : 178–183.

Raj GV, Moreno JG, Gomella LG: Utilization of polymerase chain reaction technology in the detection of solid tumors. Cancer 1998; 82(8): 1419–1442.

Reese DM, Slamon DJ: HER-2/neu signal transduction in human breast and ovarian cancer. Stem Cells 1997; 15 : 1–8.

Ried T: Interphase cytogenetics and its role in molecular diagnostics of solid tumors. Am J Pathol 1998; 152(2):325–327.

Scriver CR, Beaudet AL, Sly WS, Valle D, eds: Metabolic and Molecular Bases of Inherited Disease, 8th edn. McGraw-Hill, New York, 2001.

Sreekantaiah C: The cytogenetic and molecular characterization of benign and malignant soft tissue tumors. Cytogenet Cell Genet 1998; 82 : 13–29.

Shuster S: Recent advances in the application of immunohistochemical markers for the diagnosis of soft tissue tumors. Semin Diagn Pathol 2000; 17 : 225–235.

Vogelstein B, Kinzler K, eds: The Genetic Basis of Human Cancers, 2nd edn. McGraw-Hill, New York, 1999.

Wick MR: Immunohistology of neuroendocrine and neuroectodermal tumors. Semin Diagn Pathol 2000; 17 : 194–203.

Radiographic evaluation of cancer

Kitt Shaffer, Annick D. van den Abbeele

2

IMAGING GOALS

Goals of radiographic imaging vary in patients with malignancies depending upon whether the specific malignant diagnosis is already known, if the imaging is performed to stage disease or to follow disease. Each type of malignancy has its own spectrum of findings on imaging studies, which will be covered in detail in subsequent chapters. In this chapter, generalized imaging principles will be reviewed, with some attention to new imaging techniques which may have greater application in diagnosis and follow-up of malignancies in the future. Nuclear medicine, lymphangiography, angiography and myelography will not be covered specifically in this chapter, but often make valuable contributions to oncologic diagnoses. More

detailed information regarding these more specialized studies may be obtained in a variety of oncoradiologic texts (Vanel and Stark, 1993; Stomper, 1993).

Imaging findings in cancer patients may be very non-specific or very specific (*see* Fig. 2.1). In choosing a particular method for imaging cancer patients, the specificity and sensitivity of the imaging modality must be considered with particular reference to the type of malignancy suspected. The risk to the patient for the imaging modality must also be weighed, along with the actual cost of the study. The strengths and weaknesses of many common studies will be considered individually, with a discussion of imaging assistance for biopsy, which is often the final path to conclusive diagnosis of malignancy.

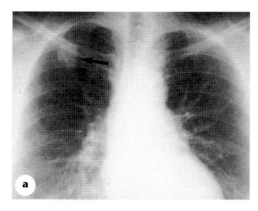
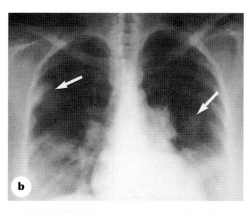
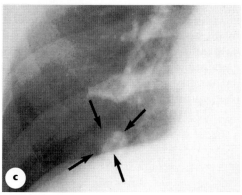
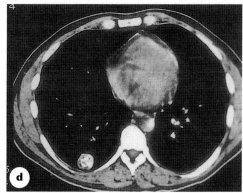

Fig. 2.1 While the chest radiograph is very sensitive for detection of lung abnormalities, findings may or may not be specific. (**a**) Frontal view of the chest in the PA projection in an asymptomatic 42-year-old female shows a slightly lobular 2 cm mass in the right upper lobe, projecting behind the right clavicle. At surgery, *a non-calcified granuloma* was removed. This lesion radiographically could not be distinguished from other solitary pulmonary nodules, such as lung carcinoma, pulmonary amyloid or a rheumatoid nodule. (**b**) Frontal view of the chest in the PA projection in a 39-year-old female with a cough shows bilateral ill-defined lung nodules (arrows), with bilateral hilar enlargement. At open-lung biopsy, *alveolar sarcoidosis* was found. Many other processes could have caused a similar appearance on the chest radiograph, such as bilateral pneumonia, lung metastases, pulmonary lymphoma, or bronchoalveolar carcinoma. (**c**) Close-up from a frontal view of the chest in the PA projection in an asymptomatic 33-year-old male obtained as part of a pre-employment physical examination shows a 1 cm smoothly rounded nodule at the right lung base (arrows). Calcification is present in a characteristic chunky, curved distribution indicating a specific benign diagnosis. (**d**) CT image at the right lung base in the same patient as Fig. 2.1**c**, displayed with mediastinal windows, shows this calcification more clearly, resembling 'popcorn', diagnostic of a *pulmonary hamartoma*. In this case, the chest radiograph (and CT) were both sensitive and specific in making the correct diagnosis.

PLAIN RADIOGRAPHY

Plain films are often the most cost-effective method to begin a diagnostic search for malignancy or to follow effects of treatment. Table 2.1 compares cost, radiation dose and practical limitations for various plain film examinations. Cost estimates are for a large tertiary care teaching institution in New England and will vary in other types of institutions and other parts of the country. Dose information is given as skin entry dose, which is at best a crude estimate of actual absorbed dose. Specific absorbed doses to particularly sensitive organs should also be considered and will vary depending on the specific views obtained. For example, the breast glandular dose from an anteroposterior (AP) chest film (where the beam enters the front of the patient) is about 70 times greater than the breast glandular dose from a posterior–anterior (PA) chest film. Overall, approximately 50% of the average radiation dose to the general public is from radon gas and only about 15% from medical imaging, including nuclear medicine (Broadbent and Hubbard, 1992).

CHEST FILMS

The chest radiograph provides an excellent survey of the lungs, mediastinum, bony thorax and pleura in a very short exam time and at a relatively low radiation dose. Because of the natural contrast between air in the lungs and soft tissue in other parts of the chest, the chest radiograph is particularly sensitive for diagnosis of many pulmonary malignancies, although usually not very specific. Chest radiographs may also provide adequate staging of lung tumors in some cases, since bone metastases and mediastinal adenopathy may be demonstrated along with the primary tumor. Chest films are also useful in detection of many treatment-related problems, such as infections, fluid overload and misplaced support lines. Problems with support lines are one of the most common abnormalities detected on portable radiographs. Even a subtle abnormality may have clinical importance. A finding of an abnormally placed line on a chest radiograph may require additional studies, such as CT or digital subtraction angiography, to determine the exact line position and whether it can be used for infusion of chemotherapy.

Chest radiographs in obese patients will show decreased contrast, but even in patients in excess of 160 kg, diagnostically useful films can usually still be obtained. For solving specific problems in the chest, additional views may be useful, such as oblique views (helpful for detection of rib, pleural or chest wall lesions and for confirming presence of questionable lung nodules), decubitus views (for demonstrating loculation of pleural fluid and for improving visualization of the lung base in the presence of large non-loculated pleural effusions), apical lordotic views (for projection of the apical portion of the lung free of overlying bony structures) or apical kyphotic views (for examination of the pleural apex). Chest radiography can be performed at the bedside; however, the quality of these exams is limited by certain fixed technical factors. The portable X-ray machine does not generate the same kVp as a standard chest unit (60–90 kVp vs 120 kVp for standard chest radiography). Also, the distance from the tube to the film is shorter (0.9–1.2 m vs 1.8 m for standard chest radiography) which increases distortion and geometric unsharpness. Radiography may also be limited by patient condition and difficulty in properly positioning the film and X-ray tube.

ABDOMINAL FILMS

Plain films of the abdomen provide a less sensitive diagnostic study for abdominal organs than the chest radiograph provides for the lung, since the air in the bowel provides the only natural contrast among the abdominal contents. Detection of retroperitoneal and solid organ abnormalities is limited, unless calcification is present. Fat planes within the abdomen may provide enough contrast to allow delineation of some solid organ contours, but is variable among patients. However, for detection of abnormalities of the bowel, plain abdominal films can be very helpful and again, are inexpensive, can be obtained at relatively low radiation dose, can be performed at the bedside and require only minimal patient co-operation. Special views which may be helpful include decubitus views (left side down for detection of minimal pneumoperitoneum outlined by the liver), prone views (to move gas into the rectum and rule out distal colonic obstruction) and upright views (to detect air–fluid levels, which are only normal in the stomach and duodenal bulb, but can be seen in the colon in patients with diarrhea or in the small bowel in cases of ileus or obstruction). Upright abdominal films can also be used to detect pneumoperitoneum, but the upright chest film is preferable because the X-ray beam is centered closer to the dome of the diaphragm and therefore will more clearly demonstrate very small collections of air. Abdominal fluoroscopy is not usually performed without contrast administration.

BONE FILMS

Bone plain films are moderately sensitive in detection of many primary and metastatic malignancies, but are most useful when interpreted in conjunction with results of nuclear medicine bone scans. Interpretation of bone films can be confounded by a variety of normal variants and benign lesions and experience in interpretation of bone films is essential. In surveying the body for bone metastases, nuclear medicine scanning is preferred to skeletal surveys, since the bone scan is more sensitive, less expensive and gives a lower radiation dose. The exception to this rule is in multiple myeloma or in very aggressive purely lytic bone metastases, where bone scanning may be negative (Woolfenden *et al.*, 1980). In these cases, skeletal surveys or plain films of long bones, skull, spine and pelvis are preferred. Consultation with a radiologist may often be helpful in limiting any bone examination to the most appropriate films. For certain bones, such as the sacrum, scapula and sternum, CT or tomography is required for best visualization of the entire bone. The particular views included in a standard study of any bone or joint will vary from department to department. Therefore, if a specific question is to be answered regarding a bone or joint, adequate clinical information must be given to the radiologist to decide if additional views must be obtained to supplement the standard views.

Table 2.1 A comparison of cost and dose of common radiographic studies

Exam[+]	Cost	Radiation Dose**
PA/lat CXR	1 cost unit*	0.007–0.01 cG (PA) 0.02–0.03 cG (lat)
Portable AP CXR	1.25	0.01–0.02 cG
KUB	0.5	0.06–0.1 cG
Decubitus abdomen	0.5	0.06–0.1 cG
AP & lat C-spine	1	0.06 cG (AP) 0.05 cG (lat)
AP & lat T-spine	1	0.2 cG (AP) 0.3–0.6 cG (lat)
AP & lat L-spine	1	0.07–0.1 cG (AP) 0.2–0.3 cG (lat)
Femur, humerus	0.75	0.08–0.2 cG each view
Pelvis	0.85	0.05–0.06 cG
Ribs	0.75	0.15 cG (two views)
Knee, shoulder, hip	1	0.07–0.1 cG each view
AP & lat skull	1	0.1–0.3 cG (AP) 0.1–0.3 cG (lat)
Barium swallow	1.4	3–5 cG
UGI (air-contrast)	2.25	8–15 cG
UGI/SBFT	2.75	10–25 cG
SBFT	2.25	3–5 cG
Enteroclysis	3	10–15 cG
BE (air-contrast)	3.1	15–30 cG
Head CT	3.25 (1–) 3.75 (1+) 4 (1–/1+)	4–6 cG (14 slices)
Chest or abdomen CT	3.6 (1–) 3.9 (1+) 4.25 (1–/1+)	1–3 cG (28 slices)
Pelvis CT	3.25 (1–) 3.75 (1+) 4 (1–/1+)	1–3 cG (14 slices)

[+]PA, posterior-anterior; lat, lateral; AP, anterior-posterior; CXR, chest radiograph; KUB, plain film of kidney urinary bladder; C, cervical; T, thoracic; L, lumbar; UGI, upper gastrointestinal series; SBFT, small bowel follow-through; BE, barium enema; CT, computed tomography; 1–, without intravenous contrast infusion; 1–/1+, without intravenous contrast followed by images with intravenous contrast infusion; 1+, with intravenous contrast infusion.

*One cost unit, for comparison purposes, is defined as the cost for a PA and lateral CXR, including both technical and professional fees.

**Doses are given as skin entry doses; actual absorbed dose will vary considerably depending on radiographic technique, body habitus and site examined. These doses also assume use of state-of-the-art image receptors and optimal radiographic technique. cG = centiGray.

GASTROINTESTINAL CONTRAST STUDIES

Care must be taken in planning the sequence of gastrointestinal studies when staging a cancer patient, particularly if contrast studies are needed. If a barium enema, bone scan, upper GI series and CT are all planned, the CT or bone scan should usually be done first (since barium from the other two studies will severely limit the ability to perform the CT or nuclear medicine studies for varying lengths of time, up to a week). The barium enema should then be performed before the upper GI series, since residual contrast will hamper either study, and contrast from a barium enema is usually eliminated more rapidly than that from an upper GI study. When in doubt about how best to schedule a series of different types of radiologic studies, consultation with a radiologist or nuclear medicine physician is often helpful.

INTRAVENOUS CONTRAST STUDIES

Intravenous contrast used in radiology can be divided into agents which are hyperosmolar relative to blood (ionic agents) and those that are iso-osmolar to blood (non-ionic agents). Ionic contrast agents produce more local effects on injection, such as pain, flushing and nausea. Non-ionic contrast agents are more expensive (over 20 times as expensive as ionic material for a single-dose, 100 ml bottle) and have a lower incidence of non-fatal contrast reactions. The incidence of fatal contrast reactions with either type of agent is approximately 1 : 100 000 uses (Caro *et al.*, 1991). The nephrotoxic effect of non-ionic agents may be less than with ionic agents. Therefore, choice of contrast agent must be based on weighing of patient comfort and safety against cost. In many institutions, specific criteria are used to select patients for non-ionic contrast material, such as age and history of asthma or other allergies. All contrast agents must be used with caution in patients with multiple myeloma, diabetes, sickle cell disease or chronic renal insufficiency.

In patients with a history of prior serious reactions to intravenous contrast material, a premedication protocol using steroids and histamine blockers is often used before a planned contrast administration (Kelly *et al.*, 1978). Whenever possible, intravenous contrast should be administered after the patient has taken nothing by mouth for several hours as food or liquids in the stomach may increase the risk of vomiting. As venous access is often a problem in cancer patients, placement of an intravenous catheter prior to a planned study is often helpful to prevent delays or cancellation of the study. In both CT and intravenous urography, optimal examinations require rapid bolus contrast administration. Therefore, the largest caliber catheter which can be inserted should usually be used.

INTRAVENOUS UROGRAPHY

The advent of CT and ultrasound has narrowed the range of indications for intravenous urography. In an intravenous pyelogram (IVP), after injection of a bolus of intravenous contrast material, films and tomograms are obtained rapidly to demonstrate the enhancement of the renal parenchyma, followed by more delayed films to show the contour of the collecting systems, ureters and bladder. Filling of the collecting systems is highly variable and it is not uncommon for small segments of the ureters to be poorly visualized. If small mucosal lesions of the collecting system are suspected, retrograde studies may be preferable. Residual barium from prior oral or rectal contrast studies will obscure the kidneys and ureters and this contrast should be allowed to pass before performing an IVP. Prior history of allergy to intravenous contrast material is a contraindication, unless the patient has been adequately pretreated with steroids. Patients should be well hydrated prior to the study, as dehydration may increase the risk of nephrotoxic effects after intravenous contrast administration. The examination requires the patient to take nothing by mouth for several hours prior to the study, preferably from the evening before. With rapid injection of ionic contrast material, flushing, nausea and vomiting are not uncommon. The cost is approximately 3.25 cost units and the radiation dose is 3–6 cG.

RETROGRADE UROLOGIC STUDIES

Contrast material can also be introduced into the urinary system via the urethra. Cystography involves filling the bladder with contrast via catheter, usually under fluoroscopic guidance. Little patient co-operation is required for this examination, other than for insertion of the catheter. To visualize the urethra, the catheter can be withdrawn after filling of the bladder and films obtained during urination in a voiding cystourethrogram (VCUG). Considerable patient co-operation is required for this examination. In conjunction with cystoscopy, the ureters can also be cannulated and retrograde injections may be performed into the collecting systems under fluoroscopic guidance. This provides the best visualization of the entire collecting system. Again, little patient co-operation is required other than for initial catheterization. The cost of a cystogram is approximately 1.5 cost units, a VCUG is 2.25 cost units and a retrograde cystourethrogram is 2.5–3 cost units. Radiation dose is 3–6 cG, with particularly high gonadal doses for the VCUG.

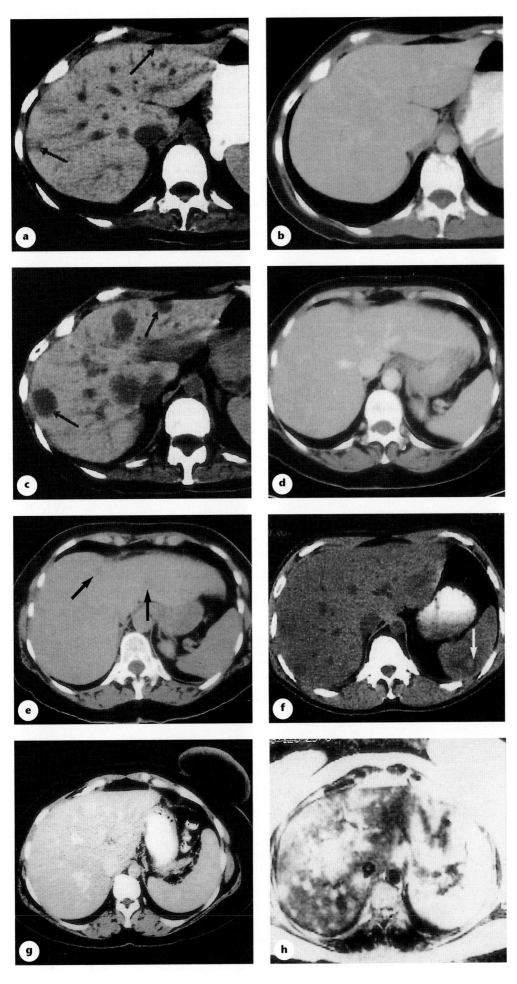

Fig. 2.2 Detection of liver and spleen abnormalities with CT and MRI use of IV contrast (**a**) CT image through the liver, without IV contrast, obtained for staging in a 35-year-old patient with breast cancer. Two small, low-attenuation lesions are visible in the liver periphery (arrows), consistent with metastases. (**b**) CT image in the same patient as Fig. 2.2**a**, obtained at a similar level in the liver on the same day, after IV contrast administration. The liver lesions are no longer visible. Good opacification of hepatic vessels is evident, indicating adequate injection rate and prompt imaging. This study demonstrates that occasionally relatively vascular metastases in the liver may be better seen without IV contrast. (**c**) CT image in the same patient as in Fig. 2.2**a**, obtained at a similar level in the liver several months later, confirming growth of the two lesions initially detected (arrows), as well as documenting the appearance of new lesions. (**d**) CT image through the liver in a 70-year-old male with carcinoid tumor of the cecum, after IV contrast administration. Good opacification of hepatic vessels and aorta is evident. No liver lesions are visible. (**e**) CT image in the same patient as Fig. 2.2**d**, at a similar level in the liver obtained 45 minutes after the previous image. Two low-attenuation liver lesions are now evident (arrows), consistent with metastases. This study demonstrates that timing of imaging after IV contrast administration can be crucial in detection of liver metastases, with some metastases less visible immediately after contrast administration. (**f**) CT images through the upper abdomen without IV contrast in a 45-year-old patient with lymphoma and new left upper quadrant pain. An irregular low-attenuation lesion is evident in the spleen and contains central areas of faint higher attenuation (arrow) consistent with hemorrhage. This faint density was not visible after IV contrast administration. This study demonstrates the usefulness of non-contrast scanning for detection of subtle high-attenuation abnormalities, such as blood or calcification. (**g**) CT image through the liver in a 35-year-old woman with breast cancer, obtained after IV contrast administration. Adequate opacification of hepatic vessels is evident. No discrete liver lesions are seen, although contrast enhancement is somewhat heterogeneous throughout the liver. (**h**) Axial T_2-weighted MR image through the liver in the same patient as in Fig. 2.2g obtained 5 days later. Many discrete, rounded liver lesions are evident, consistent with metastases. This study demonstrates that MRI may sometimes demonstrate lesions which are not visible on CT.

MAMMOGRAPHY

The quality of imaging in mammography has improved rapidly in recent years. The two goals of maximizing spatial and contrast resolution and minimizing patient dose have led to many technical innovations. Early mammography was performed with standard radiographic equipment and one view of each breast. Current mammographic standards require dedicated mammographic equipment, strict quality control standards and two views of each breast, usually in the craniocaudal and mediolateral oblique projections. Specialized views may also be obtained, such as spot compression (to search for nodules or architectural distortion), rolled or rotated (to help localize a lesion within the breast) or magnification views (to detect and characterize microcalcifications). When a mass is present which may represent a cyst, breast ultrasound may be useful. The mean glandular dose from modern film/screen mammography is under 0.3 cG for each view, which would yield approximately 10/1000 000 excess cases of breast cancer in 50-year-old patients due to the radiation from a standard four-view examination (Gofman and O'Connor, 1985). This produces a risk of dying from a radiation-induced breast carcinoma comparable to the risk of dying due to smoking 14 cigarettes, breathing the air of an industrialized Northeastern city for one month or living in Denver for 2 years (Wilson, 1979). Mammographic dose varies with breast size, density, degree of compression and type of X-ray target used and radiation risk from mammography decreases with increasing patient age.

It is very important when ordering a mammogram that any prior mammograms be available to the radiologist at the time of the examination. Comparison with such studies may be extremely helpful in determining what additional views are needed and whether other studies, such as ultrasound, may be indicated.

Findings on mammography generally can be grouped into categories based on the likelihood of malignancy, with varying followup recommendations based on this classification (Table 2.2). A normal mammogram does not exclude malignancy, as the false-negative rate of mammography ranges from 10% to 20% (Holland and Hendricks, 1983; Bird *et al.*, 1992). Mammography may be uncomfortable for the patient, because firm compression of the breast is needed for best diagnostic image quality (Feig, 1987). Patients are instructed not to use deodorant on the day of their exam, as it may be radiopaque. If patients experience cyclic changes in sensitivity of their breasts, it is helpful to schedule their mammogram at a time when they anticipate the least sensitivity. Mammograms are not generally recommended for women under the age of 30, but with newer equipment, adequate studies may be obtained even in young women if the clinical situation is sufficiently worrisome.

If the clinician feels a palpable lesion which is to be evaluated, the exact location of that lesion should be clearly communicated to the radiologist and may ideally be marked on the skin to further help in planning the examination. Mammography in patients with breast implants is more complicated and requires a total of four views of each breast in most cases (Eklund *et al.*, 1988). Breast size does not alter the technical ability to perform an adequate mammogram and high-quality images can be obtained in small-breasted women as well as in most men. Patient immobility can compromise the examination, as this may limit the ability of the technologist to bring the entire breast into the X-ray field. Other features of oncologic patients which may compromise mammography include massive ascites, recent breast, axillary or chest wall surgery and implanted reservoir catheters overlying the upper breast.

Table 2.2 Classification of common mammographic findings

Finding	Significance	Follow-up	Additional procedures
Vascular calcification	Benign	Routine*	None
Skin calcification	Benign	Routine	Tangential films
Simple cysts	Benign	Routine	Aspirate, if painful
Intramammary lymph nodes	Benign	Routine	Ultrasound, to rule out cyst
Complex cyst	Indeterminate	Depends on results of aspiration	Aspirate or excise
Multiple bilateral clusters of microcalcifications	Indeterminate	6-month f/up	Needle localization, if any one group is more worrisome in morphology
Solid smoothly marginated nodule on initial study	Indeterminate	6-month f/up	Consider core biopsy or excision; ultrasound to rule out cyst
Multiple nodules	Indeterminate	6-month f/up	Consider core biopsy or excision if any are irregular in outline
Asymmetric parenchymal densities	Indeterminate	6-month f/up	Spot compression films to exclude underlying architectural distortion
Single cluster of microcalcifications	Possibly malignant	Depends on results of biopsy	Biopsy, with needle localization
New solid nodule	Possibly malignant	Depends on results of biopsy	Biopsy, with needle localization if not palpable
Architectural distortion	Possibly malignant	Depends on results of biopsy	Biopsy, with needle localization if not palpable
Spiculated mass	Probably malignant	Depends on results of biopsy	Biopsy, with needle localization if not palpable

*Routine mammographic followup, as recommended by the American College of Radiology, consists of yearly or biennial mammography for women between the ages of 40 and 49 and yearly mammography for women aged 50 or older (Smart, 1992).

ULTRASOUND

Ultrasound offers many advantages as an imaging modality for the cancer patient. The study is generally painless and can be performed rapidly at the bedside. Ultrasound does not involve ionizing radiation and no oral or intravenous contrast materials are generally needed. The study is particularly attractive for frequent follow-up examinations for these reasons. Ultrasound can be used as a guide for biopsy or for drainage of pleural, pericardial or peritoneal fluid. Using intracavity probes, very detailed images of pelvic organs can be obtained, as well as biopsies. Ultrasound can be combined with endoscopy for examination of the heart or esophagus (Botet *et al.*, 1991) and can also be performed intraoperatively to assist in accurate tumor localization (Clarke *et al.*, 1989). With color flow and Doppler capability, venous thrombosis can be detected non-invasively. Vascular imaging of the upper extremity with ultrasound is more difficult than the lower extremity due to the sound-dampening qualities of the bony thorax and clavicle. In any ultrasound examination, an acoustic 'window' is needed to allow the sound beam to pass into the area to be examined. Bone and air do not transmit sound waves and therefore ultrasound of the chest is limited to the heart (which can be approached through the mediastinal tissues just lateral to the sternum for evaluation of cardiac chamber size, wall motion and pericardial fluid) and pleural fluid collections which touch the inner chest wall. The cost of ultrasound examinations ranges from 1.75 cost units for a breast ultrasound to 3.25 cost units for bilateral lower extremity venous ultrasounds.

BREAST ULTRASOUND

Breast ultrasound may be a helpful adjunct to mammography but is not useful as a screening tool (Jackson, 1990). Ultrasound can demonstrate the cystic quality of some breast lesions, eliminating the need for further workup. The exam is very operator dependent and images may be difficult to reproduce due to variable transducer position and settings from one exam to the next. Therefore, breast ultrasound is best used in evaluating specific lesions, such as nodules visible on mammography or palpable lesions. Ultrasound may be used as a guide for cyst aspiration as well as for fine needle or core biopsy of the breast. Ultrasound is also useful in detection of rupture of breast implants.

ABDOMINAL ULTRASOUND

Abdominal ultrasound in the cancer patient may detect liver metastases, dilated bile ducts, hydronephrosis and masses. Some liver metastases may be better seen with ultrasound than with CT. Measurement of liver and spleen size can be obtained, but may be difficult to reproduce. Measurements are particularly difficult in patients with marked organomegaly, which moves the borders of the organ beyond the range of the transducer, requiring multiple images to encompass the entire organ. Ultrasound is very sensitive in detection of ascites and may be useful in guiding paracentesis. It can also be used to guide percutaneous biopsies of abdominal lesions and for placement of nephrostomy tubes. Evaluation of the pancreas can be limited in some patients by gas in the stomach and duodenum, which blocks sound waves. Ultrasound of the abdomen may also be limited in very obese patients, as the transducers have fixed depths of penetration and fat is relatively attenuating to the sound beam. Presence of barium in the GI tract can severely limit abdominal ultrasound, as the barium blocks sound. Only minimum patient co-operation is required for most abdominal ultrasound examinations, which can be performed at the bedside.

PELVIC ULTRASOUND

Pelvic ultrasound is generally useful to detect small amounts of ascites or to detect tumors of the pelvic organs. For examination of the uterus and ovaries, either a transabdominal or transvaginal approach may be used. Many patients prefer the transvaginal approach, since the transabdominal approach requires pressing the transducer against a full bladder to provide an acoustic 'window' onto the pelvis. For prostate examination, similarly, a transabdominal or transrectal approach may be used. More patient co-operation is required for transvaginal or transrectal ultrasound than for the abdominal approach, which can be performed at the bedside. Biopsies can be performed using special needle guides on the rectal and vaginal probes. As in the abdomen, obesity can limit imaging using the transabdominal approach.

COMPUTED TOMOGRAPHY (CT)

CT scans have become the most common method of diagnosis and follow-up in cancer patients. CT offers many advantages over other imaging methods, including accurate, reproducible measurement of tumors, detection of bone metastases and enlarged lymph nodes. Most mucosal lesions of the GI tract are better examined fluoroscopically, although large lesions may be well seen on CT. CT is relatively expensive, with many examinations costing over 3.5 cost units. Examinations of contiguous portions of the body require separate exams, so that the bill for a head, chest, abdomen and pelvis study can total over 15 times the cost of a PA and lateral chest exam. Cost is even higher if intravenous contrast is used. However, for many areas of the body, such as the abdomen or mediastinum, no other imaging modality offers such complete information.

The primary imaging modality in oncology remains CT (Hopper *et al.*, 2000). Its role has expanded to include complex three-dimensional imaging of tumors for radiation planning. CT in the setting of radiation planning does not always optimally demonstrate the extent of active tumor and superimposition of CT with more functional imaging, such as PET or MR spectroscopy, may allow more accurate targeting of active tumor in the future (Rosenman, 2001; Zakian *et al.*, 2001).

USE OF IV CONTRAST

Administration of intravenous contrast for CT scanning is useful in certain specific instances, but is not required for all imaging. Most chest lesions can be detected without IV contrast, due to the inherent contrast provided by air in the lungs and fat in the mediastinum. For specific problems in the chest, such as detection of small hilar masses, vascular dissection or thrombi, bolus contrast administration is needed. In the brain, increased doses of contrast and delayed imaging may increase detection of metastases (Davis *et al.*, 1991). CT imaging of the neck generally requires IV contrast, as it is difficult to discriminate between vessels and nodes without vascular enhancement due to the frequency of anatomic variations in the veins of the neck.

In the liver, the appearance and size of metastatic lesions may vary considerably when comparing studies performed after IV contrast injection to non-contrast enhanced studies. But even in comparisons between two different contrast-enhanced scans, considerable variation may still be based on differences in size of catheter used to inject the contrast, location of vein used for injection, amount of contrast administered, cardiac output of the patient at the time of contrast administration and any delays between completion of injection and initiation of scanning (technical problems, emesis). Therefore, in following cancer patients with liver metastases, non-contrast scans (for those lesions visible without IV contrast) may provide a more reproducible image for tumor measurement. In some very vascular tumors, the exact timing of imaging after contrast administration may be particularly crucial, as some relatively vascular lesions in the liver may actually become less conspicuous after contrast administration, either transiently or for prolonged periods (Bressler *et al.*, 1987).

Intravenous contrast administration can also obscure tiny areas of hemorrhage of calcifications, such as might be present in the kidneys. Therefore, in cancer patients it is often helpful to begin any CT examination without intravenous contrast and then to assess the need for contrast injection on a case-by-case basis (*see* Fig. 2.4). For more accurate detection of very small liver lesions, as in planning resection of limited hepatic metastatic disease, more invasive procedures may be required, such as CT arterial portography, with direct injection of contrast material into the superior mesenteric artery during CT, using an angiographically placed catheter (Soyer *et al.*, 1993).

ORAL CONTRAST

For most CT examinations of the abdomen and pelvis, oral contrast is essential. Dilute barium or water-soluble material must be administered beginning at a time sufficiently before the planned examination to allow transit through the bowel. In particular, when cystic tumor collections or abscesses are suspected, meticulous care must be taken in adequately filling the GI tract with contrast. This process takes 1–4 hours in most cases and overnight preparation may sometimes be required. In detection of masses near the pancreatic head, additional imaging after further oral contrast administration may sometimes be needed to allow separation of pancreas from duodenum. If esophageal abnormalities are suspected, a thicker barium paste may be given orally, which remains in the lumen of the esophagus long enough to provide contrast for imaging. When pelvic masses are evaluated, rectal contrast administration is often useful and is usually well tolerated, as much less contrast is needed than for a barium enema. Insertion of a tampon into the vagina may be useful in evaluation of uterine or vaginal masses, as the air within the tampon is clearly visible on CT. Placement of external markers may be useful when CT is used for radiation therapy planning (*see* Fig. 2.3).

RADIATION DOSE

Calculation of radiation dose from CT scans is a complex task. The dose of a single slice cannot be simply multiplied by the number of slices to obtain the total dose, as there is some radiation delivered outside the imaging section and radiation is also scattered within the patient (Rothenberg and Pentlow, 1992). Table 2.3 gives dose information for various types of CT examinations. Dose varies among CT machines, based on types of detectors used and other technical parameters. Dose on a given machine can also vary from day to day and from patient to patient.

TECHNICAL FACTORS IN CT

The radiologist controls many technical parameters in planning a CT scan, which can alter duration of exam, radiation dose and quality of images. Most imaging parameters which increase the quality of the image do so at the expense of increasing the patient dose (Rothenberg and Pentlow, 1992). The reconstruction algorithm and brightness/contrast settings ('windows') of the image can be changed without effect on dose and may alter conspicuity of lesions (*see* Fig. 2.4). For detection of interstitial lung processes, high-resolution imaging is recommended, consisting of thin sections (1–1.5 mm thickness) and reconstruction with a high-resolution algorithm (Swensen *et al.*, 1992). In spiral (or helical) scanning the X-ray beam is constantly rotated around the patient while the patient continuously moves through the gantry. This allows acquisition of volumetric data in short time intervals and is particularly helpful in the chest, as it eliminates problems with misregistration due to variations in breathing (Costello *et al.*, 1992). Spiral scanning is also useful in rapid imaging of vascular areas (kidneys, carotids) after bolus IV contrast administration in order to capture all the enhanced images during the peak of the contrast bolus (Napel *et al.*, 1992) or to best capture arterial contrast injections during invasive procedures like liver portography (Soyer *et al.*, 1994). Disadvantages of spiral scanning include increased equipment cost and some blurring of the image, with slight resultant decrease in spatial resolution. Ultrafast CT uses a specially designed machine with no moving parts, and allows scans to be obtained in milliseconds. This provides the most detailed examination of rapidly moving structures, such as the heart (Stanford *et al.*, 1991).

Most CT examinations require only minimal patient co-operation. Breath holding is needed for optimal chest examination, but an adequate study can usually be obtained during quiet breathing. In searching for adenopathy, it must be remembered that lymphadenopathy is diagnosed on CT scans based only on nodal size, which is at best a crude method for detection of metastases (Stomper *et al.*, 1987). Even normal-sized-nodes may contain micrometastatic deposits. CT is generally not reliable for detection of invasion of the mediastinum or body wall, unless clear-cut bony erosion or growth into vascular structures is present (Pennes *et al.*, 1985). Invasion may be suspected but not proven when a tumor has a wide area of contact with an adjacent structure (*see* Fig. 2.5). Magnetic resonance imaging may provide more specific information in questions of invasion (*see* section on magnetic resonance imaging). Dense barium from prior fluoroscopic contrast studies or metallic hardware, such as hip replacements or spinal rods, will seriously degrade CT images. Most CT tables have a patient weight limit of 135–160 kg. Agitated patients must be sedated, as no useful imaging can be obtained in a moving patient. In patients with pain, consideration must be made of the length of time the patient will be required to lie still for the examination. A chest CT scan on a fourth-generation scanner takes 15–20 minutes without IV contrast. A scan of the abdomen and pelvis, with and without IV contrast, takes 30–60 minutes. If a patient cannot lie in one position for this length of time, more limited studies or other imaging modalities should be considered.

CT AS A SCREENING TOOL

With the advent of spiral CT, allowing the entire chest to be imaged in a matter of seconds, the role of CT as a screening tool for lung tumors has been reconsidered (Tockman and Mulshine, 2000). Special techniques must be used to decrease radiation dose (which also decreases image quality), but this method may become more widespread in the future. Careful cost–benefit analyses are needed and several large trials are under way to determine if early detection with CT actually has an impact on survival (Henschke, 2000; Sone *et al.*, 2001). The problem of false-positive findings of small non-specific nodules can be significant, particularly in parts of the country where histoplasmosis or coccoidomycosis is endemic. In these regions, most patients screened may have nodules, requiring difficult management decisions.

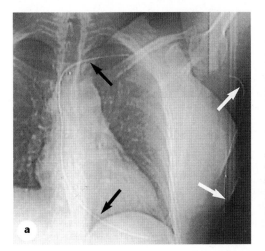
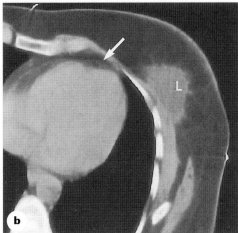
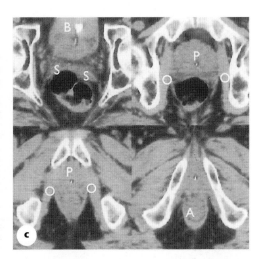

Fig. 2.3 Use of CT for planning radiation therapy. (**a**) Digital chest radiograph obtained at the start of a CT planning study in a 48-year-old woman with left breast cancer. Metallic wire markers (arrows) were placed at the margins of the planned XRT field, in the XRT simulator. The patient was then placed on the CT table in the planned XRT treatment position. (**b**) CT image through the lower chest in the patient in Fig. 2.3**a**. Skin wire markers are visible, as is the location of the left anterior descending coronary artery (arrow), allowing dose to this structure to be minimized during XRT. L = lumpectomy site. CT may also be useful in determining the location of the internal mammary vessels for planning radiation to the internal mammary node groups. (**c**) CT images through the pelvis in a 70-year-old male with prostate cancer, obtained for planning of pelvic XRT. A catheter was placed in the bladder prior to the scan to mark the course of the urethra through the treatment field. Thin sections through the pelvis allow very precise planning of the radiation ports to maximize dose to the intended areas and minimize dose to adjacent, radiation-sensitive structures. S = seminal vesicles; B = bladder; P = prostate; A = anus; O = obturator internus muscles.

Table 2.3 Organ-specific radiation doses from CT examinations*				
Site	Head CT	Chest CT	Abdomen CT	Pelvic CT
Bone marrow	0.3–0.4 cG*	0.4–0.6 cG	0.6–1.0 cG	0.5–0.8 cG
Lens of the eye	3.2–3.8 cG	–	–	–
Thyroid	0.05–0.12 cG	0.2–0.3 cG	–	–
Breast	–	2.3–2.7 cG	–	–
Lungs	–	1.9–2.5 cG	–	–
Avg total skin entry	2.2–6.8 cG	2.0–2.5 cG	2.0–2.5 cG	2.0–2.5 cG
*centiGray				
From Wagner, 1991				

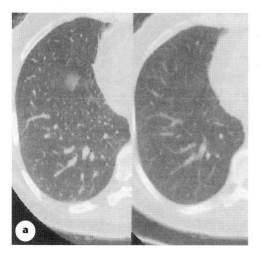

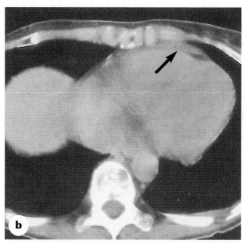

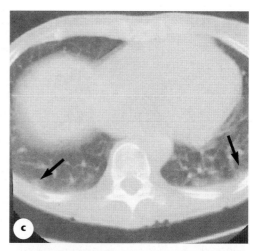

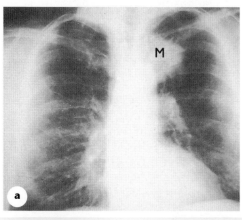

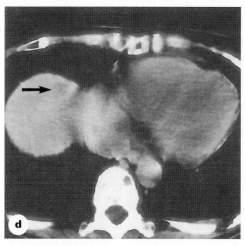

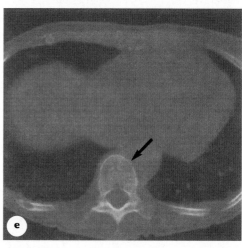

Fig. 2.4 Technical parameters in CT: slice thickness, reconstruction algorithm and windows. (**a**) Two CT images through the same portion of the right lung base in a 40-year-old female with a history of thyroid carcinoma. The image on the left was obtained using 1.5 mm slice thickness and high-resolution reconstruction algorithm and is preferable for detection of interstitial processes in the lung, such as lymphangitic carcinomatosis. Image on the right was obtained using 10 mm slice thickness and standard reconstruction algorithm and is preferable for detection of nodular processes in the lung, such as hematogenous metastasis. No metastases or interstitial abnormalities are evident on these images. (**b**) CT image through the lung base in a 45-year-old female patient, performed for staging of breast cancer, and viewed with contrast and brightness settings optimum for mediastinal structures (mediastinal windows). A small amount of pericardial fluid is seen on this image (arrow). (**c**) Same CT image, viewed with brightness and contrast settings optimum for lung (lung windows). Several ill-defined peripheral lung nodules are now visible (arrows),

consistent with metastases. (**d**) Same CT image, viewed with brightness and contrast settings optimum for the liver (liver windows). A single liver metastasis is now visible (arrow). (**e**) Same CT image, viewed with brightness and contrast settings optimum for bony structures (bone windows). A lytic metastasis in the vertebral body is now visible (arrow). It is likely that viewing of the CT image with only one or two windows would have missed at least some of these abnormalities.

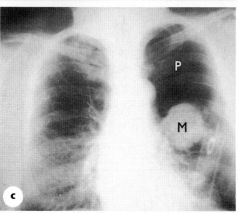

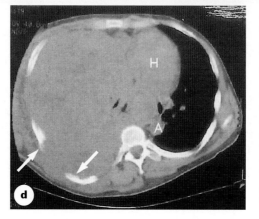

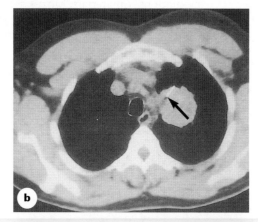

Fig. 2.5 CT is generally not specific in detection of invasion of adjacent structures by tumor, unless destruction, erosion or replacement of structures is seen. (**a**) Frontal chest radiograph in the PA projection in a 53-year-old male with hemoptysis showing a large left upper lobe mass (M) abutting the upper left mediastinum in the region of the aortic arch. Emphysema is noted in both upper lobes. (**b**) CT image in the same patient as in Fig. 2.5a obtained during a percutaneous needle biopsy shows the biopsy needle tip within the mass (arrow), and possible infiltration of the adjacent mediastinal fat by the mass. Detection of such invasion is important, as it may alter surgical therapy. (**c**) Frontal chest radiograph in the PA projection after completion of the biopsy in the same patient shows a large left pneumothorax (P), with the mass (M) freely falling away from the mediastinum, proving that the mass does not invade the mediastinum. Risk of pneumothorax after percutaneous needle biopsy of the lung is increased in patients with adjacent emphysema. (**d**) CT can only conclusively diagnose invasion of adjacent structures by tumor in advanced disease, such as this CT image through the lower chest in a 25-year-old male with a large, recurrent malignant schwannoma. Tumor fills the right hemithorax and displaces the heart (H) to the left. The tumor is destroying ribs posteriorly (arrows), which is definitive evidence of chest wall invasion. The patient clinically had chest wall pain and compromised cardiac output due to compression of the right atrium by tumor. A = descending aorta.

MAGNETIC RESONANCE IMAGING (MR)

Use of magnetic resonance (MR) imaging in cancer patients is becoming more common as equipment becomes more sophisticated and new pulse sequences and specialized detection apparatus are developed. Imaging in MR depends on electromagnetic properties of nuclei which vary depending on their bonding to other atoms and their local electromagnetic environment (Smith and McCarthy, 1992). The patient is placed in a high field strength magnet (0.3–1.5 tesla) and radiofrequency energy is introduced, which is absorbed by the patient. As time passes this energy is lost and radiofrequency energy is emitted by the patient as a signal, which is detected by receivers called 'coils'. Imaging signal can be obtained from a variety of nuclei, but hydrogen is most often used because it is so abundant, producing a strong signal at a relatively low field strength. MR is particularly useful in evaluation of the brain and spinal cord and has replaced CT and myelography in many instances.

Much research in MR focuses on methods to image function rather than simple anatomy. Use of macromolecular contrast media may allow direct assessment of microvascularity, which may have important implications for treatment with antitumor agents which act on angiogenesis (Brasch and Turetschek, 2000). More sophisticated use of MR spectroscopy may allow analysis of *in vivo* metabolic changes of apoptosis and other signs of tumor response to therapy (Evelhoch *et al.*, 2000). More detailed analysis of vascular patterns in tumors with MR, even using existing contrast agents, may allow better diagnosis of viable tumor within masses and more precise measurement of response to therapy (Taylor and Reddick, 2000). Several new MR techniques show promise for imaging of the oxygen status of tissues, which is important in many pathologic states and may have particular implications for radiation therapy (Krishna *et al.*, 2001).

MR PHYSICS

Two properties of nuclei combine to produce MR signal: T_1 and T_2, which are relaxation times or decay times for nuclei to return to their baseline state after excitation by a radiofrequency pulse. Two operator-determined variables are altered in basic MR examinations (called spin/echo imaging) to change the contribution of T_1 and T_2 to the imaging data: TR (repetition time between cycles of radiofrequency excitations) and TE (time to echo). Therefore, most spin-echo MR imaging includes at least two types of pulse sequences: those designed to most clearly demonstrate contrast due to differences in T_1 (T_1-weighted images) and those demonstrating contrast due to differences in T_2 (T_2-weighted images). T_1-weighted sequences have short TR and short TE, while T_2-weighted sequences have long TR and long TE. Other sequences may also be obtained, including those which are most dependent on actual quantity of hydrogen present (rather than on T_1 or T_2), called proton density images. Varying of other parameters, such as flip angle or adding pulses to saturate certain specific types of nuclei, can also alter image appearance. In general, T_1-weighted images display more fine anatomic detail and water (CSF, edema, effusions, ascites) appears low in signal (black) in the image. T_2-weighted images display more contrast between normal and pathologic tissues and water appears high in signal (white) in the image (Fig. 2.6).

Objects which move into and out of the section plane during the time of the scan, such as flowing blood, appear low in signal (black) in T_1- and T_2-weighted spin-echo sequences. Special sequences may be used, such as gradient echo imaging, time-of-flight or phase-contrast imaging, which will cause flowing blood to appear high in signal (white) in the image, without requiring administration of IV contrast material (*see* Table 2.3). Such imaging is sometimes called MR angiography, or MRA, and may yield information regarding flow velocity and direction as well as delineating the anatomy of vascular structures, thrombi and caliber of vessels (Atlas, 1994). MR data, which are generated by electrically modifying a magnetic field, can be obtained in any plane, unlike CT which is limited by the fixed mechanical orientation of the X-ray detectors in the scanning gantry. Coronal, sagittal or oblique imaging can be particularly advantageous in certain parts of the body, such at the lung apex or diaphragm (Fig. 2.7). True volumetric acquisitions are possible, which can be useful in surgical and radiation therapy planning. Unlike CT contrast material which contains iodine, MR contrast agents contain gadolinium. Gadolinium alters the T_1 of nearby tissues, so only T_1-weighted images are generally obtained after gadolinium administration (Hendrick and Haacke, 1993). Gadolinium is particularly useful in detection of lesions in the brain, spinal canal and breast.

IMAGING COILS

Specialized MR coils have been designed which allow more detailed examination of specific areas of the body. Breast coils allow high resolution examination of the breast parenchyma (Fig. 2.8) (Harms *et al.*, 1993). Endorectal coils are useful in detection of small lesions of the prostate (Schnall *et al.*, 1991). Phased array coils or specialized arrangements of multiple detector coils are particularly useful for pelvic imaging (Kier *et al.*, 1993). MR is not currently used for examination of the lung parenchyma, since air does not generate adequate signal, and MR also may be less useful than CT in demonstration of some bony abnormalities, since dense bone does not produce a strong signal either. Strong signal is obtained from the bone marrow and MR is the most sensitive study available for surveying marrow involvement by tumor (Negendank and Soulen, 1993). Since MR does not use ionizing radiation, it is an attractive modality for patients requiring frequent repeated imaging. MR is also useful in evaluation of vascular lesions in patients with allergy to CT contrast materials. Most MRI examinations cost from 5 to 6 cost units per study, with extra charges for contrast-enhanced studies.

MR requires placing the patient in a long, cylindrical gantry, which limits the usefulness of the study in patients with severe claustrophobia. Since the strong magnetic field will have effects on any ferromagnetic metals present within the gantry, the ability to use many patient monitoring devices is somewhat limited, although newer, non-ferromagnetic monitoring devices may solve this problem (Holshouser *et al.*, 1993). Moderate patient co-operation is required for MR studies, as the images are easily degraded by even minimal patient motion and examinations can take up to 1–2 hours to complete. MR is contraindicated in patients with certain internal metallic objects (lens implants, intraocular metallic shards, cerebral aneurysm clips, abdominal vascular clips for 3–6 months after surgery, cochlear implants) or particularly in patients with pacemakers. Like CT, MR tables have patient weight limits of 135–160 kg and patient diameter may also limit entry of certain patients into the gantry opening. Unlike CT, MR images are much less degraded by large metallic objects within the patient, such as hip replacements or spinal stabilization rods. In many areas of the body, there is considerable controversy regarding use of CT vs MR for imaging and follow-up. Often, either can be used and other considerations such as cost or ease of scheduling may become the deciding factor. It is important to keep in mind that comparisons between studies will be easier in the same imaging modality is used each time a patient is examined (Table 2.4).

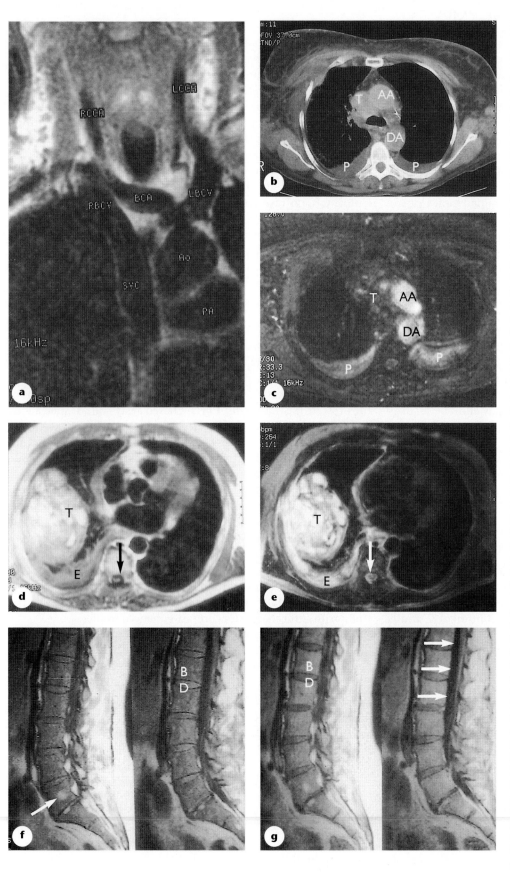

Fig. 2.6 Technical factors in MR imaging (**a**) Coronal T_1-weighted image through a normal mediastinum, demonstrating vascular structures, without the use of IV contrast. On this pulse sequence, flowing blood appears low in signal (black). SVC = superior vena cava: RBCV = right brachiocephalic vein: LBCV = left brachiocephalic vein; RCCA = right common carotid artery; LCCA = left common carotid artery; BCA = brachiocephalic artery; Ao = aorta; PA = main pulmonary artery. (**b**) CT image at a level just below the aortic arch, without IV contrast, in a 64-year-old patient with neck and facial swelling indicative of SVC syndrome. Tumor is seen in the region of the superior vena cava (T) and inseparable from it, which revealed small cell lung carcinoma on biopsy. Small bilateral pleural effusions are also present (P). AA = ascending aorta; DA = descending aorta (**c**) Axial gradient echo MR image in the same patient, at approximately the same level in the chest as in Fig. 2.6 **b**. No IV contrast was used and flowing blood appears high in signal (white) with this pulse sequence. No normal flow is detected in the expected region of the superior vena cava, which is obliterated by tumor (T). AA = ascending aorta: DA = descending aorta; P = pleural effusion. (**d**) Axial T_1-weighted MR image in a 59-year-old male with chest pain and a large right pleural mass. Biopsy revealed pleural leiomyosarcoma. Heterogeneous tumor (T) is seen in the peripheral right lower chest, along with pleural disease (E), which does not have the expected low signal of simple effusion on this pulse sequence. Note high signal (white) appearance of fat in the subcutaneous regions and mediastinum, as expected on a T_1-weighted sequence. Since fluid is typically low signal on T_1-weighted images, the CSF space appears as a black ring surrounding the higher signal spinal cord (arrow). (**e**) Axial T_2-weighted MR image in the same patient, at a similar level in the chest. The tumor (T) is again heterogeneous in appearance, but of higher signal than on the T_1-weighted image. Signal in the pleural space (E) is similar to that of the tumor, again suggesting pleural spread. Note lower signal (gray) appearance of subcutaneous fat in comparison to the T_1-weighted image, as expected on a T_2-weighted sequence. Fluid is typically high in signal on T_2-weighted images, and therefore the CSF space appears as a white ring surrounding the lower signal spinal cord (arrow). (**f**) Sagittal T_1-weighted images of the lumbar spine in a 52-year-old female with anemia and low back pain. Normally, the signal in the vertebral bodies is relatively high on T_1-weighted images, due to fat within the marrow. The signal in the vertebral bodies (B) in this patient is similar to that of the intervertebral discs (D). indicating a diffuse infiltrative marrow abnormality. Focal high signal in the L5 vertebral body (arrow) is a hemangioma. (**g**) Sagittal T_1-weighted images of the lumbar spine in the same patient, after IV administration of gadolinium. The marrow signal in the vertebral bodies does not normally change after IV contrast administration. The signal in the vertebral bodies (B) has increased and is now higher than the signal in the intervertebral discs (D), indicating diffuse enhancement, also suggestive of a diffuse infiltrative process. Bone marrow biopsy revealed evidence of Waldenstrom's macroglobulinemia. Note low signal in CSF (arrows), as expected on all T_1-weighted images.

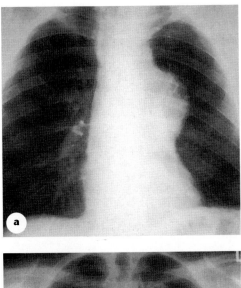

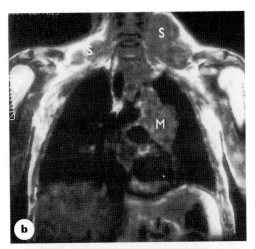

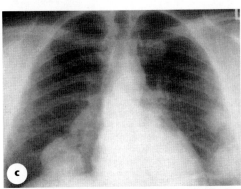

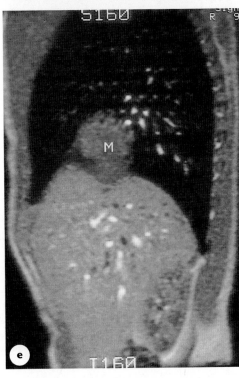

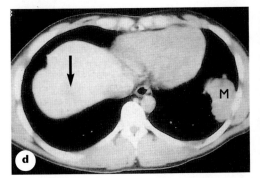

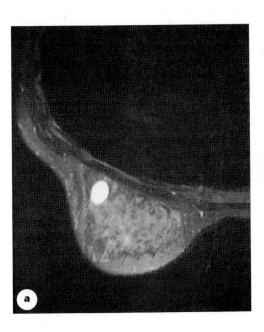

Fig. 2.7 Clinical application of multiplanar capabilities of MR. (**a**) Frontal radiograph of the chest in the PA projection in a 43-year-old male with a history of testicular teratoma. A smoothly marginated left mediastinal mass is evident overlying the left hilum. (**b**) Coronal T_1-weighted MR image in the same patient, showing a mediastinal mass (M) and also extensive bilateral supraclavicular disease (S). Biopsy revealed recurrent teratoma. (**c**) Frontal chest radiograph in the PA projection in a 29-year-old male with a history of malignant sweat gland tumor several years earlier. Large lung nodules are evident bilaterally. (**d**) CT image in the same patient, being performed for staging prior to planned resection of pulmonary metastases. A low-attenuation lesion is evident in the liver (arrow), suggesting more widespread metastatic disease which would preclude surgery. A large left lung metastasis is also evident (M). (**e**) Sagittal gradient echo MR image in the same patient. The questioned lesion in the dome of the liver represents indentation of the diaphragm by one of the lower lobe lung lesions (M). No liver metastases were detected and the patient went on to resection of his lung metastases. Note the high signal indicating flowing blood within vessels in the lung and liver, as expected on gradient echo MR sequences.

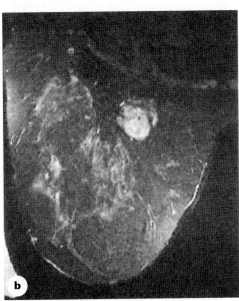

Fig. 2.8 Utility of MR imaging in the breast. (**a**) T_2-weighted breast MR in a 41-year-old patient with a palpable mass. A special pulse sequence was used, called 'fat saturation', to decrease the amount of signal from fat in the breast, and increase conspicuity of other tissues. A single, homogeneously high-signal, smooth rounded lesion is evident, consistent with a cyst, which was also confirmed with ultrasound. (**b**) T_2-weighted breast MR in a 37-year-old patient with a palpable mass. Fat saturation was also used in this patient to decrease signal from fat within the breast. A slightly lobular mass is seen deep in the breast with more heterogeneous internal signal than in the lesion in Fig. 2.8 **a**. At surgery, a fibroadenoma was removed. Use of MRI in the breast is still at an investigational stage, but may prove particularly useful in patients with very dense breast stroma on mammography or with extensive surgical scarring in which sensitivity of mammography is decreased. At present, MRI of the breast is not a substitute for mammography, but is useful in a problem-solving approach to specific mammographic abnormalities.

Table 2.4 Uses and limitations of various imaging procedures in oncologic patients

Study	Clinical Utility	Clinical Limitations
Ultrasound	1. Detection of cystic nature of superficial lesions (as in breast) 2. Guidance of biopsy 3. Guidance of thoracocentesis/pericardio-centesis 4. Detection of liver lesions, some characterization (hemangiomas) 5. Real-time imaging 6. Relatively low cost (2–3 cost units for most studies) 7. Can be done portably, intraoperatively 8. No Ionizing radiation 9. Does not require IV contrast to demonstrate flowing blood, thrombus 10. Images can be obtained in any plane	1. Limited view of mediastinum 2. Limited view of the pancreas in many patients 3. Low spatial resolution 4. Images very operator dependent 5. Limited depth of penetration 6. Not useful in detection of bone lesions 7. Abdominal studies limited in presence of barium in the GI tract from prior fluoroscopy
Computed tomography	1. Better contrast resolution than plain films, sensitive detection of fat and calcification 2. High spatial resolution 3. Guidance of biopsy/drainages 4. Detection of liver lesions, some characterization (using IV contrast and delayed imaging) 5. Sensitive in detection of abnormalities of cortical bone 6. Reproducible size measurements (not very operator dependent) 7. Very rapid imaging possible with ultrafast unit, approaching real-time imaging 8. Moderate cost (4–15 cost units, depending on areas included and use of contrast)	1. Uses ionizing radiation 2. Cannot be performed portably 3. Moderate claustrophobia 4. Limited in the presence of metallic hardware 5. Somewhat limited by patient motion 6. Requires IV contrast to detect flowing blood, thrombus 7. Requires adequate bowel opacification for most abdominal studies (up to 6 hours of preparation time required) 8. Sensitive to misregistration of scans due to respiratory variation unless SPIRAL is used 9. Scans limited to axial plane 10. Abdominal studies limited in presence of barium in the GI tract from prior procedures
Magnetic resonance imaging	1. No ionizing radiation 2. Less risk of contrast reaction than with CT contrast agents 3. Sensitive in detection of bone marrow infiltration 4. Excellent for survey of spinal cord (cord compression) 5. Most sensitive for detection of CNS metastatic disease 6. Only minimally limited by metallic hardware 7. Does not require IV contrast to detect flowing blood, thrombus 8. Scans can be obtained in any plane	1. Cannot be performed portably 2. Limited ability to monitor patients with older equipment 3. Very limited in patients with severe claustrophobia 4. Very limited by patient motion 5. Limited examination of the bowel 6. High cost (10–20 cost units) 7. Not sensitive in detection of calcification 8. Studies may take 45 min–2 hours to complete 9. Utility for biopsy guidance limited to investigational units

IMAGE-GUIDED BIOPSY

Interventional radiology is a rapidly changing field, with many procedures which previously required surgical intervention (such as inferior vena cava filter or gastrostomy tube placement) now performed by radiologists using ultrasound, angiographic or CT guidance. A description of the many interventional radiologic procedures which may be useful in cancer patients is beyond the scope of this chapter. This section will focus instead on a discussion of biopsy using image guidance.

Percutaneous biopsy can be performed with fine-gauge needles (18–22 gauge) for cytologic aspiration specimens. Using such small needles, safe entry can be made into very deep structures, sometimes passing through bowel, liver or vessels without complications (Wittenberg *et al.*, 1982). Larger caliber cutting needles (18–20 gauge) can be used to collect tissue specimens for histologic exami- nation, but are only safe, for relatively peripheral lesions. Automated core or biopsy guns use 14–18 gauge needles to collect even larger specimens and may be particularly useful in breast lesions, lymphoma or mesothelioma. Such large needles are not suitable for many deeper lesions.

For most percutaneous procedures, certain laboratory values are checked, similar to those for bronchoscopy: platelets usually must be >50 000 with normal PT and PTT. For biopsy of lesions in the lung, most nodules must be ≥1 cm in diameter, although smaller lesions may sometimes be biopsied if they are peripheral in location. Biopsy of basilar lesions is more difficult than lesions in the upper lungs, as the lung bases move more with respiration and relatively small inconsistencies in breath holding may move a lower lobe lesion out of the scan plane and needle track. Consultation with an interventional radiologist with review of all imaging is useful prior to scheduling percutaneous biopsies, to assess accessibility of lesions and to plan the approach. In most cases, it is helpful to obtain a complete cross-sectional imaging series through the lesion (CT or MR) prior to the biopsy to localize any nearby structures which should be avoided, such as nerves, vessels or pleural fissures. Either CT or fluoroscopy can be used for guidance of biopsies in the chest. Fluoroscopy is generally easier and faster but may not be appropriate for very central lesions. Most abdominal biopsies use CT or ultra- sound guidance (Vassiliades and Bernardino, 1991). Ultrasound has the advantage of providing real-time visualization of the needle

position (see Fig. 2.9). Ultrasound is limited by requirement for an acoustic 'window' to allow imaging and sometimes by depth of pen- etration of the transducer, particularly in large or obese patients.

Considerable patient co-operation is required for image-guided biopsy procedures. In the chest in particular, the patient must remain still for up to one hour and also suspend respiration repeat- edly when the needle is in place. If the patient is restless, coughing uncontrollably or in extreme pain, any image-guided biopsy may be impossible, since each time the patient moves on the scan table, the entire procedure for localizing the lesion must begin again. Most image-guided biopsy procedures can be performed on an outpatient basis. For outpatient chest biopsies, patients are usually monitored for 2–4 hours after the procedure for pneumothorax before being sent home. Ultrasound-guided biopsies may be performed at the bedside. Radiation dose will vary depending on the modality used for guidance. Cost will also vary, with ultrasound generally the least expensive. A cytologic wet reading is often obtained at the time of sample collection, to determine if more samples are needed. This increases the rate of success in obtaining a diagnosis and may also decrease complications through decrease in the total number of samples collected (Johnsrude et al., 1985).

Interventional radiology's role in the care of cancer patients con- tinues to expand with development of safer and less invasive biopsy techniques, such as transjugular liver biopsy, as well as less invasive treatment methods, such as chemoembolization, radiofrequency or ultrasonic ablation and gene therapy (Ray, 2000).

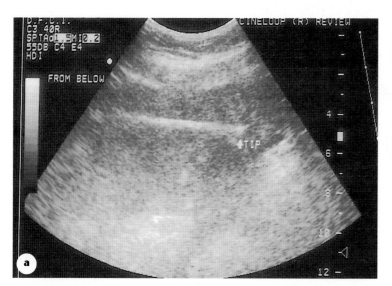
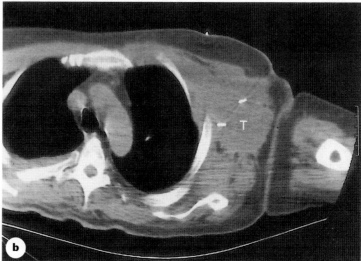

Fig. 2.9 Utility of CT and US in guiding interventional procedures. (**a**) Real- time ultrasound image obtained during placement of temperature-sensing probes within a large axillary mass for research hyperthermia protocol in a 58- year-old male with metastatic squamous cell carcinoma of the lung. Continuous monitoring is possible during the entire procedure, with color flow imaging used to locate vascular structures. (**b**) CT image through the left axillary mass in the same patient. The position of two of the probes within the mass is evident, with one near the deepest margin of the tumor (T), just outside the ribcage.

NEWER IMAGING MODALITIES

POSITRON EMISSION TOMOGRAPHY (PET)

Positron emission tomography (PET) is a non-invasive diagnostic imaging modality that provides whole-body functional imaging capability and holds great promise for cancer patients. It uses positron-emitting isotopes of elements such as carbon (C-11), nitrogen (N-13), oxygen (O-15) and fluorine (F-18) to label compounds that are similar to naturally occurring substances in the body. These radiopharmaceuticals can be used as tracers for physiologic and pathophysiologic processes that correlate with various disease states.

2-[F-18]-Fluoro-2-deoxy-d-glucose (F-18-FDG) is a FDA-approved positron-emitting glucose analog, which is transported into tumor cells, phosphorylated by hexokinase into FDG-6-phosphate, but does not go further along the glycolytic pathway and remains trapped within the cell. This 'metabolic trapping' leads to progressive intracellular accumulation of F-18-FDG over time, with preferential accumulation in tissues with higher glucose metabolism (Fig. 2.10).

Tumor cells show an increased expression of glucose transporter messenger RNA and glucose transporter molecules (GLUT-1 and GLUT-3), as well as an increased activity of hexokinase II (the isoenzyme associated with anaerobic glycolysis) and downregulation of glucose-6-phosphatase enzymes. This increased glycolytic activity is the rationale for the use of F-18-FDG in the functional imaging of cancer.

The positron emitted by the radionuclide travels a short distance (~1 mm) in human tissue, combines with an electron and annihilates. This reaction results in the production of two 511 keV photons that are emitted very close to 180° from each other. These high-energy photons can be detected at the same time (in 'coincidence') defining a line of response along which lies the site of the annihilation reaction. The resulting information can be reconstructed to produce a three-dimensional map of the tracer concentration throughout the body. There are a variety of cameras able to perform PET, ranging from modified traditional nuclear medicine cameras to systems dedicated solely to coincidence imaging. The image quality and performance of the latter tend to be much better than that of the former (Fig. 2.11).

A disadvantage of PET is the short half-life of the positron emitters. The 110-min half-life of F-18 is sufficiently long that tracers can be labeled with it and shipped from a location outside a PET facility. However, other positron emitters have a much shorter half-life ranging from 2 min for O-15 to 20 min for C-11, which requires on-site production. This is a limitation since most hospitals cannot afford the expense of an on-site cyclotron and radiopharmaceutical production facility. F-18 is therefore likely to remain the workhorse clinical PET radionuclide in the near future.

For a typical whole-body imaging protocol, the patient is asked to fast for 4 h or preferably overnight. F-18-FDG (10–20 mCi (370–740 MBq)) is injected intravenously and images are obtained 40–60 min later. Images are usually interpreted qualitatively but quantitative analysis can also be performed based on a region of interest (ROI) corrected for injected dose and body weight. Quantitative indices include standardized uptake value (SUV), distribution absorption ratio (DAR), differential uptake ratio (DUR), tumor-to-normal tissue ratio (T/NT) and regional metabolic rate of glucose (rMRglu). The normal distribution of F-18-FDG one hour post-injection of the tracer includes the brain, the blood pool, urinary activity within the renal collecting system and the bladder, as well as uptake in smooth and striated muscles. Myocardial uptake is highly dependent on the fasting state and is enhanced in the presence of insulin, as is the uptake in skeletal muscle (Fig. 2.12).

PET offers a number of significant advantages over other diagnostic technologies. It can differentiate between benign and malignant tissue with a high degree of accuracy (Fig. 2.13). It is the best imaging modality to evaluate an indeterminate solitary pulmonary nodule (Lowe et al., 1998; Gould et al., 2001) and it can differentiate tumor recurrence from scar (Flamen et al., 1999; Valk et al., 1999). PET has a better overall diagnostic accuracy than CT or MRI for staging and restaging, in part because of its ability to detect disease in normal-sized nodes (Patz et al., 1995; Jerusalem et al., 1999; Dwamena et al., 1999; Magnami et al., 1999; Dietlein et al., 2000; Pieterman et al., 2000; Lerut et al., 2000; Lowe et al., 2000). Most studies report sensitivities between 80% and 100% and specificity estimates between 76% and 100%. F-18-FDG false-positive uptake can be seen in areas of inflammation (such as sarcoidosis) and in infections (such as histoplasmosis, coccoidomycosis and tuberculosis). When PET is discordant with other modalities, PET is correct in 40–96% of cases (Zinzani et al., 1999). Splenic involvement in lymphomas may be better defined on F-18-FDG than on gallium scintigraphy. PET affects patient management decisions in 5–23% of cases mainly by either upstaging or downstaging disease (Fig. 2.14; Valk et al., 1996; Moog et al., 1998; Kalff et al., 2001). It is helpful in assessing surgical eligibility (Fong et al., 1999) and is cost effective (Gould and Lillington 1998). It is also useful in the evaluation of therapeutic response (Rege et al., 2000) and may be a better prognostic factor compared with CT in lymphoma (Okada et al., 1994; Jerusalem et al., 1999). It may also more accurately predict the likelihood of long-term survival in patients with NSCLC (Dunagan et al., 2001).

The Centers for Medicine and Medicaid Services (CMS) have approved reimbursement for PET scans for the diagnosis staging and restaging of non-small cell lung cancer, melanoma, esophageal cancer, colorectal cancer, Hodgkin's and non-Hodgkin's lymphomas and head and neck cancers other than CNS and thyroid cancers. CMS also approved reimbursement for the evaluation of indeterminate solitary pulmonary nodule, locoregional recurrence, distant metastasis, and evaluation of therapeutic response in breast cancer. Third-party payers have approved reimbursement in other tumors as well.

PET may soon become the major imaging modality for oncology (Mankoff and Bellon, 2001) and has already shown particular utility in neuro-oncology (Roelcke and Leenders, 2001). The potential power of PET imaging will be greatly expanded in the future through development of new positron-emitting radiopharmaceuticals which may offer even more specificity than FDG. Agents which target cellular proliferative markers and steroid receptors show great promise for more detailed metabolic imaging (Mankoff et al., 2000). As more specific peptide and antibody markers for tumors are discovered, these will have roles both as treatment agents and potentially as imaging agents if they can be labeled with either positron emitters or γ-emitters for SPECT imaging (Chester et al., 2000). As more specific drugs are developed for treatment of cancer, PET may also be used to assess their suitability for a particular patient and to follow the progress of therapy if radiolabeling can be accomplished with an appropriate isotope (Phelps, 2000). The introduction of combined PET and CT scanners will also have a major impact on the management of patients with cancer by allowing precise localization of abnormal findings on PET, optimal characterization of masses, and radiation therapy planning.

INTERVENTIONAL MR AND MR SPECTROSCOPY

Several recent developments in MR technology may have potential clinical utility in the cancer patient. A new open configuration MR design (Jolesz and Blumenfeld, 1994) creates the potential for interventional MR (see Fig. 2.15). In combination with non-ferromagnetic needles and innovative coil designs such new magnet configurations allow use of MR for guiding biopsies, drainages and other interventional procedures (Orel *et al.*, 1994). Another area of investigation in MR is use of spectroscopy *in vivo* to detect signal generated by isotopes other than hydrogen, including phosphorus, nitrogen, sodium and fluorine. The abundance of these isotopes is less than that of hydrogen in the body and the signal which they generate is also lower, limiting the quality of the images which can be generated with current equipment (Partain and Patton, 1994). Use of higher field strength magnets may increase the signal detectable from these isotopes and improve clinical imaging. MR spectroscopy using phosphorus may give insight into energy metabolism in tumors (Barker *et al.*, 1993).

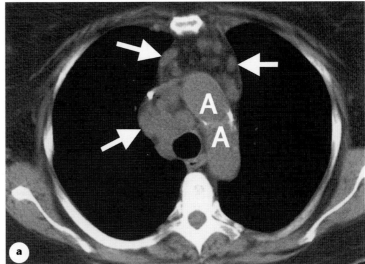

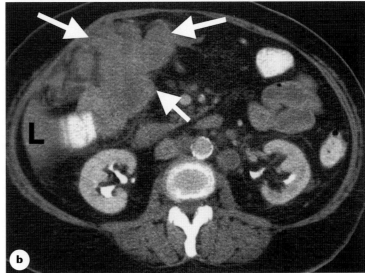

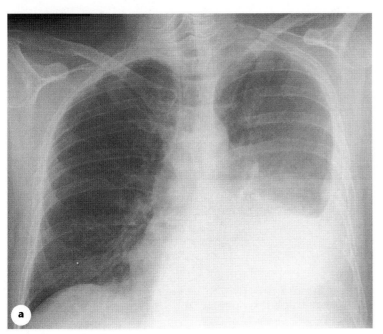

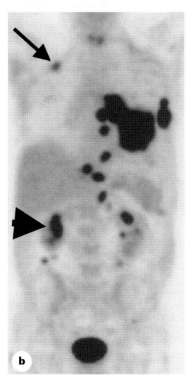

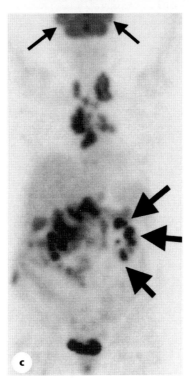

Fig. 2.10 PET imaging depends on accumulation of F-18-FD6 in tissues with high rates of glucose metabolism and often demonstrates disease sites not suspected on routine imaging. (**a**) Chest radiograph in a 77-year-old man with known poorly differentiated lung cancer and new shortness of breath. A large left pleural effusion obscures most of the left chest. (**b**) The projection image from the patient's PET scan shows extensive abnormal uptake in the left lower lobe in a mass-like configuration not typical for malignant effusion. This large lung mass was obscured by the pleural effusion on the chest film. Areas of abnormal uptake near the midline are consistent with metastases to mediastinal nodes and there is also left lateral chest wall uptake suspicious for skeletal invasion. A focal area of uptake on the right (small black arrow) indicates unsuspected contralateral supraclavicular spread. Uptake in the renal collecting systems (large black arrow) is normal.

Fig. 2.11 PET imaging with a dedicated scanner allows staging of the entire body in a single scan, detecting disease in many different sites. (**a**) Image from a non-enhanced CT scan of the chest at the level of the aortic arch (AA) showing extensive adenopathy in the anterior mediastinum and right paratracheal regions (white arrows) in a 58-year-old patient with colon adenocarcinoma. (**b**) Image from the abdominal portion of the patient's CT scan shows an irregular mass in the right upper quadrant adjacent to the lowermost tip of the liver (L) that could be mistaken for unopacified bowel loops. (**c**) Projection image from the patient's whole-body FDG-PET scan shows extensive abnormal uptake in the mediastinum and upper abdomen corresponding to the abnormalities seen on CT. Uptake in the brain (small black arrows) is normal. Focal activity in the collecting systems of the kidneys (large black arrows) can be discriminated from disease sites by its characteristic configuration and location.

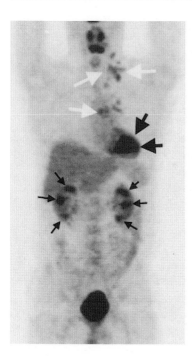

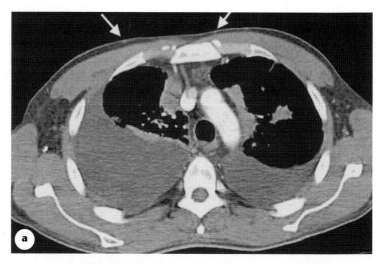

Fig. 2.12 Cardiac and brain uptake of F-18-FD6 is normal in the non-fasting state. Projection image of a whole-body PET scan of a patient with nodular sclerosis Hodgkin's disease shows abnormal uptake in the left supraclavicular area and left mediastinum (white arrows). Intense uptake over the heart (large black arrows) is normal in a non-fasting patient. Uptake over the calyces of the kidneys (small black arrows) and in the bladder is normal due to renal excretion of the radiotracer.

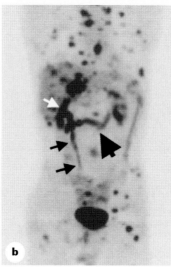

Fig. 2.13 PET imaging with a dedicated system can distinguish between benign and malignant processes in many cases. (**a**) Image from a contrast-enhanced CT scan of the chest in a 50-year-old man with diffuse large B-cell lymphoma. Large bilateral pleural effusions and patchy lung disease are evident along with tiny skin lesions (tip of white arrows), which are barely visible on CT. (**b**) The projection image from the patient's PET scan shows much more extensive skin involvement than was evident on the CT scan. Normal activity in the right renal pelvis (white arrow) and right ureter (small black arrows) as well as in bowel (large black arrow) should not be mistaken for disease.

DIGITAL RADIOGRAPHY

Digital radiographic imaging will probably ultimately replace analog imaging for most plain film radiography. In digital radiography, a phosphor-coated plate is substituted for the photographic film used in routine radiography. This plate is exposed using standard X-ray equipment and is then read out electronically in the form of digital imaging data. The plate can be erased and reused. The digital imaging data can be used to print images on transparent film or paper or displayed on a monitor. Digital imaging has many advantages over routine radiography, including fewer under- or overpenetrated films, ability to change contrast and brightness of the image after acquisition, existence of edge-enhancing algorithms for image processing and digital storage, allowing electronic transfer of imaging information (Cowen et al., 1993). Drawbacks include slightly lower spatial resolution, slow display of images on some monitors and initial expense of installation. Combination of digital imaging systems with radiology scheduling and reporting systems allows progression to a 'film-less' radiology department, utilizing a totally integrated 'picture archiving and communication system' or PACS (Choplin et al., 1992). Particularly with newer, faster computer systems and improvements in rate of data transfer, this goal appears to be attainable in the near future.

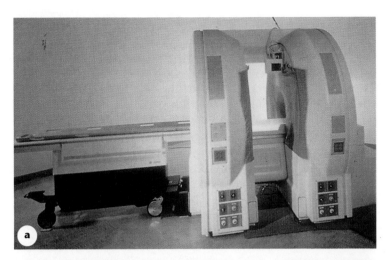

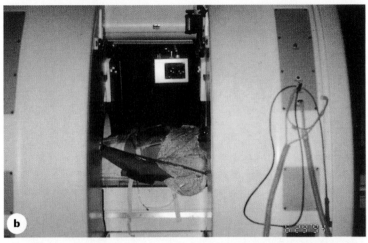

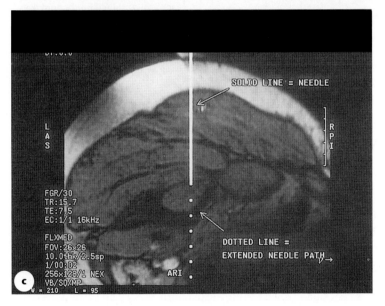

Fig. 2.14 Interventional MR. (**a**) The open configuration interventional MR scanner at Brigham and Women's Hospital in Boston, Massachusetts. The magnet gantry is constructed to provide access to the patient during scanning. (**b**) Open configuration MR scanner with patient in place, demonstrating degree of access available to the radiologist for interventional procedures. (**c**) Specialized rapid MR acquisition (spoiled gradient echo) obtained during an interventional procedure, showing planned needle path for biopsy of a lesion in the left iliac bone. The MR biopsy was non-diagnostic, yielding only bloody material. At final pathology after a surgical biopsy, a primary vascular tumor of bone was diagnosed, an epithelioid hemangio-endothelioma. In such tumors, needle aspirates are rarely diagnostic as they will only yield bloody fluid, as seen here.

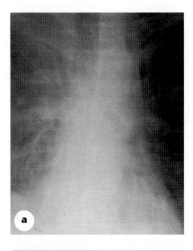
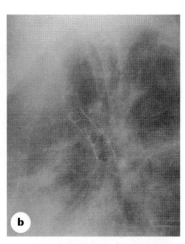

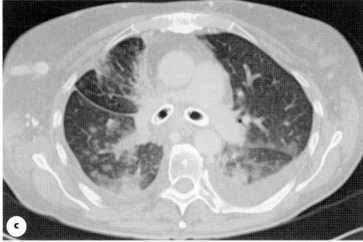

THE FUTURE

Other new technologies may offer innovative methods of visualization of tumor involvement, such as optical coherence tomography (Fujimoto *et al.*, 2000). In this experimental method, visible light is used in a manner similar to ultrasound to obtain tomographic characterization of tissues on the micron scale *in situ* over short distances. This technology may have a role in the future in conjunction with endoscopy to allow multiple followup studies of mucosal and submucosal tumors to determine response or in actual diagnosis in cases where biopsy is not technically possible.

Fig. 2.15 Digital radiography allows post-image capture manipulation to maximize visualization of subtle findings. This patient with poorly differentiated non-small cell lung carcinoma had bilateral mainstem bronchial stents placed to manage airway compression. The stents were difficult to see on routine films, but with adjustment of contrast and edge enhancement, they were easily seen. (**a**) Close-up of frontal view of the chest showing clear demonstration of stent position. (**b**) Close-up of lateral view of the chest, also showing stents clearly in spite of limited penetration. Edge-enhancing algorithms were used to accentuate fine details of sharply defined structures, such as the stents, and make them more easily visible. (**c**) Image from the patient's chest CT scan showing the stents in place. (Case courtesy of Dr Raphael Bueno, Thoracic Surgery Division, Brigham and Women's Hospital.)

REFERENCES

Atlas SW: MR angiography in neurologic disease. Radiology 1994; 193 : 1–16.

Barker PB, Glickson JD, Bryan RN: In vivo magnetic resonance spectroscopy of human brain tumors. Topics MRI 1993; 5 : 32–45.

Bird RE, Wallace TW, Yankaskas BC: Analysis of cancers missed at screening mammography. Radiology 1992; 184 : 613–617.

Botet JF, Lightdale CJ, Zauber AG, Gerdes H, Urmacher C, Brennan MF: Preoperative staging of esophageal cancer: comparison of endoscopic US and dynamic CT. Radiology 1991; 181 : 419–425.

Brasch R, Turetschek K: MRI characterization of tumors and grading angiogenesis using macromolecular contrast media: status report. Eur J Radiol 2000; 34(3): 148–155.

Bressler EL, Alpern MB, Glazer GM, Francis IR, Ensminger WD: Hypervascular hepatic metastases: CT evaluation. Radiology 1987: 162 : 49–51.

Broadbent MV, Hubbard LB: Science and perception of radiation risk. Radiographics 1992; 12 : 381–392.

Caro JJ, Trinidade E, McGregor M: The risks of death and of severe nonfatal reactions with high- vs. low-osmolality contrast media: a meta-analysis. AJR 1991; 156 : 825–832.

Chester KA, Mayer A, Bhatia J, *et al.*: Recombinant anti-carcinoembryonic antigen antibodies for targeting cancer. Cancer Chemo Pharmacol 2000; 46 (suppl):S8–12.

Choplin RH, Boehme JM, Maynard CD: PACS mini refresher course: picture archiving and communication systems: an overview. Radiographics 1992; 12 : 127–129.

Clarke MP, Kane RA, Steele G. *et al.*: Prospective comparison of preoperative imaging and intraoperative ultrasonography in the detection of liver tumors. Surgery 1989; 106 : 849–855.

Costello P, Dupuy DE, Ecker CP, Tello R: Spiral CT of the thorax with reduced volume of contrast material: a comparative study. Radiology 1992; 183 : 663–666.

Cowen AR, Workman A, Price JS: Physical aspects of photostimulable phosphor computed radiography. Br J Radiol 1993; 66 : 332–345.

Davis PC, Hudgins PA, Peterman SB, Hoffman JC Jr. Diagnosis of cerebral metastases: double-dose delayed CT vs. contrast-enhanced MR imaging. Am J Neuroradiol 1991; 12 : 293–300.

Dietlein M, Weber K, Gandjour A, et al.: Cost-effectiveness of FDG-PET for the management of potentially operable non small cell lung cancer: priority for a PET-based strategy after nodal-negative CT results. Eur J Nucl Med 2000; 27: 1598–1609.

Dunagan D, Chin R Jr, McCain T, et al.: Staging by positron emission tomography predicts survival in patients with non-small cell lung cancer. Chest 2001; 119: 333–339.

Dwamena BA, Sonnad SS, Angobaldo JO, Wahl RL: Metastases from non-small cell lung cancer: mediastinal staging in the 1990s – meta-analytic comparison of PET and CT. Radiology 1999; 213: 530–536.

Eklund GW, Busby RC, Miller SH, Job JS: Improved imaging of the augmented breast. AJR 1988; 151 : 469–473.

Evelhoch JL, Gillies RJ, Karczmar GS, et al.: Applications of magnetic resonance in model systems: cancer therapeutics. Neoplasia 2000; 2(1–2):152–165.

Feig SA: Mammography equipment: principles, features, selection. Radiol Clin N Am 1987; 25 : 897–911.

Flamen P, Stroobants S, van Cutsem E, et al.: Additional value of whole-body positron emission tomography with fluorine-18–2-fluoro-2-deoxy-D-glucose in recurrent colorectal cancer. J Clin Oncol 1999; 17: 894–901.

Fong Y, Saldinger PF, Akhurst T, et al.: Utility of 18F-FDG positron emission tomography scanning on selection of patients for resection of hepatic colorectal metastases. Am J Surg 1999; 178: 282–287.

Fujimoto JG, Pitris C, Boppart SA, Brezinski ME: Optical coherence tomography: an emerging technology for biomedical imaging and optical biopsy. Neoplasia 2000; 2 : 9–25.

Gofman JW, O'Connor E: X-rays: Health Effects of Common Exams. Sierra Club Books, San Francisco, 1985.

Gould MK, Lillington GA: Strategy and cost in investigating solitary pulmonary nodules. Thorax 1998; 53:S32–37.

Gould MK, Maclean CC, Kuschner WG, Rydzak CE, Owens DK: Accuracy of positron emission tomography for diagnosis of pulmonary nodules and mass lesions: a meta-analysis. JAMA 2001; 285: 936–937.

Harms SE, Flamig DP, Hesley KL, et al.: Fat-suppressed three-dimensional MR imaging of the breast. Radiographics 1993; 13 : 247–267.

Hendrick RE, Haacke EM: Basic physics of MR contrast agents and maximization of image contrast. J MRI 1993; 3 : 137–148.

Henschke CI: Early lung cancer action project: overall design and findings from baseline screening. Cancer 2000; 89(11 suppl):2474–2482.

Holland R, Hendricks JH, Mravunac M: Mammographically occult breast cancer: a pathologic and radiologic study. Cancer 1983; 52 : 1810–1819.

Holshouser BA, Hinshaw DB, Shellock FG: Sedation, anesthesia, and physiologic monitoring during MR imaging: evaluation of procedures and equipment. J MRI 1993; 10 : 287–298.

Hopper KD, Singapuri K, Finkel A: Body CT and oncologic imaging. Radiology 2000; 215(1):27–40.

Jackson VP. The role of US in breast imaging. Radiology 1990; 177 : 305–311.

Jerusalem G, Beguin Y, Gassotte MF, et al.: Whole-body positron emission tomography using F-18-fluorodeoxyglucose for post-treatment evaluation in Hodgkin's disease and non-Hodgkin's lymphoma has higher diagnostic and prognostic value than classical computed tomography scan imaging. Blood 1999; 94 : 429–433.

Johnsrude IS, Silverman JF, Weaver MD, McConnal RW: Rapid cytology to decrease pneumothorax incidence after percutaneous biopsy. AJR 1985; 144 : 793–794.

Jolesz F, Blumenfeld S: Interventional use of magnetic resonance imaging. Magnet Res Quart 1994; 10(2):85–96.

Kalff VV, Hicks RJ, MacManus M, et al.: Clinical impact of (18)F-fluorodeoxyglucose positron emission tomography in patients with non-small cell lung cancer: a prospective study. J Clin Oncol 2001; 19: 111–118.

Kelly JF, Patterson R, Lieberman P, Mathison DA, Stevenson DD: Radiographic contrast media studies in high-risk patients. J Allergy Clin Immunol 1978; 62 : 181–184.

Kier R, Wain S, Troiano R: Fast spin-echo MR images of the pelvis obtained with a phased-array coil: value in localizing and staging prostatic carcinoma. AJR 1993; 161(3):601–606.

Krishna MC, Subramanian S, Kuppusamy P, Mitchell JB: Magnetic resonance imaging for in vivo assessment of tissue oxygen concentration. Semin Radiat Oncol 2001; 11(1):58–69.

Lerut T, Flamen P, Ectors N, et al.: Histopathologic validation of lymph node staging with FDG-PET scan in cancer of the esophagus and gastroesophageal junction: a prospective study based on primary surgery with extensive lymphadenectomy. Ann Surg 2000; 232 : 743–752.

Lowe VJ, Boyd JH, Dumphy FR, et al.: Surveillance for recurrent head and neck cancer using positron emission tomography. J Clin Oncol 2000; 18: 651–658.

Lowe VJ, Fletcher JW, Gobar L, et al.: Prospective investigation of positron emission tomography in lung nodules. J Clin Oncol 1998; 16: 1075–1084.

Magnami P, Carretta A, Rizzo G, et al.: FDG/PET and spiral CT image fusion for mediastinal lymph node assessment of non-small cell lung cancer patients. J Cardiovasc Surg 1999; 40 : 741–748.

Mankoff DA, Bellon JR: Positron-emission tomographic imaging of cancer: glucose metabolism and beyond. Semin Radiat Oncol 2001; 11(1): 16–27.

Mankoff DA, Dehdashti F, Shields AF: Characterizing tumors using metabolic imaging: PET imaging of cellular proliferation and steroid receptors. Neoplasia 2000; 2(1–2):71–88.

Moog F, Bangertner M, Diederichs CG, et al.: Extranodal malignant lymphoma detection with FDG PET versus CT. Radiology 1998; 206 : 475–481.

Napel S, Marks MP, Rubin GD, et al.: CT angiography with spiral CT and maximum intensity projection. Radiology 1992; 185 : 607–610.

Negendank W, Soulen RL: Magnetic resonance imaging in patients with bone marrow disorders. Leukemia Lymphoma 1993; 10 : 287–298.

Okada J, Oonishi H, Yoshikawa K, et al.: FDG PET for predicting the prognosis of malignant lymphoma. Ann Nucl Med 1994; 8 : 187–191.

Orel SG, Schnall MD, Newman RW, Powell CM, Torosian MH. Rosato EF: MR imaging-guided localization and biopsy of breast lesions: initial experience. Radiology 1994; 193 : 97–102.

Partain CL, Patton JA: Magnetic resonance imaging systems. In: Taveras JM, Ferrucci JT, eds: Radiology: Diagnosis-Imaging-Intervention, vol X. Lippincott, Philadelphia, 1994; p. 33.

Patz EF Jr, Lowe VJ, Goodman PC, et al.: Thoracic nodal staging with PET imaging with 18 FDG in patients with bronchogenic carcinoma. Chest 1995; 108 : 1617–1621.

Pennes DR, Glazer GM, Wimbish KJ, Gross BH, Long RW, Orringer MB: Chest wall invasion by lung cancer: limitations of CT evaluation. AJR 1985; 144 : 507–511.

Phelps ME: PET: the merging of biology and imaging into molecular imaging. J Nucl Med 41(4):661–681.

Pieterman RM, van Putten JW, Meuzlaar JJ, et al.: Preoperative staging of non-small-cell lung cancer with positron emission tomography. N Engl J Med 2000; 343 : 254–261.

Ray CE Jr: Interventional radiology in cancer patients. Am Family Physician 2000; 62(1):95–102.

Rege S, Safa AA, Chaiken L, Hoh C, Juillard G, Withers HR: Positron emission tomography: an independent indicator of radiocurability in head and neck carcinomas. Am J Clin Oncol 2000; 23 : 164–169.

Roelcke U, Leenders KL: PET in neuro-oncology. J Can Res 2001; 127(1):2–8.

Rosenman J: Incorporating functional imaging information into radiation treatment. Semin Radiat Oncol 2001; 11(1):83–92.

Rothenberg LN, Pentlow KS: Radiation dose in CT. Radiographics 1992; 12 : 1225–1243.

Schnall MD, Imai Y, Tomaszewski J, Pollack HM, Lenkinski RE: Prostate cancer: local staging with endorectal surface coil MR imaging. Radiology 1991; 178 : 797–802.

Smart CR: Mammographic screening: efficacy and guidelines. Curr Opin Radiol 1992; 4(5):108–117.

Smith RC, McCarthy S: Physics of magnetic resonance. J Reprod Med 1992; 37(1):19–26.

Sone S, Li F, Yang ZG, et al.: Results of three-year mass screening programme for lung cancer using mobile low-dose spiral computed tomography scanner. Br J Cancer 2001; 84(1):25–32.

Soyer P, Bluemke DA, Hruban RH, Sitzmann JV, Fishman EK: Hepatic metastases from colorectal cancer: detection and false-positive findings with helical CT during arterial portography. Radiology 1994; 193 : 71–74.

Soyer P, Levesque M, Caudron C, Elias D, Seitoun G, Roche A: MRI of liver metastases from colorectal cancer vs. CT during arterial portography. J Computer Assisted Tomography 1993; 17 : 67–74.

Stanford W, Galvin JR, Weiss RM, Hajduczok ZD, Skorton DJ: Ultrafast computed tomography in cardiac imaging: a review. Semin Ultrasound CT MR 1991; 12 : 45–60.

Stomper PC, Cancer Imaging Manual. Lippincott, Philadelphia, 1993.

Stomper PC, Fung CY, Socinski MA, Jochelson MS, Garnick MB, Richie JP: Detection of retroperitoneal metastases in early-stage nonseminomatous testicular cancer: analysis of different CT criteria. AJR 1987; 149:1187–1190.

Swensen SJ, Aughenbaugh GL, Douglas WE, Myers JL: High-resolution CT of the lungs: findings in various pulmonary diseases. AJR 1992; 158:971–979.

Taylor JS, Reddick WE: Evolution from empirical dynamic contrast-enhanced magnetic resonance imaging to pharmacokinetic MRI. Adv Drug Delivery Rev 2000; 41:91–110.

Tockman MS, Mulshine JL: The early detection of occult lung cancer. Chest Surg Clin N Am 2000; 10(4):737–749.

Valk PE, Abella-Columna E, Haseman MK, et al.: Whole-body PET imaging with {18F}fluorodeoxyglucose in management of recurrent colorectal cancer. Arch Surg 1999; 134:503–511.

Valk PE, Pounds TR, Tesar RD, et al.: Cost-effectiveness of PET imaging in clinical oncology. Nucl Med Biol 1996; 23:737–743.

Vanel D, Stark D, eds: Imaging Strategies in Oncology. John Wiley, New York, 1993.

Vassiliades VG, Bernardino ME: Percutaneous renal and adrenal biopsies. Cardiovasc Interventional Radiol 1991; 14(1):50–54.

Wagner LK: Absorbed dose in imaging: why measure it? Radiology 1991; 178:622–623.

Wilson R: Analyzing the daily risks of life. Technol Rev 1979; Feb: 41–46.

Wittenberg J, Mueller PR, Ferrucci JT, et al.: Percutaneous core biopsy of abdominal tumors using 22 gauge needles: further observations. AJR 1982; 139:75–80.

Woolfenden JM, Pitt MJ, Burie BGM, Moon TE: Comparison of bone scintigraphy and radiography in multiple myeloma. Radiology 1980; 134:723–728.

Zakian KL, Doutcher JA, Ballon D, et al.: Developments in nuclear magnetic resonance imaging and spectroscopy: application to radiation oncology. Semin Radiat Oncol 2001;11(1):3–15.

Zinzani PL, Magagnoli M, Chierichetti F, et al.: The role of positron emission tomography (PET) in the management of lymphoma patients. Ann Oncol 1999; 10: 1181–1184.

Cancer of the head and neck region

A. Dimitrios Colevas, John R. Clark, James N. Suojanen, Marshall Posner

3

Cancers of the lips, oral cavity, the oro-, naso- and hypopharynx, the larynx, the nasal and paranasal sinuses and the neck, ear and salivary glands, as well as those of regional soft tissues and supporting bones, are customarily grouped as cancers of the head and neck. Consequently, a large variety of neoplasms may be encountered, including sarcomas of any type, adenocarcinomas of major or minor salivary gland origin and squamous cell carcinomas of the mucosal lining of the upper aerodigestive tract. Squamous cell carcinoma (SCCHN) is the most common head and neck cancer, occurring in over 90% of cases. Thus, the term head and neck cancer is most often equated with squamous cell carcinoma.

Estimates provided by the American Cancer Society suggest that more than 40 000 new cases of head and neck cancer were diagnosed in the United States in 2000 and approximately 30% of these patients will die of their disease (Greenlee et al., 2000). SCCHN represents approximately 5% of cancers in men and 2% of cancers in women. Despite the fact that more than 70% of patients present with disease apparently confined to the head and neck region, 5-year survival rates for whites and blacks are 56% and 34% respectively for cancers of the oral cavity and pharynx. Because disease of the larynx tends to become apparent at an earlier stage, 5-year survival rates at this site are slightly better – 66% and 53% for whites and black respectively. There has been no change in these survival statistics over the past 25 years. These percentages may change, however, given the increasing use of tobacco products (including smokeless tobacco) by women and young adults and the decreasing use of tobacco by men (MMWR 1998).

Squamous cell carcinoma of the aerodigestive tract is directly related to tobacco and alcohol use. Of these two substances, tobacco is the more important but they appear to be synergistic. Individuals who consume substantial quantities of both tobacco and alcohol are 20 times more likely to develop SCCHN than non-users of these substances (Lewin et al., 1998). The cessation of both alcohol and tobacco consumption is associated with a decreased subsequent risk for all upper aerodigestive neoplasms.

Additional risk factors for cancer of the upper aerodigestive tract include exposure to ionizing radiation and occupational and environmental exposure to carcinogens other than tobacco. For instance, workers involved in plastic fabrication, metal working and textile processing, as well as individuals occupationally or environmentally exposed to asbestos, exhibit an increased incidence of head and neck cancers. Similarly, nasal and sinus cancers are more common in workers in the furniture industry exposed to the dust of hardwoods. Given that the entire mucosa of the upper aerodigestive tract is exposed in such instances, multicentric lesions are not uncommon and may occur either simultaneously or sequentially. With time, the risk for a second, related cancer can exceed that for direct recurrence of the original tumor. The concept that a focus of cancer is but part of a generally 'sick mucosa' is essential to the management of these tumors.

Recent data suggest a possible etiological role of human papilloma virus infection in a subset of SCCHN (Snyderman, 1998; Gillison et al., 2000).

HISTOLOGY

Epithelial lesions

Two types of premalignant epithelial lesions are recognized based on their clinical appearance: leukoplakia and erythroplasia. Leukoplakia, commonly referred to as smoker's keratosis, is marked by raised, white patches that microscopically represent hyperkeratosis or parakeratosis with varying degrees of atypia and associated mucosal atrophy. The atypia can be graded, in a manner similar to changes seen in the uterine cervix, as mild, moderate or severe, based on the degree of mucosal involvement by disorderly cells with nuclear abnormalities. There are many causes of leukoplakia. While the majority of such lesions are innocent and secondary to chronic irritation such as tobacco exposure or dental trauma, 3–15% of persistent raised white lesions within the oral cavity and oropharynx represent premalignant dysplastic leukoplakia. Therefore, even leukoplakia on mucous membranes should be considered dysplastic and potentially premalignant until proved otherwise. These lesions always contain some degree of cellular atypia, the severity of which is impossible to determine without biopsy.

Erythroplasia is a mucosal abnormality of greater concern. Visually, the lesions consist of superficial or slightly depressed areas of denuded mucosa where cellular atypia has reached the mucosal surface; they appear red and velvet-like. It should be assumed that they represent at least carcinoma in situ, because over 80% of such lesions at the time of biopsy exhibit pleomorphic squamous cells with full-thickness atypia of the mucosa. With in situ lesions, the basement membrane separating the mucosa from the underlying stroma is intact, but early microinvasion of the basement membrane with extension into the adjacent stroma can also clinically present as erythroplasia. Locations at high risk for erythroplasia include the central floor of the mouth, the ventrolateral surface of the tongue, the buccal mucosa, the anterior tonsillar pillars and the soft palate.

In the vast majority (90%) of cases, malignant neoplasms of the head and neck arise from the surface epithelium and are therefore squamous cell carcinomas or one of its many variants, including undifferentiated carcinoma, lymphoepithelioma, spindle cell carcinoma and verrucous carcinoma (see Table 3.1). Malignant transformation is accompanied by varying degrees of differentiation of the squamous cells, ranging from well- and moderately well-differentiated to poorly differentiated and anaplastic lesions. As a general rule, less differentiated tumors have a higher incidence of infiltration into neighboring glands, muscles and loose connective tissue, as well as regional spread to lymph nodes of the neck. Bone, cartilage, ligaments, vessels and nerves, however, offer higher resistance to tumor infiltration. In advanced cancers, the morphologic picture may vary considerably in different regions of the lesion. Therefore, surface biopsy specimens may not necessarily represent the entire lesion.

SALIVARY GLAND TUMORS

Salivary gland neoplasms may arise from any of the paired major salivary glands – the parotid, submandibular or sublingual glands – or from one of the many minor salivary glands present throughout the mucosal surfaces of the upper aerodigestive system. These tumors may be benign or malignant and the probability that a given lesion is malignant varies among sites (*see* Table 3.2). Parotid gland tumors, which are relatively common, are usually benign, pleomorphic adenomas being the most frequently encountered. Other benign salivary tumors include papillary cystadenoma lymphomatosum (Warthin's tumor or adenolymphoma) and benign lymphoepithelial lesions, such as Godwin's tumor. Malignant parotid tumors are less common, but a spectrum of malignant histologic types may be encountered (*see* Table 3.3). Histological classification of salivary gland cancers is difficult because of the wide extent of morphological variation within each tumor type (van der Wal *et al.*, 1998). The same spectrum of benign and malignant histologic types of neoplasms as are found in the parotid gland may be encountered in the other major salivary glands and the minor salivary glands.

LESS FREQUENTLY ENCOUNTERED NEOPLASMS

Esthesioneuroblastomas (olfactory neuroblastomas) arise from the respiratory epithelium about the cribriform plate and nasal septum. They may occur at any age, but are most commonly seen in the second and third decades. Histologically, these lesions are composed of rather uniform small blue cells of neuroectodermal origin. They may be confused with undifferentiated carcinoma, undifferentiated lymphoma or rhabdomyosarcoma (*see also* discussions and illustrations of PNET in Chapter 12 and non-CNS PNET in Chapter 16).

Chemodectomas or non-chromaffin paragangliomas are a group of uncommon, slow-growing neoplasms that may originate wherever glomus bodies are found. Most often they arise from the carotid artery and temporal bone and only rarely from the orbit, nasopharynx, larynx, nasal cavity, paranasal sinuses, tongue, jaw and trachea. In 10–20% of cases, glomus tumors may occur in multiple sites, especially in families with a history of this tumor. The histologic picture of these benign lesions is marked by nests of epithelioid cells within stroma containing thin-walled blood vessels and non-myelinated nerve fibers; the relative amounts of epithelioid and vascular tissue may vary. The criterion of malignancy is based on the clinical progress of the disease rather than the histologic appearance. Metastases are infrequent (less than 5% of cases). Endocrine activity has been reported and serotonin has been identified on histochemical staining, thus confirming the tumor's origin from primitive neuroectodermal cells.

Extramedullary plasmacytomas may occur throughout the body, but 80% of these malignancies are located in the head and neck, most notably in the upper air passages and associated structures: nasopharynx, tonsil, maxillary sinus, nasal vestibule and trachea. The majority of patients are in their sixth to eighth decades. Up to 25% of patients present with cervical lymph node involvement and 10–40% eventually progress to multiple myeloma. Histologically identical to the osseous form of plasmacytoma, these extramedullary tumors consist of sheets and aggregates of plasma cells.

Inverting papillomas are low-grade neoplasms that are generally considered to be benign. Most frequently affecting the nasal cavity and paranasal sinuses, they are clinically aggressive lesions characterized by extensive bone destruction, intracranial extension and multiple recurrences. There is an association with squamous cell carcinoma in 10–15% of cases. The histologic picture is that of a papilloma that is growing into the stroma rather than outward.

Mucosal melanomas of the head and neck represent 0.5–2% of all malignant melanomas. The most common location within the head and neck is the nasal cavity, where melanomas represent up to 18% of all malignant tumors. Although varying in their gross appearance, they are usually solid, polypoid lesions about 3.5 cm in diameter. Approximately one-third are amelanotic. The histologic picture is similar to that of cutaneous melanoma, although lymphocytic infiltration is rare.

Midline lethal non-healing granuloma is a non-specific term encompassing a variety of histologic and clinical entities that lead to progressive destruction of the nose, paranasal sinuses, hard palate and contiguous structures. Midline lethal granuloma has been subdivided into three different entities: midline malignant (polymorphic) reticulosis, malignant lymphoma (usually diffuse large cell lymphoma) and Wegener's granulomatosis. (Text on Staging of Head and Neck Cancers and Clinical Manifestations begins on page 40.)

MOLECULAR BIOLOGY

The molecular biology of head and neck cancers has not been defined systematically except for lesions arising from squamous epithelium. Efforts are being made to determine the genetic events associated with, and perhaps responsible for, the conversion of normal squamous epithelium to dysplastic leukoplakia or erythroplasia, to carcinoma *in situ* and, finally, to invasive cancer. These studies attempt to define environmental and genetic differences between patients with isolated mucosal lesions and those with multiple neoplastic abnormalities, so-called 'field carcinogenesis'. Related studies are under way to define the incidence of known oncogenes and tumor suppressor genes in invasive epithelial tumors and to determine their influence on clinical events such as tumor growth rate, potential for metastatic spread, response to therapy and prognosis after treatment.

The most commonly deleted chromosomal region in SCCHN is 9p21. This region encodes for the tumor suppressor p16 (INK4A/MTS-1/CDKN2A), a cyclin-dependent kinase inhibitor (Reed *et al.*, 1996). The loss of p16 is seen early in the evolution of SCCHN, suggesting it may play a part in the early carcinogenic process. Additionally, mutations of the tumor suppressor gene *p53* are also common both in malignant and premalignant mucosal lesions of the head and neck, as well as the histologically normal mucosa of patients with treated squamous cell cancers of the oral cavity and oropharynx (Boyle *et al.*, 1993).

Mutations of *p53* within invasive head and neck squamous carcinomas are frequent, but to date they have not generally been associated with clinical outcome. This may be due to the relatively proximal position of this lesion in the multistep molecular process of carcinogenesis. In contrast, gene amplifications of known oncogenes, while less frequently encountered than *p53* mutations, have been associated with poor prognosis.

Cytogenetic evidence for genetic instability and gene amplification of DNA markers on chromosome 11 band q13 has been identified in many invasive head and neck cancers. Moreover, the presence of 11q13 rearrangements has been associated with poor clinical outcome and younger patient age at presentation. This is of interest since amplification of several oncogenes located in 11q13, such as *int*-2, *bcl*-1, *prad*-1 and cyclin D1, has been reported in this cancer. Amplification of cyclin D1 in particular has been identified in up to 20% of head and neck cancers and is independently associated with tobacco exposure and poor prognosis (Jares *et al.*, 1994).

Several studies have reported overexpression of epidermal growth factor receptor (EGFR) and transforming growth factor α (TGF-α) in many invasive head and neck squamous cancers. These findings suggest growth stimulation in these tumors by autocrine or paracrine mechanisms and overexpression of EGFR family members is associated with a worse prognosis (Todd and Wong, 1999; Almadori *et al.*, 1999). While tobacco and alcohol environmentally induce the majority of head and neck cancers, viral infection has been suggested as contributory in many patients. Human papilloma virus 16 has been detected by polymerase chain reaction (PCR) in 36% of 95 oropharyngeal and laryngeal cancers (Snyderman, 1998; Gillison *et al.*, 2000). Epstein–Barr virus DNA has similarly been detected in most nasopharyngeal carcinomas and in some non-nasopharyngeal squamous head and neck cancers (Raab-Traub *et al.*, 1987; Kieff, 1995). In addition, human herpesvirus 6, previously isolated from patients with lymphoproliferative disorders and acquired immunodeficiency syndrome, can be detected in up to 80% of oral SCCHN (Yadav *et al.*, 1997). Oral carcinogenesis is probably a multistep process with a multifactorial etiology. Some oncogenic viruses, perhaps acting synergistically with chemical carcinogens and a patient's underlying genetic predisposition, could facilitate the transformation process to carcinoma.

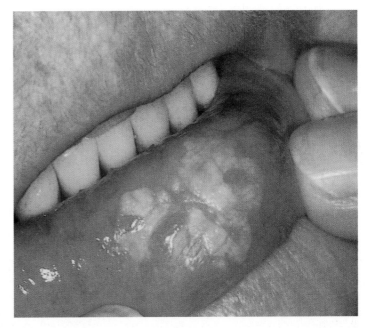

Fig. 3.1 Leukoplakia. Also known as smoker's keratosis, this premalignant tumor is marked by extensive, irregular, white thickening or plaques. The woman shown here habitually allowed cigarettes to burn down to the end against her lip. A carcinoma subsequently developed in this area.

Table 3.1 Classification of premalignant and malignant epithelial tumors

Tumor Type	Typical Location
Premalignant lesions	
Leukoplakia	Floor of mouth Ventral and lateral surfaces of tongue Buccal space
Erythroplasia	Same as for leukoplakia
Malignant lesions	
Squamous cell carcinoma	
Well differentiated	All sites, especially oral cavity
Moderately well differentiated	All sites
Poorly differentiated	All sites
Verrucous carcinoma (variant of well differentiated)	Oral cavity
Spindle cell carcinoma*	All sites
Undifferentiated carcinoma (includes lymphoepithelioma)	Nasopharynx and Waldeyer's ring
Nonkeratinizing epithelial carcinoma	Nasopharynx and Waldeyer's ring

*Spindle cell carcinoma is also known as pleomorphic carcinoma, pseudosarcoma, and sarcomatoid squamous cell carcinoma.

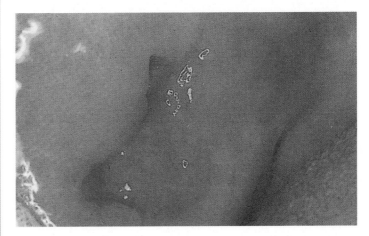

Fig. 3.2 Erythroplasia. An extensive red lesion of the buccal mucosa lies either level with or depressed below the surface of the surrounding epithelium due to atrophy of the overlying tissue layers. Biopsy showed severe dysplasia.

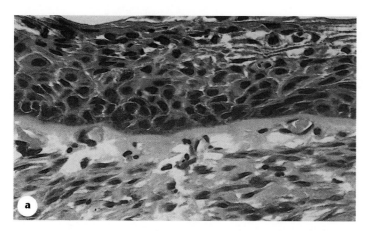

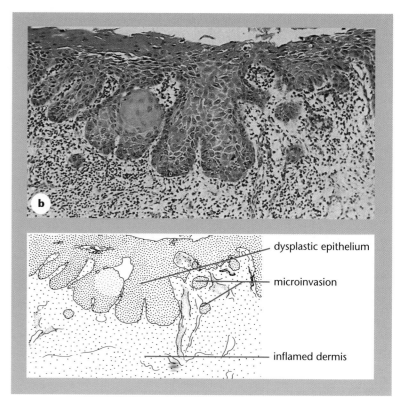

Fig. 3.3 Erythroplasia. The microscopic presentation of this lesion is variable, ranging from (**a**) maturation disarray of the mucosal surface with complete disorder of the squamous cells (dysplasia of atrophic epithelium) to (**b**) early finger-like extension into the underlying stroma (microinvasion or early carcinoma *in situ*).

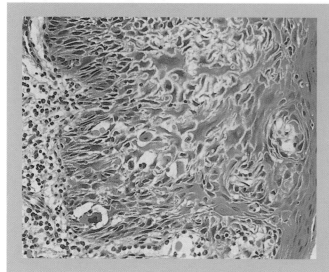

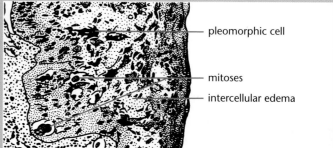

Fig. 3.4 Severe dysplasia. There is total loss of differentiation between basal and prickle cells, with many irregular pleomorphic hyperchromatic, including giant, nuclei. The dysplastic changes are confined to the epithelium, which is completely disorganized. Since there is no invasion, this appearance can also be called carcinoma *in situ*.

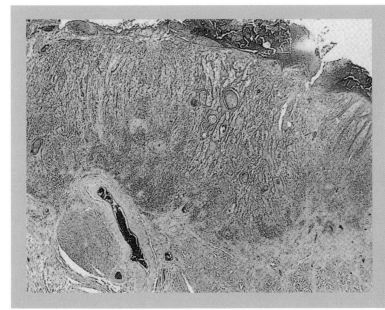

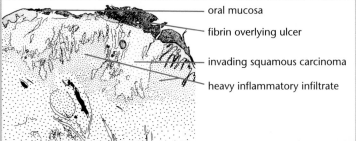

oral mucosa

fibrin overlying ulcer

invading squamous carcinoma

heavy inflammatory infiltrate

Fig. 3.5 Squamous cell carcinoma. Low-power microscopic section shows an early invasive lesion of the lip. Note the epithelial proliferation and invasion of the underlying tissue by strands and islands of tumor cells.

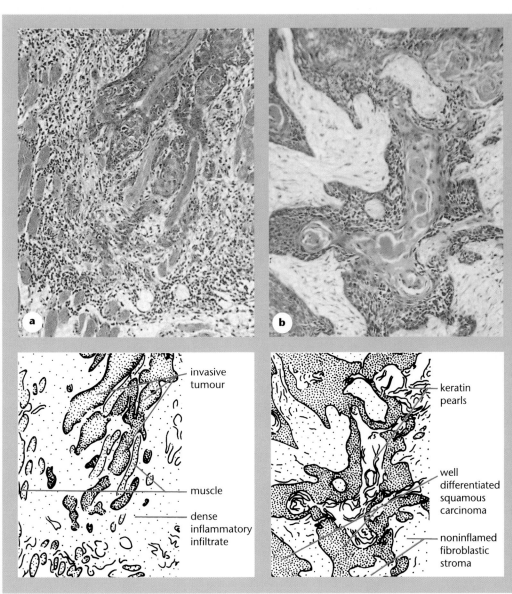

Fig. 3.6 Squamous cell carcinoma. These well-differentiated tumors demonstrate the variable stromal response that may be encountered, ranging from (**a**) a heavy, chronic inflammatory infiltrate surrounding the invasive tumor to (**b**) an inflammation-free stroma marked by fibroblastic proliferation. Note the presence of numerous keratin pearls.

a

b

invasive tumour

muscle

dense inflammatory infiltrate

keratin pearls

well differentiated squamous carcinoma

noninflamed fibroblastic stroma

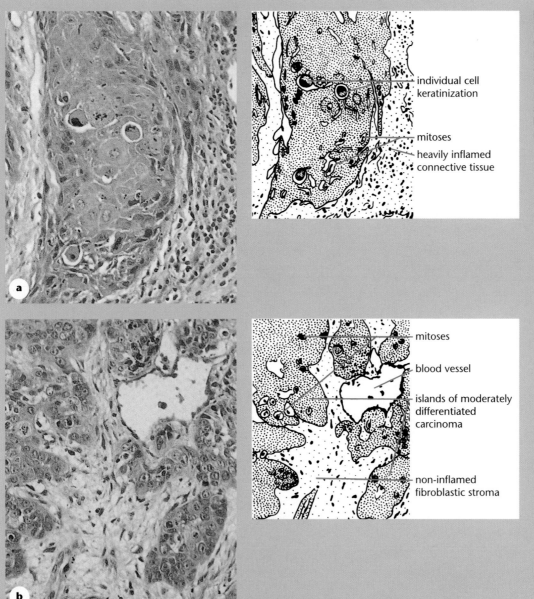

Fig. 3.7 Squamous cell carcinoma. In moderately well-differentiated tumors (**a**) individual cell keratinization may be present; in this instance the stroma also shows a heavy inflammatory infiltrate. (**b**) A moderately high mitotic rate is a common feature. In this section, there is no evidence of keratinization or an inflammatory response.

individual cell keratinization

mitoses

heavily inflamed connective tissue

mitoses

blood vessel

islands of moderately differentiated carcinoma

non-inflamed fibroblastic stroma

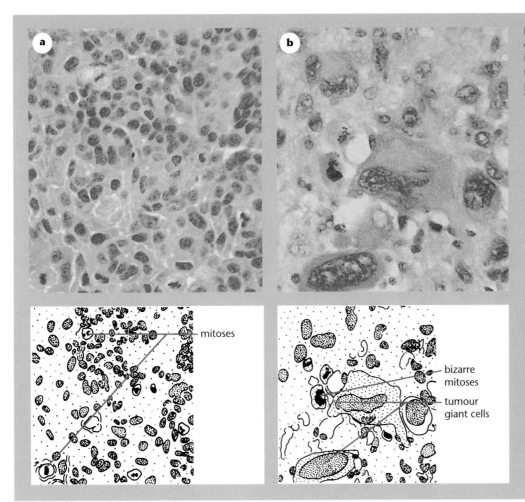

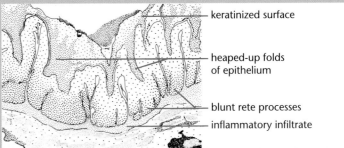

Fig. 3.8 Squamous cell carcinoma. Poorly differentiated tumors are marked by (**a**) sheets of immature cells and no evidence of keratinization. (**b**) Neoplastic cells show extreme degrees of pleomorphism, often with bizarre mitoses. Tumor giant cells may also be observed

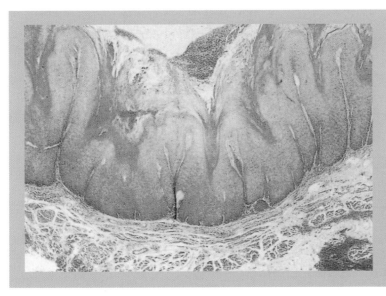

Fig. 3.9 Verrucous carcinoma. This variant of well-differentiated squamous cell carcinoma is marked by papillary masses of heaped-up folds of heavily keratinized epithelium separated by deep cleft-like spaces. The advancing edge of the lesion consists of blunt rete ridges forming a characteristic 'pushing margin'. An intact basement membrane makes this by definition an *in situ* lesion. Below the tumor is a dense chronic inflammatory infiltrate.

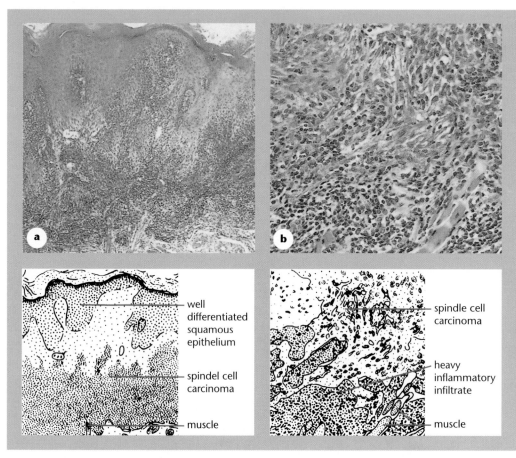

Fig. 3.10 Spindle cell carcinoma. (**a**) Low-power photomicrograph shows sheets of neoplastic cells arising from dysplastic epithelium. (**b**) At high power, the lesion is composed of uniform spindle-shaped cells. This variant of a poorly differentiated carcinoma is also referred to as a pleomorphic carcinoma, pseudocarcinoma or a sarcomatoid squamous cell carcinoma. Its reputation as 'radiation resistant' is probably unfounded; its natural history is that of a poorly differentiated squamous cell carcinoma.

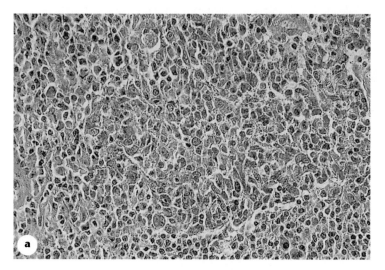

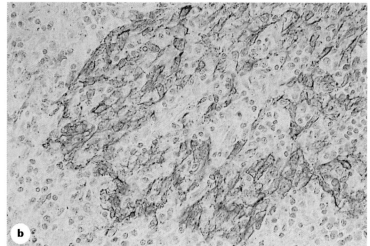

Fig. 3.11 Undifferentiated carcinoma (anaplastic carcinoma). (**a**) Undifferentiated epithelial tumors of the head and neck are frequently encountered in the nasopharynx, but may also occur in the oropharynx from within Waldeyer's ring. Lesions exhibiting abundant lymphotropism have traditionally been referred to as lymphoepitheliomas, whereas similar lesions without lymphocytes are designated as anaplastic carcinomas. (**b**) Positive immunoperoxidase staining for keratin confirms the epithelial origin of the tumor.

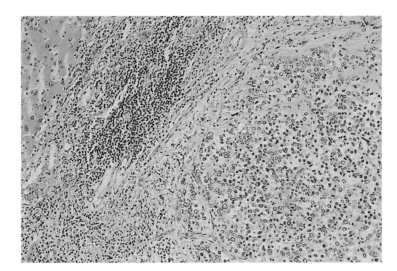

Fig. 3.12 Undifferentiated carcinoma (lymphoepithelioma). This metastatic lesion in the liver, composed of undifferentiated epithelial cells and numerous small lymphocytes, is identical to that of the primary tumor. Its lymphotropism is remarkable and supports the contention that a lymphoepithelioma of the nasopharynx is more than an undifferentiated carcinoma passively infiltrating neighboring lymphoid tissue.

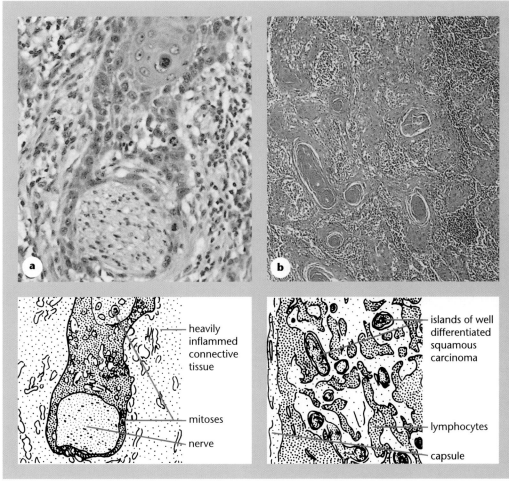

Fig. 3.13 Squamous cell carcinoma. These tumors are locally aggressive lesions, frequently invading (**a**) regional nerves, blood vessels or (**b**) lymphatic channels. Perineural invasion by tumor accounts for the rare pattern of relapse along the course of an invaded nerve proximal to the site of the original lesion.

Table 3.2 Salivary gland tumors and their frequency.

Type	Location	Type	Frequency (%)
Major	Parotid	Benign	75
		Malignant	25
	Submandibular	Benign	40
		Malignant	60
	Sublingual	Benign	15
		Malignant	85
Minor	Throughout mucous membranes of upper aerodigestive tract	Benign	45
		Malignant	55

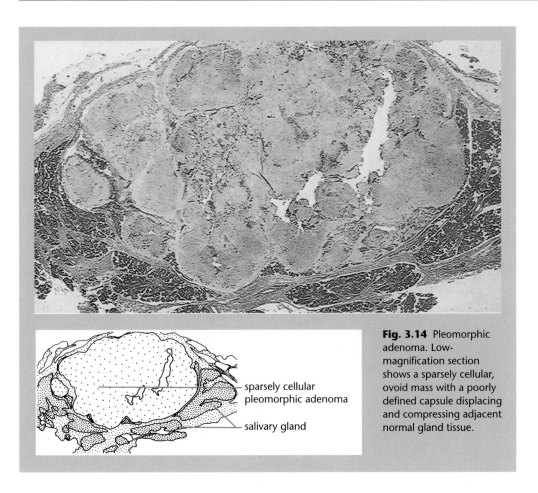

sparsely cellular
pleomorphic adenoma

salivary gland

Fig. 3.14 Pleomorphic adenoma. Low-magnification section shows a sparsely cellular, ovoid mass with a poorly defined capsule displacing and compressing adjacent normal gland tissue.

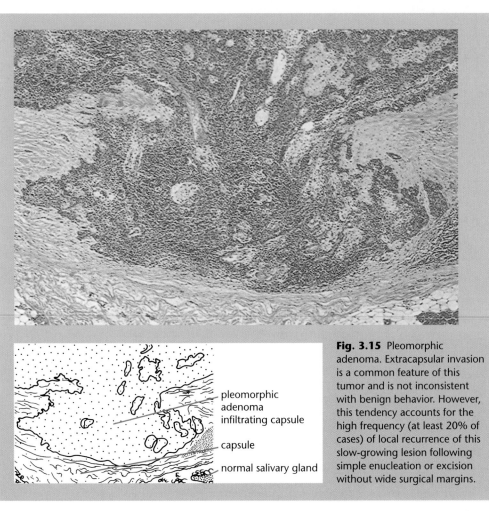

pleomorphic adenoma infiltrating capsule

capsule

normal salivary gland

Fig. 3.15 Pleomorphic adenoma. Extracapsular invasion is a common feature of this tumor and is not inconsistent with benign behavior. However, this tendency accounts for the high frequency (at least 20% of cases) of local recurrence of this slow-growing lesion following simple enucleation or excision without wide surgical margins.

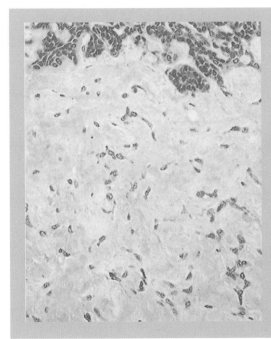

Fig. 3.16 Pleomorphic adenoma. Strands of epithelium and individual cells in a myxoid stroma are very common in these tumors. Other morphologic variants include areas of cartilage-like tissue, double-layered ductlike structures and spindle cells; the latter are probably the result of the proliferation of myoepithelial cells.

— strands and sheets of epithelial cells

— sparsely cellular myxoid stroma

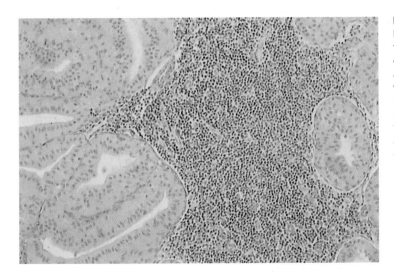

Fig. 3.17 Papillary cystadenoma lymphomatosum (Warthin's tumor). Microscopically, both epithelial and lymphoid elements are present in this benign lesion, which probably arises from ductal inclusions in intra- or periparotid lymph nodes. Epithelial cells form tubules, cysts and solid nests that are arranged in a characteristic double layer. The lymphoid component represents lymph node. Accounting for 5–10% of all parotid neoplasms, it occurs predominantly in the tail of the gland in older men. In about 10% of cases it is bilateral and may be multiple in one or both sides. Recurrence is rare after excision.

Table 3.3 Classification of malignant parotid tumors and their frequency

Type	Frequency (%)
Mucoepidermoid carcinoma	29
High grade (26%)	
Low grade (74%)	
Adenocarcinoma	14
Adenoid cystic carcinoma	13
Malignant mixed tumor	13
Undifferentiated carcinoma	11
Squamous cell carcinoma	8
Acinic cell carcinoma	6
Malignant lymphoma	2
Melanoma	<1
Other	3

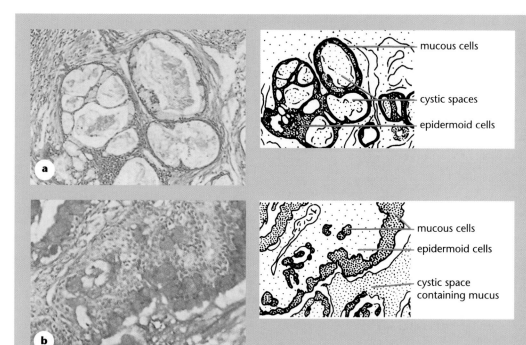

Fig. 3.18
Mucoepidermoid carcinoma. (**a**) Tumors of low-grade malignancy consist predominantly of mucous and epidermoid cells, as seen here forming well-defined microcysts in a fibrous stroma. (**b**) The mucous cells are obvious with PAS staining. Although these tumors are generally well circumscribed (and thus readily cured by wide excision), in this instance there is little or no capsule about the lesion. Occasionally, mucoepidermoid tumors act aggressively, widely infiltrating the normal gland or becoming fixed to skin. Cervical metastases are rare.

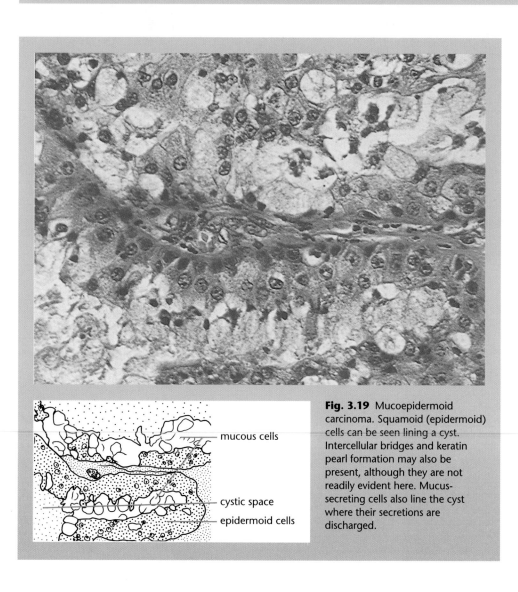

Fig. 3.19 Mucoepidermoid carcinoma. Squamoid (epidermoid) cells can be seen lining a cyst. Intercellular bridges and keratin pearl formation may also be present, although they are not readily evident here. Mucus-secreting cells also line the cyst where their secretions are discharged.

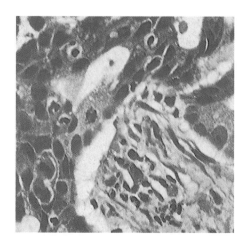

Fig. 3.20 Adenocarcinoma of parotid gland. The infiltrative growth pattern of this tumor is marked by gland and tubule formation. This moderately well-differentiated tumor has a brisk mitotic rate.

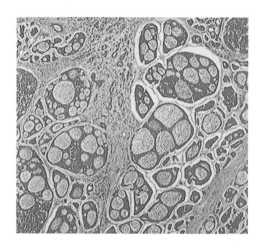

Fig. 3.21 Adenoid cystic carcinoma. This neoplasm is relatively uncommon in the parotid gland, but it is the most common malignant tumor of the submandibular and sublingual glands and the minor salivary glands. It is composed of small, dark-staining myoepithelial cells and cells resembling the lining of normal ducts arranged around cystic spaces. Lesions with a predominance of the cribriform pattern, as shown here, appear to have a more favorable natural history.

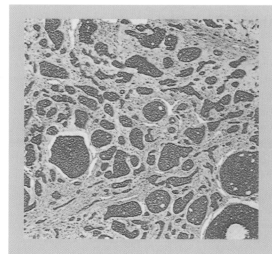

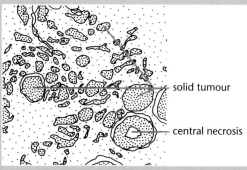

Fig. 3.22 Adenoid cystic carcinoma. A variant histologic presentation shows solid masses of cells, often with central necrosis. The absence of a predominant cribriform pattern in this instance suggests a less favorable natural history than that for the tumor shown in Fig. 3.21.

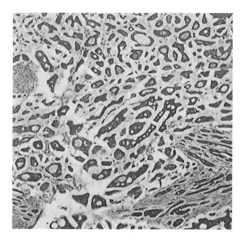

Fig. 3.23 Adenoid cystic carcinoma. Perineural and intraneural spread is typical of this tumor.

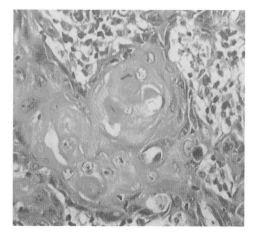

Fig. 3.24 Squamous cell carcinoma of parotid gland. The absence of mucus and the abundance of keratin characterize this well-differentiated tumor. A rare salivary lesion, squamous cell carcinoma probably arises from salivary ducts, a Warthin's tumor or a lymphoepithelial lesion. It tends to recur locally or in regional lymph nodes (70% of cases); distant metastases are rare.

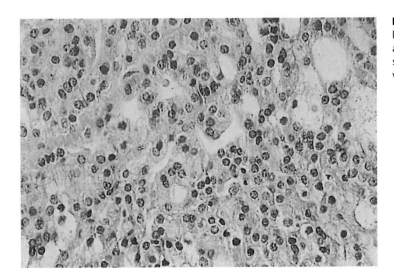

Fig. 3.25 Acinic cell carcinoma. This slow-growing, low-grade variant of a well-differentiated adenocarcinoma arises from the terminal acinus of a salivary duct. Note the groups of closely packed cells with clear or finely granular cytoplasm and small nuclei.

STAGING OF HEAD AND NECK CANCERS

Tumors of the head and neck are staged according to a site-specific TNM system (*see* Figs 3.26, 3.27, 3.28) (Flemming *et al.*, 1997) (Cancer 1997). The multiple TNM combinations are ultimately grouped into four stages (Table 3.4), each having a progressively lower survival rate. At best, this anatomically dependent system provides a rapid estimate of a patient's prognosis, facilitates the formation of a treatment plan and assures the uniform reporting of treatment outcomes. Unfortunately, TNM staging is rather complex and the concordance in staging between any two physicians is low. The greatest utility of this imperfect measure of disease potential is restricted to the definition of patients with limited lesions and a good prognosis.

Recommended staging procedures for determining a patient's TNM classification include direct and indirect (mirror or fiberoptic) inspection and palpation of all accessible mucosal surfaces in the head and neck and radiologic investigation. Radiographs or radionuclide scanning of the mandible may be appropriate in selected cases; however, CT or MRI is standard for exact anatomic localization of primary lesions and facilitates quantification of regional lymph node involvement and parapharyngeal spread of disease. In addition, CT scanning and MRI may be helpful in identifying the site of an occult primary lesion in patients with a solitary neck mass.

There is considerable debate about the necessity for 'triple endoscopy' in staging patients with head and neck cancers. The addition of bronchoscopy and esophagoscopy to direct laryngoscopy may be appropriate for patients with tumors of the oropharynx, hypopharynx or larynx that are inadequately evaluated by indirect means. The time, risk and expense of these additional procedures are negligible given the incidence (as high as 5% in some series) for multiple synchronous primary tumors of the head and neck, lung and esophagus. On the other hand, the value of 'triple endoscopy' remains controversial in most patients with localized lesions of the oral cavity that can adequately be staged by indirect, non-invasive means (Forastiere *et al.*, 1998). 'Triple endoscopy' is particularly important for patients with intraoral lesions associated with diffuse mucosal abnormalities such as leukoplakia or erythroplasia, who are more likely to have multiple primary tumors.

CLINICAL MANIFESTATIONS

The clinical manifestations and natural history of head and neck cancers depend on the site from which they arise. Thus, considerable variability exists and certain characteristic features for the several primary anatomic locations are discussed separately.

Occasionally, patients present with solitary, asymptomatic cervical adenopathy, usually in the upper neck. The primary cancer may be asymptomatic, but will usually be discovered on a detailed head and neck examination. Pain may be the first manifestation, usually representing more locally advanced disease. Surprisingly, some patients have large lesions that cause minimal, if any, symptoms.

LIPS

Cancer of the lips accounts for 15% of all head and neck cancers. In 95% of cases, the lesion occurs on the lower lip and may involve the vermilion and mucosal surfaces. It typically presents as a recurrent scab or a persistent or slow-growing sore, blister or ulcer. Owing to its location, it is discovered early and lymphatic spread of squamous cell carcinoma to submental and submaxillary lymph nodes occurs in only 5–10% of patients. The approximate 5-year survival after standard treatment is greater than 90% for all stages, as most lesions are quite limited. Survival falls to 65% for patients with locally advanced lesions of the upper lip or with regional adenopathy.

ORAL CAVITY

The oral cavity encompasses the floor of the mouth, oral tongue, buccal mucosa, gingiva, retromolar trigone and hard palate. Cancers involving these structures account for 20% of all head and neck malignancies. Typically, cancers of the oral cavity present as asymptomatic lesions noted on routine dental examination, as painful ulcers with or without referred otalgia or in association with ill-fitting dentures, difficulty in swallowing or chewing or altered speech. The principal sites of involvement are the ventrolateral surface of the tongue and the floor of the mouth. In up to 40% of patients, adenopathy may be present in the upper jugular and submandibular lymph nodes. Carcinomas of the middle and posterior thirds of the mobile tongue have the greatest metastatic potential.

NASOPHARYNX

Cancers of the nasopharynx are unique in their histology (frequently an undifferentiated or non-keratinizing epithelial cancer), biology and epidemiology. They are minimally associated with tobacco use, but are 25 times more prevalent in patients of southern Chinese descent. The Epstein–Barr virus (EBV) serum titer is typically elevated and molecular biologic techniques reveal EBV incorporation into the genome in the majority of tumors. These lesions occur in a younger population than patients with SCCHN at other sites and are best known for their propensity for early spread to regional and distant sites and their relative sensitivity to chemotherapy and radiotherapy.

Nasopharyngeal cancers of epithelial origin typically arise from the lateral pharyngeal wall adjacent to the orifice of the eustachian tube. Cancers similar to those of the nasopharynx may occur in other areas of Waldeyer's ring (a ring of lymphoid tissue encircling the naso- and oropharynx). Although many of these lesions are asymptomatic and found incidentally during evaluation of an upper neck mass of unknown origin, limited lesions may present in association with epistaxis, nasal obstruction or unilateral hearing loss due to eustachian tube obstruction. More advanced lesions may present with headache, direct osseous involvement of the parasphenoid region or multiple cranial neuropathies due to tumor extension behind the sphenoid (cranial nerves II through VI) or along the base of the skull about the hypoglossal foramen (cranial nerves XI and XII). The metastatic potential of these lesions is well known. Malignant adenopathy involving the retropharynx and lateral pharyngeal wall is present in 80% of patients at presentation. Bilateral adenopathy is common and involvement of the posterior cervical chain is characteristic.

The nasopharynx may also be involved in non-epithelial malignancies, including sarcomas, minor salivary gland carcinomas, esthesioneuroblastomas or other neuroectodermal lesions, and unusual tumors such as angiofibromas. Presenting features may mimic those of the more common squamous cell carcinoma and therefore adequate biopsy specimens must be obtained in all cases.

OROPHARYNX

Accounting for 10% of all head and neck malignancies, oropharyngeal cancers may involve the tonsillar fossa or pillars, soft palate, base of the tongue or lateral or posterior pharyngeal wall. They may be clinically silent until they present as advanced tumors with local pain, odynophagia, dysphagia, referred otalgia or trismus. Tonsillar and base-of-tongue carcinomas have the greatest metastatic potential, with upper jugular (subdigastric or jugulodigastric) lymphadenopathy present in up to 70% of cases. These areas therefore require careful visual inspection and digital palpation during evaluation of a patient with either pharyngeal symptoms consistent with carcinoma or an upper neck mass of unknown origin. CT scanning is standard for tumors presenting at this site.

The oropharynx is rich in lymphatic tissue belonging to Waldeyer's ring. Occasionally, primary Waldeyer's ring lymphomas arise, typically non-Hodgkin's lymphomas of the diffuse large cell type. These tumors are often difficult to distinguish from epithelial tumors on clinical grounds. After histologic and immunologic confirmation, staging procedures for a Waldeyer's ring lymphoma should include bone marrow aspiration and biopsy, CT scan of the chest, abdomen and pelvis and, given the high incidence of concurrent gastric involvement, radiographic or endoscopic visualization of the stomach.

HYPOPHARYNX

Hypopharyngeal carcinomas, which occur primarily in the pyriform sinus, account for 5% of head and neck cancers. At presentation, patients typically have locally advanced lesions, with odynophagia, dysphagia, referred otalgia or evidence of laryngeal involvement, including cough, hoarseness or repeated aspirations. Hypopharyngeal cancers are biologically aggressive; metastases to retropharyngeal or midjugular lymph nodes are common (up to 80% of patients). The 5-year survival of patients with hypopharyngeal carcinomas is reported to be as low as 20–30%.

LARYNX

Cancers of the larynx, which may arise from the supraglottic, glottic or subglottic larynx, are the most frequently encountered head and neck cancers in the United States, accounting for 33% of cases. They affect men more commonly than women, most often in the sixth and seventh decades. Chronic inflammation and cigarette smoking are known risk factors. Hoarseness is the most common presenting symptom but otalgia, dysphagia or odynophagia may occur. The natural history of these lesions is variable.

The supraglottic structures include the epiglottis, the arytenoid cartilage, the aryepiglottic folds and the false vocal cords, all of which are rich in lymphatic channels. Tumors of the supraglottic larynx present late in comparison with other laryngeal tumors and are associated with malignant middle or upper jugular adenopathy in 40% of patients. The glottis, on the other hand, which is rich in elastic tissue, has few lymphatic channels and nodal metastases are rare (less than 5% of cases) with either limited or advanced primary lesions. Glottic carcinomas arise from the true vocal cords, which anatomically represent a modified tracheal ring. These tumors tend to be well-differentiated lesions presenting early due to hoarseness or a change in voice. Subglottic carcinomas, the least common tumors of the larynx, are essentially tracheal lesions that arise immediately beneath the true vocal cords. They commonly present with hemoptysis, change in voice or dyspnea. Lymph node metastases to the low neck or retrosternal region are occasionally present in patients with limited lesions, but they may be found in up to 40% of patients with advanced tumors.

NASAL CAVITY AND PARANASAL SINUSES

Squamous cell carcinomas of the nasal cavity and paranasal sinuses are uncommon, constituting less than 5% of head and neck cancers. Sarcomas, plasmacytomas, lymphomas, minor salivary gland carcinomas and esthesioneuroblastomas may also occur at these sites, as well as histologically benign lesions, such as mucoceles and inverted papillomas that mimic carcinomas. The maxillary antrum is the most frequently involved location within the paranasal sinuses. Tumors at this site typically present with signs and symptoms suggesting inflammatory sinusitis, such as local pain and tenderness, toothache, nasal discharge or nasal obstruction. Evidence for more invasive disease would include looseness of teeth, ill-fitting dentures, visual disturbances or proptosis, ulcerations of the hard or soft palate or cheek swelling. Lymph node involvement is present in 15% of patients, a relatively low percentage given the aggressiveness of many primary lesions.

MAJOR AND MINOR SALIVARY GLANDS

Tumors of the parotid, submandibular and sublingual glands account for 3–4% of all head and neck neoplasms. About 80% of major salivary gland lesions occur in the parotid but the majority of these tumors are benign. In contradistinction are the tumors of the minor salivary glands. While less common than tumors of the parotid, the majority of these tumors are malignant. Most malignant tumors present as painless masses. With time, local pain, referred pain along the path of an adjacent nerve or nerve palsy may develop. The latter symptom strongly suggests malignancy.

Malignant salivary gland tumors are heterogeneous in their tendency to infiltrate neighboring tissues and to spread to regional lymph nodes or distant sites. High-grade tumors frequently metastasize to the neck or distantly. For example, up to 25% of patients with salivary adenocarcinomas, which are aggressive tumors, have clinical (20%) or occult (5%) lymph node metastases at presentation. In patients with adenoid cystic carcinomas, metastases to regional nodes are much less common than distant metastases, which may develop in up to 75% of cases. Perineural involvement is a characteristic finding with these tumors, leading to infiltration along nerve trunks; in the case of parotid lesions, facial nerve paralysis may be present at the time of presentation. In patients with slow-growing tumors, adenoid cystic carcinomas may recur months to years after primary treatment. Similarly, acinic cell carcinomas, which microscopically invade contiguous bone, nerve, skin and blood vessels, are known to recur locally in up to 35% of cases following inadequate excision; relapse may occur as long as 25–30 years after initial treatment.

Minor salivary gland tumors are uncommon, accounting for less than 2% of malignant tumors of the head and neck. They may occur anywhere throughout the upper aerodigestive system, but they are typically located in the oral cavity, nasal cavity and paranasal sinuses. Benign mixed tumors are the most common benign lesions and adenoid cystic carcinomas account for two-thirds of malignant minor salivary gland tumors. Although presenting symptoms depend on the site of origin and local extension, they are usually those of a mass lesion.

Fig. 3.26 T categories for cancer of the lip and oral cavity (Flemming et al., 1997).

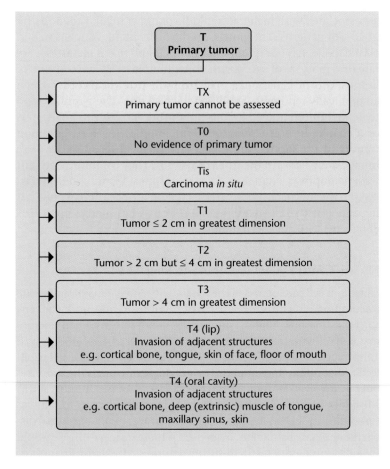

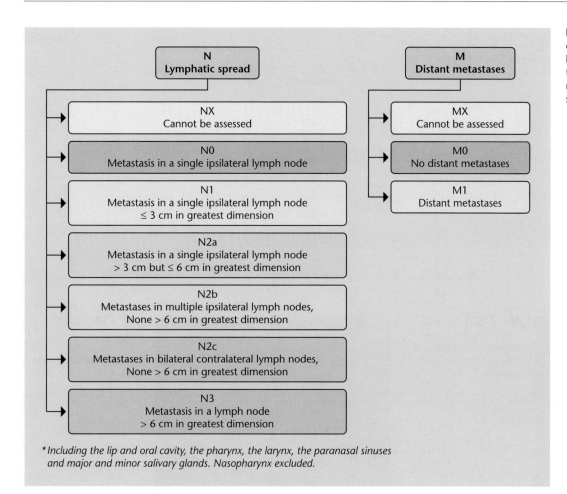

Fig. 3.27 N and M categories for cancer of the head and neck sites, including the lip and oral cavity, the pharynx, the larynx, the paranasal sinuses and the major and minor salivary glands. For nasopharynx, see Fig. 3.28 (Flemming *et al.*, 1997).

Including the lip and oral cavity, the pharynx, the larynx, the paranasal sinuses and major and minor salivary glands. Nasopharynx excluded.

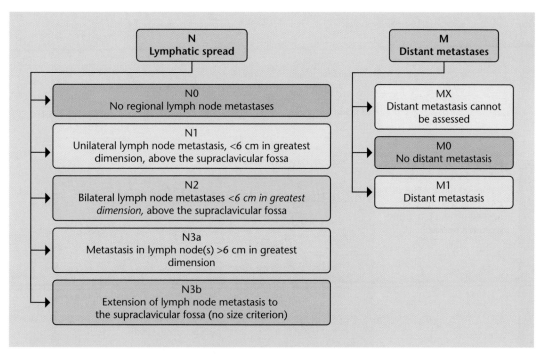

Fig. 3.28 N and M categories for nasopharyngeal cancer (Flemming *et al.*, 1997).

Table 3.4 Stage grouping for cancer of the head and neck sites excluding nasopharynx (Flemming *et al.*, 1997)

Stage	T (primary tumor)	N (regional nodes)	M (metastases)
0	Tis	N0	M0
I	T1	N0	M0
II	T2	N0	M0
III	T3	N0	M0
	T1, T2, or T3	N1	M0
IV	T1, T2, or T3	N2 or N3	M0
	T4	Any N	M0
	Any T	Any N	M1

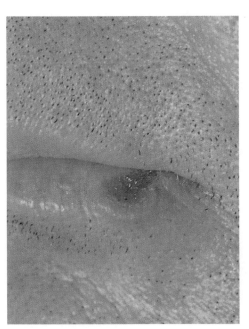

Fig. 3.29 Squamous cell carcinoma. A central ulcer with an indurated margin is present on the lower lip.

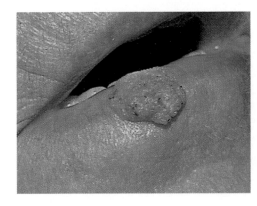

Fig. 3.30 Squamous cell carcinoma. This lesion had a warty, crusted surface, but the base was firm and suspicious for malignant disease.

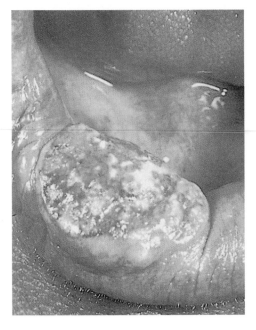

Fig. 3.31 Squamous cell carcinoma. Although this lesion has a white surface at the rim, it is heaped up and forms an ulcerated nodule.

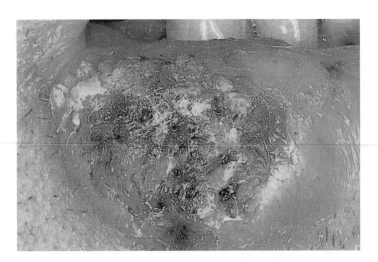

Fig. 3.32 Squamous cell carcinoma. Neglected by the patient for about a year, this advanced lesion exhibits the typical thickened, rolled edge and necrotic, scabbing floor.

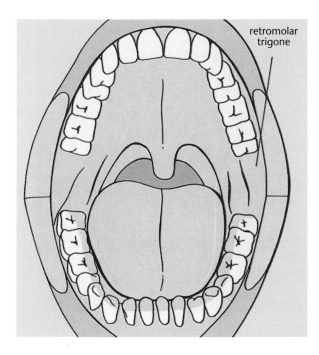

Fig. 3.33 Intraoral carcinoma. The majority of intraoral tumors are concentrated in the relatively small 'drainage' areas (highlighted in blue) where saliva pools.

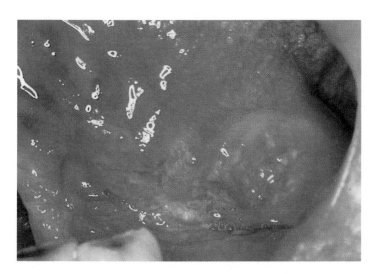

Fig. 3.34 Squamous cell carcinoma of tongue. Located on the lateral border of the tongue, as is common with these tumors, this nodular lesion was painless despite its being a well-established invasive tumor.

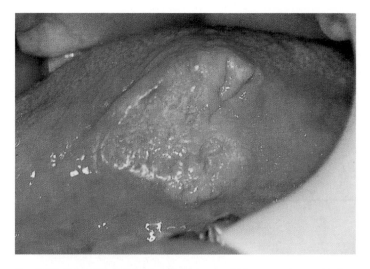

Fig. 3.35 Squamous cell carcinoma of tongue. This more advanced lesion shows the classic but late features of this malignancy, namely raised, rolled margins and a granulating floor.

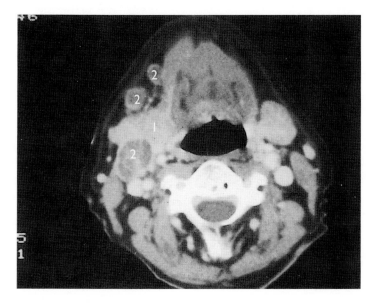

Fig. 3.36 Squamous cell carcinoma of tongue. The patient was a 57-year-old man who presented with tongue swelling. This contrast-enhanced CT reveals extension of the tumor mass (1) into the submandibular region and several lymph nodes (2). The size and peripheral enhancement of the nodes suggest metastatic spread. Surgery confirmed the latter.

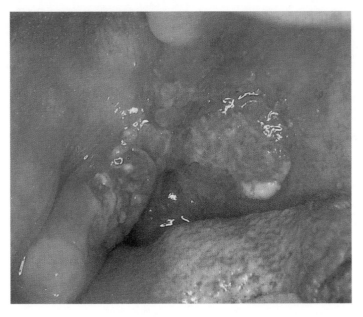

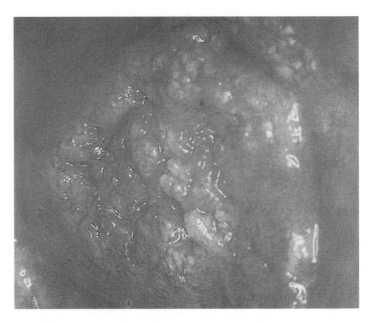

Fig. 3.37 Squamous cell carcinoma of retromolar region and soft palate. The lesion on the alveolar ridge shows the typical features of a malignant ulcer, but that of the soft palate appears only as a white patch.

Fig. 3.38 Squamous cell carcinoma of buccal mucosa. The characteristic features of an extensive malignant ulcer, in particular the rough granulating floor, are apparent.

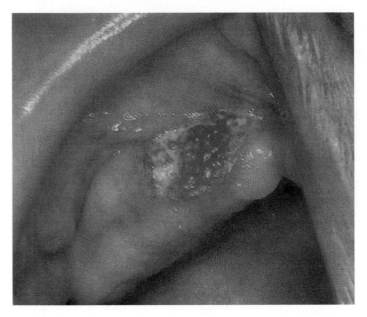

Fig. 3.39 Squamous cell carcinoma of alveolar ridge. This relatively early lesion is marked by a predominantly red area without obvious ulceration at this stage.

Fig. 3.40 Squamous cell carcinoma of floor of mouth. This typical malignant ulcer erodes the base of the lingual frenulum.

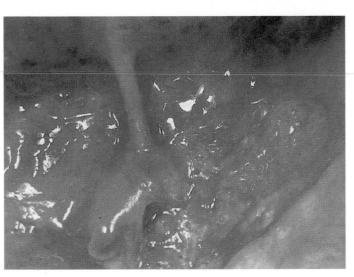

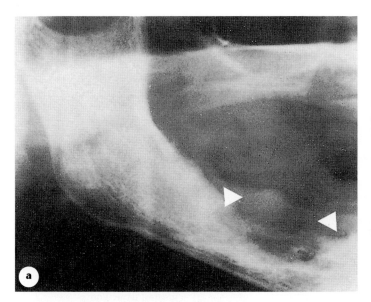

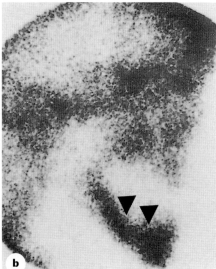

Fig. 3.41
Squamous cell carcinoma of floor of mouth. (**a**) Panoramic tomogram shows a localized area of bone destruction (arrowheads) in the body of the mandible. (**b**) Bone scan reveals the true extent of the tumor. The photodeficient area (arrowheads) corresponds to the area of bone destruction seen on the tomogram. The area of increased uptake, indicating the actual extent of bone invasion, is much greater, encompassing most of the mandible. (Reproduced with permission from Noyek *et al.*, 1987.)

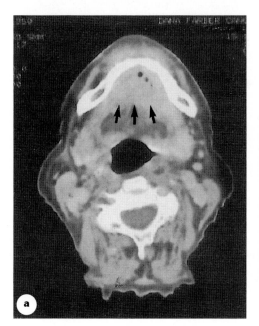

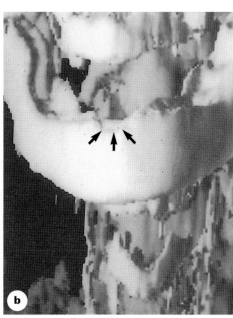

Fig. 3.42 (**a**) CT scan of squamous cell carcinoma involving the mandible (arrows). (**b**) Spiral CT reconstruction of the lesion localizes the extent of bone involvement and facilitates planning for surgical resection (arrows).

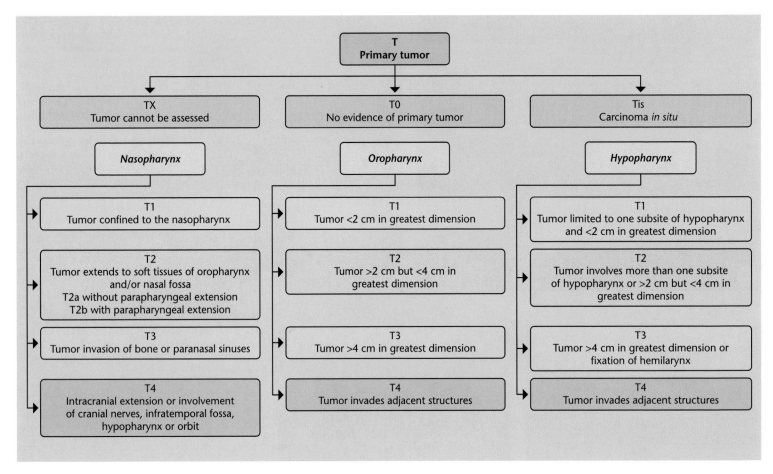

Fig. 3.43 T categories for cancer of the pharynx (*see* Fig. 3.27 and Table 3.4 for N and M categories and stage grouping of head and neck cancers) (Flemming *et al.*, 1997).

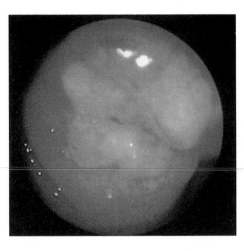

Fig. 3.44 Squamous cell carcinoma of nasopharynx. Persistent or recurrent serous effusion of the middle ear in adults is suspicious for a nasopharyngeal tumor. A Hopkins rod nasopharyngeal telescope reveals a carcinoma arising from the posterior wall of the nasopharynx.

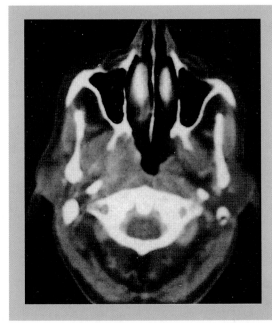
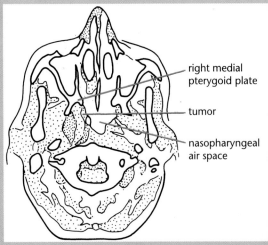

right medial
pterygoid plate

tumor

nasopharyngeal
air space

Fig. 3.45 Squamous cell carcinoma of nasopharynx. A 64-year-old woman presented with a persistent serous effusion of the right middle ear. An axial CT scan demonstrates a soft tissue mass in the right lateral aspect of the nasopharynx in the region of the fossa of Rosenmuller. The tumor infiltrates deeply and involves the eustachian tube. Note that the fascial planes have been destroyed by the advancing neoplasm (compare with normal left side).

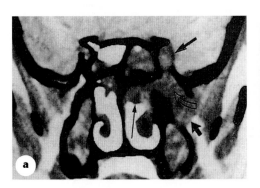
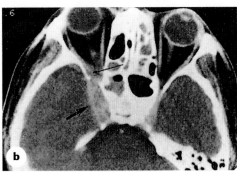

Fig. 3.46 Squamous cell carcinoma of nasopharynx. (**a**) Coronal CT section shows a tumor extending into the middle cranial fossa (medium arrow) and inferiorly through the inferior orbital fissure (short, thick arrow), which is markedly widened (open arrow). Tumor is also present in the superior aspect of the nasal cavity (thin arrow). There is a soft tissue thickening within the sphenoid sinus. (**b**) The axial projection shows tumor at the apex of the right orbit (thin arrow) and extending as an enhancing mass into the right cavernous sinus (thick arrow). (Courtesy of EE Kassel.)

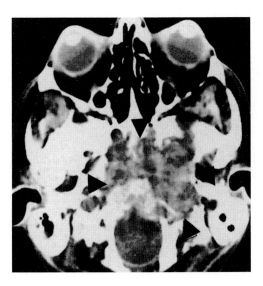

Fig. 3.47 Squamous cell carcinoma of nasopharynx. A 57-year-old woman presented with chronic headaches and dysfunction of cranial nerves IX through XI. This CT scan demonstrates extensive erosion of the base of the skull, with destruction of the petrous bone and the greater wing of the sphenoid by a soft tissue lesion (arrowheads).

Table 3.5 Stage grouping for nasopharyngeal cancer

Stage	T (primary tumor)	N (regional nodes)	M (metastases)
0	Tis	N0	M0
I	T1	N0	M0
IIA	T2a	N0	M0
IIB	T1, T2a, or T2b	N1	M0
	T2b	N0	M0
III	T1, T2a, or T2b	N2	M0
	T3	N0, N1 or N2	M0
IVA	T4	N0, N1, or N2	M0
IVB	Any T	N3	M0
IVC	Any T	Any N	M1

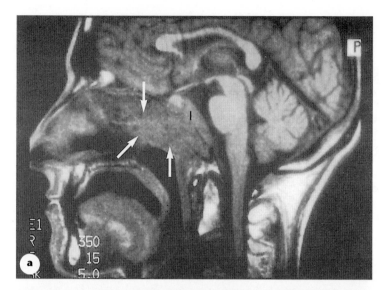

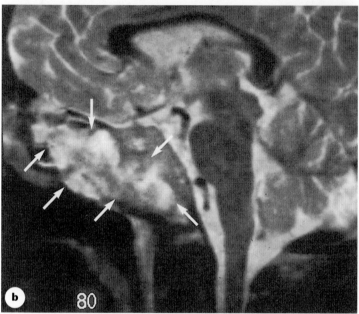

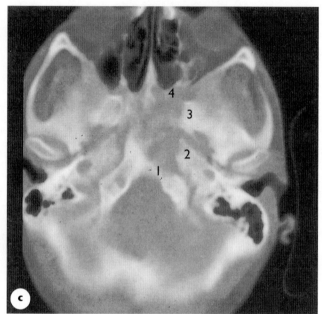

Fig. 3.48 Squamous carcinoma of nasopharynx. A 35-year-old woman complained of nasal stuffiness. (**a**) Sagittal T_1-weighted MRI image shows a large soft tissue mass (arrows) involving the sphenoid sinus, ethmoid sinus and clivus (1). (**b**) Sagittal T_2-weighted MRI image shows the extent of the primary tumor mass (arrows) with destruction of local structures. (**c**) CT scan shows the extent of bony involvement of clivus (1); petrous temporal bone (2); sphenoid bone (3); and ethmoid (4).

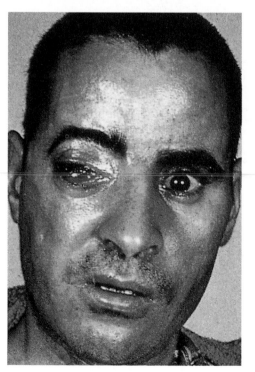

Fig. 3.49 Squamous cell carcinoma of nasopharynx (parasellar syndrome). Parasellar structures are frequently affected by invasive nasopharyngeal tumors. In this instance, the lesion has invaded the orbit via the superior orbital fissure, leading to severe right proptosis.

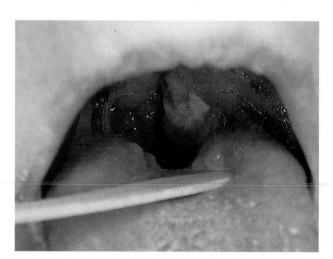

Fig. 3.50 Squamous cell carcinoma of oropharynx. A 56-year-old woman presented with chronic pharyngeal pain and difficulty in swallowing of several months' duration. Clinical examination reveals a bulging necrotic lesion of the left tonsil with involvement of the neighboring soft palate and displacement of the uvula. Biopsy yielded the histologic diagnosis.

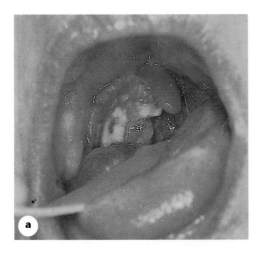

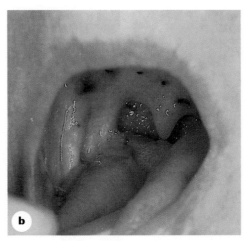

Fig. 3.51 Squamous cell carcinoma of oropharynx. A 63-year-old woman presented with difficulty in swallowing and otalgia. (**a**) Examination reveals an extensive lesion of the right tonsil that involves the lateral pharyngeal wall, as well as the soft palate and uvula. After biopsy, which confirmed the diagnosis, the lesion was outlined (tattooed) with India ink and treated with combination chemotherapy and radiotherapy. (**b**) This photograph, taken after chemotherapy but before radiotherapy, shows complete clinical regression of the tumor.

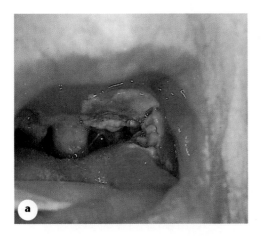

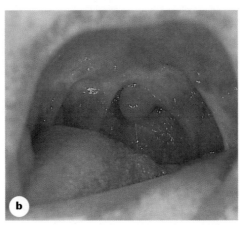

Fig. 3.52 Squamous cell carcinoma of oropharynx. A 53-year-old woman presented with odynophagia and nasal regurgitation of food. (**a**) Examination reveals a large, exophytic, ulcerative lesion of the left tonsil that diffusely involves the soft palate and uvula. Palatal insufficiency resulted from a fistula in the right soft palate extending into the nasopharynx. (**b**) After treatment with combination chemotherapy, the lesion completely regressed, replaced by fibrous tissue, and the fistula closed. Treatment continued with definitive radiotherapy. The patient remains free of disease in long-term followup.

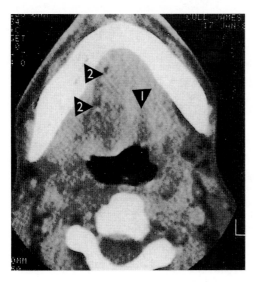

Fig. 3.53 Squamous cell carcinoma of oropharynx. A 48-year-old man presented with unilateral otalgia. Clinical examination revealed no obvious tumor. Axial CT scan through the base of the tongue shows an ill-defined T4 mass (1) in the left side of the tongue that obliterates the normal fat planes on the right (2). The tumor crosses the midline. Biopsy of the lesion yielded the histologic diagnosis.

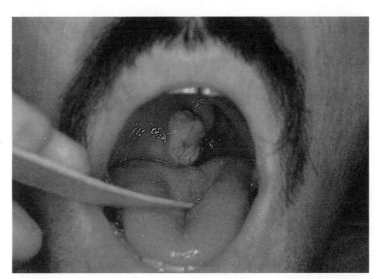

Fig. 3.54 Diffuse large cell lymphoma of oropharynx. A 24-year-old man, a non-smoker, presented with a 3-week history of odynophagia and fatigue refractory to a trial of antibiotics. A massive necrotic lesion of the right tonsil is apparent. Intraoral biopsy yielded the histologic diagnosis.

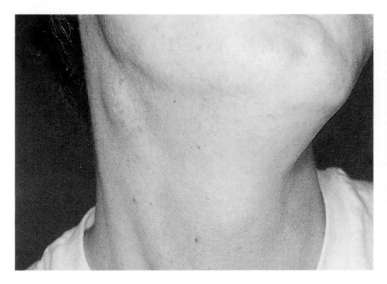

Fig. 3.55 Diffuse large cell lymphoma of oropharynx. Additional evaluation of this 33-year-old man who presented with right tonsillar enlargement revealed only this jugulodigastric mass; biopsy yielded the histologic diagnosis. For clinical stage II disease, he received six cycles of combination chemotherapy, which resulted in a complete response. He remains disease free 8 years after treatment.

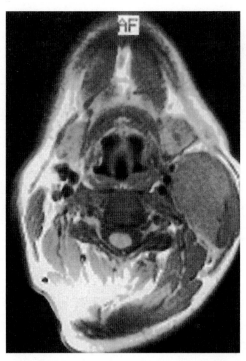

Fig. 3.56 Diffuse large cell lymphoma involving the neck, clinical stage I disease. This axial MR scan reveals a soft tissue mass within the neck consistent with malignant regional adenopathy. The homogeneous texture of the lesion favors a diagnosis of lymphoma which was confirmed after an initial, unremarkable, evaluation of the head and neck mucosal surfaces under anesthesia by a head and neck surgeon and subsequent excisional biopsy of the neck lesion.

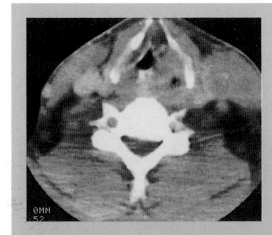

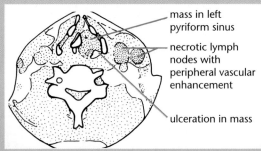

mass in left pyriform sinus

necrotic lymph nodes with peripheral vascular enhancement

ulceration in mass

Fig. 3.57 Squamous cell carcinoma of hypopharynx. Contrast-enhanced axial CT scan in a 45-year-old man shows that the left pyriform sinus is filled with necrotic tumor (note the central ulceration). In addition, two large, centrally necrotic lymph nodes are apparent, with minimal but definite peripheral vascular enhancement.

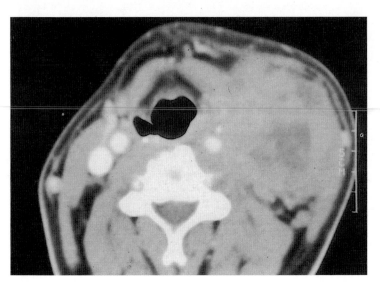

Fig. 3.58 Squamous cell carcinoma of the hypopharynx. A 56-year-old man presented with a bulky cervical mass. Indirect laryngoscopy revealed bulging of the lateral pharyngeal wall with obliteration of the pyriform sinus. An axial CT revealed a massive neck lesion involving the carotid sheath and the parapharyngeal space. A primary site lesion was suggested on CT. Needle aspiration of the neck mass showed squamous cell carcinoma. Direct laryngoscopy confirmed a small primary site tumor in the pyriform sinus.

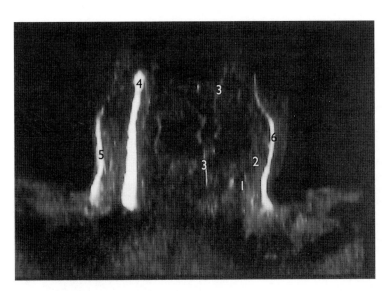

Fig. 3.59 Squamous cell carcinoma of the hypopharynx. MR venography reveals obstruction of the ipsilateral internal jugular vein (1) by tumor (2). Note collateral veins (3) and normal right internal jugular vein (4), right external jugular vein (5) and left external jugular vein (6).

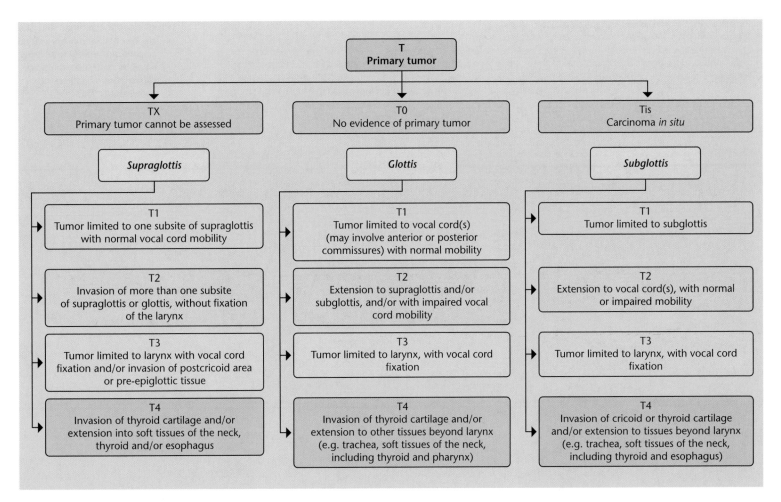

Fig. 3.60 T categories for cancer of the larynx (see Fig. 3.27 and Table 3.4 for the N and M categories and stage grouping of head and neck cancers) (Flemming *et al.*, 1997).

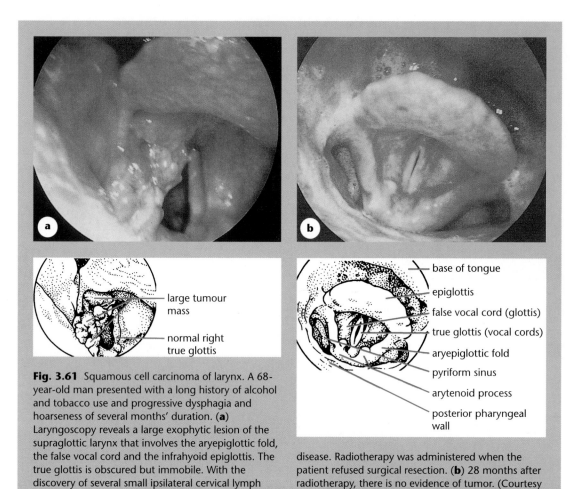

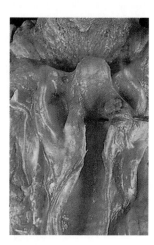

large tumour mass

normal right true glottis

base of tongue

epiglottis

false vocal cord (glottis)

true glottis (vocal cords)

aryepiglottic fold

pyriform sinus

arytenoid process

posterior pharyngeal wall

Fig. 3.61 Squamous cell carcinoma of larynx. A 68-year-old man presented with a long history of alcohol and tobacco use and progressive dysphagia and hoarseness of several months' duration. (**a**) Laryngoscopy reveals a large exophytic lesion of the supraglottic larynx that involves the aryepiglottic fold, the false vocal cord and the infrahyoid epiglottis. The true glottis is obscured but immobile. With the discovery of several small ipsilateral cervical lymph nodes, the patient was felt to have stage IV (T3N2b)

disease. Radiotherapy was administered when the patient refused surgical resection. (**b**) 28 months after radiotherapy, there is no evidence of tumor. (Courtesy of Dr J Parsons, University of Florida, Gainesville, FL.)

Fig. 3.62 Squamous cell carcinoma of larynx. The trachea and larynx have been opened posteriorly to reveal a small fungating supraglottic tumor arising in the right aryepiglottic fold.

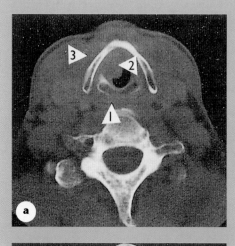

Fig. 3.63 Squamous cell carcinoma of larynx. (**a**) Axial CT scan at the level of the posterior lamina of the cricoid cartilage (arrow 1) in a 58-year-old man shows subglottic extension of an intralaryngeal tumor mass (arrow 2). The thyroid cartilage is indicated (arrow 3). (**b**) Section through the glottis (about 1 cm cephalad to the previous scan) shows that necrotic tumor extends anteriorly into the soft tissue of the neck. The central portion of the thyroid cartilage has been destroyed. The tumor encroaches on the airway and has obliterated the anterior commissure. This is classified as a T4 lesion.

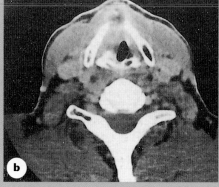

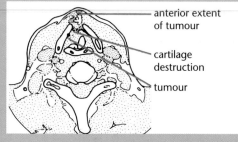

anterior extent of tumour

cartilage destruction

tumour

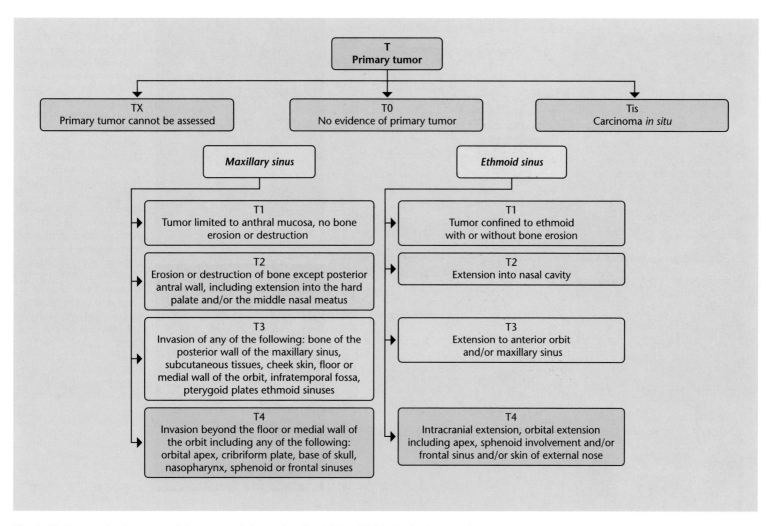

Fig. 3.64 T categories for cancer of the paranasal sinuses (*see* Fig. 3.27 and Table 3.4 for the N and M categories and stage grouping of head and neck cancers (Flemming *et al.*, 1997).

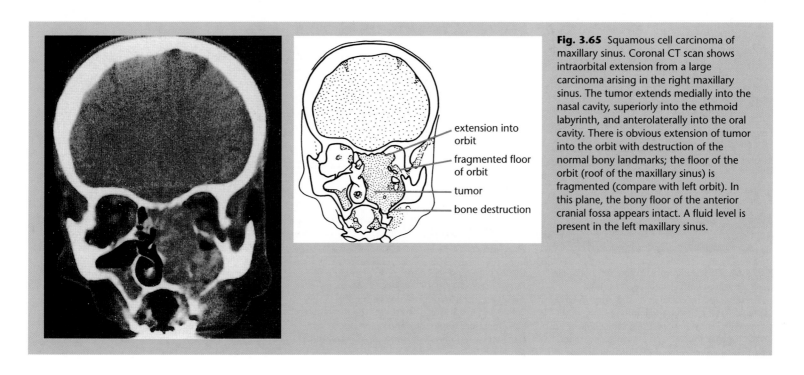

Fig. 3.65 Squamous cell carcinoma of maxillary sinus. Coronal CT scan shows intraorbital extension from a large carcinoma arising in the right maxillary sinus. The tumor extends medially into the nasal cavity, superiorly into the ethmoid labyrinth, and anterolaterally into the oral cavity. There is obvious extension of tumor into the orbit with destruction of the normal bony landmarks; the floor of the orbit (roof of the maxillary sinus) is fragmented (compare with left orbit). In this plane, the bony floor of the anterior cranial fossa appears intact. A fluid level is present in the left maxillary sinus.

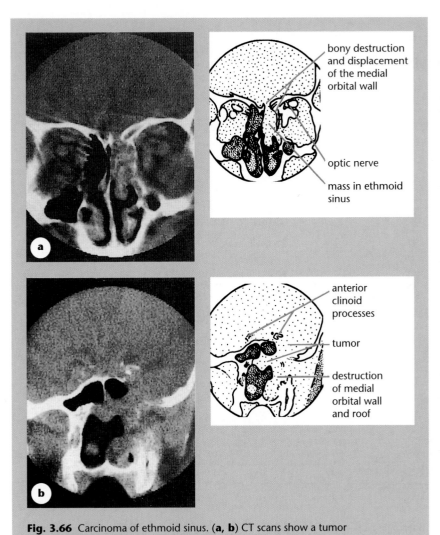

bony destruction
and displacement
of the medial
orbital wall

optic nerve

mass in ethmoid
sinus

anterior
clinoid
processes

tumor

destruction
of medial
orbital wall
and roof

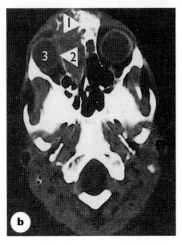

Fig. 3.67
Esthesioneuroblastoma. A 16-year-old boy presented with nasal obstruction of recent onset. (**a**) Axial CT scan shows a large expansile mass (arrows) in the right nasal cavity. The medial wall of the orbit is bowed outward, displacing the globe laterally. The anteromedial wall of the maxillary sinus is displaced but appears intact. (**b**) A more cephalad cut shows expansion of the entire ethmoid labyrinth by tumor with extensive bone destruction (1) anteriorly. The lamina papyracea (2), a portion of which has been destroyed by the tumor, is displaced laterally and abuts the globe (3).

Fig. 3.66 Carcinoma of ethmoid sinus. (**a, b**) CT scans show a tumor expanding the ethmoid sinus, destroying the medial orbital wall and invading posteriorly into the middle cranial fossa.

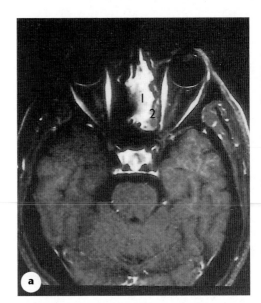

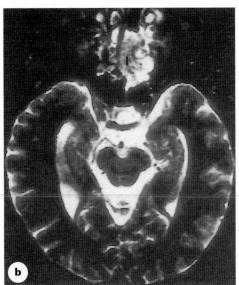

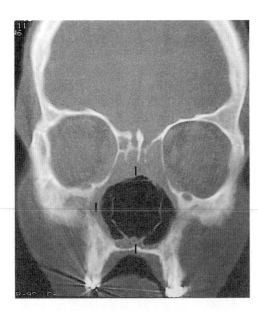

Fig. 3.68 Esthesioneuroblastoma. A 55-year-old male presented with several years of nasal congestion and recent unilateral change in vision. (**a**) Axial T_1-weighted gadolinium-enhanced MR image with fat saturation shows enhancing tissue within the ethmoid air cells (1) with a posterior area of non-enhancement (2). The enhancing tissue could represent either normal mucosa or tumor mass. (**b**) Axial T_2-weighted MR image shows a central low-signal area within the enhancing tissue which represents the tumor mass (1). The bright tissue surrounding it represents retained secretions within surrounding ethmoidal air cells.

Fig. 3.69 Wegener's granulomatosis. This 39-year-old female presented with nasal congestion and epistaxis. Examination revealed an erosive nasal cavity mass. Coronal CT scan revealed gross destruction of the nasal septum by a mass lesion (1).

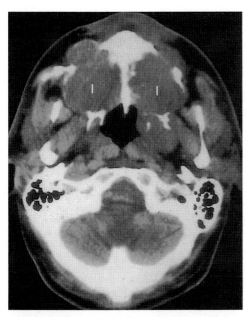

Fig. 3.70 Solitary plasmacytoma of paranasal sinuses. This 69-year-old female presented with head and nasal congestion and clear nasal discharge. Examination revealed a nasal cavity mass. (1) Axial CT scan indicated an extensive lesion involving both maxillary sinuses as well as the nasal cavity. Biopsy of the nasal cavity mass confirmed the diagnosis. Subsequent bone marrow aspiration and biopsy failed to reveal evidence for multiple myeloma.

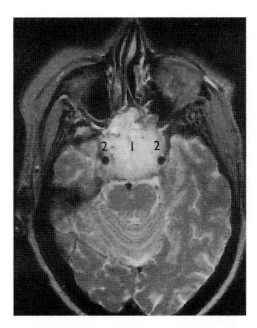

Fig. 3.71 Breast carcinoma metastatic to sphenoid sinus. This 62-year-old patient with known breast carcinoma metastatic to the axial skeleton presented with bitemporal headache of several months' duration. Axial T_2-weighted MRI shows an expansile mass within the sphenoid sinus (1) extending into the cavernous sinuses (2).

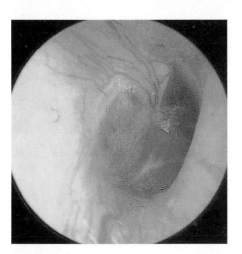

Fig. 3.72 Glomus jugulare tumor of middle ear. Otoscopic view shows a non-ulcerated, smooth tumor filling the inferior half of the right middle ear; it is beginning to extend through the tympanic membrane. Note the adjacent dilated blood vessels.

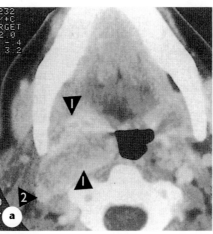

Fig. 3.73 Glomus vagale tumor of parapharyngeal space. (**a**) Contrast-enhanced axial CT scan demonstrates a large mass (1) in the right parapharyngeal space that encroaches on the nasopharynx and extends into the deep fascial spaces of the neck, displacing the internal carotid artery laterally (2). The periphery of the mass enhances but the central portion is relatively hypodense. (**b**) Conventional carotid arteriogram shows a tangle of small vessels (3) supplied by branches of the external carotid artery. The vascular tumor abuts the internal carotid artery, which is bowed anteriorly (4).

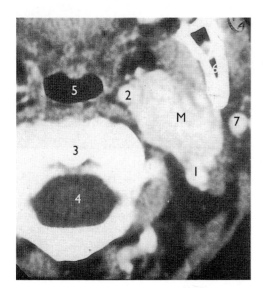

Fig. 3.74 Glomus jugulare tumor involving the neck. Axial contrast-enhanced CT image demonstrates an intensely enhancing mass (M) which separates the internal (1) and external (2) carotid arteries. Note the cervical spine (3), spinal cord (4), oropharynx (5), angle of mandible (6) and jugular vein (7).

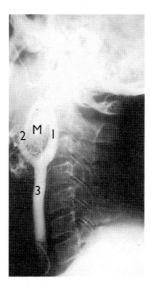

Fig. 3.75 Glomus jugulare tumor involving neck (*see* Fig. 3.74). Angiogram showing displacement of the internal and external carotid arteries by a hypervascular mass (M). Note the internal (1), external (2) and common (3) carotid arteries.

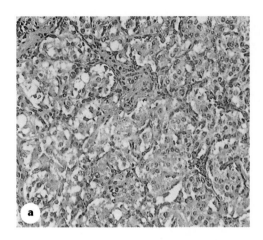

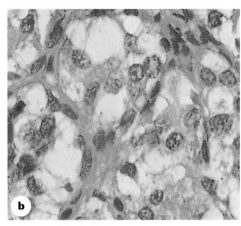

Fig. 3.76 Glomus jugulare tumor. (**a**) This tumor consists of a dense network of thin-walled sinusoidal capillaries that surround glomerular or alveolar-like nests of tumor cells ('Zellballen'). (**b**) The nests or groups of tumor cells contain 5–20 epithelioid cells, which have a moth-eaten, clear or eosinophilic granular cytoplasm and round vesicular nuclei with prominent nucleoli.

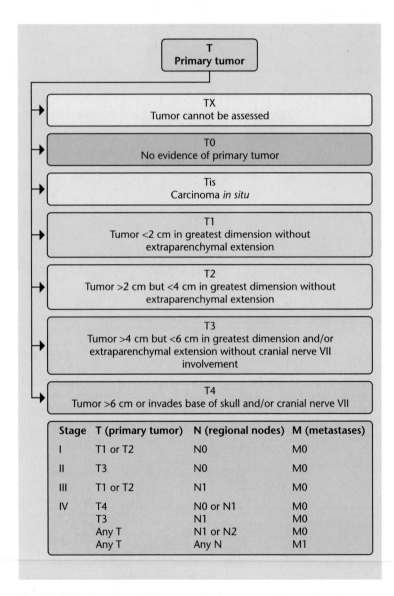

| | **T** | | |
| **Primary tumor** | | | |

TX
Tumor cannot be assessed

T0
No evidence of primary tumor

Tis
Carcinoma *in situ*

T1
Tumor <2 cm in greatest dimension without extraparenchymal extension

T2
Tumor >2 cm but <4 cm in greatest dimension without extraparenchymal extension

T3
Tumor >4 cm but <6 cm in greatest dimension and/or extraparenchymal extension without cranial nerve VII involvement

T4
Tumor >6 cm or invades base of skull and/or cranial nerve VII

Stage	T (primary tumor)	N (regional nodes)	M (metastases)
I	T1 or T2	N0	M0
II	T3	N0	M0
III	T1 or T2	N1	M0
IV	T4	N0 or N1	M0
	T3	N1	M0
	Any T	N1 or N2	M0
	Any T	Any N	M1

Fig. 3.77 T categories and stage grouping for cancer of the major salivary glands (*see* Fig. 3.27 for N and M categories) (Flemming *et al.*, 1997).

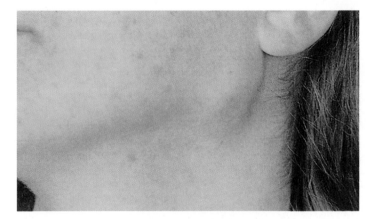

Fig. 3.78 Pleomorphic adenoma of parotid gland. Clinically, as is common with these tumors, there is a painless swelling; in this instance, the tumor involves the lower pole of the gland.

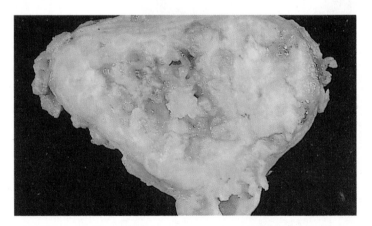

Fig. 3.79 Pleomorphic adenoma of parotid gland. The cut surface of this fairly well-circumscribed, multinodular tumor has a myxoid cartilaginous appearance and there are small foci of cystic change and hemorrhage. These tumors tend to recur locally, most often as a consequence of spread through the capsule, which results in incomplete surgical excision.

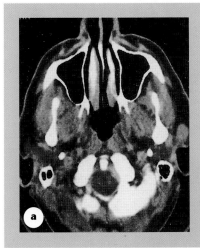

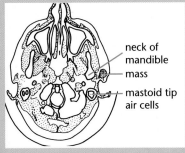

neck of
mandible
mass

mastoid tip
air cells

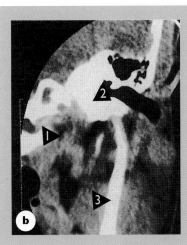

Fig. 3.80 Pleomorphic adenoma of parotid gland. (**a**) Axial CT scan shows a well-circumscribed mass within the left parotid gland of a 57-year-old man. (**b**) Coronal CT section shows that the tumor (arrow 1) is sharply demarcated from the rest of the parotid gland and does not involve deeper structures. The internal auditory canal (arrow 2) and the mandibular ramus (arrow 3) are indicated.

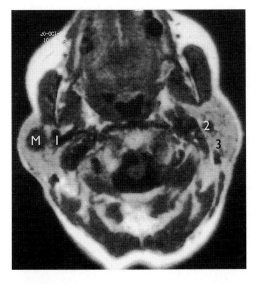

Fig. 3.81 Pleomorphic adenoma of parotid gland. Pleomorphic adenoma in the right parotid (M) is a well-defined, low-signal intensity mass on the axial T$_1$-weighted MRI. Note displacement of the retromandibular vein (1) medially by the mass compared with the normal left retromandibular vein (2). The left facial nerve (3) branching through the normal left parotid is seen.

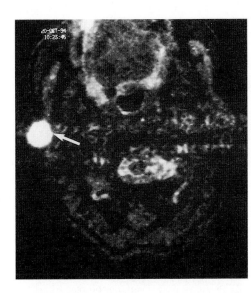

Fig. 3.82 Pleomorphic adenoma of parotid gland. Same patient as Fig. 3.81; the lesion has high but slightly mixed signal intensity on the axial T$_2$-weighted image with fat saturation (arrow).

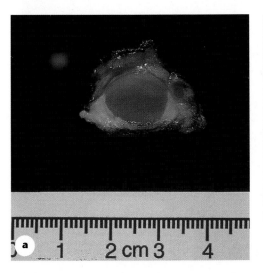

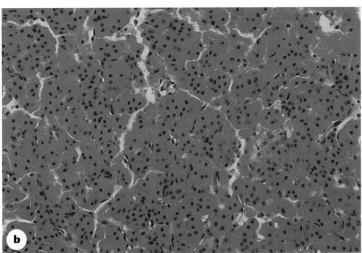

Fig. 3.83 Oncocytoma of salivary gland. (**a**) Gross photo of a resected parotid gland oncocytoma. It is a benign tumor of elderly patients characterized by a solid or organoid proliferation of polygonal cells with deeply eosinophilic granular cytoplasm. (**b**) This characteristic cytoplasmic staining pattern is due to abundant mitochondria, which may be demonstrated by electron microscopy or staining with phosphotungstic acid-hematoxylin (PTAH). The tumor may occasionally recur after excision, especially when multifocal at presentation.

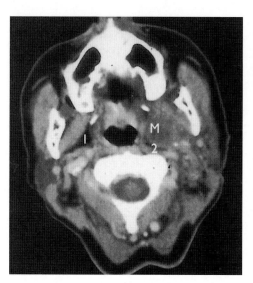

Fig. 3.84
Adenocarcinoma of parotid gland. This 72-year-old male complained of jaw pain and had some left parotid fullness. Poorly differentiated adenocarcinoma of the parotid gland appears on axial CT scan image as a large heterogeneous mass (M) projecting from the deep lobe of the parotid into the parapharyngeal space. Note the normal right parapharyngeal space (1) compared with the effaced space on the left (2).

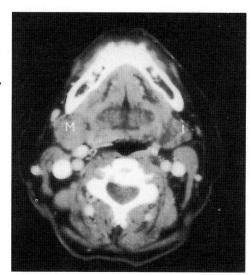

Fig. 3.85
Myoepithelial carcinoma of parotid gland. This 55-year-old-woman presented with swelling underneath her jaw. The enlarged, slightly heterogeneous right submandibular gland (M) seen on CT scan contained a myoepithelial carcinoma. Note the normal avoid-shaped left submandibular gland (1).

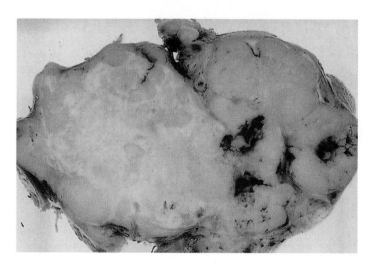

Fig. 3.86 Carcinoma arising in pleomorphic adenoma of submandibular gland. This specimen was excised from a 73-year-old man who noticed a small lump under the jaw for 25 years. A rapid increase in size of the lesion prompted him to see his doctor. The tumor, measuring $10 \times 7 \times 6$ cm in the fresh state, appears encapsulated, is multinodular and contains gelatinous and hemorrhagic foci. Although it exhibits features very similar to a benign pleomorphic adenoma, there was unequivocal histologic evidence of malignancy.

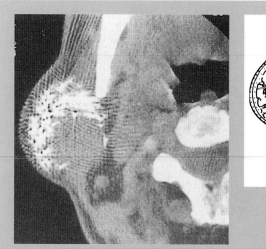
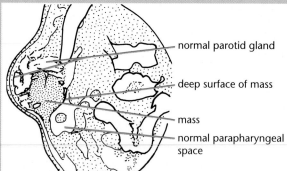

normal parotid gland

deep surface of mass

mass

normal parapharyngeal space

Fig. 3.87 Papillary cystadenoma lymphomatosum (Warthin's tumor) of parotid gland. Axial CT-sialogram demonstrates a mass in the right parotid gland of a 78-year-old man. Normal glandular tissue (opacified by the contrast agent) surrounds the mass. The deep surface of the parotid tumor is sharply demarcated from the fat-containing parapharyngeal space.

REFERENCES

Almadori G, Cadoni G, Galli J, *et al*.: Epidermal growth factor receptor expression in primary laryngeal cancer: an independent prognostic factor of neck node relapse. Int J Cancer 1999; 84(2): 188–191.

Boyle J, Hakim J, Koch W, *et al*.: The incidence of p53 mutations increases with progression of head and neck cancer. J Otolaryngol Head Neck Surg 1993; 53: 4477–4480.

Flemming I, Cooper J, Henson D, *et al*. (Eds) for the American Joint Committee on Cancer: AJCC Cancer Staging Manual, 5th edn. Lippincott–Raven, Philadelphia, 1997.

Forastiere A, Goepfert H, Goffinet D, *et al*.: NCCN practice guidelines for head and neck cancer. National Comprehensive Cancer Network. Oncology (Huntingt) 1998; 12 (7A):39–147.

Gillison ML, Koch WM, Capone RB, *et al*.: Evidence for a causal association between Human Papillomavirus and a subset of head and neck cancers. J Natl Cancer Inst 2000; 92 : 709–702.

Greenlee RT, Murray T, Bolden S, Wingo PA: Cancer statistics. CA Cancer J Clin 2000; 50(1):13–30.

Jares P, Fernandez P, Campo E, *et al*.: PRAD-1/cyclin D1 gene amplification correlates with messenger RNA overexpression and tumor progression in human laryngeal carcinomas. Cancer Res 1994; 54 (17):4813–4817.

Kieff E: Epstein–Barr virus – increasing evidence of a link to carcinoma. N Engl J Med 1995; 333 (11):724–726.

Lewin F, Norell SE, Johansson H, *et al*.: Smoking tobacco, oral snuff, and alcohol in the etiology of squamous cell carcinoma of the head and neck. Cancer 1998; 82 : 1367–1375.

MMWR: Tobacco use among high school students – United States, 1997. Morbidity and Mortality Weekly Report 1998; 47(12):229–233.

Noyek A, Wortzman G, Kassel E: Diagnostic imaging in rhinology. In: Goldman J, ed: Modern Rhinology. John Wiley, New York, 1987.

Raab-Traub N, Flynn K, Pearson G, *et al*.: The differentiated form of nasopharyngeal carcinoma contains Epstein–Barr virus DNA. Int J Cancer 1987; 39 (1):25–29.

Reed A, Califano J, Cairns P, *et al*.: High frequency of p16 (CDKN2/MTS-1/INK4A) inactivation in head and neck squamous cell carcinoma. Cancer Res 1996; 56 : 3630–3633.

Snyderman CH: Human papillomavirus and head and neck cancer: epidemiology and molecular biology. Head and Neck 1998; 20 : 250–265.

Todd R, Wong D: Epidermal growth factor receptor (EGFR) biology and human oral cancer. Histol Histopathol 1999; 14 (2):491–500.

van der Wal JE, Leverstein H, Snow G, Kraaijenhagen H, van der Waal I: Parotid gland tumors: histologic reevaluation and reclassification of 478 cases. Head and Neck 1998; 20 : 204–207.

Yadav M, Arivananthan M, Chandrashekran A, Tan B, Hashim B: Human herpesvirus-6 (HHV-6) DNA and virus-encoded antigen in oral lesions. J Oral Pathol Med 1997; 26(9):393–401.

FIGURE CREDITS

The following books published by Gower Medical Publishing are sources of figures in the present chapter. The figure numbers given in the listing are those of the figures in the present chapter. The page numbers (or slide numbers) given in parentheses are those of the original publication.

Cawson RA, Eveson JW: Oral Pathology and Diagnosis. Heinemann Medical Books/Gower Medical Publishing, London, 1987: Figs 3.1 (p. 12.8), 3.2 (p. 12.11), 3.3 (p. 12.22), 3.4 (p. 12.25), 3.5 (p. 13.8), 3.6 (p. 13.13), 3.7 (p. 13.12), 3.8 (p. 13.12), 3.9 (p. 13.14), 3.10 (p. 13.14), 3.13 (p. 14.13), 3.14 (p. 14.13), 3.15 (p. 14.13), 3.16 (p. 14.15), 3.18 (p. 14.19), 3.19 (p. 14.19), 3.20 (p. 14.22), 3.21 (p. 14.21), 3.22 (p. 14.21), 3.23 (p. 14.22), 3.24 (p. 14.22), 3.32 (p. 13.8), 3.33 (p. 13.6), 3.34 (p. 13.9), 3.35 (p. 13.9), 3.36 (p. 13.9), 3.37 (p. 13.10), 3.38 (p. 13.10), 3.39 (p. 13.10), 3.66 (p. 14.12).

du Vivier A: Atlas of Clinical Dermatology. Churchill Livingstone/Gower Medical Publishing, Edinburgh/London, 1986: Figs 3.29 (p. 7.16), 3.30 (p. 7.16), 3.31 (p. 4.13).

Fletcher CDM, McKee PH: An Atlas of Gross Pathology. Edward Arnold/Gower Medical Publishing, London, 1987: Figs 3.56 (p. 13), 3.67 (p. 23).

Hawke M, Jahn AF: Diseases of the Ear: Clinical and Pathologic Aspects. Lea and Febiger/Gower Medical Publishing, Philadelphia/New York, 1987: Figs 3.42 (p. 3.49), 3.62 (p. 3.100), 3.64 (p. 3.102).

Kassner EG, ed: Atlas of Radiology Imaging. Lippincott/Gower Medical Publishing, Philadelphia/New York, 1989: Figs 3.40 (p. 12.27), 3.43 (p. 12.19), 3.44 (p. 12.23), 3.50 (p. 12.40), 3.53 (p. 12.45), 3.53 (p. 12.45), 3.57 (p. 12.38), 3.59 (p. 12.20), 3.61 (p. 12.26), 3.63 (p. 12.43), 3.68 (p. 12.31), 3.70 (p. 12.30).

Perkin GD, Rose FC, Blackwood W, *et al*.: Atlas of Clinical Neurology. Lippincott/Gower Medical Publishing, Philadelphia/London, 1986: Fig. 3.46 (p. 12.12).

Price AB, Morson BC, Scheuer PJ, eds: Alimentary system. In: Turk JL, Fletcher CDM, eds: RSCI Slide Atlas of Pathology. Gower Medical Publishing, London, 1986: Fig. 3.69 (slide 35).

Spalton DJ, Hitchings RA, Hunter PA: Atlas of Clinical Ophthalmology. Lippincott/Gower Medical Publishing, Philadelphia/New York, 1984: Fig. 3.60 (p. 29.19).

4 Lung cancer and tumors of the heart and mediastinum

Ravi Salgia, Ramon Blanco, Arthur T. Skarin

LUNG CANCER

INCIDENCE AND ETIOLOGY

Lung cancer is the most common cancer in the world with about 900,000 new cases per year (1994 statistics). The estimate for new cases of lung cancer in the USA in men for 2002 is 100 700 and among women, 82 500 (Jemal *et al.*, 2002). Lung cancer will still be the leading cause of death from malignancy in both sexes in the United States, resulting in 67 300 estimated deaths in women in 2002 and 94 100 deaths in men. Lung cancer is responsible for 25% of all cancer deaths and for 5% of all deaths in the USA. The vast majority of cases (85% or more) are due to chronic cigarette smoking. Other etiologic factors include asbestos (shipyard workers, insulators, etc.), radon gas (underground mining, etc.), ionizing radiation and certain industrial agents and compounds (chloromethyl ether, arsenic, nickel-cadmium and chromium). Tobacco smoking is thought to be synergistic with the latter elements. Tobacco smoke contains oxidants which are believed to be important in biological damage of DNA, proteins and lipids, leading to lung cancer. Genetic abnormalities as well as underlying lung disease (chronic obstructive pulmonary disease) also predispose patients to lung cancer.

Whereas lung cancer is one of the easiest cancers to prevent, it is one of the most difficult to cure, owing to the early dissemination in many cases and therapeutically refractory disease when metastases occur. The overall rate of cure for all patients is about 10%, although there is a wide range of cure rates related mainly to stage of disease. If a patient survives the initial cancer the risk of subsequent lung cancer increases to 3–7% per year. By discontinuing cigarette smoking, the patient lowers the risk for primary lung cancer as well as subsequent cancer, but it takes 15–20 years before the risk approaches that of non-smokers. Still, at 15 years after quitting smoking the risk is 1.5 times that of a person who never smoked. Passive smoking accounts for 3–5% of all cases of lung cancer. According to the Surgeon General, 5000–10 000 of the 156 900 deaths due to lung cancer each year occur in patients exposed to sidestream smoke.

LUNG CANCER, GENDER AND AGE

Lung cancer rates in women have risen dramatically, both worldwide and in the United States. Population-based data by the National Cancer Institute (NCI) Surveillance, Epidemiology and End Results (SEER) Program have shown that the age-adjusted rate for lung cancer for all race/sex groups has risen sharply since 1950. The incidence started rising in the mid-1930s and overtook breast cancer as the leading cause of cancer deaths among women in the late 1980s. This observation correlates with the increase in the number of women who smoke. The male to female ratio is 3.47 in patients over 45 years of age and 1.7 in patients younger than 45. Adenocarcinoma is the most common type in young patients and squamous cell carcinoma in the older age group.

HISTOPATHOLOGY

Over 95% of lung neoplasms are of epithelial origin (carcinomas), comprising four main types (Table 4.3). Based on clinical features and biologic properties from studies of cultured malignant cells, these carcinomas can be separated into two major categories: non-small cell lung cancer (squamous cell, adenocarcinoma and undifferentiated large cell types) and small cell lung cancer (Minna *et al.*, 1989). About 5% of lung cancers are composed of rare mixed epithelial types or neoplasms arising from bronchial glands and other tissues (Table 4.3).

Preinvasive lesions

In the new World Health Organization (WHO)/International Association for the Study of Lung Cancer (IASLC) 1999 classification, preinvasive lesions include squamous dysplasia/carcinoma *in situ* (leading to squamous cell carcinoma), atypical adenomatous hyperplasia (AAH, characterized by discrete ill-defined bronchioloalveolar proliferation, leading to adenocarcinomas) and diffuse idiopathic pulmonary neuroendocrine cell hyperplasia (DIPNECH, characterized by proliferation of neuroendocrine cells throughout the peripheral airways, leading to carcinoids) (Travis *et al.*, 1999).

Non-small cell lung cancer

Non-small cell lung cancer (NSCLC) comprises about 75% of all lung cancers. They are subdivided in three groups. Squamous cell carcinoma (SCC) is characterized by keratin formation (cytokeratin proteins are intermediate filaments). Keratin may appear under the light microscope as 'keratin pearls' (*see* Fig. 4.3) or as desmosomes (a type of tight junction seen as 'intercellular bridges' Fig. 4.3). The incidence of this type of lung cancer is decreasing in the United States for unknown reasons. Most squamous cell carcinomas arise from the central or proximal tracheal-bronchial tree in areas of squamous cell metaplasia, dysplasia and carcinoma *in situ*. Squamous cell carcinomas grow slowly and tend to cavitate in about 20% of cases. About one-third of squamous cell carcinomas are poorly differentiated and, as such, show a greater potential for distant spread, especially to the liver and small intestine. Poorly differentiated squamous cell carcinomas may acquire a spindle cell morphology that may mimic a sarcoma; identification of such tumors is based on finding a transition zone between the epithelial-appearing tumor cells and the spindle cells and/or on the demonstration of keratin in the spindle cells by immunohistochemistry.

Adenocarcinoma is characterized by definite gland formation (well and moderately differentiated) or by the presence of mucus production in a solid tumor (poorly differentiated) as determined by mucin stains (mucicarmine and D-PAS) (*see* Fig. 4.7). Adenocarcinomas are increasing in frequency in the United States: at most medical centers they are now more common than squamous cell carcinomas. In about two-thirds of cases, adenocarcinomas originate in peripheral airways and alveoli. Classically, they were thought to arise from scars ('scar carcinoma'). This view is no longer accepted: the 'scar tissue' (desmoplasia) is now thought to be induced by the neoplastic cells (*see* Fig. 4.6). Around one-third of cases arise centrally, in larger bronchi, from either the surface epithelium or the submucosal glands. Adenocarcinomas frequently present as subpleural nodules, often with a malignant effusion. These cases must be differentiated by means of special stains from malignant mesothelioma, which lacks mucin (*see* Fig. 10.97). Metastases from adenocarcinoma to distant sites occur early (e.g. before symptoms or diagnosis) in most patients. Adenocarcinoma arising from sites other than lung can also look very similar to adenocarcinoma arising in the lung. Cytokeratins (7 versus 20) can aid in distinguishing adenocarcinoma from lung versus other sites (in the case of lung, cytokeratin 7 is usually positive and cytokeratin 20 usually negative). A new marker, TTF-1 (thyroid transcription factor-1), is found almost exclusively in adenocarcinoma of the lung and thyroid cancer and is useful in the differential diagnosis of metastatic adenocarcinoma from an unknown primary site (Ordonez, 2000).

Bronchioloalveolar carcinoma (BAC) is a subtype of well-differentiated adenocarcinoma, constituting about 3% of cases, that appears to be increasing in frequency and is the one subtype of lung carcinoma (in addition to carcinoid tumors) that is not associated with cigarette smoking. BAC arises from the peripheral bronchioles or alveoli. About 50% are mucin-secreting tumors consisting of tall columnar cells, whereas the remaining 50% have little or no mucin and consist of peg-shaped ('hobnail') cells with variable degrees of pleomorphism. They are thought to arise from Clara cells or type II pneumocytes. Some adenocarcinomas may contain a small proportion of tumor cells with BAC morphology, typically in the periphery of the tumor. In the new WHO classification, true BAC has growth in a lepidic fashion with lack of invasive growth (Travis *et al.*, 1999). BAC tends to spread throughout air passages, while preserving (or recapitulating) the septal and lobular architecture. The tumor is slow growing and usually metastasizes late in the course of the disease. It characteristically induces a voluminous clear sputum production (bronchorrhea). Prognosis is related to stage of disease, but because BAC may be mistaken for chronic infection or diffuse interstitial disease, there may be a long delay in diagnosis. Five-year survival is only about 5%.

Undifferentiated large cell carcinoma is characterized by large cells with vesicular nuclei, prominent eosinophilic nucleoli, moderate to abundant cytoplasm, distinct cytoplasmic membrane and no evidence of squamous or glandular differentiation by light microscopy. Some of these tumors may contain features of either squamous and/or glandular differentiation as evidenced by immunohistochemistry or electron microscopy, implying some heterogeneity in this group. Giant cell and clear cell variants are uncommon. A giant cell variant may mimic an anaplastic large cell lymphoma (Ki-1 lymphoma). Clinically, most patients present with large, bulky, peripheral tumors. Metastases occur early, preferentially to the CNS, and the 5-year survival is under 5%.

Small cell lung cancer

Small cell lung cancer (SCLC) represents about 20% of all lung tumors, is extremely aggressive, is frequently associated with distant metastases and has the poorest prognosis of all lung neoplasms. SCLC has a central origin in most cases, although 10% of these tumors are found in the peripheral lung field. The tumor has a white-tan appearance, is friable and shows extensive necrosis.

Histologically, they are characterized by scant cytoplasm or high nuclear: cytoplasmic (N/C) ratio, fine chromatin and 'nuclear molding'. Small cells are characterized as 'small blue cell tumor' and need to be distinguished from lymphoma, carcinoid tumors, Ewing's sarcoma and PNET. The rapid growth and scanty cytoplasm of small cell carcinomas make them unusually susceptible to ischemic necrosis, as well as crush artefact, during handling and fixation. Although not pathognomonic, the so-called Azzopardi effect (crushed DNA material encrusted around blood vessels) is very characteristic (Fig. 4.18b). The subclassification of small cell carcinoma into oat cell, intermediate cell and combined oat cell carcinoma has been dropped from the new WHO classification and the only subtype of SCLC is combined SCLC. Less than 10% of SCLC is admixed with NSCLC components (with large cells 4–6%, 1–3% with adenocarcinoma or squamous cell carcinoma).

Data (Kimura *et al.*, 1993) indicate that nuclear DNA measurements may be useful in predicting the likelihood of metastases and response to chemotherapy. Most (but not all) small cell carcinomas contain dense-core granules (containing amines, peptide products, L-dopa decarboxylase), indicating neuroendocrine differentiation. Immunohistochemical studies demonstrate the presence of neuron-specific enolase (NSE), chromogranin A, Leu-7 (a natural killer cell antigen also present in some neuroendocrine cells) and synaptophysin. Other antigens that may also be expressed are carcinoembryonic antigen (CEA), adrenocorticotrophin hormone (ACTH) and 'big' ACTH. SCLC cells, as with most carcinomas, express keratin proteins.

Small cell carcinomas produce and release into the circulation a variety of functioning polypeptide hormones that can result in paraneoplastic syndromes (Fig. 4.86). They also grow in a submucosal pattern with a high frequency of lymphatic and vascular invasion. Prominent mediastinal adenopathy is often present. Almost 70% of patients have metastatic disease at the time of diagnosis. Almost any organ can be involved, but preferential sites include the liver, bone, bone marrow, CNS, adrenal glands, abdominal lymph nodes, pancreas, skin and endocrine organs.

Carcinoid tumor and the spectrum of neuroendocrine tumors of the lung

The classification of neuroendocrine neoplasms of the lung has evolved substantially over the past two decades. Initially there were only two categories: carcinoid and SCLC. The latter is discussed above.

Typical carcinoid (TC) or carcinoid tumors (bronchial carcinoid tumors) are similar to tumors arising in the GI tract and elsewhere. They are characterized by small (0.7–3.5 cm), well-circumscribed solid tan/yellow nodules with no necrosis or hemorrhage. Usually they are centrally seen, less commonly peripheral in location. By light microscopy, tumor cells are round, uniform in size, with finely granular eosinophilic cytoplasm. The nucleus is centrally placed with finely granular or stippled chromatin and small nucleoli. The cells arrange themselves in an organoid pattern (cords, nests and acini may be formed). Mitoses are rare and necrosis is not seen. By electron microscopy numerous cytoplasmic membrane-bound, dense-core granules (90–450 nm) are usually seen. By immunohistology they are usually positive for NSE, chromogranin A, Leu-7, synaptophysin, bombesin, CEA, ACTH, calcitonin and keratin. Carcinoid tumors may be responsible for ectopic hormone secretion, particularly 5-hydroxytryptamine, ACTH, vasopressin and insulin. Typical carcinoid have low malignant potential.

Atypical carcinoid (AC) is a third category described in 1972. AC is similar to TC, but usually larger (1.5–2.3 cm) and contains foci of necrosis and mitoses (usually 3–4/10 HPF, always 10/10 HPF).

Atypical carcinoids can follow a more aggressive clinical course than TC and have metastatic potential. AC represent approximately 10% of all carcinoid tumors.

The fourth category proposed is large cell neuroendocrine carcinoma (LCNEC). LCNEC is a malignant neuroendocrine neoplasm composed of large polygonal cells with relatively low N/C ratio, coarse nuclear chromatin, frequent nucleoli, high mitotic rate (>10/10 HPF) and frequent necrosis. The cells in LCNEC are larger than cells in SCLC and have more abundant eosinophilic cytoplasm. Although the concept of LCNEC is attractive, it is still controversial and not fully accepted. Clinicopathologic correlation and long-term followup studies will determine the validity of this concept.

CHROMOSOMES, GENES AND LUNG CANCER

The evolution to cancer in general is currently understood as a multistep process. Insight into this evolution has been gained through recent advances in cytogenetics, cell biology and mainly molecular biology. It has become apparent that mutations in a limited number of genes, which control cell proliferation and differentiation, are key events in this process. Proto-oncogenes ('activated' by a particular mutation) and tumor suppressor genes ('deactivation' unleashes unregulated proliferation of cells) play major roles in malignant transformation of cells and may be prognostic forms (see Table 4.5).

Chromosomal abnormalities and telomerase activation

Using both actual tumor specimens and cell lines, various chromosomal and oncogene abnormalities have been identified. In NSCLC, chromosomal aberrations have been described on 3p, 8p, 9p, 11p, 15p and 17p with deletions of chromosomes 7, 11, 13 or 19. Also, in SCLC, chromosomal abnormalities have been described on 1p, 3p, 5q, 6q, 8q, 13q or 17p. One of the most consistent chromosomal abnormalities in lung cancer has been the loss of the short arm of chromosome 3 (3p(14–25)). The loss of alleles at 3p is observed in >90% of SCLC tumors and approximately 50% of NSCLC tumors. As many as three tumor suppressor genes may contribute to SCLC pathogenesis. Most recently, the FHIT gene (for fragile histidine triad) has been localized to 3p 14.2 and about 80% of SCLC tumors show abnormalities of this gene. The protein product of the FHIT gene is involved in the metabolism of diadenosine tetraphosphate into ATP and AMP (Sozzi et al., 1996).

Other genetic losses have, although not consistently, been identified in lung cancer. In NSCLC, these include genetic loss at chromosome 8p (21.3–22) and may be abnormal in 50% of tumor samples. Genetic loss at 9p(21–22) could potentially involve the p16 (MTS1/p16INK4A) and p15 (MTS2/p15INK4B) tumor suppressor genes, which are involved in cell cycle regulation at the G_1 checkpoint by inhibiting cyclin-dependent kinase CDK4 and may be affected in 67% of tumor samples. Genetic loss at 11p (p13 and p15) may involve the Wilms' tumor suppressor gene at region p13 and can be affected in 20–46% of tumor samples.

Telomeres, which are genetic elements at the ends of linear eukaryotic chromosomes consisting of tandem repeats of simple DNA sequences, are important in stabilizing chromosomes from degradation, illegitimate recombination or cellular senescence. Longer telomeres are present in germ cells and in most cancer cells, via the telomerase enzyme, and these maintain the ability of the cells to divide indefinitely. Telomerase activity has been directly correlated with malignant and metastatic phenotype of a wide array of solid tumors. In one study, 80% of tumor tissue from lung cancer had telomerase activity (Hiyama et al., 1995).

Proto-oncogenes in NSCLC

Amplification of the ras genes (K-ras, H-ras and N-ras) is frequent in NSCLC. The level and frequency vary with the tumor type, ranging from about 30% in adenocarcinoma compared to 10% in other cell types. There is some evidence of linking mutations in the ras family with a poor prognosis in patients undergoing surgery. Several investigators have found a correlation between K-ras mutations in adenocarcinomas and smoking history. In particular, mutations of the K-ras oncogene involving codon 12 may be a specific target of tobacco smoke and may occur early and irreversibly during carcinogenesis in adenocarcinomas of the lung (Westra et al., 1993). Amplification of c-myc is found in about 10% of NSCLC of all types. Although activated L-myc is not found in NSCLC in general, its presence has been correlated with poor prognosis in Japanese patients. Such correlation is not found in non-Japanese patients.

The erbB-1 (epidermal growth factor receptor) protein is overexpressed in approximately 50% of NSCLC, with high expression in squamous cell carcinomas.

The c-erbB-2 (HER-2/neu) gene encodes a transmembrane tyrosine-specific protein kinase, p185neu. Frequency of abnormal expression of c-erbB-2 is approximately 25%. This gene is frequently amplified in adenocarcinomas and squamous cell carcinomas; in adenocarcinomas, p185neu expression tends to be found in older patients and is usually associated with shorter survival.

The c-fos and c-jun genes encode nuclear proteins that form the complex AP-1, which acts as a transcriptional factor for genes possessing a specific DNA recognition site. AP-1 may be implicated in signal transduction. Adenocarcinomas and squamous cell carcinomas have been reported to have increased nuclear AP-1. The significance of this finding is unknown at present.

Tumor suppressor genes in NSCLC

The p53 gene encodes a 53 kDa nuclear phosphoprotein identified as a transcriptional activator. High levels of the wild-type gene product inhibit growth, possibly by acting as a checkpoint for DNA damage at the G_0–G_1 transition in cell division. Mutations in p53 are very common features in different types of cancer and are present in NSCLC and have been detected in preinvasive lesions of the bronchus (Sundaresan et al., 1992). The frequency of mutations varies with the type of NSCLC: about 67% of squamous cell carcinomas and 37% of adenocarcinomas contain p53 mutations. Mutations are also present in undifferentiated large cell carcinomas. No significant correlation has been found between p53 mutations and age, sex, histopathology, clinical stage or lymph node involvement. G:C to T:A transversions, found in about 50% of NSCLC, are remarkably uncommon in other types of human cancer. Since one of the components of cigarette smoking is benzo[a]pyrene, a potent mutagen that causes G:C to T:A transversions, the implication is that smoking may be responsible for these mutations. Interestingly, mutations in both p53 and K-ras are most commonly G to T transversions in lung cancer versus G to A transitions in other cancers (Johnson and Kelley, 1993). Although the correlation between smoking and p53 mutations has been verified in Japanese patients, it has not been confirmed in American lung cancer patients. The cause of these contradictory results is unknown, but it has been speculated that differences in the genetic make-up of the two populations might be responsible. Initially, it was believed that lung cancer has an adverse correlation with p53 protein overexpression (Mitsudomi et al., 1993). However, recent data suggest that high expression of the p53 oncoprotein may be a favorable prognostic factor in a subset of patients with NSCLC (Lee et al., 1995).

The retinoblastoma gene (Rb-1) encodes a DNA-binding protein of 110 kDa that is involved in important events of cell division. Inactivation of this gene by deletion and loss of heterozygosity has been found in several cancers, with abnormalities in NSCLC approximately 15%. In NSCLC, an inverse correlation exists between p16INK4A expression and Rb-1 expression, thereby implicating a key role of these proteins in growth suppression.

The expression of neural cell adhesion molecules and the blood group antigen A are reportedly both signs of favorable prognosis. Loss of ABH blood group antigens in lung carcinomas seems to correlate with their metastatic potential. Apparently the loss of blood group B antigens more significantly affected both hematogenous metastasis and prognosis than that of A and H antigens (Matsumoto et al., 1993). Also, bcl-2, the proto-oncogene involved in the follicular lymphoma 14:18 translocation, may be abnormally expressed in some NSCLC and its expression may have favorable prognostic significance (Pezzella et al., 1993).

Proto-oncogenes in SCLC

Mutations in ras genes are absent in SCLC. Gene amplification of all three types of myc genes have been observed in SCLC. Amplification of myc genes has been observed more frequently in patients who have undergone chemotherapy, but cell lines established from SCLCs before and after chemotherapy did not alter their status of myc gene copy number. It is unclear whether chemotherapy can actually cause myc gene amplification. Increased expression of N-myc gene has been reported to correlate with poor subsequent response to chemotherapy, rapid tumor growth and short survival times.

Tumor suppressor genes in SCLC

The Rb gene (chromosome 3q) is absent or aberrant in over 90% of patients. This was the first identification of a recessive oncogene participating in the pathogenesis of lung cancer (Otterson et al., 1992). Rb gene protein has important functions in the regulation of growth stages of cell cycle events, by maintaining cells in a quiescent or growth-arrested state.

Mutations of the p53 gene are present in over 75% of SCLCs and are considered an early event in carcinogenesis. Structural abnormalities have been detected in some cell lines, but in the absence of Rb mRNA and p105 Rb protein.

Chromosomal abnormalities in SCLC mainly consist of chromosome 3 short-arm deletions, in three different regions between 3p21 and 3p25, occurring in over 90% of cases.

Growth factor abnormalities in SCLC

In SCLC, many of the tumor cells produce neuroendocrine peptides, such as gastrin-releasing peptide (GRP), and respond to them in an autocrine or paracrine fashion. GRP binds to the receptor (G-protein family member) and transduces intracellular signal with proliferation of SCLC cells. Another growth factor, insulin-like growth factor I, is elevated in >95% SCLC and modulates mitogenic signaling. Also, Steel factor, the ligand for the proto-oncogene tyrosine kinase receptor c-Kit, supports growth and survival of immature hematopoietic cells of multiple lineages. In SCLC, c-Kit and Steel factor are simultaneously expressed, thus forming an autocrine loop.

Metastatic mechanisms in lung cancer

Paget initially observed that metastasis of tumor cells occurred when certain tumor cells ('seed') had special affinity for the growth environment provided by certain specific organs ('soil'). Tumor cells are heterogeneous and have different angiogenic, invasive and metastatic properties. Inducing angiogenesis may be an important mechanism for a tumor cell to proliferate and eventually metastasize. Angiogenesis has been shown to be a prognostic factor in stage I NSCLC (Harpole et al., 1996). Tumor cells can also penetrate preexisting vessels, thereby leading to metastasis. In one study, 15% of patients with tumor invasion had a poor survival and higher recurrence rate in patients with peripheral, node-negative NSCLC (Macchiarini et al., 1992).

Staging of lung cancer

The most widely used system is the International Staging System (ISS) using TNM, categories to place patients into stages I–IV, each having a progressively lower survival rate (Fig. 4.28). It was revised in 1997 with additional stage subgroupings (Mountain, 1997; see also Figs 4.30 and 4.31). Only 30% of patients present with stage I or II disease; 15–20% have potentially resectable stage IIIA disease and the remainder have advanced unrespectable stage IIIB or metastatic stage IV disease. Although the ISS can be applied to all cell types, SCLC is often categorized as limited disease (stage I, II or III) or extensive disease (stage IV) for therapeutic purposes. Survival for patients with SCLC appears to have improved over the last 15 years. However, 2–3-year survival still occurs in only 10–25% of patients with limited disease and 1–2% of patients with extensive disease. Moreover, relapse of SCLC and development of other neoplasms are common in patients surviving beyond 2 years. Prognostic indicators (disease stage) should help target individual SCLC patients for specific intensive treatments designed to prolong survival and achieve cure (Skarin, 1993).

Staging procedures consist of CT scan of the chest and upper abdomen to include liver and adrenals. Assays for tumor markers (e.g. CEA, CA 125 and NSE; Salgia et al., 2001), if elevated, may be of prognostic value and also allow for monitoring of disease status. A bone scan and head CT scan with contrast MRI should be performed in all patients except for those with stage I NSCLC who are asymptomatic with normal chemistries. In these patients, the likelihood of early (occult) metastases is under 5%. PET scans are also of value in initial assessment and followup restaging or search for metastases (see Chapter 2). Whole-body positron-emission tomography (PET) using ^{18}F-fluordeoxyglucose as a tracer is a new imaging technique based upon the increased metabolism of glucose in malignant cells. PET has a 95% sensitivity for detecting primary lung cancers and mediastinal lymph node involvement (Pieterman et al., 2000). The threshold of detection is around 3–5 mm. It may more accurately predict the likelihood of long-term survival than chest CT does (Dunagan et al., 2001). It is also useful to differentiate benign from malignant pulmonary nodules, assess response to treatment and recurrence and assist in radiography planning (Marom et al., 2000). Bone marrow involvement as the only stage IV manifestation is unusual, however, and occurs in approximately 5% of cases with limited thoracic disease in SCLC.

Invasive staging procedures include thoracoscopy, cervical (suprasternal) mediastinoscopy and anterior mediastinoscopy (Chamberlain procedure). One or more may be carried out to evaluate mediastinal nodal stations (see Fig. 4.27) or suspicious sites of disease in resectable patients, particularly when multimodality treatment protocols are utilized. Video-assisted thoracoscopic surgery (VATS) is being utilized for staging as well as management in selected cases (see Fig. 4.50). VATS has minimal mortality and greatly reduces hospitalization time compared to traditional thoracotomy (Mentzer and Sugarbaker, 1994).

CLINICAL MANIFESTATIONS

The signs and symptoms of lung cancer are related directly to the primary malignancy or to distant metastases. Indirect signs and symptoms may be encountered as a result of the secretion of biologically active polypeptides and hormones.

Manifestations of early thoracic disease depend on the location of the primary cancer. Central (proximal) lesions such as squamous cell carcinoma often erode the bronchus, causing hemoptysis and cough. Chest pain is a common symptom in early-stage lung cancer. As the tumor spreads, bronchial obstruction with atelectasis and pneumonia often occurs. Hilar adenopathy and cavitation of the primary cancer may also develop. Although small cell cancers are central in origin, they grow submucosally and thus rarely cause hemoptysis. Due to lymphatic invasion, mediastinal adenopathy occurs in most cases. Extension into the recurrent laryngeal nerve results in hoarseness and involvement of the phrenic nerve causes a paralyzed (elevated) diaphragm. Stridor, caused by invasion of the trachea or bilateral vocal cord paralysis, results from compromise of the lumen of the trachea. Invasion and compression of the superior vena cava leads to the SVC syndrome (see Fig. 4.55); this can occur either with isolated stage IIIB disease or as part of stage IV (metastatic) disease. Extension of malignancy into the pericardium results in pericardial effusion and acute cardiac tamponade.

Cancers that arise in the peripheral lung fields, such as adenocarcinoma and large cell carcinoma, cause chest pain and cough due to involvement of the pleura, often with malignant pleural effusion and resultant dyspnea. Undifferentiated large cell tumors may reach enormous size before symptoms occur. Widespread metastases develop in most cases.

Cancers arising in the apex of the lung grow into the adjacent soft tissues, resulting in a Pancoast tumor or superior sulcus tumor syndrome, the features of which may vary. Histologically, Pancoast tumors are usually squamous cell carcinomas, although other non-small cell types of cancer can occur; the rarest cause is small cell (oat cell) lung cancer. Persistent symptoms can result from early lesions that may be missed on routine radiographs, unless apical views or tomograms are obtained. CT scans can detect early lesions and define the extent of regional disease. The advanced syndrome is marked by shoulder pain radiating to the ulnar nerve distribution, rib and vertebral body destruction and Horner's syndrome (enophthalmos, ptosis, miosis and ipsilateral loss of sweating) due to invasion of the sympathetic nerves. With early involvement, mydriasis (pupillary dilatation) may be the first clue. Unilateral supraclavicular adenopathy is a sign of advanced local disease.

Metastatic disease can occur to any organ and thus a variety of clinical and laboratory manifestations may be encountered. At autopsy, the frequency of extrathoracic metastases related to histologic type of lung cancer is as follows: squamous cell carcinoma, 25–54%; adenocarcinoma, 50–82%; large cell carcinoma, 48–86%; and small cell carcinoma, 74–96%. With advanced disease, there are no particular selective sites for metastases related to histologic type. Lymphangitic spread of the tumor through the parenchyma of the lung is characterized by progressive dyspnea, cough and hypoxia.

Indirect manifestations of lung cancer vary from severe weight loss and cachexia, seen in up to one-third of patients, to one or more of several paraneoplastic syndromes. The latter are due to the secretion of biologically active polypeptide hormones or to unknown factors often related to certain histologic cell types (see Fig. 4.86). Patients may initially present with these problems, which can be misinterpreted, for example, joint pains due to clubbing being mistaken for arthritis. Hypertrophic osteoarthropathy can occur with symptoms of swelling and pain in the joints and extremities. These manifestations, however, should also be viewed as clues to an underlying lung cancer. In some patients, the initial chest film may fail to show an obvious lesion, a scenario occasionally seen in SCLC. In this situation, CT scanning may reveal a small tumor mass or bronchoscopy may yield the correct diagnosis.

Table 4.1 Lesions causing a mass on chest radiography

Neoplastic	Infective	Miscellaneous
Malignant	Bacterial	Sarcoidosis
Primary lung carcinoma	Pneumonia	Rheumatoid nodules
Carcinoid tumor	Lung abscess	Pseudolymphoma
Lymphoma	Empyema	Wegener's grahulomatosis
Plasmacytoma		Bronchocentric granulomatosis
Thymoma	Tuberculous	Echlnococcal cyst
Germ cell tumor	Tuberculoma	Pseudotumor (fluid)
Sarcoma		Bronchial lymph node
Metastatic carcinoma	Fungal	
	Aspergilloma	
Benign	Allergic aspergillosis	
Neurofibroma	Histoplasmoma	
Hamartoma	Mycetoma	
Thymoma		
Cyst		
Arteriovenous malformation		

Table 4.2 Diagnostic methods for assessment of mass lesions

Fiberoptic bronchoscopy	Radiology	Transthoracic biopsy
Bronchial tree secretions, bacteriology and cytology	Plain PA and lateral views	Fine needle aspiration
Bronchial biopsy	Computed tomography (CT)	Cutting needle biopsy
Transbronchial biopsy	Magnetic resonance imaging (MRI)	Video assisted thoracoscopic biopsy/resection
Transbronchial needle aspiration	Galtium citrate Ga 67 scanning	
Selective bronchial brushing	Angiography (not often used)	
Bronchioalveolar lavage		

*When the biopsy studies given here are negative, madiastinoscopy or mediastinotomy may be indicated in selected patients

Table 4.3 Histopathologic classification of lung carcinoma, with relative frequencies (modified from Mountain *et al.*, 1987; Hirsch *et al.*, 1988)

Type	Subtype*
Non-small cell carcinoma (75%)	• Squamous cell (epidermoid) carcinoma (40%) WD, MD, PD and PD spindle-cell variant • Adenocarcinoma** (47%) WD, MD, PD and WD BAC • Large cell undifferentiated carcinoma (13%) giant cell and clear cell
Small cell carcinoma (20–25%)	• Pure small cell (90%) • Mixed small/large cell type (about 5%) • Combined small cell/squamous cell or small cell/adenocarcinoma (about 5%)
Others (5%)	• Adenosquamous carcinoma • Adenoldcystic carcinoma • Mucoepidermold carcinoma • Carcinoid tumor • Miscellaneous

*WD = well differentiated
MD = moderately differentiated
PD = poorly differentiated
BAC = bronchioloalveolar cell carcinoma
**World Health Organization subtypes: acinar papillary, bronchioloalveolar, solid with mucin production

Table 4.4 Prognostic factors in stage I non-small cell lung cancer (Strauss *et al.*, 1995)

Histopathologic markers

Variable	Favorable	Unfavorable
1. T. (tumor) status	T1	T2
2. Histologic subtype	Squamous	Large cell[1]
3. Degree of tumor differentiation (diff)	Well diff	Poorly diff[2]
4. Lymphatic and/or blood vessel invasion	Absent	Present
5. Mitotic index	Low	High
6. Plasma cell infiltration	Present	Absent or minimal
7. Tumor giant cells	Absent	Present
8. World Health Organization subtype of adenocarcinoma	Bronchoalveolar or acinar or papillary	Solid tumor with mucus formation

Molecular genetic markers

Variable	Favorable	Unfavorable
1. K-*ras* oncogene activation	No point mutation	Point mutation at codon 12
2. *Ras* gene protein product expression	Absent p21 staining	Strong p21 staining[3]
3. C-*erb*-2 protein expression	Normal	Increased
4. p53 Tumor supressor gene	No mutation	Gene mutation present
5. p53 Protein product expression	Normal p53	Overexpression of p53
6. Retinoblastoma (Rb) protein expression	Rb positive	Rb negative
7. *bcl*-2 Protein expression	*bcl*-2 Positive	*bcl*-2 Negative

Differentiation markers

Variable	Favorable	Unfavorable
1. Expression of blood group antigen on tumor cells	Conserved expression of blood group antigens	Altered expression of blood group antigens
2. Expression of H/Ley/Leb antigens	Negative staining with MIA-15-5	Positive staining with MIA-15-5

Proliferation markers

	Favorable	Unfavorable
1. DNA content (flow cytometry)	Diploid	Aneuploid
2. S-phase fraction (flow cytometry)	Low	High
3. Mitotic Index	<13 mitoses per 10 high powered fields	≥ 13 mitoses per 10 high powered fields
4. Proliferation index using KI-67 nuclear antigen	PI <3.5	PI >3.5
5. Thymidine labeling Index	TLI <2.9	TLI >2.9
6. Number of nucleolar organizing regions	Mean <3.80/cell	Mean >3.80/cell
7. Proliferating cell nuclear antigen (PCNA)	< 5% of tumor cells stained with PCNA	>5% of tumor cells stained with PCNA

Markers of Metastatic Propensity in Stage I NSCLC

Variable	Favorable	Unfavorable
1. Intensity of angiogenesis	Low microvessel count and density grade	High microvessel
2. Basement membrane deposition (squamous cell carcinoma)	Extensive deposition	Limited deposition[4]
3. Ability to establish in vitro cell lines	In vitro cell lines not established	Independent cell lines
4. Soluble Interleukin 2 receptor	Post-operative value less than preoperative	Post-operative value greater than preoperative

1 Adenocarcinoma is intermediate prognosis
2 Moderately diff is intermediate prognosis
3 Moderate staining is intermediate prognosis
4 Moderate deposition is intermediate prognosis

Table 4.5 Chromosomes, genes and lung cancer

Type	Subtype	Cytogenic abnormalities	Proto-oncogenes	Onco-suppressor genes
NSCLC	Not specified	1p13, 3p13 8p11-q11 8p11-q11 15p11-q11 17p11 chrs. 7, 13, 19	c-*myc* (10%) *bcl*-2	p53 (50%)
	Squamous cell carcinoma	Chr. 11 3p17q	*erb*B-1 c-*erb*B-2 c-*fos* c-*jun* (AP-1)	p53 (67%)
	Adenocarcinoma	3p21.3 (<50%) 3p14.1–12.1	k-*ras* (30%) c-*erb*B-2 (25%) c-*fos* c-*jun* (AP-1)	p53 (37%)
Small cell carcinoma		3p21.3–3p25 (90%) 3p14 5q21 (APC) 6q24 8q24 1p32 13q14 17q13	c-*raf*-1 c-*fms* c-*myb* c-*myc* L-*myc*	 p53 (80%) RB (90%)

*Frequency (%) of abnormalities among the types of lung cancer is indicated
(Data adapted from Anderson, 1993)

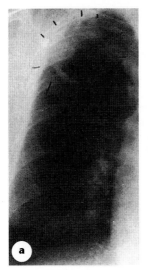
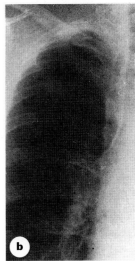
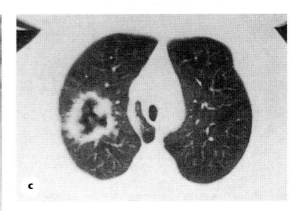

Fig. 4.1 Squamous cell carcinoma. A 58-year-old man who presented with increasing cough was found to have a large cavitating lesion in the right upper lung (**a**). (**b**) Chest film obtained four years earlier shows a small nodule that most likely represents the primary cancer. (**c**) CT scan shows a localized cavitating lesion. Squamous cell carcinoma often presents with cavitation due to tumor necrosis.

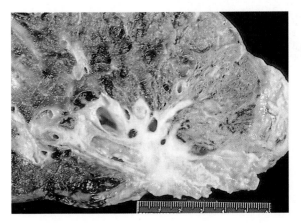

Fig. 4.2 Squamous cell carcinoma. A 66-year-old woman had a long-standing history of cigarette smoking and presented with metastatic disease. Bronchoscopy was positive for squamous cell carcinoma. Death resulted from widespread metastases. Mid-coronal section of the left lung shows local invasion of the large bronchi and hilum. Most squamous cell lung tumors are of central origin. (Courtesy of Pathology Department, Brigham and Women's Hospital, Boston, MA).

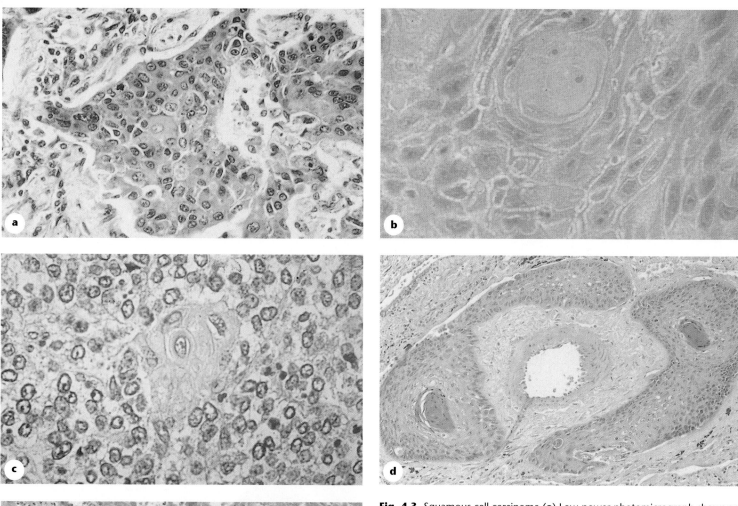

Fig. 4.3 Squamous cell carcinoma (**a**) Low-power photomicrograph shows an invasive squamous cell carcinoma. Note the distinction between the cells at the periphery and the keratinized cells in the center of the island of tumor. (**b**) This high-power view exhibits the classic appearance of a keratin pearl and intercellular bridges diagnostic for squamous cell carcinoma. (**c**) This poorly differentiated tumor shows a focal central keratinized area. Immunoperoxidase staining for keratin protein was positive (not shown). (**d**) Squamous cell carcinoma invading and extending through lymphatic vessels surrounding a small blood vessel. (**e**) Squamous cell carcinoma in blood vessels.

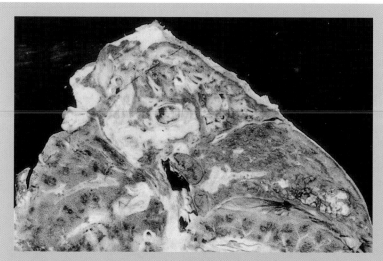

Fig. 4.4 Hematite pneumoconiosis with squamous cell carcinoma and tuberculosis. This postmortem lung specimen was taken from a 61-year-old man who had been an iron-ore miner for 20 years and had required numerous hospital admissions for deteriorating respiratory function.

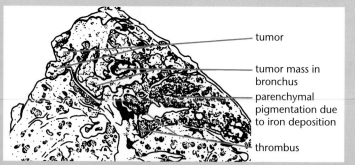

tumor

tumor mass in bronchus

parenchymal pigmentation due to iron deposition

thrombus

A section through the upper lobe shows a variety of features: Brick-red parenchymal pigmentation with focal fibrosis, a pale mass arising in the upper lobe bronchus that has infiltrated the upper lobe, small foci of caseous necrosis at the base of the upper lobe and an organized thrombus in the upper lobe branch of the pulmonary artery. Tuberculosis, as well as bronchial carcinoma, is a not uncommon complication of hematite lung. The carcinoma may frequently develop away from the bronchial wall in an area of scarring. It is thought that the increased radioactivity in hematite mines may be responsible for this neoplastic change.

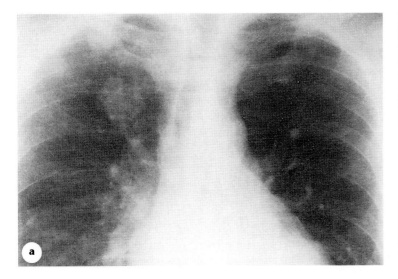

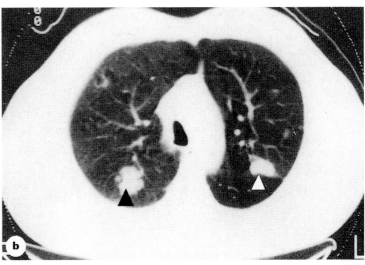

Fig. 4.5 Adenocarcinoma. (**a**) On routine medical examination, the chest film of a 64-year-old man shows bilateral primary lung tumors in the upper lobes; the lesion on the left side is partly obscured by the clavicle. (**b**) CT scan clearly defines the irregularly shaped primary lesions (arrows). Synchronous primary lung cancers occur in about 3–5% of patients and can be of different histologic subgroups.

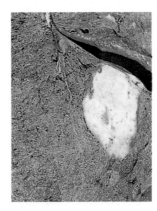

Fig. 4.6 Adenocarcinoma. Just beneath the pleura of the oblique interlobar fissure of this lung specimen is an irregular, well-demarcated, pale tumor situated well away from the main bronchial tree. Most peripheral primary pulmonary malignancies are adenocarcinomas, which constitute about 30–35% of all lung cancers. Some peripheral lesions may be associated with scarring, mainly considered to be induced by the tumor itself.

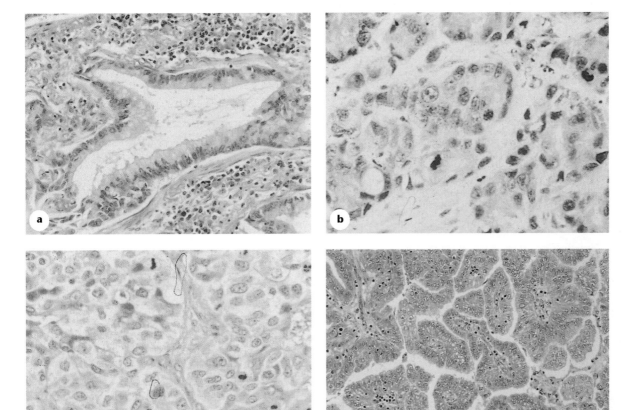

Fig. 4.7 Adenocarcinoma. (**a**) Microscopic section shows the typical appearance of a gland formation. (**b**) On high-power view, this poorly to moderately differentiated adenocarcinoma exhibits clusters of cells with eccentric nuclei and abundant cytoplasm. Note a cluster of tumor cells with a central lumen in the lower left of the field. (**c**) This poorly differentiated adenocarcinoma shows positive mucicarmine staining for intra- and extracytoplasmic mucin. (**d**) Papillary adenocarcinoma of lung. Low-power view of a moderately well-differentiated adenocarcinoma with papillary features. Metastases from ovary, thyroid, breast or kidney cancer should be considered in the differential diagnosis of papillary adenocarcinoma.

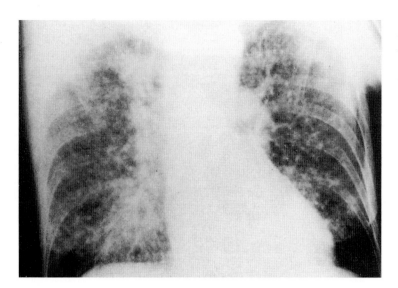

Fig. 4.8 Bronchioloalveolar carcinoma. A 60-year-old female presented with the classic features of advanced disease: increasing dyspnea on exertion with a frequent cough that produced large amounts of frothy sputum. Chest radiograph shows extensive metastases throughout the lung fields with hilar and mediastinal adenopathy.

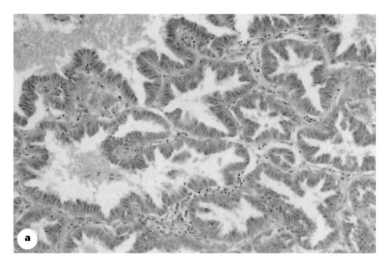

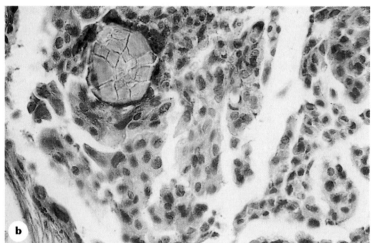

Fig. 4.9 Bronchioloalveolar carcinoma. (**a**) Lower-power photomicrograph shows tall columnar peg-shaped cells growing in a 'picket-fence' pattern on the alveolar walls. (**b**) On high-power view, a typical psammoma body, characterized by concentric laminations, is evident.

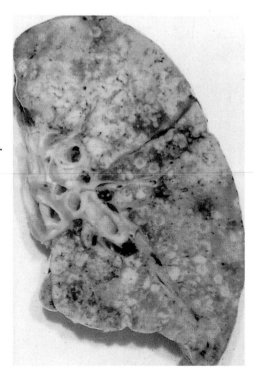

Fig. 4.10 Bronchioloalveolar carcinoma. This is a postmortem specimen from a 45-year-old man who presented with a 2-year history of cough and malaise. Chest radiography suggested tuberculosis. Despite empirical treatment, his condition deteriorated with increasing dyspnea and hemoptysis and he died. At autopsy, except for a single involved lymph node at the carina, there was no evidence of metastasis elsewhere. A coronal section through the right lung shows widespread, diffuse infiltration by pale tumor, which has a nodular appearance in places. Very little normal parenchyma remains.

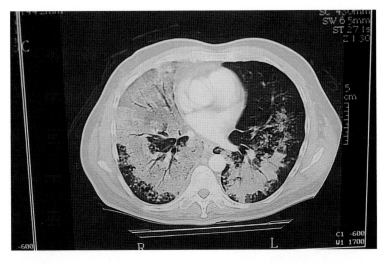

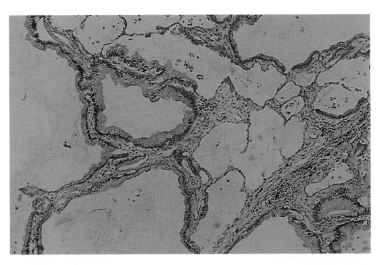

Fig. 4.11 Bronchioloalveolar carcinoma. CT scan shows bilateral lung lesions in this 48-year-old woman with cough and excessive sputum production. Note the classic air bronchograms (arrows).

Fig. 4.12 Bronchioloalveolar cell carcinoma. Microscopic view shows lepidic (scale-like) growth along alveolar septa.

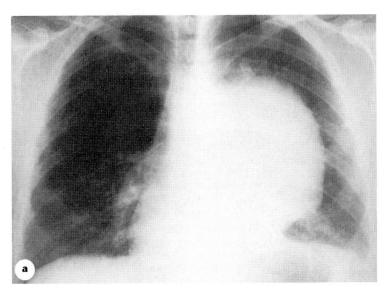

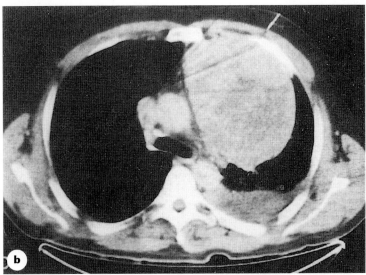

Fig. 4.13 Large cell carcinoma. A 45-year-old man with a history of chronic cigarette smoking developed increasing chest pain and cough. (**a**) Radiograph shows a huge primary mass. (**b**) CT scan shows the mass extending into the left anterior chest wall; a small pleural effusion is also apparent. Note the biopsy needle.

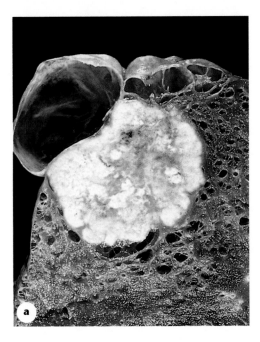

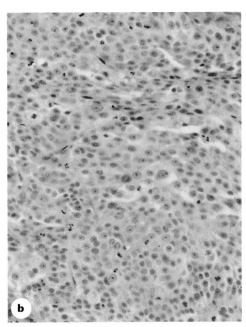

Fig. 4.14 Large cell carcinoma. (**a**) Surgical specimen from a 60-year-old man shows a primary malignancy arising in the periphery of the lung. In this case, the tumor, which is well circumscribed with focal central areas of necrosis, is associated with subpleural cyst formation. (**b**) Microscopic section reveals mainly undifferentiated large cells with ovoid to spindly shapes. Note the discrete cell borders and prominent nucleoli. In some patients with the giant cell variant of large cell undifferentiated carcinoma, a diagnosis of Ki-1 anaplastic large cell lymphoma must be considered. Appropriate immunoperoxidase stains will establish the correct diagnosis (*see* Fig. 14.56).

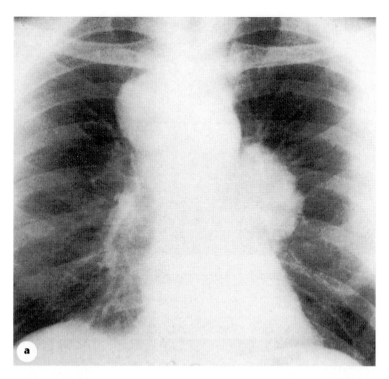

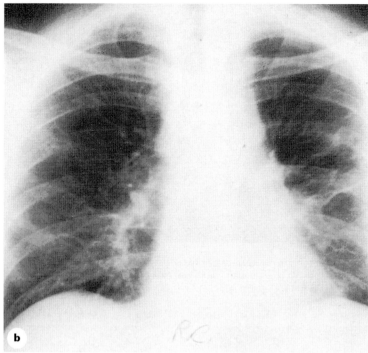

Fig. 4.15 Small cell carcinoma. (**a**) Chest radiograph of a 46-year-old man who presented with a cough and chest pain shows bilateral mediastinal nodal metastases. Bronchoscopy was positive for small cell lung cancer. Combination chemotherapy followed by mediastinal irradiation resulted in complete remission. (**b**) On followup examination 18 months later, a chest film shows continuing remission.

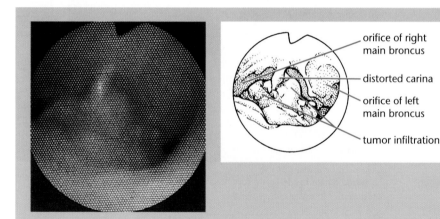

orifice of right main broncus

distorted carina

orifice of left main broncus

tumor infiltration

Fig. 4.16 Small cell carcinoma. A 66-year-old woman presented with a 5-month history of wheeze, sputum-producing cough and episodic right-sided chest pain. In addition she had lost 6 kg in weight in that period and had recently experienced upper abdominal pain; her liver was enlarged. She had smoked 30 cigarettes a day for over 40 years. Her chest radiograph showed signs of right lower lobe collapse. Laboratory findings revealed elevated liver enzymes, as well as severe airway obstruction. On fiberoptic bronchoscopy, the upper airway appeared normal but, as seen in this view, the carina is involved posteriorly by tumor. The tumor has broadened the carina and infiltrated it bilaterally, making it immobile. Tumor occluded the right upper lobe bronchus and partially obstructed the main bronchus, which could not be entered. The histology of the biopsy specimen showed a small cell (oat cell) carcinoma.

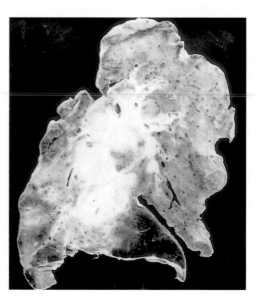

Fig. 4.17 Small cell carcinoma. This specimen was excised from a 40-year-old man who presented with a 6-week history of a dry cough and pleuritic chest pain. Radiographs showed collapse and consolidation of the left lower lobe and bronchoscopy showed rigid infiltration of the left lower lobe bronchus. Mediastinal lymph node involvement was noted during a left pneumonectomy. This coronal section through the left lung shows a large, irregularly infiltrative, pale neoplasm arising at the lung hilum. The lower lobe bronchus is virtually obliterated and the hilar lymph nodes are invaded in continuity with the main tumor mass. Extensive infarction of the remainder of the lower lobe suggests vascular occlusion or disruption by tumor. Microscopic examination of the tumor revealed a small cell anaplastic (oat cell) carcinoma.

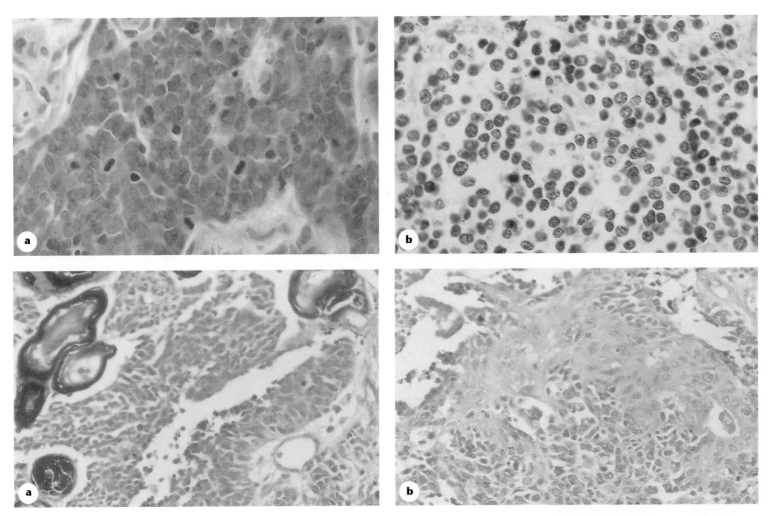

Fig. 4.18 Small cell carcinoma. (**a**) Photomicrograph shows the classic appearance of 'oat-like' cells. Each cell is approximately twice the size of a lymphocyte and has scant cytoplasm, finely dispersed chromatin and an inconspicuous nucleolus. Note characteristic 'molding' of cells and a high mitotic rate. (**b**) In another case, the cells have a 'lymphocyte-like' appearance. Such tumors are included in the category of small cell lung cancer. Other malignancies that have a 'small cell' appearance include lymphomas, Merkel cell tumor, carcinoid tumors, rhabdomyosarcoma, Ewing's sarcoma and neuroblastoma. (**c**) Small cell carcinoma. This low-power view shows the Azzopardi effect, due to crushed DNA material encrusted around blood vessels, which is characteristic although not pathognomic of small cell carcinoma. (**d**) Small cell carcinoma, mixed sub-type. This tumor shows small cell and squamous cell components.

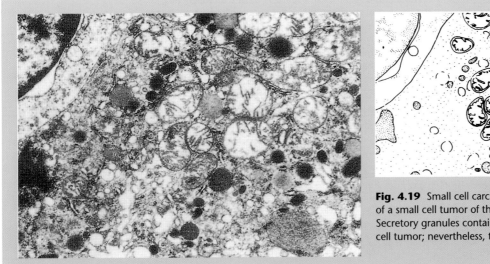

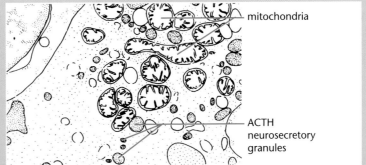

Fig. 4.19 Small cell carcinoma. Electron micrograph shows the ultrastructure of a small cell tumor of the lung associated with Cushing's syndrome. Secretory granules containing ACTH are less frequent than they are in the islet cell tumor; nevertheless, they are also characteristic of neuroendocrine cells.

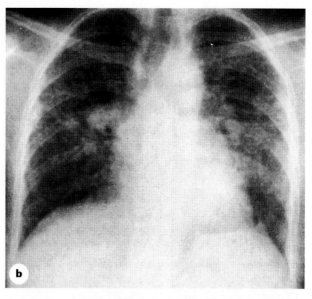

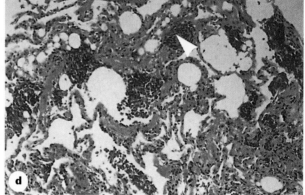

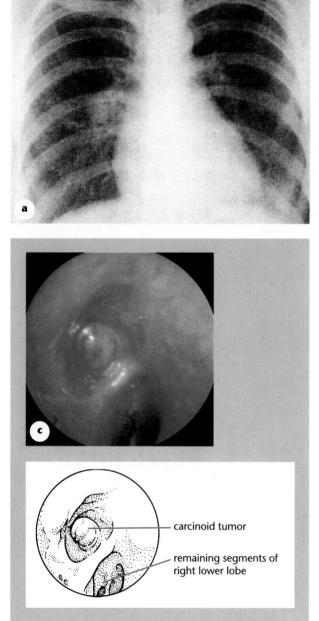

carcinoid tumor

remaining segments of
right lower lobe

Fig. 4.20 Carcinoid tumor. (**a**) Routine chest radiograph of an 18-year-old woman reveals a prominence in the right hilar region. Three years later she was treated for tuberculosis, although test results were negative. Four years afterward she developed increased breathlessness and backache and on examination was found to have abnormal facial hair, dyspnea at rest and signs of mitral incompetence. Echocardiography showed a thickened interventricular septum, reduced left ventricular cavity size and systolic posterior cusp prolapse. Pulmonary function tests indicated a marked restrictive defect. (**b**) Chest radiograph at this time shows a prominent right hilum and diffuse bilateral pulmonary metastases. (**c**) Fiberoptic bronchoscopy, using a rigid bronchoscope for clarity, reveals a lesion in the apical segment of the right lower lobe bronchus exhibiting the typical appearance of a carcinoid tumor (bronchial 'adenoma'). Bronchial and transbronchial biopsies were performed, revealing a carcinoid tumor infiltrating the lung. (Courtesy of Dr P Stradling.) (**d**) Transbronchial specimen shows lymphatic infiltration by tumor (arrow). The diagnosis was supported by finding a whole blood 5-hydroxytryptamine level of 705 ng/ml (normal range: 100–250 ng/ml) and an elevated 24-hour urinary 5-hydroxyindoleacetic acid level of 56 mg (normal range: <20 mg).

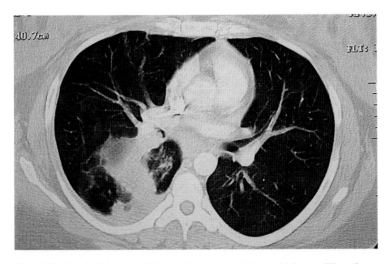

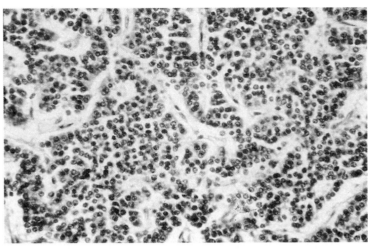

Fig. 4.21 Carcinoid tumor. CT scan shows an endobronchial mass filling the bronchus intermedius (arrow) of this 24-year-old woman with a history of recurrent asthma and episodes of pneumonia. Note large area of consolidation due to the obstructing lesion.

Fig. 4.22 Carcinoid tumor. High-power photomicrograph shows a uniform population of small, bland 'blue' cells with delicate nuclear chromatin and small amounts of cytoplasm. Note the organized arrangement of the tumor cells.

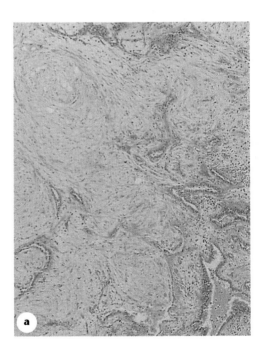

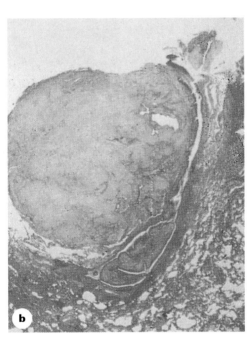

Fig. 4.23 Bronchial hamartoma. A 70-year-old man with a history of cigarette smoking and a cough presented with a nodule in the left lower lung. A video-assisted thoracoscopic resection revealed a bronchial hamartoma. (**a**) Low power at right reveals nodular growth. (**b**) High power at left displays benign cartilaginous growth with embedded epithelial elements. The term hamartoma means 'tumor-like malformation,' indicating a benign proliferation composed of tissue normally found in a location but present in excess or disarray. Recently, cytogenetic abnormalities have been observed in bronchial hamartomas involving chromosomes 18 and 6p21, suggesting a clonal origin (Fletcher *et al.*, 1992).

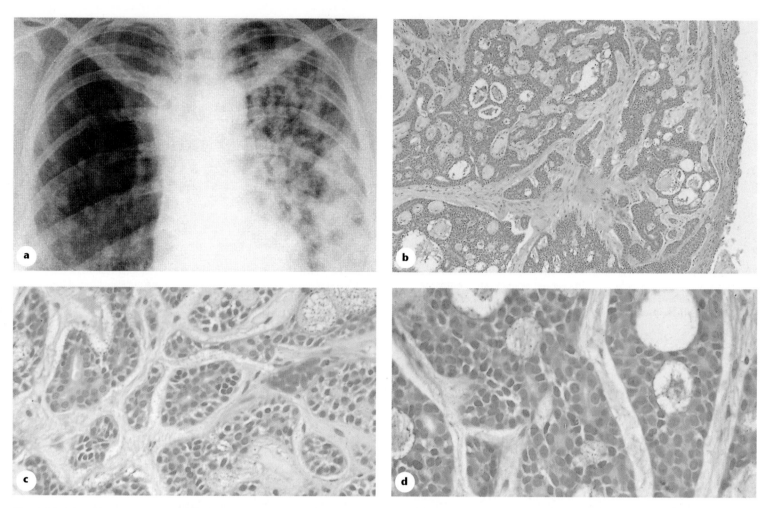

Fig. 4.24 Adenoid cystic carcinoma. (**a**) Chest film of a 40-year-old woman, who had resection of a primary adenoid cystic carcinoma of the right upper lobe 4 years earlier and developed multiple bilateral metastases with slowly progressive increase in size of the lesions. The upper mediastinum is slightly widened, suggesting adenopathy. Her symptoms were only mild dyspnea on exertion. (**b**) Adenoid cystic carcinoma may arise in bronchial mucous glands of the lung. The tumor cells form branching ductal structures with round, 'punched-out' spaces, giving the tumor a lace-like pattern. (**c**) In this case the stroma separating cell clusters contains dense homogeneous eosinophilic basement membrane-like material, (**d**) but may also contain bubbly, bluish, mucoid material. The round spaces are filled by either material and surrounded by tumor cells with round to ovoid nuclei, coarse chromatin and scant cytoplasm. Adenoid cystic carcinoma (also called cylindroma) occurs mainly in the upper aerodigestive tract (*see* Figs 3.22 and 3.23). Involvement of the lung is unusual. The tumor shows histologic features that resemble salivary glands but are more aggressive than salivary gland cylindromas. Metastases to regional nodes and distant sites are common and perineural involvement is characteristic. Occurrence in the respiratory tract may result in obstructive symptoms including recurrent wheezing, often leading to a misdiagnosis of asthma (which also occurs in the bronchial carcinoid tumors).

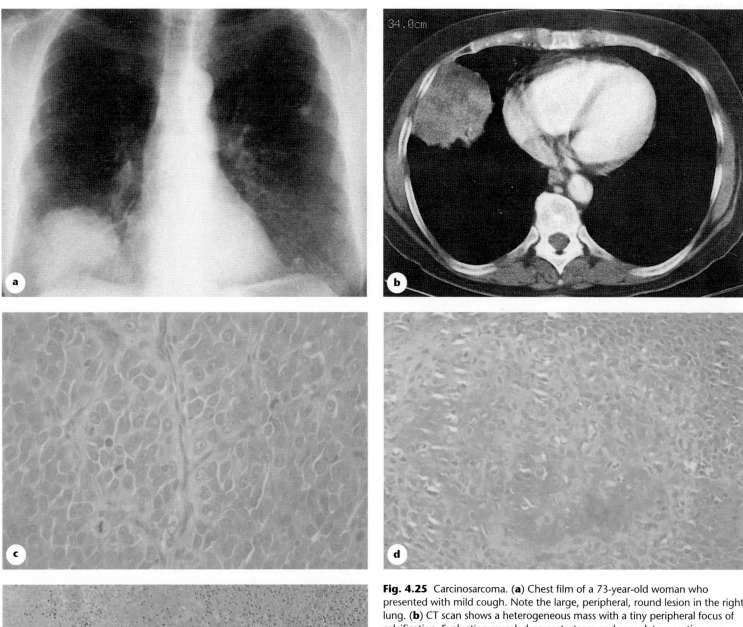

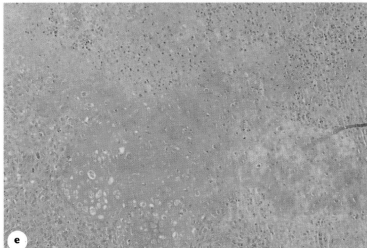

Fig. 4.25 Carcinosarcoma. (**a**) Chest film of a 73-year-old woman who presented with mild cough. Note the large, peripheral, round lesion in the right lung. (**b**) CT scan shows a heterogeneous mass with a tiny peripheral focus of calcification. Evaluation revealed no metastases and complete resection was carried out. (**c**) High-power view of the tumor mass reveals large epithelial cells with abundant cytoplasm, large vesicular nuclei and occasionally prominent nucleoli. (**d**) High-power view of a different area reveals a malignant mesenchymal component (chondrosarcoma). (**e**) High-power view of malignant mesenchymal component stained with mucicarmine highlights in red the cartilaginous ground substance (rich in mucopolysaccharides). Carcinosarcoma is an uncommon lung malignancy, generally with a poor prognosis unless completely resected. The mesenchymal component may be fibrosarcoma, osteosarcoma and, less frequently, chondrosarcoma or rhabdosarcoma. Metastases may consist of either carcinomatous and/or sarcomatoid elements. Historically, carcinosarcomas were thought to arise from primitive cells which can differentiate into carcinomatous and sarcomatous elements. However, current ultrastructural, cell culture and immunohistochemical data support a monoclonal origin and suggest that 'sarcomatoid carcinoma' is a more accurate designation for this neoplasm (Wick and Swanson, 1993).

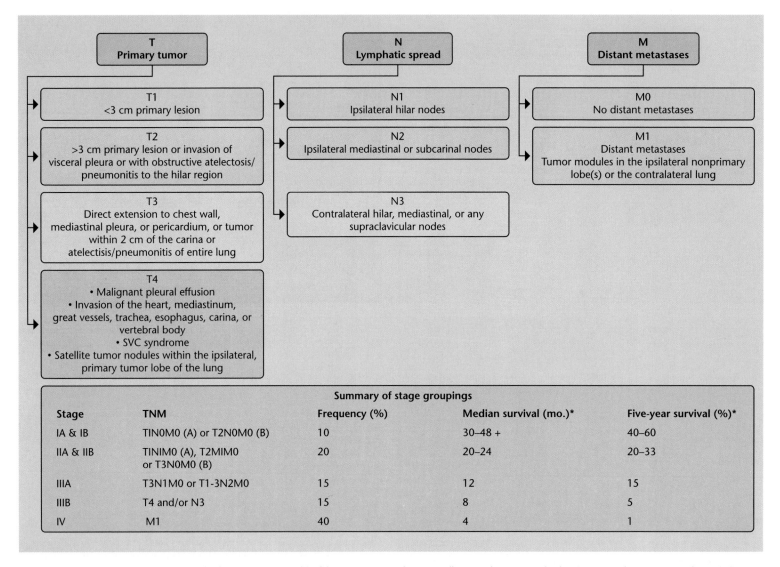

Fig. 4.26 International Staging System for lung cancer (simplified from Mountain, 1986, 1993). The frequency of each clinical stage varies, depending upon patient referral patterns. Survival is based upon clinical staging. Survival for surgically staged patients is higher in resected cases. Not indicated above: TX – malignant cells in bronchopulmonary secretions but primary cancer not otherwise visualized; T0 – no evidence of primary tumor; Tis – carcinoma *in situ*.

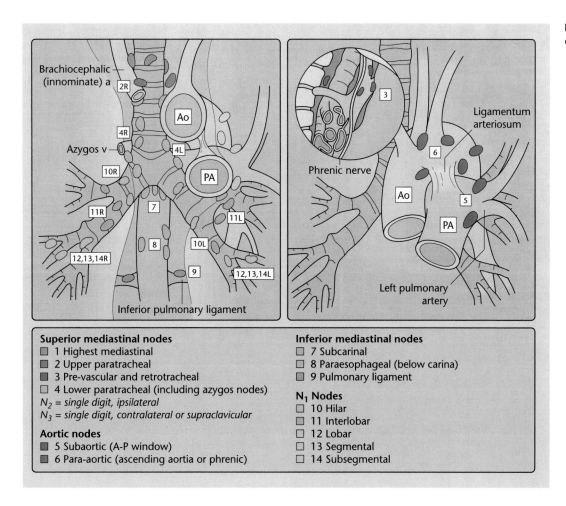

Fig. 4.27 Regional nodal stations for lung cancer staging (from Mountain, 1997).

Superior mediastinal nodes
- ☐ 1 Highest mediastinal
- ☐ 2 Upper paratracheal
- ☐ 3 Pre-vascular and retrotracheal
- ☐ 4 Lower paratracheal (including azygos nodes)
- N₂ = single digit, ipsilateral
- N₃ = single digit, contralateral or supraclavicular

Aortic nodes
- ☐ 5 Subaortic (A-P window)
- ☐ 6 Para-aortic (ascending aortia or phrenic)

Inferior mediastinal nodes
- ☐ 7 Subcarinal
- ☐ 8 Paraesophageal (below carina)
- ☐ 9 Pulmonary ligament

N₁ Nodes
- ☐ 10 Hilar
- ☐ 11 Interlobar
- ☐ 12 Lobar
- ☐ 13 Segmental
- ☐ 14 Subsegmental

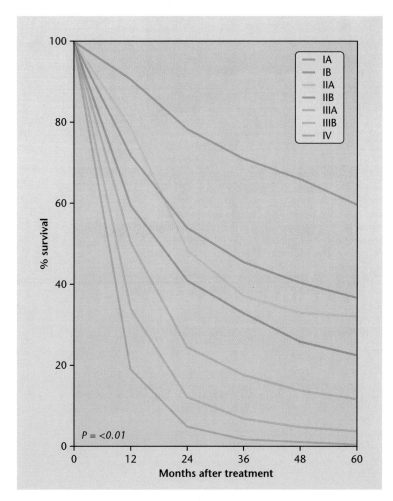

Fig. 4.28 Cumulative proportion of patients expected to survive following treatment according to clinical estimates of the stage of disease (from Mountain et al., 1997).

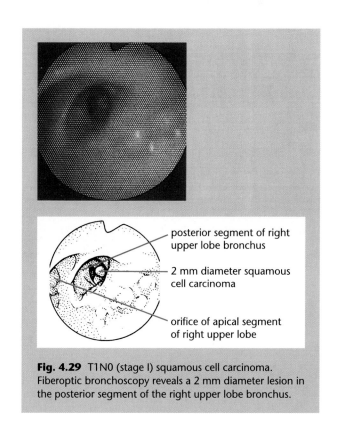

Fig. 4.29 T1N0 (stage I) squamous cell carcinoma. Fiberoptic bronchoscopy reveals a 2 mm diameter lesion in the posterior segment of the right upper lobe bronchus.

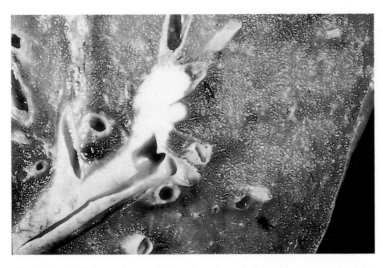

Fig. 4.30 T1N0 (stage I) squamous cell carcinoma. Surgical specimen from a 60-year-old woman who presented with hemoptysis shows the bronchial origin of the tumor. No regional or distant metastases were present.

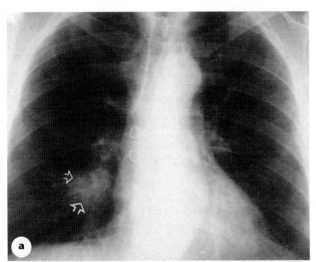

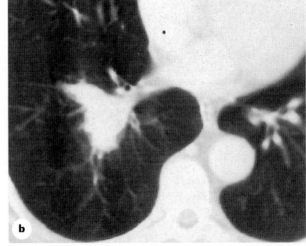

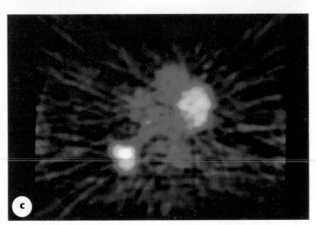

Fig. 4.31 T1N0 (stage I) adenocarcinoma. (**a**) PA chest film in a 60-year-old man with hemoptysis demonstrates a poorly defined, spiculated 2.5 cm mass in the right lower lobe (RLL) (arrows). The patient had a prior sternotomy and CABG. (**b**) CT confirms the radiographically indeterminate RLL mass. (**c**) Axial PET image at the level of the mass demonstrates significantly increased uptake within the tumor which was proven to be an adenocarcinoma by bronchoscopy. Note the normal increased activity in the left ventricle myocardium. Staging studies showed no metastases and a successful lobectomy was carried out. (Courtesy of Dr EF Patz Jr.)

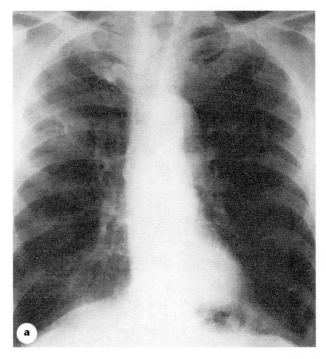

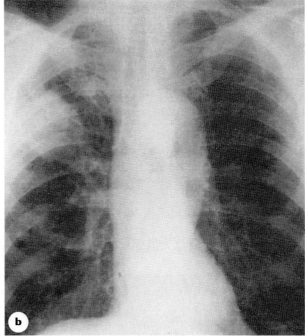

Fig. 4.32 T2N0 (stage IB) squamous cell carcinoma. A 77-year-old man had a history of heavy alcohol intake and presented with right-sided pleuritic pains. (**a**) Chest radiograph shows right upper lobe shadowing, which in view of the patient's heavy smoking was provisionally diagnosed as peripheral bronchial carcinoma. As there was no obvious evidence of metastatic disease, a transbronchial biopsy was attempted under radiographic screening. At fiberoptic bronchoscopy, a hard, irregular mass was found in the orifice of the right intermediate bronchus; it was not possible to inspect the distal lobar bronchi. Superficially, the mass resembled a tumor but as attempts were made to take a biopsy, it became clear that it was a foreign body embedded in granulation tissue. The mass was removed using a rigid bronchoscope with general anesthesia. The foreign body was subsequently identified as a vertebra from a rabbit. The patient had no explanation for its presence in his bronchial tree, but he had presumably inhaled it during one of his drinking bouts. The diagnosis was therefore revised to a pneumonic process in the right upper lobe resulting from proximal obstruction by a foreign body. Paradoxically, the initial diagnosis proved to be correct. (**b**) Chest film obtained 1 year later shows enlargement of the peripheral shadow despite removal of the foreign body. Subsequent investigations indicated the presence of a 4 cm squamous cell carcinoma.

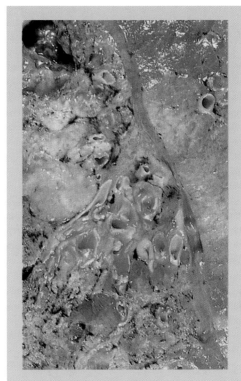

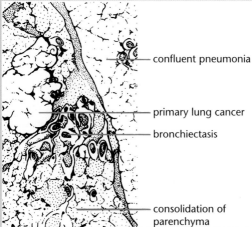

confluent pneumonia

primary lung cancer

bronchiectasis

consolidation of parenchyma

Fig. 4.33 T2N0 (stage I) lung cancer. At the apex of the left lower lobe of this pneumonectomy specimen is a partly necrotic, pale 3.5 cm neoplasm that has obliterated the lower lobe bronchus. Distally, the smaller bronchi are grossly dilated (bronchiectasis) and the remaining parenchyma shows consolidation; the adjacent middle lobe shows confluent bronchopneumonia. These common complications of obstructive bronchial carcinoma may also be accompanied by collapse or abscess formation.

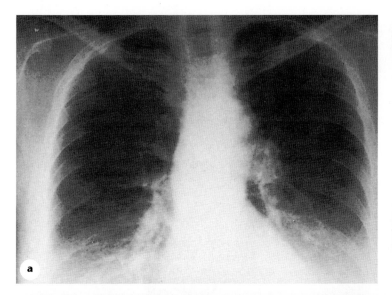

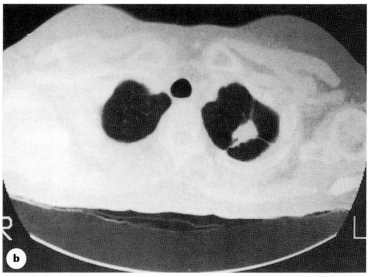

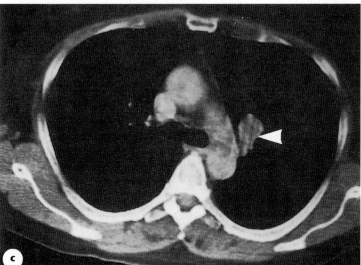

Fig. 4.34 T1N1 (stage II) poorly differentiated adenocarcinoma. This 56-year-old woman presented with recent onset of cough. (**a**) Chest radiograph shows left hilar adenopathy and a small lesion in the left upper lobe. CT scans confirm (**b**) a 1.5–2.0 cm primary lesion in the left upper lobe and (**c**) an enlarged left hilar node (arrow). No mediastinal adenopathy was present and the tumor was successfully resected.

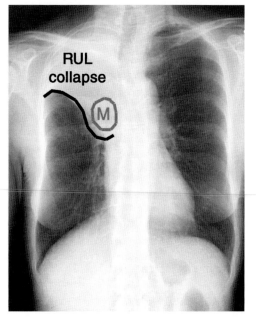

RUL
collapse

(M)

Fig. 4.35 T1N1 (stage IIA) adenocarcinoma. This PA chest radiograph shows classic features of right upper lobe collapse due to a central obstructing hilar mass (M). The combination of lobar volume loss sharply outlined by the elevated minor fissure and the rounded density of the hilar mass results in the reverse S-sign of Golden, as seen in this case.

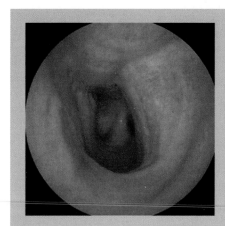

Fig. 4.36 T3 (stage IIIA) lung cancer. Bronchoscopy demonstrates extrinsic compression of the left lower trachea and distortion of the carina and right bronchus by tumor. The cancer was within 2 cm of the carina but without invasion of the carina or trachea. This image was made via a rigid bronchoscope for clarity; it is oriented for a bronchoscopist standing in front of the subject. (Courtesy of Dr P Stradling.)

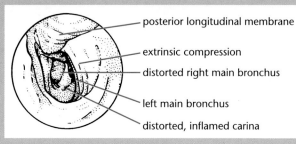

posterior longitudinal membrane

extrinsic compression

distorted right main bronchus

left main bronchus

distorted, inflamed carina

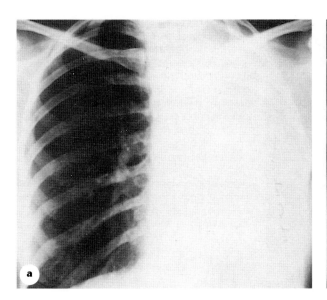

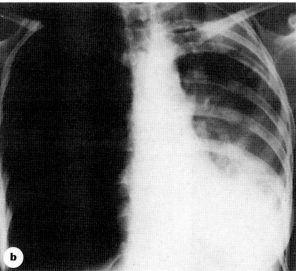

Fig. 4.37 T3 (stage IIB) lung cancer. A 27-year-old woman presented with increasing cough and sudden shortness of breath. (**a**) Chest radiograph shows complete collapse of the left lung. At bronchoscopy, a tumor was identified at the orifice of the left main bronchus. (**b**) Chest film following treatment shows re-expansion of the upper lobe. Involvement of the proximal bronchus within 2 cm of the carina, but not involvement of the carina itself, constitutes T3 (stage IIB) disease that is marginally resectable.

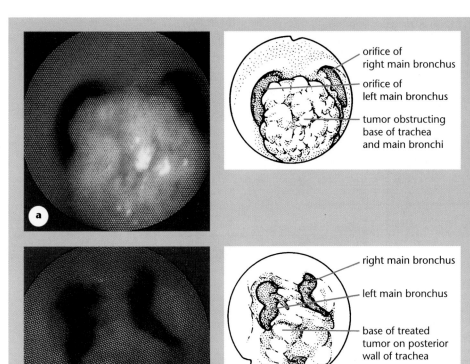

Fig. 4.38 T4 (stage IIIB) tracheal carcinoma. A 66-year-old man presented with a 6-week history of rapidly increasing breathlessness which had originally been attributed to asthma. As his stridor became more obvious, bronchoscopy was performed and tumor was found at the main carina, causing severe obstruction of the orifices of both main bronchi (**a**). The tumor was cut back by laser photoresection to its base on the carina and posterior tracheal wall, resulting in substantial improvement in the airway (**b**). Both main bronchi are now clearly seen. Pulmonary function tests showed great improvement. Subsequent investigations showed that the tumor was confined to the base of the trachea and main carina. Eventually, the patient underwent surgery for resection of the carina and lower trachea with anastomosis to the main bronchi. Unfortunately, overall prognosis for squamous cell carcinoma of the trachea is poor due to recurrent regional disease as well as distant metastases. Adenoid cystic carcinomas are less common and less aggressive with improved survival after surgery and/or irradiation (Allen, 1993).

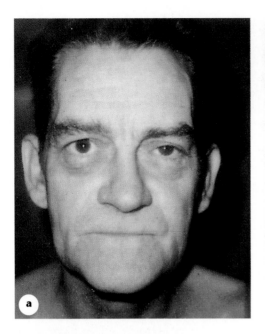

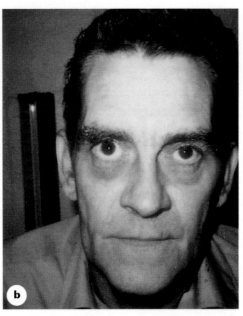

Fig. 4.39 T3 (stage IIIA) Pancoast tumor. (**a**) This 58-year-old man presented with chronic left arm and shoulder pain along with progressive weakness of his lower arm and hand. Physical examination showed clinical findings of a superior sulcus (Pancoast) tumor: ptosis of the left eyelid, miosis of the pupil and decreased sweating of the left face, arm and upper chest (Horner's syndrome) and a tumor mass in the lung apex that involved the brachial plexus and adjacent rib. (**b**) After radiotherapy, the manifestations of Horner's syndrome have resolved. There was also improvement in his pain and neurologic symptoms. Survival is poor with Pancoast tumors (under 30% at 5 years) due to progressive regional disease, but also distant metastases.

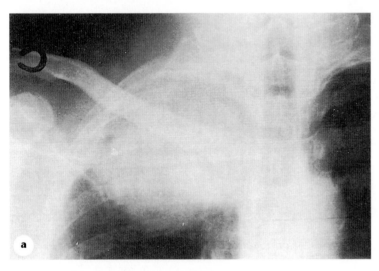

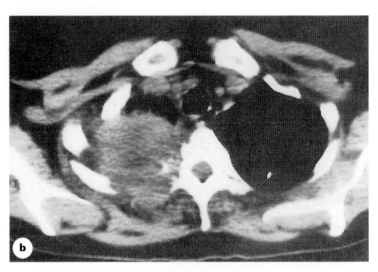

Fig. 4.40 T4 (stage IIIB) Pancoast tumor. A 52-year-old woman presented with long-standing right shoulder and back pain. (**a**) Her chest film shows a large tumor of the right upper lobe that has destroyed the adjacent rib. (**b**) CT scan reveals rib and soft tissue involvement as well as destruction of an adjacent vertebral body. Biopsy showed a squamous cell carcinoma. While in the past

Pancoast (superior sulcus) tumors were mostly squamous cell carcinomas, many centers are now reporting more adenocarcinomas than squamous cell type, similar to other lung cancers (*see* Table 4.3). Large cell carcinoma is third in frequency while small cell carcinoma rarely presents as a Pancoast tumor.

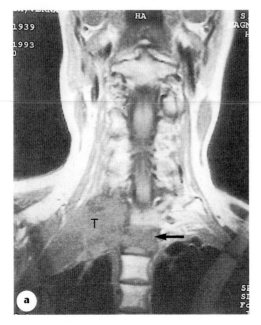

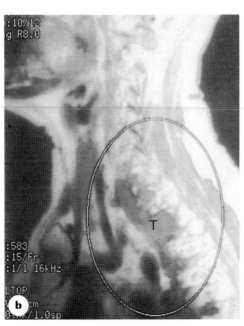

Fig. 4.41 T4 (stage IIIB) Pancoast tumor. (**a**) A 60-year-old man developed increasing right shoulder, back and arm pain. Chest radiograph (not shown) revealed a mass in the right lung apex. Fine-needle aspiration was positive for poorly differentiated adenocarcinoma. T_1-weighted MR image in the coronal plane through the region of the thoracic inlet shows a Pancoast tumor on the right (T). The tumor directly invades one of the upper thoracic vertebral bodies (arrow). (**b**) A 48-year-old woman presented with severe pain in the shoulder and arm with marked arm weakness. T_1-weighted MR image in the sagittal plane to the right of midline shows tumor (T) growing into the region of several adjacent neural foramina.

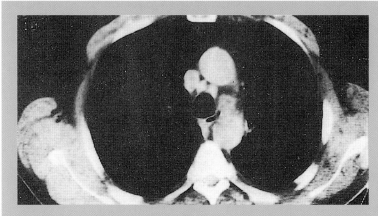

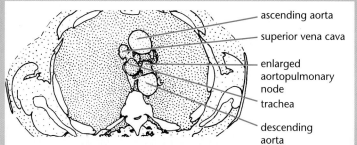

ascending aorta
superior vena cava
enlarged aortopulmonary node
trachea
descending aorta

laryngoscopy showed paralysis of the left vocal cord. This CT scan reveals an enlarged lymph node in the aortopulmonary window which was not seen on chest radiography. Anterior mediastinotomy (Chamberlain procedure) confirmed a metastatic tumor in the mediastinal node that compressed the recurrent laryngeal nerve, resulting in hoarseness.

Fig. 4.42 N2 (stage IIIA) adenocarcinoma. A 47-year-old man with a primary tumor of the left upper lobe presented with hoarseness. Indirect

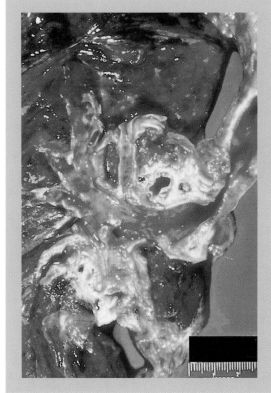

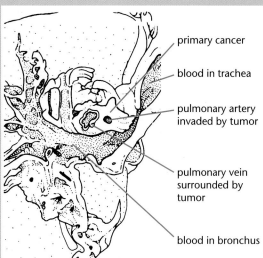

primary cancer

blood in trachea

pulmonary artery invaded by tumor

pulmonary vein surrounded by tumor

blood in bronchus

Fig. 4.43 T4 (stage IIIB) squamous cell carcinoma (pulmonary artery invasion). This autopsy specimen was taken from a 64-year-old man who died 1 day after a diagnosis was established by bronchoscopy. Exsanguination occurred when the malignancy eroded into the pulmonary artery. It is interesting to note that this patient was cured of a diffuse large cell lymphoma after combination chemotherapy 4 years earlier. He was a heavy cigarette smoker.

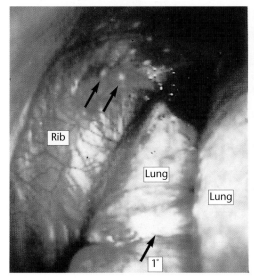

Rib

Lung

Lung

1°

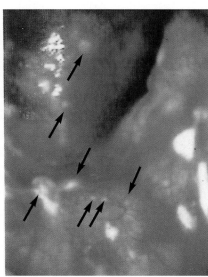

Fig. 4.44 T4 (stage IIIB) adenocarcinoma. A 44-year-old woman presented with increasing cough and chest radiograph (not shown) revealed a 2 cm infiltrative lesion in the left lower lobe (left panel, 1° tumor). CT scan showed no mediastinal adenopathy but some small pleural densities were present (not shown). VATS (video-assisted thoracoscopic surgery) was carried out and revealed multiple small visceral and parietal pleural nodules (arrows; right panel). Biopsies were positive for metastatic adenocarcinoma unresectable stage IIIB disease. The patient was spared a formal thoracotomy by the staging VATS procedure.

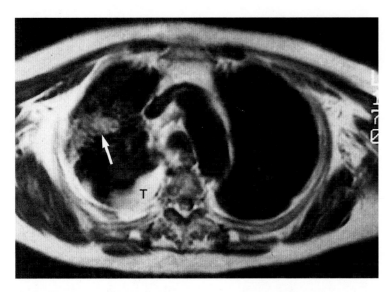

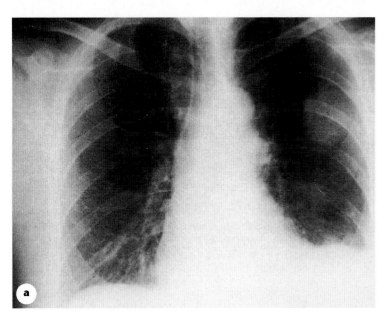

Fig. 4.45 T4 (stage IIIB) adenocarcinoma. A 76-year-old man with COPD and previous asbestos exposure presented with increasing pulmonary complaints. Chest radiographs showed chronic scarring and infiltrates in the right lung along with multiple pleural lesions (not shown). In this patient, a T$_1$-weighted MR image in the axial plane at the level of the aortic arch shows tumor in the pleural space posteriorly (T) with extension into the major fissure on the right (arrow). Fine-needle aspiration biopsy with special immunoperoxidase stains (see Figs 4.47, 4.67) was diagnostic for poorly differentiated adenocarcinoma of the lung. The lesion originated in the peripheral lung and extended throughout the pleura.

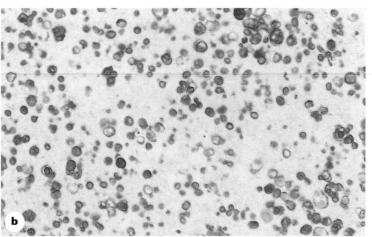

Fig. 4.46 T4 (stage IIIB) adenocarcinoma. A 61-year-old woman developed increasing left chest wall pain with dyspnea on exertion. (a) Chest radiograph shows a pleural-based tumor mass with a pleural effusion. (b) CT scan confirms these findings and reveals a second small pleural metastasis. CT-guided needle biopsy showed a non-small cell lung cancer; thoracocentesis was positive for a poorly differentiated adenocarcinoma. Mammograms and other staging studies were normal.

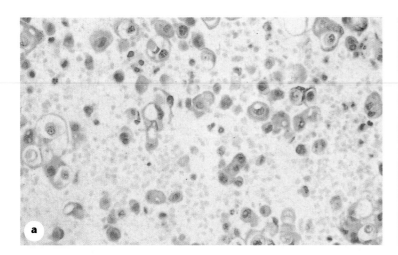

Fig. 4.47 T4 (stage IIIB) adenocarcinoma. Histopathologic studies of the same patient as shown in Figure 4.46 reveal (a) positive mucicarmine stain (red) for intracytoplasmic mucin and (b) positive immunoreactive immunoperoxidase stain (brown) for callus cytokeratin. The peripheral pattern of staining is characteristic of adenocarcinoma, as opposed to mesothelioma, which has perinuclear and cytoplasmic staining. Immunoperoxidase stains were also positive for epithelial membrane antigen and CEA, confirming the epithelial origin of the tumor (see also Fig. 1.3).

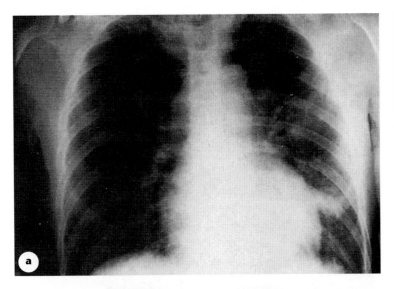

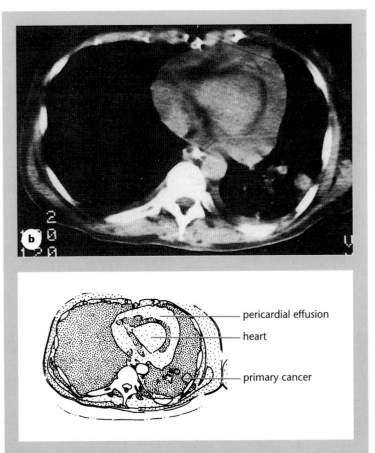

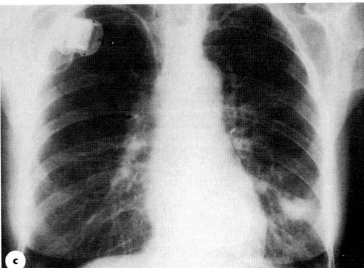

Fig. 4.48 T4 (stage IIIB) adenocarcinoma. A 62-year-old woman presented with severe dyspnea at rest. (**a**) Chest film shows a tumor mass in the left lower lobe associated with cardiomegaly due to pericardial effusion with acute tamponade, findings that are confirmed on CT scan (**b**). Histopathologic specimens obtained by pericardiocentesis showed poorly differentiated adenocarcinoma cells. Radiotherapy was administered. (**c**) Followup chest film reveals improvement in heart size but persistence of the primary tumor mass.

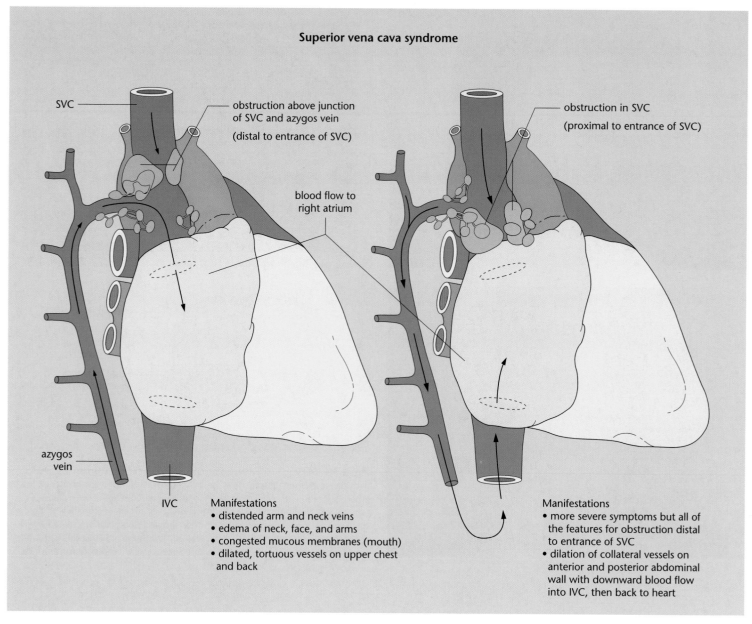

Superior vena cava syndrome

SVC

obstruction above junction of SVC and azygos vein
(distal to entrance of SVC)

obstruction in SVC
(proximal to entrance of SVC)

blood flow to right atrium

azygos vein

IVC

Manifestations
• distended arm and neck veins
• edema of neck, face, and arms
• congested mucous membranes (mouth)
• dilated, tortuous vessels on upper chest and back

Manifestations
• more severe symptoms but all of the features for obstruction distal to entrance of SVC
• dilation of collateral vessels on anterior and posterior abdominal wall with downward blood flow into IVC, then back to heart

Fig. 4.49 T4 (stage IIIB) lung cancer (SVC syndrome). Compression of the superior vena cava by a tumor mass or mediastinal lymph node metastases leads to increased venous pressure and a variety of manifestations depending on the level of obstruction. SVC syndrome can occur as an isolated finding in stage IIIB lung cancer or as a part of metastatic disease (stage IV). The syndrome occurs in 3–5% of patients with lung cancer. It is seen most commonly in those with small cell lung cancer (15–45%), followed by squamous cell cancer (20–25%), adenocarcinoma (5–25%) and large cell carcinoma (4–30%).

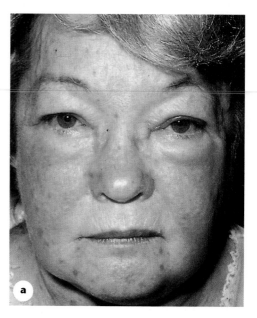
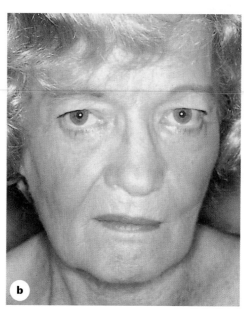

Fig. 4.50 T4 (stage IIIB) squamous cell carcinoma (SVC syndrome). (**a**) A 56-year-old woman with diagnosed lung cancer presented with marked facial edema characteristic of SVC syndrome. (**b**) After radiotherapy, the swelling regressed dramatically.

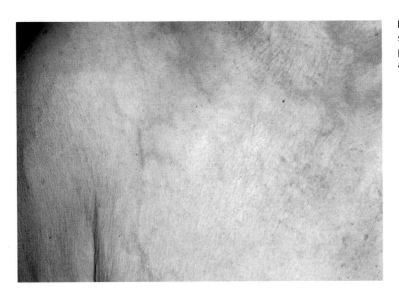

Fig. 4.51 T4 (stage IIIB) large cell carcinoma (SVC syndrome). Dilatation of superficial collateral veins, as noted on the chest wall of this 70-year-old patient, is a common clinical finding in SVC syndrome. Collateral veins may also develop in the lower chest wall and upper abdomen.

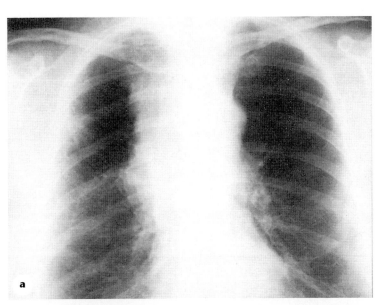

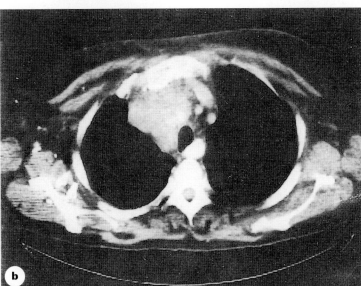

Fig. 4.52 T4 (stage IIIB) squamous cell carcinoma (SVC syndrome). A 45-year-old woman developed increasing facial edema, distended neck veins, enlarged breasts and shortness of breath. (**a**) Chest radiograph reveals a large mass in the right upper lung and mediastinum. (**b**) CT scan shows encasement of the superior vena cava by the primary tumor mass. For MRI findings in SVC syndrome *see* Figure 14.84.

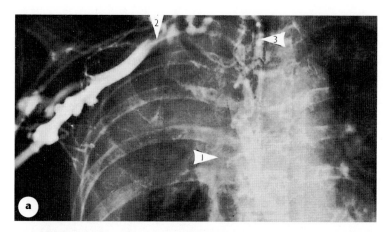

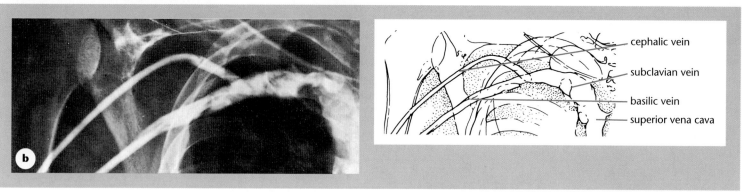

Fig. 4.53 T4 (stage IIIB) bronchogenic carcinoma (SVC syndrome). (**a**) Upper extremity venogram performed on a patient with SVC syndrome due to large bronchogenic tumor (arrow 1) in the right lung shows complete obstruction of the subclavian vein (arrow 2) and filling of venous collaterals (arrow 3) bypassing the obstructed superior vena cava. (**b**) By contrast, this normal right subclavian venogram demonstrates filling of the basilic and cephalic veins, which then fill the subclavian vein and finally the normal superior vena cava. The lucent defects within the contrast-filled subclavian vein represent inflow of unopacified blood from venous tributaries.

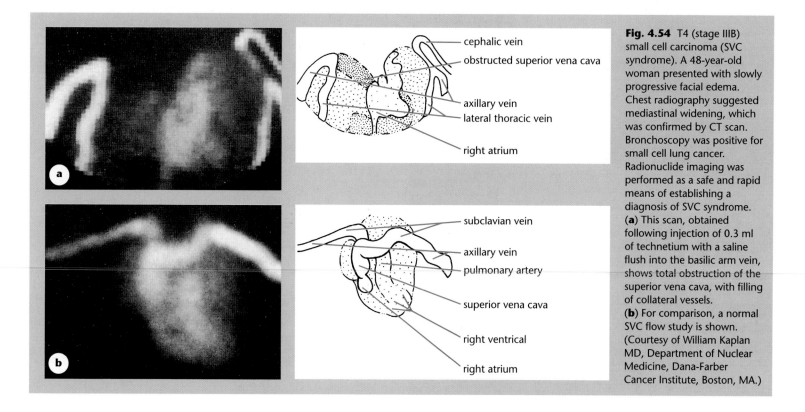

Fig. 4.54 T4 (stage IIIB) small cell carcinoma (SVC syndrome). A 48-year-old woman presented with slowly progressive facial edema. Chest radiography suggested mediastinal widening, which was confirmed by CT scan. Bronchoscopy was positive for small cell lung cancer. Radionuclide imaging was performed as a safe and rapid means of establishing a diagnosis of SVC syndrome. (**a**) This scan, obtained following injection of 0.3 ml of technetium with a saline flush into the basilic arm vein, shows total obstruction of the superior vena cava, with filling of collateral vessels. (**b**) For comparison, a normal SVC flow study is shown. (Courtesy of William Kaplan MD, Department of Nuclear Medicine, Dana-Farber Cancer Institute, Boston, MA.)

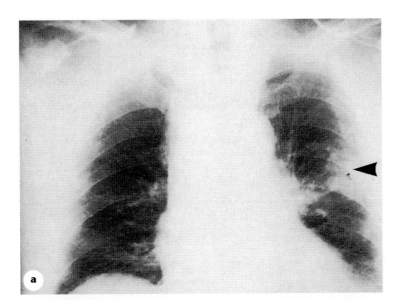

Fig. 4.55 N3 (stage IIIB) poorly differentiated adenocarcinoma. A 67-year-old man complained of increasing cough, chest discomfort and weight loss. (**a**) Chest radiograph shows a lesion (arrow) in the left upper lobe. (**b**) CT scan confirms a 2–3 cm primary lung tumor (T2) based in the pleura and reveals in addition bilateral mediastinal lymph node metastases. Bronchoscopy was negative, but needle biopsy of the primary lesion yielded the histologic diagnosis.

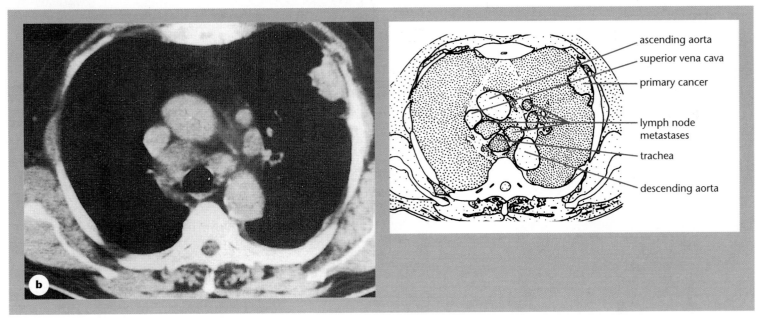

ascending aorta

superior vena cava

primary cancer

lymph node metastases

trachea

descending aorta

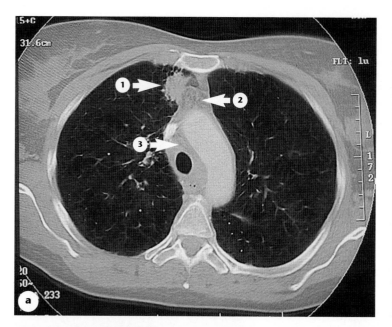

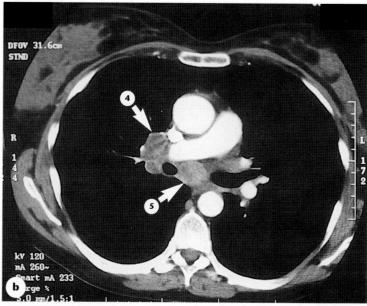

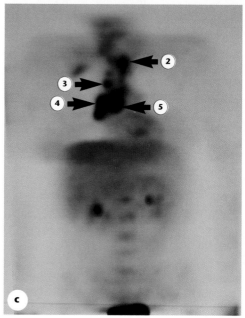

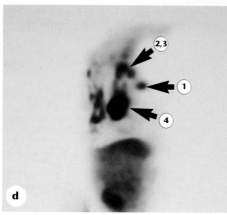

Fig. 4.56 T1N3 (stage IIIB) adenocarcinoma of the lung. A 44-year-old woman presented with an enlarged supraclavicular lymph node mass. Biopsy showed metastatic adenocarcinoma that was positive for TTF-1 (thyroid transcription factor-1) and cytokeratin 7 but negative for cytokeratin 20, consistent with lung cancer. At age 18, she was treated for stage IIIB Hodgkin's disease with MOPP chemotherapy followed by mantle field irradiation. CT scan shows: (**a**) the primary cancer in the medial right upper lobe (1), left (2) and right (3) mediastinal nodes; (**b**) right hilar (4) and subcarinal (5) nodes. A staging PET scan reveals: (**c**) coronal image: right hilar (4), subcarinal (5) and upper mediastinal (2,3) nodes; (**d**) sagittal image: primary cancer (1), upper mediastinal (2,3) and right hilar (4) nodes. Normal liver uptake and renal excretion are noted. No other metastases were evident. The diagnostic role of TTF-1 is discussed by Ordonez (2000) while the value of PET staging is reviewed by Pieterman *et al.* (2000). (Courtesy of Milos Janicek MD, PhD, Department of Radiology, Brigham and Women's Hospital and Dana-Farber Cancer Institute, Boston, MA.)

Table 4.6 Causes of interstitial lung disease. The finding of an interstitial pattern on chest radiography may be the result of numerous causes, among them lung neoplasia.

Neoplastic	Immunologic	Occupational	Infectious	Drug-related	Rare
Multiple metastatic deposits	Collagen-vascular diseases	Asbestosis	Miliary tuberculosis	Amiodarone	Hemosiderosis
Bronchio-alveolar carcinoma	Cryptogenic fibrosing alveolitis	Silicosis	Fungal infection (e.g. candidiasis)	Cytotoxic drugs	Eosinophilic granuloma
Lymphangitis carcinomatosa	Extrinsic allergic alveolitis	Siderosis	Protozoan infection (e.g. pneumocystis)	Paraquat	Alveolar proteinosis
Leukemia	Pulmonary eosinophilia	Talcosis	Viral infection (e.g. cytomegalovirus)		
Lymphoma	Granulomatous disorders				

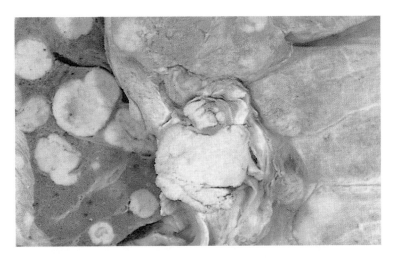

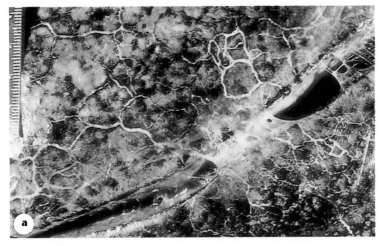

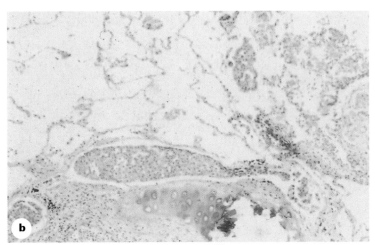

Fig. 4.57 Multiple pulmonary metastases. Beneath the pleura and in the lung parenchyma are numerous pale, umbilicated nodules of tumor. Up to a third of patients dying of malignant disease have pulmonary metastases, the most common sources of which are primary tumors of the breast, colon, stomach and lung itself. The extensive vascular and lymphatic system of the lungs is responsible for the predilection that metastases show for this site.

Fig. 4.58 Pulmonary lymphangitis carcinomatosa. (**a**) The pleural surface of this autopsy specimen from a patient who died of a poorly differentiated non-small cell lung cancer shows dilated lymphatic channels filled with tumor.

(**b**) Microscopic section of the lung demonstrates malignant cells infiltrating lymphatic channels.

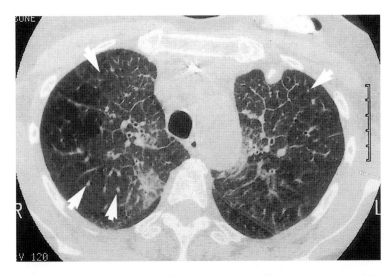

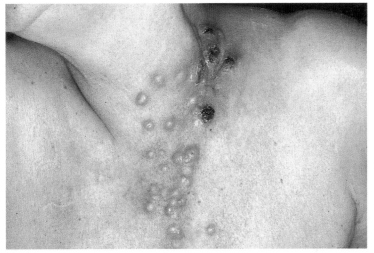

Fig. 4.59 Pulmonary lymphangitis carcinomatosa. A 49-year-old woman with previous resection of a poorly differentiated adenocarcinoma of the lung presented with increasing dyspnea on exertion. Chest radiograph showed non-diagnostic features. CT image at the level of the aortic arch displayed with lung windows shows bilateral thickening of interlobular septae consistent with lymphangitic tumor spread. The thickened septae (arrows) form polygons containing a central dot, representing a pulmonary vein.

Fig. 4.60 Cutaneous metastases. A 48-year-old woman with a small cell (oat cell) lung cancer developed numerous skin lesions. Generalized skin or subcutaneous metastases, which may be quite painful, often occur and they may be seen in all histologic subtypes. In some patients, a solitary early skin metastasis may be the presenting sign of an underlying lung tumor.

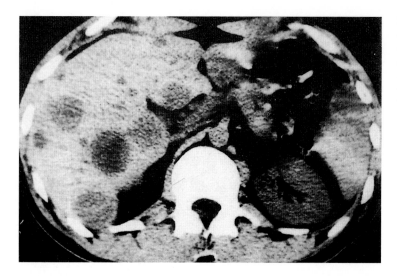

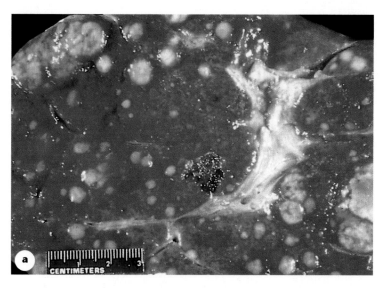

Fig. 4.61 Liver metastases. CT scan of a 28-year-old man with metastatic atypical carcinoid tumor shows numerous metastatic liver deposits which developed after control of his primary pulmonary malignancy by surgery. CT is quite accurate in detecting early metastases and use of contrast with CT helps rule out benign cysts which do not enhance with contrast. Ultrasound can also differentiate cystic from solid lesions. These lesions would also be evident by technetium sulfur colloid scanning.

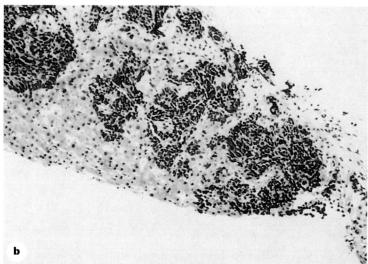

Fig. 4.62 Liver metastases. (**a**) Autopsy specimen from a patient who died of widespread small cell (oat cell) lung cancer exhibits numerous lesions ranging in size from a few millimeters to 1–2 cm. A similar pattern can be seen with non-small cell carcinomas. (**b**) Photomicrograph of a liver biopsy from a patient with small cell lung tumor shows marked involvement by clumps of undifferentiated dark-staining cells.

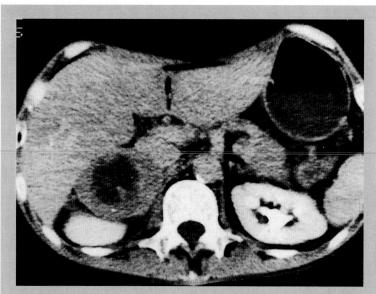

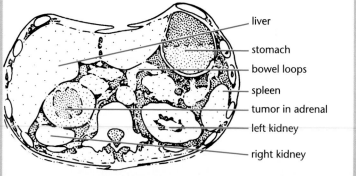

liver
stomach
bowel loops
spleen
tumor in adrenal
left kidney
right kidney

Fig. 4.63 Adrenal metastases. Abdominal CT scan of a patient with a non-small cell lung cancer shows a large metastatic lesion in the right adrenal gland; central tumor necrosis is also evident. This patient was considered for surgery before the adrenal lesion was detected. About 5–10% of patients with localized lung cancer on chest radiography have asymptomatic adrenal metastases. Carcinoma of the lung is by far the most common source of adrenal metastases, followed by carcinoma of the breast and malignant melanoma. In general, adrenal metastases are bilateral and most often appear first in the medulla. Cortical involvement is also common and in rare cases such metastatic spread may give rise to Addison's disease.

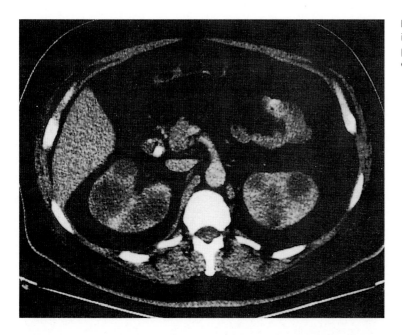

Fig. 4.64 Kidney metastases. CT scan shows bilateral renal metastases in a 63-year-old man who also had liver and bone involvement by a primary adenocarcinoma of the lung. Renal cysts can usually be ruled out by ultrasound.

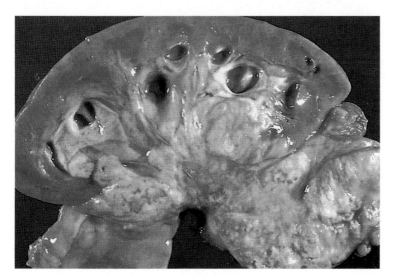

Fig. 4.65 Kidney metastases. Metastatic small cell carcinoma of the lung has extensively infiltrated the renal hilum, producing moderate hydronephrosis. Ureteral and periureteral metastases may also occur, resulting in urinary tract obstruction and infection. Since primary renal cell carcinoma is not uncommon in older patients, it should also be considered in the differential diagnosis, especially when there are no other sites of metastatic lung cancer.

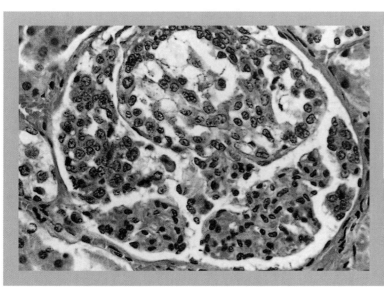

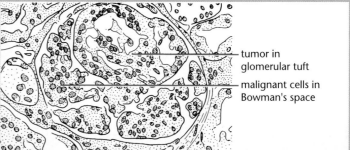

tumor in glomerular tuft

malignant cells in Bowman's space

Fig. 4.66 Kidney metastases. Hematogenous spread of a lung carcinoma is evident in this glomerulus, which contains a nodule of metastatic adenocarcinoma in the capillary tuft, as well as malignant cells in Bowman's space. (Reproduced with permission from Schumann GB, Weiss MA: Atlas of Renal and Urinary Tract Cytology and Its Histopathologic Bases. Lippincott, Philadelphia, 1981.)

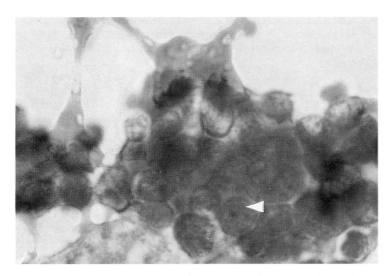

Fig. 4.67 Kidney metastases. Fine-needle aspiration biopsy specimen from the kidney shown in Figure 4.65 contains loose aggregates of small malignant cells with the cytologic characteristics typical of small cell (oat cell) carcinoma – nuclei with moderately granular chromatin, small, inconspicuous nucleoli, scant cytoplasm and prominent nuclear molding (arrow). Fine-needle aspiration is a useful diagnostic procedure for differentiating metastatic tumors from primary urinary tract malignancies (Papanicolaou stain).

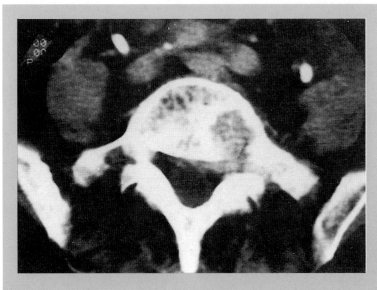

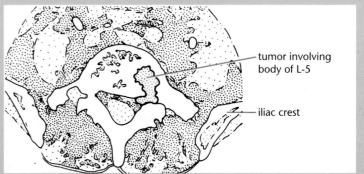

tumor involving body of L-5

iliac crest

Fig. 4.68 Bone metastases. A 74-year-old woman presented with pain and weakness of the left leg. A right lower lobe mass was noted on her chest radiograph and a diagnosis of adenocarcinoma was subsequently made by bronchoscopy. CT scan shows compression of the cauda equina by tumor involving the body of L5. Her leg pain and weakness dramatically improved after radiotherapy.

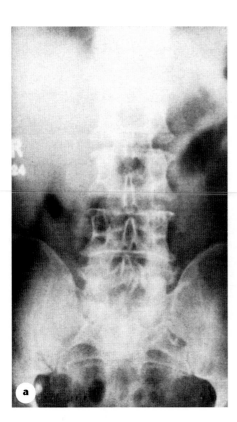

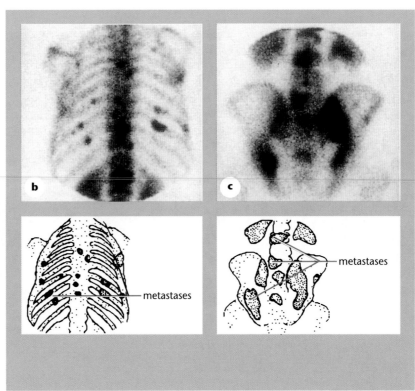

metastases

metastases

Fig. 4.69 Bone metastases. (**a**) Radiograph of the lumbar spine in a patient who had a bronchial carcinoma and complained of back pain indicates no abnormality. However, radionuclide bone scans (**b, c**) reveal multiple metastases in the lumbar spine and pelvis, as well as deposits in thoracic vertebrae and ribs.

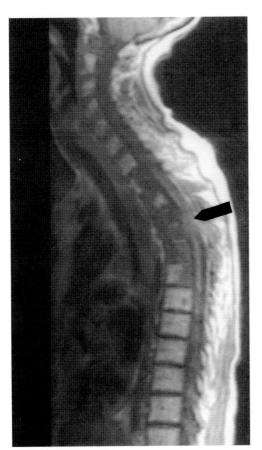

Fig. 4.70 Bone marrow metastases. A 62-year-old woman presented with upper back pain and neurological findings diagnostic of early spinal cord compression. Normal bone marrow appears white on this T_2-weighted MRI scan due to fat content, except in the upper spine where metastatic lung cancer has replaced the bone marrow and appears black. The spinal cord appears white and shows an area of displacement due to compression by tumor invading through the intervertebral space (arrow).

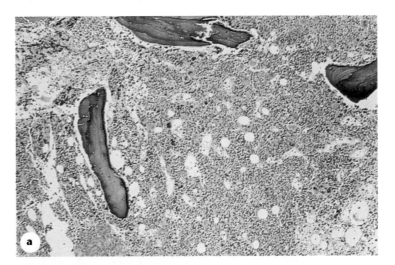

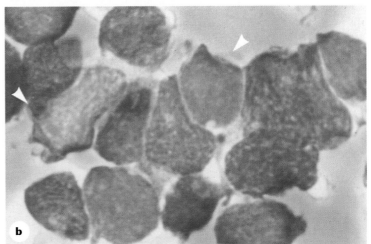

Fig. 4.71 Bone marrow metastases. (**a**) Low-power photomicrograph of a bone marrow biopsy specimen shows focal involvement by metastatic small cell (oat cell) lung cancer. (**b**) High-power view of a bone marrow aspirate shows a cluster of malignant small cells with prominent nuclear molding (arrows). The differential diagnosis of this cytology includes other small blue cell malignancies, e.g. Ewing's sarcoma, neuroblastoma, rhabdomyosarcoma, and lymphoma. Bone marrow involvement as the only site of metastatic disease occurs in 5–10% of cases; the incidence rises to 40% or greater when metastases are found at other sites.

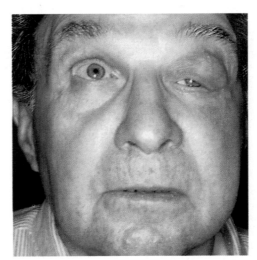

Fig. 4.72 Orbital metastases. This 62-year-old man had a lung adenocarcinoma that metastasized to the retro-orbital space, resulting in proptosis and limitation in eye motion.

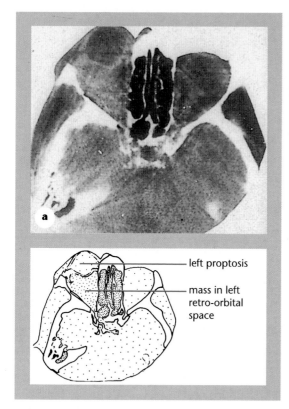

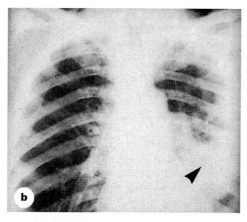

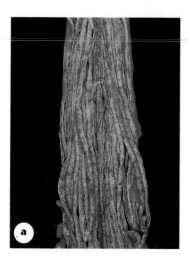

left proptosis

mass in left retro-orbital space

Fig. 4.73 Orbital metastases. A 75-year-old woman presented with retro-orbital pain and a VI cranial nerve palsy. Later, proptosis developed, with downward and outward deviation of the globe. (**a**) CT scan shows a high-density lesion in the left retro-orbital space. (**b**) Chest film demonstrates a mass below the left hilum (arrow), which on aspiration biopsy proved to be an adenocarcinoma.

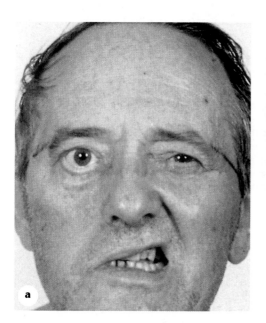

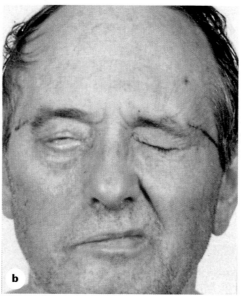

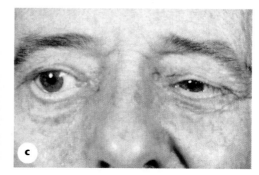

Fig. 4.74 Cranial nerve metastases. This 61-year-old man presented with loss of feeling in the left leg, left facial numbness, and ataxias. CT scan demonstrated multiple cerebral metastases of a bronchial carcinoma. Involvement of the right VI, and VII cranial nerves is reflected in the weakness of the orbicular muscle of the right eye (**a**) and that of the right side of the mouth (**b, c**). Incomplete abduction of the right eye is also apparent.

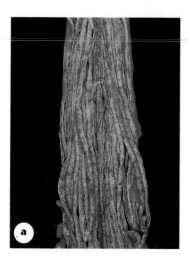

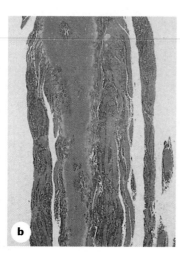

Fig. 4.75 Leptomeningeal metastases. (**a**) The red hypervascular patches on the nerve roots of the cauda equina in this fresh specimen represent leptomeningeal deposits of a metastatic lung carcinoma. The cauda equina is a favorite location for this process. (**b**) Whole-mount section of the specimen, which better demonstrates the extent of infiltration, shows ropy thickening of individual nerve roots by dense, blue-staining tumor cell nuclei. Minor extension of tumor into the spinal cord is also evident.

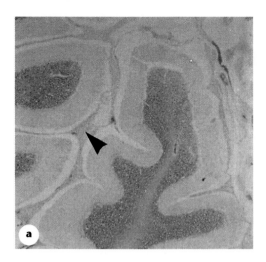

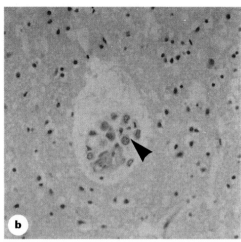

Fig. 4.76 Leptomeningeal metastases. A 55-year-old man was diagnosed with an undifferentiated large cell lung cancer. Two months later, he presented with headache followed by numbness of the hands. Examination showed diplopia, dysarthria, nystagmus, palsies of the left VI and right VII cranial nerves, bilateral limb ataxia, areflexia and gait ataxia. (**a**) Section of cerebellum shows infiltration of the leptomeninges by malignant cells (arrow) and, on high-power view (**b**), invasion of the Virchow–Robin space (arrow).

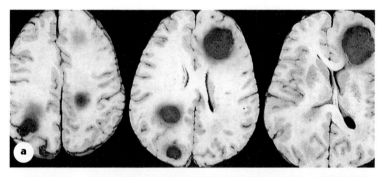

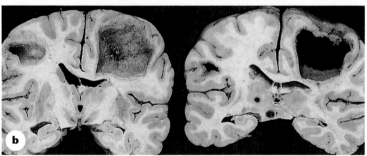

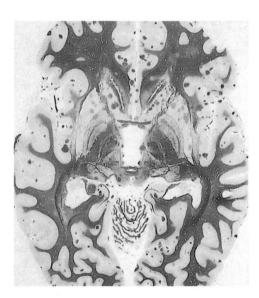

Fig. 4.77 Brain metastases. (**a**) Gross specimens show metastatic deposits of an undifferentiated large cell lung carcinoma. The metastases form essentially necrotic masses with peripheral enhancement and peritumoral edema. (**b**) Occasionally, extensive necrosis transforms metastases into cysts lined by only a thin rim of viable tumor.

Fig. 4.78 Brain metastases. Horizontal whole-mount section of a brain shows metastatic small cell lung carcinoma as miliary cerebral metastases. Many are situated in gray matter or at the gray–white matter junction. The ventricular surface is also involved. Note the relative sparing of white matter and the absence of edema.

Table 4.7 Manifestations of selected paraneoplastic syndromes in lung cancer patients by type of manifestation and frequency. (Modified from Minna *et al.*, 1989.)

Type of manifestation	Frequency (%)
Systemic	
Anorexia-cachexia	31
Fever	21
Suppressed Immunity	
Skeletal	
Digital clubbing	29
Periostitis (hypertrophic pulmonary osteoarthropathy) – commonly associated with adenocarcinoma	1–10
Endocrine	
Hypercalcemia (ectopic parathyroid hormone) – commonly associated with squamous cell carcinoma	
Hyponatremia (inappropriate secretion of ADH) – commonly associated with small cell carcinoma	
Cushing's syndrome (ectopic ACTH secretion) – commonly associated with small cell carcinoma	
Hematologic	8
Anemia	
Granulocytosis	
Eosinophilia	
Leukoerythroblastosis	
Coagulation–Thrombotic	1–4
Venous thrombosis (migratory thrombophlebitis, Trousseau's syndrome)	
Arterial embolism (non-bacterial thrombotic endocarditis)	
Hemorrhage (disseminated Intravascular coagulation)	
Neurologic–Myopathic	1
Eaton–Lambert syndrome (myasthenia) – commonly associated with small cell carcinoma	
Peripheral neuropathy	
Subacute cerebellar degeneration	
Cortical degeneration	
Polymyositis	
Neurologic – Cutaneous	1
Dermatomyositis	
Acanthosis nigricans	
Renal	< 1
Nephrotic syndrome	
Glomerulonephritis	

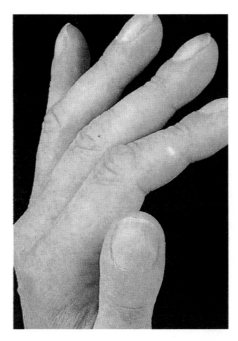

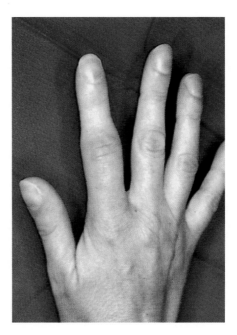

Fig. 4.79 Hypertrophic pulmonary osteoarthropathy (HPO; digit clubbing). A characteristic manifestation of HPO, digit clubbing occurs in about 10% of lung cancer patients of all histologic subgroups, but particularly in adenocarcinoma. The disease may be early or advanced. Benign tumors, inflammatory disease and liver disease are also associated with clubbing. While the pathophysiology is poorly understood, digital clubbing, painful joints and tender extremities – features commonly seen in HPO – often reverse dramatically after successful thoracotomy, radiotherapy, or chemotherapy.

Fig. 4.80 HPO and digital metastases. This 45-year-old woman presented with HPO and also pain and swelling of her right index finger. Radiographs showed lytic lesions in the middle phalanx and bone scan was positive in this area (not shown). Biopsy was positive for metastatic, poorly differentiated adenocarcinoma from the lung. Metastases to bone beyond the humerus and/or femur are unusual in any type of primary cancer.

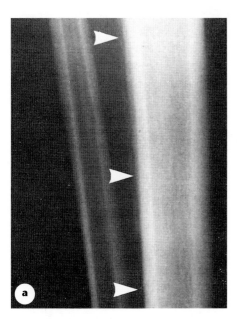

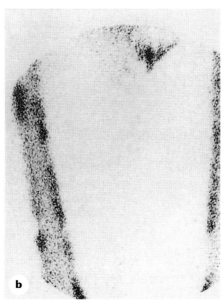

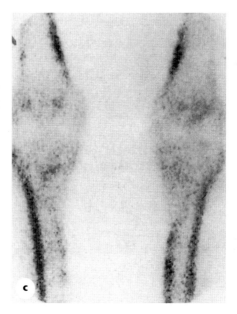

Fig. 4.81 HPO (periostitis). (**a**) Radiograph of the lower leg shows periosteal elevation (arrows) in the tibia of a patient who presented with joint pain of the lower legs and feet. Evaluation subsequently showed a primary lung adenocarcinoma of the right upper lobe (**b, c**) Bone scans show focal increased uptake of radiopharmaceutical in both legs in areas of new bone formation; no bone metastases are evident.

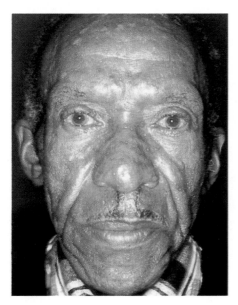

Fig. 4.82 HPO (pachydermoperiostitis). This 60-year-old man with squamous cell lung cancer developed HPO and changing facial features resembling acromegaly. His appearance became progressively coarser, with deepening facial and scalp furrows. Thickening of the legs and forearms, with the development of spade-like hands and feet, may also occur in this paraneoplastic syndrome.

TUMORS OF THE HEART

Primary tumors of the heart are rare. The incidence varies from 0.0017% to 0.28% in autopsy studies. Cardiac myxomas are by far the most common, up to 30%, arising most often in adulthood, equally in either sex. Patients with myxomas typically present either with the features of mitral valve disease or with systemic emboli; they often remain asymptomatic. Unusual clinical features include polyarthralgia, Reynaud's phenomenon, malaise and weight loss. The great majority of cardiac myxomas develop as pedunculated tumors in the left atrium (75–80%); the right atrium is the second most common site; the ventricles are only rarely affected. The precise nature of these benign lesions has been a source of controversy. Once viewed as representing simply organized, rather myxoid thrombi, myxomas are currently regarded as true neoplasms derived from subendocardial tissue. Histologically, they exhibit only primitive mesenchymal differentiation.

The most common primary malignancy of the heart is angiosarcoma, which occurs mainly in the right atrium. Most patients present with congestive heart failure and the diagnosis may not even be established until autopsy. There is no effective therapy in the vast majority of cases.

In contrast, metastatic tumors to the heart are relatively common. Lung cancer often spreads to the pericardium, resulting in malignant pericardial effusion and acute tamponade, but metastases can also develop in the endocardium and myocardium, producing arrhythmias and cardiac failure. Rarely, coronary artery metastases occur, with resultant angina or acute myocardial infarction. Other malignancies that often spread to the heart include malignant melanoma, breast cancer, lymphoma, leukemia, soft tissue sarcomas, renal cell carcinoma, choriocarcinoma and hepatocellular carcinoma. Kaposi's sarcoma may also involve the heart, particularly in AIDS patients.

**Table 4.8 Tumors and cysts of the heart and pericardium.
(Modified from McAllister and Fenoglio, 1978.)**

Type	Frequency (%)	Type	Frequency (%)
Benign Tumors		Malignant Tumors	
Myxoma	24.4	Angiosarcoma	7.3
Lipoma	8.4	Rhabdomyosarcoma	4.9
Papiliary fibroelastoma	7.9	Mesothelioma	3.6
Rhabdomyoma	6.8	Fibrosarcoma	2.6
Fibroma	3.2	Malignant lymphoma	1.3
Hemangioma	2.8	Extraskeletal osteosarcoma	*
Teratoma (dermoid cyst)	2.6	Neurogenic sarcoma	*
Mesothelioma of atrioventricular node	2.3	Malignant teratoma	*
		Thymoma	*
Granular cell tumor	*	Leiomyosarcoma	*
Neurofibroma	*	Liposarcoma	*
Lymphangioma	*	Synovial sarcoma	*
Cyst			
Pericardial cyst	15.4		
Bronchogenic cyst	1.3		

*Frequency is <1% each

**Table 4.9 General manifestations of neoplastic heart disease.
(Reproduced with permission from Hall and Cooley, 1986.)**

Pericardial Involvement	Myocardial Involvement	Intracavity Tumor
Pericarditis pain	Arrhythmias ventricular and atrial	Cavity obliteration
Pericardial effusion	Electrocardiographic changes	Valve obstruction and valve damage
Radiographic evidence of enlargement	Radiographic evidence of enlargement (generalized localized)	Embolic phenomena (systemic, neurologic, coronary)
Arrhythmia, predominantly atrial	Conduction disturbances and heart block	Constitutional manifestations
Tamponade	Congestive heart failure	
Constriction	Coronary involvement (angina, infarction)	

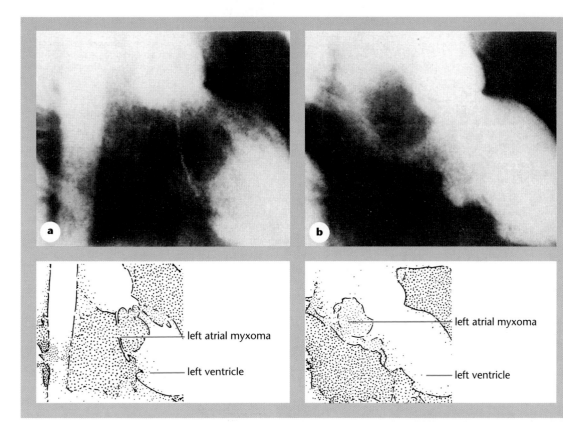

Fig. 4.83 Left atrial myxoma. (**a**) Left ventriculogram in the right anterior oblique projection shows a mobile left atrial myxoma as a space-filling defect within the mitral valve in diastole. (**b**) Sufficient mitral regurgitation is present to delineate the myxoma in the left atrium in systole. (Reproduced with permission from Hall and Cooley, 1986.)

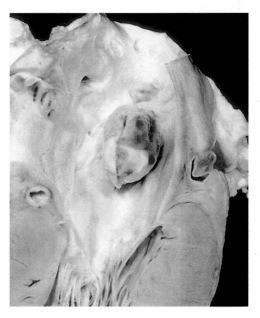

Fig. 4.84 Left atrial myxoma. The left side of the heart has been opened to show a rounded, polypoid, gelatinous tumor (1.5 cm in diameter) arising from the interatrial septum below the oval fossa. This was an incidental finding at autopsy of a 66-year-old hypertensive woman who died of a cerebral hemorrhage. Note the marked left ventricular hypertrophy, a probable consequence of hypertension.

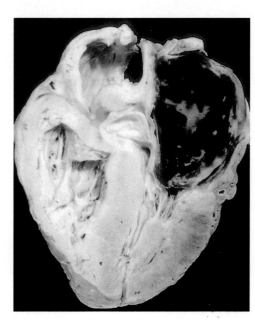

Fig. 4.85 Left atrial myxoma. This autopsy specimen from a 46-year-old woman who died after being admitted with severe congestive heart failure and atrial fibrillation has been sectioned to reveal a 7 cm hemorrhagic mass filling the left atrium. Originating near the oval fossa, the tumor occludes the mitral valve orifice and projects through it. The myocardium of both ventricles is hypertrophied.

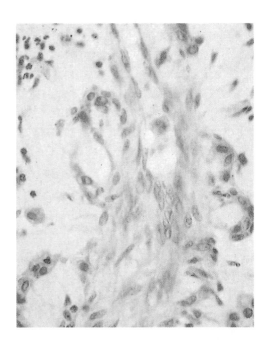

Fig. 4.86 Cardiac myxoma. Histologic section of a tumor shows polygonal cell strands within a mucoid stroma.

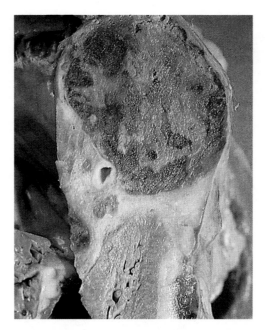

Fig. 4.87 Angiosarcoma. This specimen shows an angiosarcoma of the heart localized in the atrioventricular groove. Note the characteristic hemorrhagic appearance.

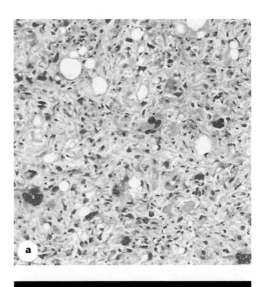

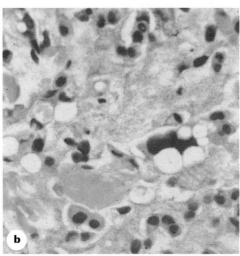

Fig. 4.88 Cardiac liposarcoma. A 23-year-old man presented with an anterior mediastinal mass. Biopsy demonstrated a high-grade sarcoma with many pleomorphic cells (**a**, low-power). At high power (**b**) a lipoblast with fat-containing intracytoplastic vacuoles, indenting on a hyperchromatic nucleus, can be seen. These features are diagnostic of liposarcoma. He had a rapid downhill course despite attempt at therapy. At autopsy, the heart and large vessels were encased in tumor (24 cm in maximal dimension). (**c, d**) The tumor appeared to arise from the epicardial/pericardial tissue. (Gross pictures courtesy of Dr Klaus Busam, Brigham and Women's Hospital, Boston, MA.)

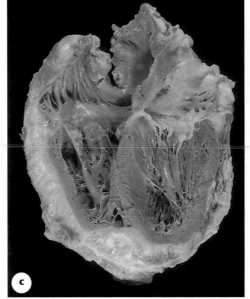

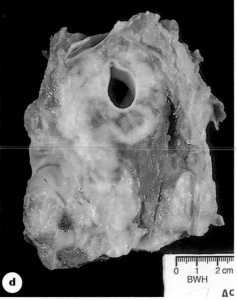

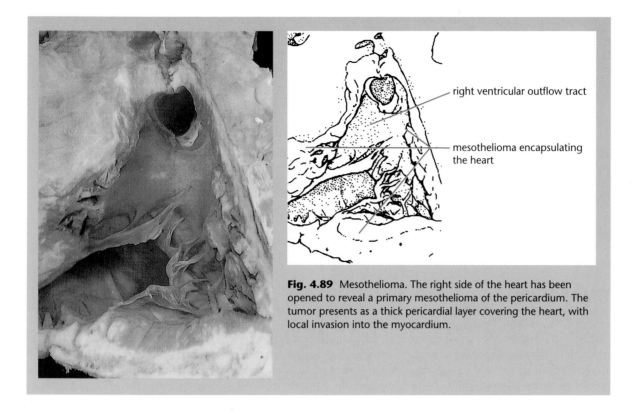

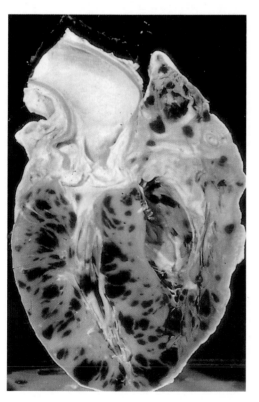

Fig. 4.89 Mesothelioma. The right side of the heart has been opened to reveal a primary mesothelioma of the pericardium. The tumor presents as a thick pericardial layer covering the heart, with local invasion into the myocardium.

Fig. 4.90 Metastatic malignant melanoma. An adult male who had undergone excision of a primary cutaneous malignant melanoma over the right iliac crest 18 months previously developed lymph node and hepatic metastases, followed by bony and cutaneous deposits with terminal melanuria. This section through the heart shows numerous pigmented deposits of metastatic melanoma throughout the myocardium.

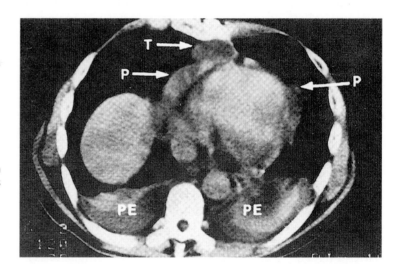

Fig. 4.91 Metastatic renal cell carcinoma. CT scan of the chest at the level of the heart in a patient with renal cell carcinoma reveals metastases to the anterior mediastinum (T) and the pericardium (P). Bilateral pleural effusions (PE) also are evident. (Courtesy of F Parker Gregg MD, Houston, TX. Reproduced with permission from Hall and Cooley, 1986.)

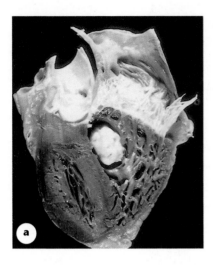

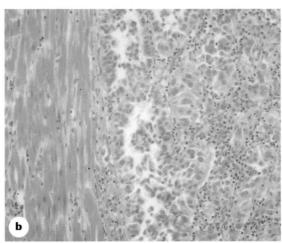

Fig. 4.92 Metastatic renal cell carcinoma. A 54-year-old man had a renal cell carcinoma with positive nodes resected 6 years previously, but subsequently developed jaundice and other evidence of widespread metastases. (**a**) Autopsy showed a single, large metastasis to the right ventricle protruding into the lumen. (**b**) High-power photomicrograph reveals the renal cell carcinoma, papillary type, invading cardiac muscle. The patient had not developed any cardiac symptoms.

TUMORS OF THE MEDIASTINUM

The mediastinum is formed laterally by the parietal pleura, anteriorly by the sternum and attached muscles and posteriorly by the thoracic spine. Its upper limit is the first thoracic vertebra and the manubrium; its lower limit is the diaphragm. For descriptive purposes, the mediastinum is usually divided into four major compartments: superior, anterior, middle and posterior (*see* Fig. 4.93). Clinical manifestations of the various disorders of the mediastinum are related mainly to pressure or invasion of the structures within each division.

The mediastinum is the site of a variety of primary and metastatic tumors. The latter are quite common, most frequently originating from lymphomas or from carcinomas of the lung, breast, intestinal tract and testes. In some cases, the original cancer may be occult. Primary tumors of the mediastinum, on the other hand, are quite rare. The majority of tumors, about 75%, are benign; of these, most are neurogenic tumors or primary cysts (bronchogenic, pericardial, enteric and others).

HISTOLOGY
Germ cell tumors

All types of germinal tumors found in the testes are known to occur in the mediastinum. Primary seminomas, less than 5% of which occur in women, constitute half of all cases. Non-seminomatous tumors may be pure or mixed germ cell tumors. About 60–70% of patients have elevated levels of β-HCG (choriocarcinomatous elements) and/or α-fetoprotein (AFP) (embryonal and endodermal sinus elements). Benign teratomas, which account for about 20% of anterior mediastinal tumors, occur with equal frequency in men and women. The teratoma, which is cystic in nature, is often referred to as a dermoid cyst and it is entirely comparable with ovarian dermoid tumors. Histologic sections usually reveal tissues arising from all three germ cell layers. The tumors contain hair, sebaceous material, bone, cartilage and other tissues. Calcifications are present in 75% of lesions and may be seen on radiographs. Malignant transition to teratocarcinoma occurs in 10–20% of cases.

Thymic tumors

Thymic tumors most frequently occur in the superior mediastinum but may develop in the anterior mediastinum as well. Thymomas are often large and encapsulated and exhibit fibrous septa on cut section. These tumors are composed of neoplastic epithelial cells with a variable admixture of T-lymphocytes. Histologically, several types are seen: mixed lymphoepithelial (43%), lymphocytic (25%), epithelial or polygonal cell (25%), spindle cell (6%) and unknown (1%). Prognosis for thymomas is generally good, with 5- and 10-year survival rates over 60% and 50% respectively. Poor prognostic features include predominantly epithelial histology, large tumor size and local invasion at surgery (about one-third of cases). About 30–40% of all patients have myasthenia gravis (most common in the mixed cell type), whereas 10% have other paraneoplastic syndromes such as pure red cell aplasia, hypogammaglobulinemia, polymyositis or positive lupus erythematosus preparation.

Other primary tumors of the thymus are rare. These include carcinomas, carcinoids and neuroendocrine tumors, as well as germ cell tumors and lipomas. Hodgkin's disease and non-Hodgkin's lymphomas may rarely arise.

Neurogenic tumors

Neurogenic tumors characteristically arise in the posterior mediastinum near the paravertebral gutter. They occur at all ages, but the malignant variants are often present in childhood. The lesions arise from nerve cells of the sympathetic nervous system, peripheral nerve sheaths or embryonal neurogenic rests. Types of tumors include neurofibromas (singly or in association with von Recklinghausen's disease), neurilemmomas (from the sheath or Schwann's membrane), ganglioneuromas (from the sympathetic chain) and neuroblastomas.

CLINICAL MANIFESTATIONS

Mediastinal tumors, even when massive, may be asymptomatic and are often detected incidentally on routine chest radiography. However, symptoms occur in about two-thirds of patients, consisting of retrosternal pain, dyspnea and other respiratory complications in anterior mediastinal tumors. In the posterior mediastinum, symptoms vary greatly. Compression of the trachea and bronchi results in cough and dyspnea, whereas esophageal compression causes dysphagia. Other presenting problems include paralysis of the diaphragm, hoarseness, Horner's syndrome and SVC syndrome in tumors involving the superior mediastinum.

Diagnostic evaluation includes standard radiologic studies, as well as esophagograms in some cases. CT scanning and MR imaging are approximately equivalent in assessing the primary lesion and any regional metastases. A specific diagnosis can be established by a number of procedures, including needle biopsy, mediastinoscopy, mediastinotomy or in some cases thoracotomy with resection of the lesion.

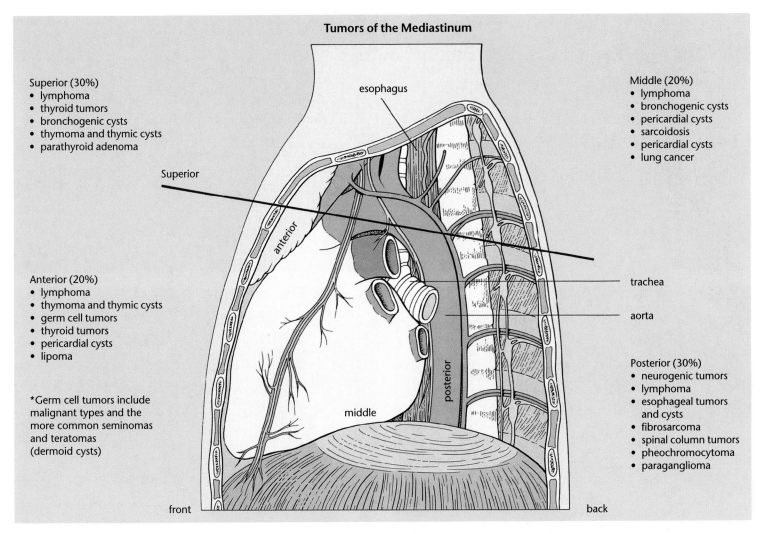

Tumors of the Mediastinum

esophagus

Superior (30%)
- lymphoma
- thyroid tumors
- bronchogenic cysts
- thymoma and thymic cysts
- parathyroid adenoma

Superior

anterior

Anterior (20%)
- lymphoma
- thymoma and thymic cysts
- germ cell tumors
- thyroid tumors
- pericardial cysts
- lipoma

*Germ cell tumors include malignant types and the more common seminomas and teratomas (dermoid cysts)

middle

posterior

front

Middle (20%)
- lymphoma
- bronchogenic cysts
- pericardial cysts
- sarcoidosis
- pericardial cysts
- lung cancer

trachea

aorta

Posterior (30%)
- neurogenic tumors
- lymphoma
- esophageal tumors and cysts
- fibrosarcoma
- spinal column tumors
- pheochromocytoma
- paraganglioma

back

Fig. 4.93 Tumors of the mediastinum. The customary subdivisions of the mediastinum are illustrated, together with a partial listing of mediastinal tumors and the relative frequency of occurrence of tumors in the various mediastinal divisions. About 25% of mediastinal tumors are malignant. There is some overlap in cell types.

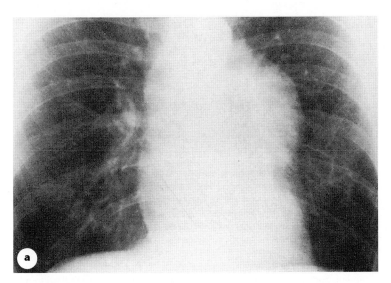

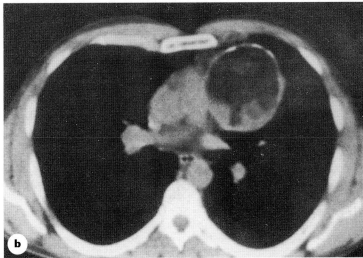

Fig. 4.94 Benign teratoma. A 30-year-old man developed mild chest discomfort. (**a**) Chest radiograph reveals a large mass in the anterior mediastinum. (**b**) CT scan shows a thin-walled cystic lesion. The tumor was completely resected at thoracotomy.

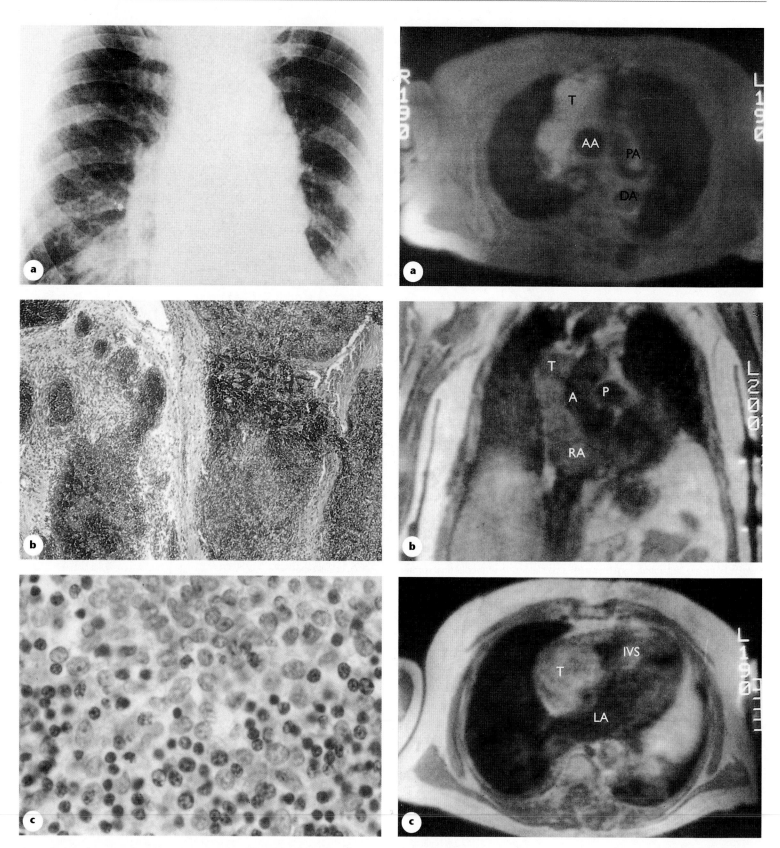

Fig. 4.95 Thymoma. A 50-year-old woman presented with severe anemia due to pure red cell aplasia. (**a**) Chest radiograph demonstrates an anterior mediastinal mass. A locally invasive thymoma was resected, but small pleural metastases were found. (**b**) Low-power photomicrograph of the lesion shows fibrous septa separating tumor nodules. (**c**) On high-power view, neoplastic epithelial cells are evident with an admixture of T-lymphocytes, which are probably non-neoplastic. The epithelial cells are positive for keratin. Metastases are uncommon within the chest and even more outside the chest. Thymic carcinomas, however, are more invasive and often metastasize to rare distant sites.

Fig. 4.96 Thymoma invading the heart. A 67-year-old man presented with early features of SVC syndrome (*see* Fig. 4.49). He also had increasing cough and several syncopal episodes. He arrested in the Emergency Room, but was resuscitated and received radiotherapy with improvement. Chest radiograph showed an anterior mediastinal mass. (**a**) T_1-weighted MR image in the axial plane at the level of the main pulmonary artery (PA) with a lobular mediastinal mass (T) on the right wrapping around the ascending aorta (AA). DA = descending aorta. (**b**) T_1-weighted image in the coronal plane through the ascending aorta (A) with tumor extending from the upper right mediastinum (T) down into and filling the right atrium (RA). P = main pulmonary artery. (**c**) T_1-weighted MR image in the axial plane at the level of the left atrium (LA) with tumor filling the right atrium (T). IVS = interventricular septum.

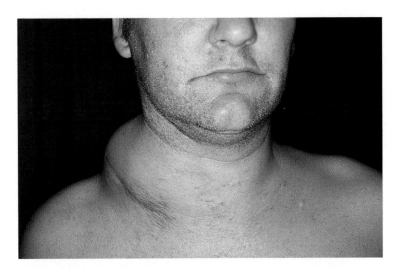

Fig. 4.97 Thymoma. This 38-year-old man with recurrent malignant thymoma had disease progression directly into the supraclavicular and cervical lymph node sites, that was refractory to both chemotherapy and radiation therapy.

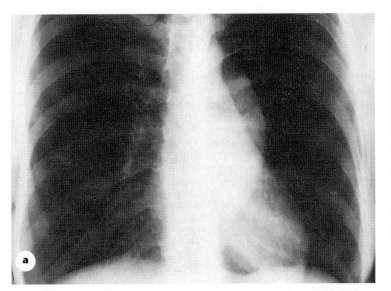

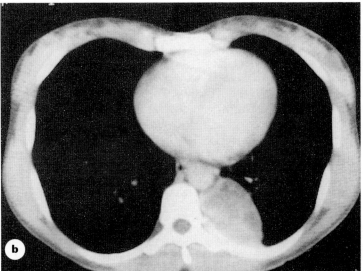

Fig. 4.98 Ganglioneuroma. (**a**) During evaluation for an unrelated problem, chest radiography in a 24-year-old woman revealed an asymptomatic posterior mediastinal mass. (**b**) CT scan shows the classic location of a neurogenic tumor in the posterior mediastinum. The lesion is multicystic. Curative resection revealed a ganglioneuroma.

REFERENCES

Allen MS: Malignant tracheal tumors. Mayo Clin Proc 1993; 68 : 680–684.

Anderson M, Spandidos D: Oncogenes and onco-suppressor genes in lung cancer. Respir Med 1993; 87 : 413–420.

Dunagan DP, Chin R Jr, McCain TW, *et al.*: Staging py positron emission tomography predicts survival in patients with non-small cell lung cancer. Chest 2001; 119 : 333–339.

Fletcher JA, Pinkus GS, Donovan K, *et al.*: Clonal rearrangement of chromosome band:6p21 in mesenchymal component of pulmonary chondroid hamartoma. Cancer Res 1992; 52 : 6224–6228.

Hall R, Cooley D: Neoplastic heart disease. In: Hurst J, ed: The Heart: Arteries and Veins, 6th edn. McGraw-Hill, New York, 1986.

Harpole D, Richards W, Herndon J, *et al.*: Angiogenesis and molecular biologic substaging in patients with stage I non-small cell lung cancer. Ann Thorac Surg 1996; 61 : 1470–1476.

Hirsch RF, Matthews MJ, Aisner S, *et al.*: Histopathologic classification of small cell lung cancer. Cancer 1988: 62 : 973–977.

Hiyama K, Ishioka S, Shirotani Y, *et al.*: Alterations in telomeric repeat length in lung cancer are associated with loss of heterozygosity in p53 and RB. Oncogene 1995; 10 : 937–944.

Jemal A, Thomas A, Murray T, *et al.*: Cancer statistics 2002. Ca Cancer J Clin 2002: 52:23–47.

Johnson BE, Kelley MJ: Overview of genetic and molecular events in the pathogenesis of lung cancer. Chest 1993; 103 : 1S–3S.

Kimura T, Sato T, Onodera K: Clinical significance of DNA measurements in small cell lung cancer. Cancer 1993; 72 : 3216–3222.

Lee J, Yoon A, Kalapurakal S, *et al.*: Expression of p53 oncoprotein in non-small cell lung cancer: a favorable prognostic factor. J Clin Oncol 1995; 13 : 1893–1903.

Macchiarini P, Fontanini G, Hardin J, *et al.*: Most peripheral, node-negative, non-small-cell lung cancers have low proliferative rates and no intratumoral and peritumoral blood and lymphatic vessel invasion. J Thorac Cardiovasc Surg 1992; 104 : 892–899.

Marom EM, Erasmus JJ, Patz EF Jr: Lung cancer and positron emission tomography with fluorodeoxyglucose. Lung Cancer 2000; 28 : 187–202.

Matsumoto H, Muramatsu H, Shimotakahara T, *et al.*: Correlation of expression of ABH blood group carbohydrate antigens with metastatic potential in human lung carcinomas. Cancer 1993; 72 : 75–81.

McAllister HA Jr, Fenoglio JJ Jr: Tumors of the Cardiovascular System. Armed Forces Institute of Pathology, Washington DC, 1978.

Mentzer SJ, Sugarbaker DJ. Thoracoscopy and video-assisted thoracic surgery. In: Brooks DC, ed: Current Techniques in Laparoscopy. Current Medicine, Philadelphia, 1994: pp 20.1–12.

Minna JD, Pass H, Glatstein EJ: Cancer of the lung. In: DeVita VT Jr, Hellman S, Rosenberg SA, eds: Cancer: Principles and Practice of Oncology, 3rd edn. Lippincott, Philadelphia, 1989: pp 591–724.

Mitsudomi T, Oyama T, Kusano T, *et al.*: Mutations of the p53 gene as a predictor of poor prognosis in patients with non-small cell lung cancer. J Natl Cancer Inst 1993; 85 : 2018.

Mountain CF: A new international staging system for lung cancer. Chest 1986: 89(suppl):225–233.

Mountain CF: Lung cancer staging classification. Clin Chest Med 1993; 14(1):48–53.

Mountain CF: Revisions in the international system for staging lung cancer. Chest 1997; 111 : 1710–1717.

Ordóñez NG: Value of thyroid transcription factor-1, E-cadherin, BG8, WT1, and CD44S immunostaining in distinguishing epithelial pleural mesothelioma from pulmonary and nonpulmonary adenocarcinoma. Am J Surg Pathol 2000; 24 : 598–606.

Otterson G, Lin A, Kaye F, *et al.*: Genetic etiology of lung cancer. Oncology 1992; 6(9):97–107.

Pezzella F, Turley H, Kuzu I, *et al.*: bcl-2 protein in non-small cell lung carcinoma. N Engl J Med 1993; 329 : 690–694.

Pieterman RM, van Putten JWG, Meuzelaar JJ, *et al.*: Preoperative staging of non-small cell lung cancer with positron-emission tomography. N Engl J Med 2000; 343 : 254–261.

Salgia R, Harpole D, Herndon D, *et al.*: Role of serum markers CA125 and CEA in non-small cell lung cancer. Anticancer Res 2001;21:1241–1246.

Skarin AT: Analysis of long-term survivors with small-cell lung cancer. Chest 1993; 103 : 440S–444S.

Sozzi G, Veronese M, Negrini M, *et al.*: The FHIT gene at 3p14.2 is abnormal in lung cancer. Cell 1996; 85 : 17–26.

Strauss GM, Kwiatkowski DJ, Harpole DH, *et al.*: Molecular and pathologic analysis of stage I non-small cell carcinoma of the lung: implications for the future. J Clin Oncol 1995; 13 : 1265–1279.

Sundaresan V, Ganly P, Hasleton P, *et al.*: p53 and chromosome 3 abnormalities, characteristic of malignant lung tumors, are detectable in preinvasive lesions of the bronchus. Oncogene 1992; 7 : 1989–1997.

Travis WD, Colby TV, Corrin B, *et al.*: Histological Typing of Lung and Pleural Tumors, 3rd edn. Springer Verlag, Berlin, 1999.

Westra WH, Slebos RJC, Offerhaus GJA, *et al.*: K-ras oncogene activation in lung adenocarcinomas from former smokers. Cancer 1993; 72 : 432–438.

Wick MR, Swanson PE: Carcinosarcomas: current perspectives and an historical review of nosological concepts. Semin Diag Pathol 1993; 10(2):118–127.

FIGURE CREDITS

The following books published by Gower Medical Publishing are sources of figures in the present chapter. The figure numbers given in the listing are those of the figures in the present chapter. The page numbers (or slide numbers) given in parentheses are those of the original publication.

Anderson RH (ed): Cardiovascular system. In: Turk JL, Fletcher CDM, eds: RCSE Slide Atlas of Pathology. Gower Medical Publishing, London, 1986: 4.84 (slide 72), 4.85 (slide 73), 4.89 (slide 76).

Becker AF, Anderson RH: Cardiac Pathology. Churchill Livingstone/Gower Medical Publishing, Edinburgh/London, 1983: Fig. 4.88 (p 8.4).

Besser GM, Cudworth AG: Clinical Endocrinology. Lippincott/Gower Medical Publishing, Philadelphia/London, 1987: Fig. 4.19 (p 19.7).

Dieppe PA, Bacon PA, Bamji AN, *et al.*: Atlas of Clinical Rheumatology. Lea & Febiger/Gower Medical Publishing, Philadelphia/London, 1986: Figs 4.69 (p 21.6), Table 4.7 (p 21.2).

du Bois RM, Clarke SW: Fibreoptic Bronchoscopy in Diagnosis and Management. Lippincott/Gower Medical Publishing, Philadelphia/London, 1987: Table 4.1 (p 3.2), Table 4.2 (p 3.2) 4.16 (p 3.12) 4.20 A,B (p 3.15), 4.20 C,D (p 3.16), 4.29 (p 3.8), 4.32 (p 6.4), 4.36 (p 3.11), 4.37 (p 6.18), 4.38 (p 6.15), Table 4.6 (p 4.2).

Fletcher CDM, McKee PH: An Atlas of Gross Pathology. Edward Arnold/Gower Medical Publishing, London, 1987: Figs 4.6 (p 21), 4.33 (p 21), 4.57 (p 21).

Hurst JW, ed: Atlas of the Heart. McGraw-Hill/Gower Medical Publishing, New York, 1988: Table 4.8 (p 13.2), Table 4.9 (p 13.2), Figs 4.88 (p 4.31), 4.8 (p 13.9), 4.89 (p 13.9), 4.91 (p 3.11).

Kassner, EG, ed: Atlas of Radiologic Imaging. Lippincott/Gower Medical Publishing, Philadelphia/New York, 1989: Fig. 4.53 (p 8.8).

Okazaki H, Scheithauer BW: Atlas of Neuropathology. Lippincott/Gower Medical Publishing, Philadelphia/New York, 1988: Figs 4.75 (p 168), 4.77 (p 171), 4.78 (p 170).

Perkin GD, Rose FC, Blackwood W, *et al.*: Atlas of Clinical Urology. Lippincott/Gower Medical Publishing, Philadelphia/London, 1986: Figs 4.73 (p 7.13), 4.74 (p 7.13), 4.76 (p 9.8).

Spencer H, ed: Respiratory system. In: Turk JL, Fletcher CDM, eds: RCSE Slide Atlas of Pathology. Gower Medical Publishing, London, 1986: Figs 4.2 (slide 68), 4.5 (slide 91), 4.17 (slide 87).

Weiss MA, Mills SE: Atlas of Genitourinary Tract Disorders. Gower Medical Publishing, Philadelphia/New York, 1988: Figs 4.65 (p 8.21), 4.66 (p 11.55), 4.67 (p 8.21).

Cancer of the gastrointestinal tract

Matthew H. Kulke, Jerrold R. Turner, Arthur T. Skarin

5

ESOPHAGEAL CANCERS

The prevalence of esophageal cancer varies over 20-fold throughout the world. Esophageal cancer is most common in central Asia and remains relatively rare in the United States. Approximately 13 000 new cases of esophageal cancer occur annually in the United States, where 75% of esophageal cancers develop in men and only 25% in women.

HISTOLOGY OF ESOPHAGEAL CANCER

Worldwide, 90% of esophageal cancers are squamous cell carcinomas. The risk of esophageal squamous cell carcinoma is related closely to excessive alcohol consumption and chronic cigarette smoking. The squamous cell carcinomas, including spindle cell and verrucous variants, are most prevalent in the upper esophagus. Interestingly, in the past two decades, the relative incidence of squamous cell carcinoma and adenocarcinoma of the esophagus has shifted dramatically in both the United States and Europe. In these regions, squamous cell carcinoma has become somewhat less common, whereas the incidence of esophageal adenocarcinoma has increased dramatically. In US white males, for example, the incidence of adenocarcinoma now exceeds the incidence of squamous cell carcinoma. Adenocarcinomas of the esophagus generally occur in the distal third of the esophagus and are particularly common at the gastroesophageal junction. The risk of esophageal adenocarcinoma has been closely linked to the presence of chronic gastroesophageal reflux and Barrett's esophagus.

Other risk factors for esophageal cancer include exposure to nitrosamines, aflatoxins, vitamin A and riboflavin deficiencies and fungal toxins in pickled vegetables. Mucosal damage caused by ingestion of lye or of extremely hot tea, by chronic achalasia or by radiation-induced stricture may precede the development of esophageal cancer. Both benign and malignant esophageal strictures are more common in the elderly. Finally, patients with Plummer–Vinson syndrome, celiac disease and tylosis have increased risk of esophageal carcinoma.

Rare undifferentiated small cell carcinomas occur in the lower and middle esophagus. Risk factors for these unusual lesions have not been established. These highly malignant tumors behave like small cell lung cancers, occasionally producing paraneoplastic syndromes.

STAGING OF ESOPHAGEAL CANCERS

The unique structure of the esophagus is significant to the biologic understanding and clinical management of malignant disease. There is a rich lymphatic drainage throughout the length of the esophagus and a discontinuous serosa. Therefore, 'skip areas' of micrometastases occur, necessitating wide surgical resection of operable tumors. Lymph node drainage varies within the esophagus (cervical vs thoracic). Nodal metastases frequently develop in mediastinal, para-aortic and celiac lymph nodes.

In the TNM staging system commonly used for esophageal carcinoma, stages I and II represent operable disease, stage III denotes marginally resectable disease and stage IV signifies inoperable cancer. The last stage is characterized by metastases (M1). About 15% of cancers originate in the upper third of the esophagus (cervical and upper thoracic esophagus), 50% in the middle third and 35% in the lower third. The site of the primary tumor is critically important, as it relates to prognosis, clinical behavior (adjacent organ involvement, nodal metastases) and technical resectability. Primary surgical resection is possible in about 40–50% of cases. About one-third of patients are candidates for palliative surgery and 20–30% present with resectable stage III or IV disease. The 5-year survival rate is only 5% for stage IV disease, but is about 70% for stage I cancers.

Staging procedures involve triple endoscopy, including detailed ENT examination as well as bronchoscopy and esophagoscopy, owing to a high potential for development of other aerodigestive cancers because of similar risk factors. Mediastinoscopy, laparoscopy and CT scanning of the chest, liver and upper abdomen are important to determine the presence of nodal or visceral metastases. PET scanning has been shown to be highly sensitive in detecting occult metastases from esophageal cancer and is being increasingly used as a staging procedure.

CLINICAL MANIFESTATIONS

About 90% of patients present with dysphagia and weight loss, often accompanied by pain on swallowing (odynophagia). These symptoms characteristically appear with advanced disease, because difficulty in swallowing arises when at least 60% of the esophageal circumference is infiltrated by cancer. Other symptoms include regurgitation or emesis and discomfort in the throat, substernal area or epigastrium. In advanced disease, local invasion of the trachea, bronchi, lung or even aorta may result in aspiration pneumonia, massive hemorrhage, pleural effusion or SVC syndrome. Moreover, the development of one or more tracheo- or bronchoesophageal fistulae may also occur, as well as esophageal perforation and mediastinitis. Occasionally, patients present with supraclavicular lymph node, bone or liver metastases (*see* section on Gastric Cancers).

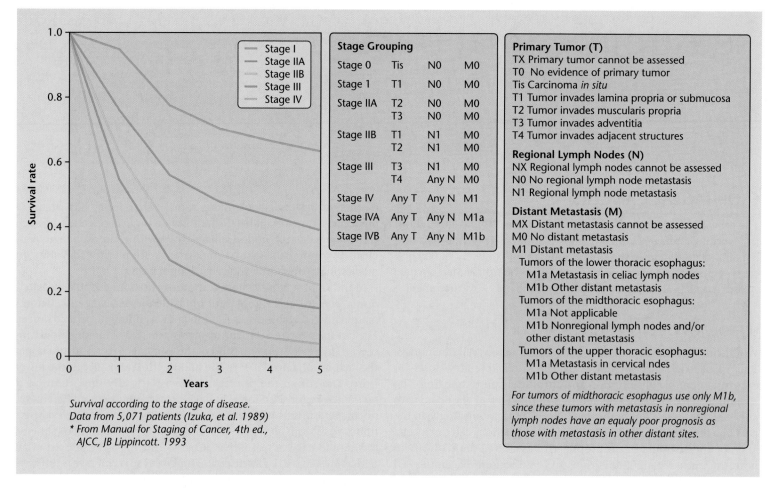

Stage Grouping			
Stage 0	Tis	N0	M0
Stage 1	T1	N0	M0
Stage IIA	T2	N0	M0
	T3	N0	M0
Stage IIB	T1	N1	M0
	T2	N1	M0
Stage III	T3	N1	M0
	T4	Any N	M0
Stage IV	Any T	Any N	M1
Stage IVA	Any T	Any N	M1a
Stage IVB	Any T	Any N	M1b

Primary Tumor (T)
TX Primary tumor cannot be assessed
T0 No evidence of primary tumor
Tis Carcinoma *in situ*
T1 Tumor invades lamina propria or submucosa
T2 Tumor invades muscularis propria
T3 Tumor invades adventitia
T4 Tumor invades adjacent structures

Regional Lymph Nodes (N)
NX Regional lymph nodes cannot be assessed
N0 No regional lymph node metastasis
N1 Regional lymph node metastasis

Distant Metastasis (M)
MX Distant metastasis cannot be assessed
M0 No distant metastasis
M1 Distant metastasis
    Tumors of the lower thoracic esophagus:
        M1a Metastasis in celiac lymph nodes
        M1b Other distant metastasis
    Tumors of the midthoracic esophagus:
        M1a Not applicable
        M1b Nonregional lymph nodes and/or
        other distant metastasis
    Tumors of the upper thoracic esophagus:
        M1a Metastasis in cervical ndes
        M1b Other distant metastasis

For tumors of midthoracic esophagus use only M1b, since these tumors with metastasis in nonregional lymph nodes have an equally poor prognosis as those with metastasis in other distant sites.

*Survival according to the stage of disease.
Data from 5,071 patients (Izuka, et al. 1989)
* From Manual for Staging of Cancer, 4th ed.,
AJCC, JB Lippincott. 1993*

Fig. 5.1 Staging of esophageal carcinoma.

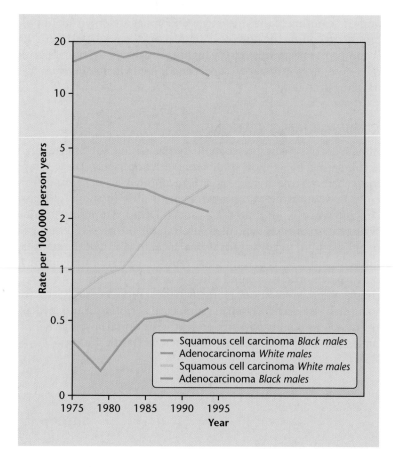

Fig. 5.2 Trends in age-adjusted incidence rates for esophageal carcinoma amongst US mates by race and cell type, 1974–76 to 1992–94 (from Devesa *et al.*, 1998).

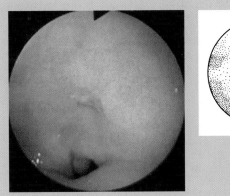
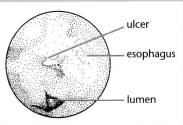

Fig. 5.3 Squamous cell carcinoma. Endoscopic view of the esophagus shows a tiny, early ulcer which proved on biopsy to be malignant.

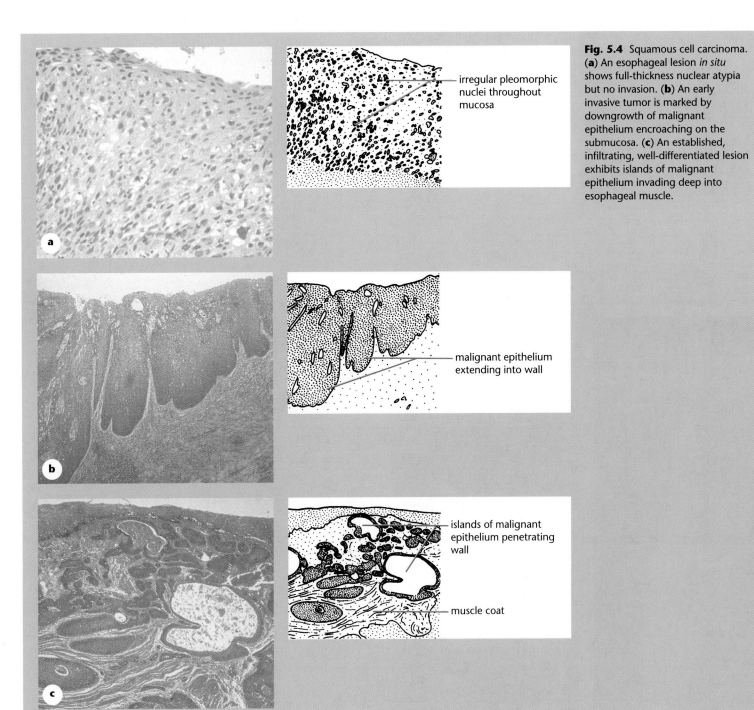

Fig. 5.4 Squamous cell carcinoma. (**a**) An esophageal lesion *in situ* shows full-thickness nuclear atypia but no invasion. (**b**) An early invasive tumor is marked by downgrowth of malignant epithelium encroaching on the submucosa. (**c**) An established, infiltrating, well-differentiated lesion exhibits islands of malignant epithelium invading deep into esophageal muscle.

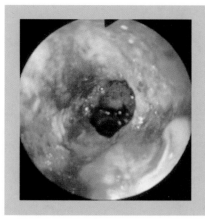

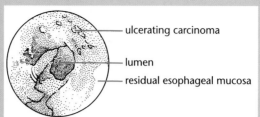

Fig. 5.5 Squamous cell carcinoma. Endoscopic view shows circumferential involvement of the esophagus with friable tumor. Note the narrowed lumen.

ulcerating carcinoma

lumen

residual esophageal mucosa

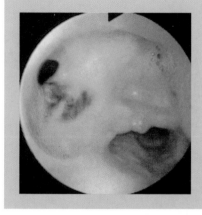

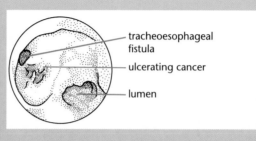

Fig. 5.6 Squamous cell carcinoma. Endoscopy shows a tracheo-esophageal fistula caused by an ulcerating esophageal squamous cancer. The orifice of the fistula tract is clearly visible.

tracheoesophageal fistula

ulcerating cancer

lumen

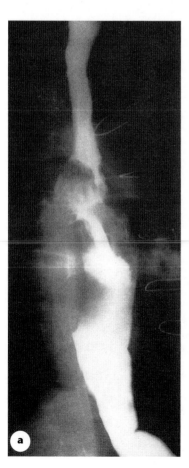

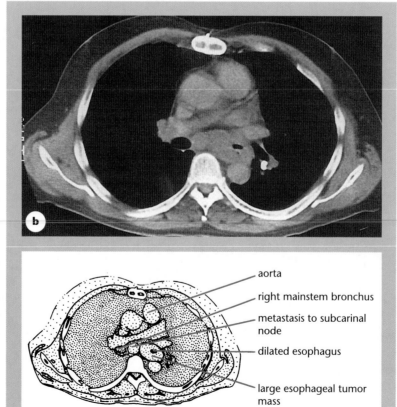

Fig. 5.7 Squamous cell carcinoma. A 62-year-old man with progressive dysphagia and marked weight loss was found on endoscopy to have a poorly differentiated tumor of the middle third of the esophagus. (**a**) Barium swallow film shows narrowing of the esophagus with mucosal destruction, consistent with esophageal cancer. (**b**) CT scan reveals regional metastases and a large primary mass obstructing the esophagus. Complete clinical remission was achieved in 3 months after combination chemotherapy plus radiotherapy. Unfortunately, liver metastases subsequently occurred.

aorta

right mainstem bronchus

metastasis to subcarinal node

dilated esophagus

large esophageal tumor mass

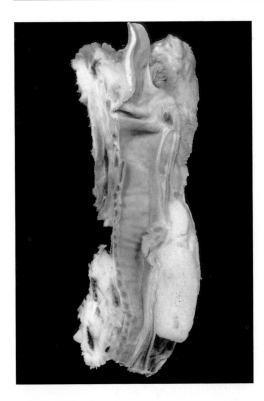

Fig. 5.8 Squamous cell carcinoma. This sagittal section through the larynx, trachea and anterior wall of the esophagus (on the right) was obtained at autopsy of a 57-year-old man who presented with a short history of dysphagia. A barium swallow revealed neoplastic obstruction of the esophagus; the patient died soon afterward from bronchopneumonia. A solid, raised, pale tumor (6 × 2 × 2 cm), arising in the esophagus, has infiltrated the posterior wall of the trachea, forming a nodular projection into the tracheal lumen. Anthracotic paratracheal lymph nodes are extensively infiltrated by pale tumor. This case clearly demonstrates the spread of esophageal carcinoma.

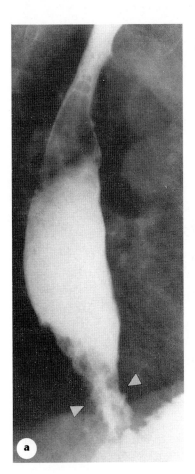

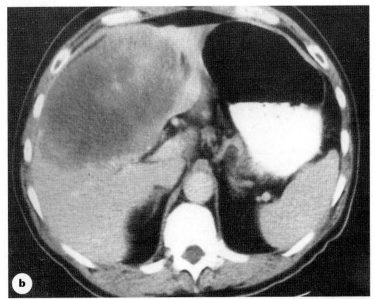

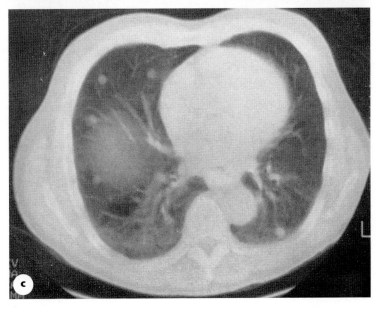

Fig. 5.9 Adenocarcinoma. Weight loss and right upper abdominal pain, with minimal dysphagia, developed in a 58-year-old man. Esophagoscopy showed a constricting, poorly differentiated lesion of the lower third of the esophagus. (**a**) Barium swallow film defines the extent of the lesion (arrows). On CT scan, (**b**) a large liver metastasis and (**c**) early pulmonary metastases are noted.

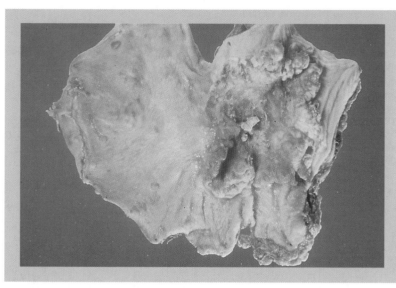
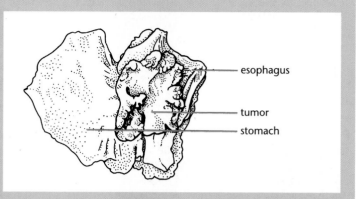

Fig. 5.10 Adenocarcinoma. This ulcerating tumor arose at the gastroesophageal junction where, as in this case, it is often impossible to distinguish an esophageal carcinoma from one arising in the gastric fundus and growing upward to involve the distal esophagus.

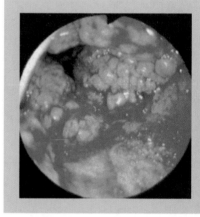
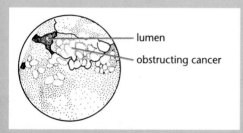

Fig. 5.11 Adenocarcinoma in Barrett's metaplasia. Endoscopic view demonstrates an extensive lesion arising in an area of Barrett's metaplasia; the lumen is obstructed by a bleeding and polypoid exophytic mass.

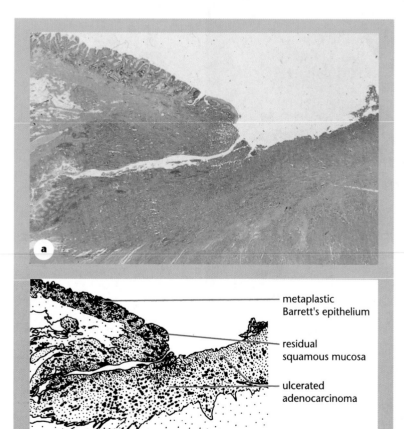
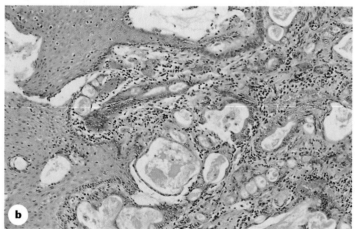

Fig. 5.12 Adenocarcinoma in Barrett's metaplasia. (**a**) Low-power photomicrograph shows esophageal tissue with metaplastic Barrett's epithelium, with columnar cells and villous changes. There is some residual esophageal squamous mucosa adjacent to an area of ulcerated adenocarcinoma. (**b**) High-power view shows glands of tumor encroaching on the squamous epithelium.

GASTRIC CANCERS

There is a marked variation in the incidence of gastric cancer worldwide. Death rates are highest in Costa Rica and Japan, where they are over 10-fold greater than those in the US. Nonetheless, both the incidence and the mortality rate of gastric cancer have decreased worldwide over the past 50 years. In 1930, gastric cancer was the leading cause of cancer-related deaths in men, with a US rate of 37 per 100 000, as compared with the current US rate of less than 6 per 100 000. In the US, the incidence of gastric cancer is higher in males than females, with reported male to female ratios as high as 2 : 1. The incidence of gastric cancer increases after age 50 and is highest in lower socio-economic groups.

Many etiologic influences have been proposed to explain the decreasing incidence of gastric cancer, mostly concerning dietary (environmental) factors and the increased availability of refrigeration, which reduces the growth of nitrate-producing bacteria in food. Another factor, loss of gastric acidity, may predispose to stomach cancer. This condition can be caused by partial gastrectomy, atrophic gastritis or achlorhydria with subsequent pernicious anemia. Chronic gastritis is frequently associated with gastric cancer and the presence of intestinal metaplasia further elevates the risk of gastric cancer. Recent studies suggest that infection with *Helicobacter pylori* is associated with gastric cancer, leading some to postulate a pathogenic role. Other premalignant lesions include adenomas, 40% of which may progress to carcinoma.

HISTOLOGY

About 90% of gastric malignancies are adenocarcinomas, with the remainder comprising malignant gastrointestinal stromal tumors (leiomyosarcomas) and lymphomas. Histologically, adenocarcinomas are classified as intestinal or diffuse. Intestinal-type cancers are characterized by cohesive neoplastic cells that form gland-like tubular structures resembling colonic adenocarcinomas. They are often preceded by premalignant changes (chronic atrophic gastritis and intestinal metaplasia) and may result in ulcerative lesions, particularly in the antrum or the lesser curvature. Diffuse-type cancers are composed of infiltrating gastric mucous or 'signet ring' cells that infrequently form masses or ulcers. They tend to occur throughout the stomach, often resulting in a linitis plastica ('leather bottle') appearance. Much of the decline in gastric cancer rates has been due to decreases in the intestinal type. Consequently, the diffuse-type adenocarcinomas have become relatively more common, accounting for up to one-third of cases. Diffuse-type malignancies are associated with a very poor prognosis, with a survival rate of less than 2%. Much of the pale 'tumor' tissue in this variant actually represents fibrosis of the submucosa and muscle.

Macroscopically, gastric cancers are classified into five categories. The ulcerative variant (25% of cases) may resemble a benign gastric ulcer. About 7% and 36% are polypoid and fungating tumors, respectively, and are nodular tumors which can reach a large size. The remaining 26% of gastric cancers show a scirrhous pattern caused by thickening and rigidity of the gastric wall due to diffuse infiltration by signet ring cells. The marked fibrous reaction results in the appearance of linitis plastica. The least common gross appearance is the superficial type, representing less than 6% of cases. The normal mucosa is replaced by sheet-like collections of malignant cells that do not invade beyond the submucosa. This type is categorized as early gastric cancer and represents potentially resectable (for cure) cancers.

STAGING OF GASTRIC CANCERS

A TNM staging system is used for gastric cancers. The 5-year survival rate is 60–90% for the uncommon cases that are detected in stage I of the disease, 30–70% for stage II, less than 20% for stage III and 3% for stage IV. A clinically useful system classifies cases as resectable, localized disease (stages I and II), regional disease (stage III) and unresectable or metastatic disease (stage IV).

Extensive local invasion by gastric cancer is common and most often involves the pancreas, omentum, transverse colon, liver or spleen; direct contiguous spread into the esophagus or duodenum is also common. Moreover, because gastric cancer so often penetrates the serosa, it is particularly prone to transperitoneal dissemination. Spread also occurs via lymphatics and blood vessels. Staging studies therefore include double-contrast radiographic evaluation and gastroscopy, with mucosal biopsy and abrasion balloon cytology of all suspicious lesions. Chest films and CT scans of liver, abdomen and pelvis should be obtained.

CLINICAL MANIFESTATIONS

Early gastric cancer is asymptomatic, thus most patients present with advanced disease. Symptoms include ulcer-related pain, anorexia, weight loss and vague epigastric distress. Development of left supraclavicular adenopathy (Virchow's node), an ovarian mass (Krukenberg tumor), hepatomegaly, ascites or anemia may be the initial manifestation. Gastric carcinoma is also a well-recognized cause of secondary pyloric stenosis in adulthood.

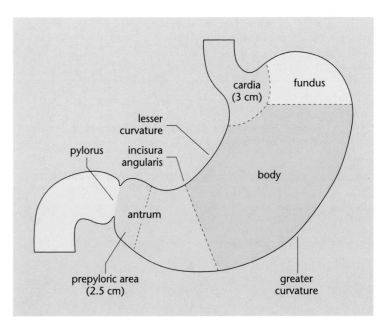

Fig. 5.13 Anatomic subdivisions of the stomach.

Table 5.1 Distribution of malignancies among subdivisions of the stomach.

Subdivision	Frequency (%)
Antrum and prepylorus	≥50
Cardia and fundus	~25
Lesser curvature	20
Greater curvature	3–5
Entire stomach	5–10

*2% of patients may have cancers in multiple sites

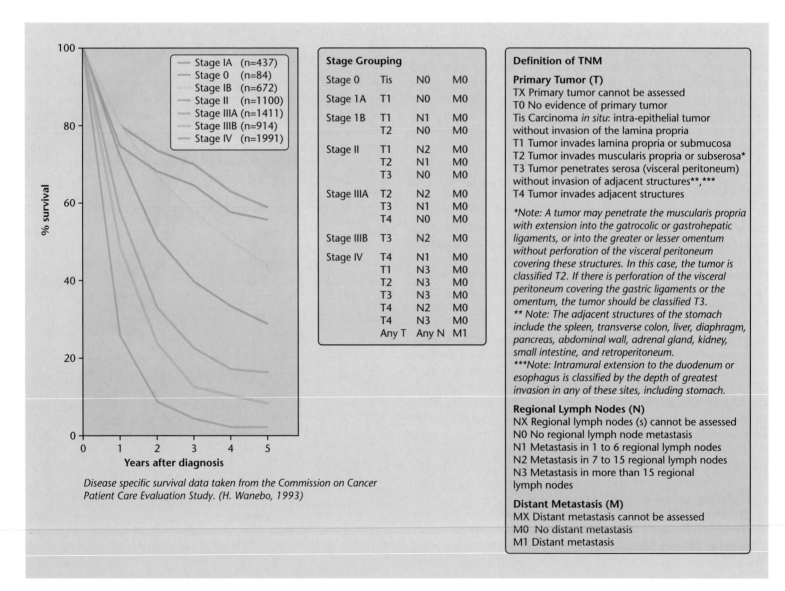

Disease specific survival data taken from the Commission on Cancer Patient Care Evaluation Study. (H. Wanebo, 1993)

Stage Grouping

Stage 0	Tis	N0	M0
Stage 1A	T1	N0	M0
Stage 1B	T1	N1	M0
	T2	N0	M0
Stage II	T1	N2	M0
	T2	N1	M0
	T3	N0	M0
Stage IIIA	T2	N2	M0
	T3	N1	M0
	T4	N0	M0
Stage IIIB	T3	N2	M0
Stage IV	T4	N1	M0
	T1	N3	M0
	T2	N3	M0
	T3	N3	M0
	T4	N2	M0
	T4	N3	M0
	Any T	Any N	M1

Definition of TNM

Primary Tumor (T)
TX Primary tumor cannot be assessed
T0 No evidence of primary tumor
Tis Carcinoma *in situ*: intra-epithelial tumor without invasion of the lamina propria
T1 Tumor invades lamina propria or submucosa
T2 Tumor invades muscularis propria or subserosa*
T3 Tumor penetrates serosa (visceral peritoneum) without invasion of adjacent structures**,***
T4 Tumor invades adjacent structures

Note: A tumor may penetrate the muscularis propria with extension into the gatrocolic or gastrohepatic ligaments, or into the greater or lesser omentum without perforation of the visceral peritoneum covering these structures. In this case, the tumor is classified T2. If there is perforation of the visceral peritoneum covering the gastric ligaments or the omentum, the tumor should be classified T3.
** Note: The adjacent structures of the stomach include the spleen, transverse colon, liver, diaphragm, pancreas, abdominal wall, adrenal gland, kidney, small intestine, and retroperitoneum.
***Note: Intramural extension to the duodenum or esophagus is classified by the depth of greatest invasion in any of these sites, including stomach.

Regional Lymph Nodes (N)
NX Regional lymph nodes (s) cannot be assessed
N0 No regional lymph node metastasis
N1 Metastasis in 1 to 6 regional lymph nodes
N2 Metastasis in 7 to 15 regional lymph nodes
N3 Metastasis in more than 15 regional lymph nodes

Distant Metastasis (M)
MX Distant metastasis cannot be assessed
M0 No distant metastasis
M1 Distant metastasis

Fig. 5.14 Staging of gastric carcinoma (from Flemming *et al.*, 1997).

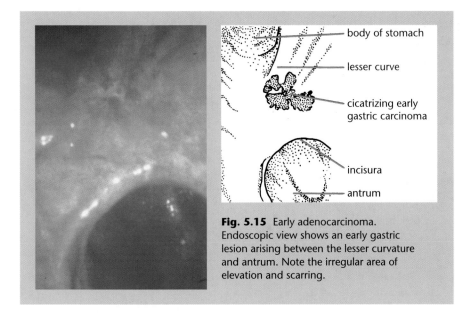

Fig. 5.15 Early adenocarcinoma. Endoscopic view shows an early gastric lesion arising between the lesser curvature and antrum. Note the irregular area of elevation and scarring.

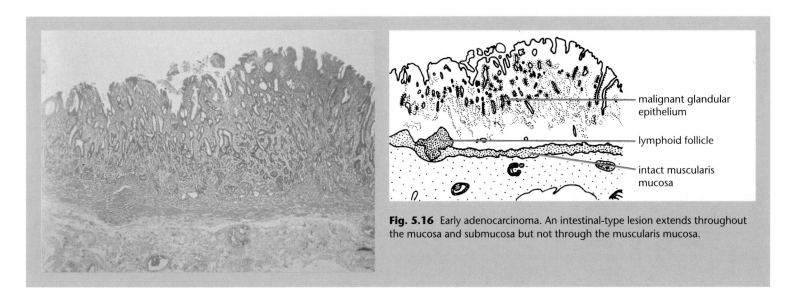

Fig. 5.16 Early adenocarcinoma. An intestinal-type lesion extends throughout the mucosa and submucosa but not through the muscularis mucosa.

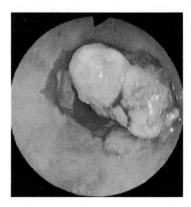

Fig. 5.17 Adenocarcinoma. Endoscopic view shows a lesion extending from the cardia into the distal esophagus.

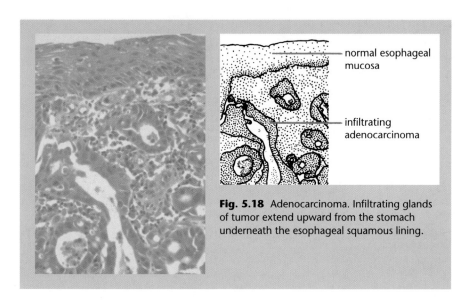

Fig. 5.18 Adenocarcinoma. Infiltrating glands of tumor extend upward from the stomach underneath the esophageal squamous lining.

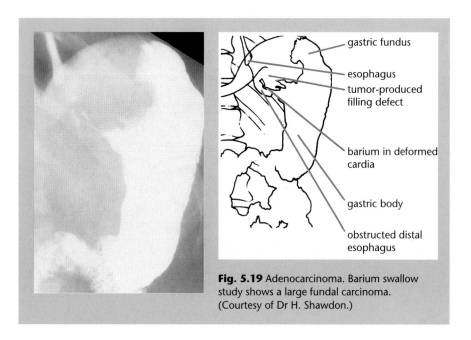

Fig. 5.19 Adenocarcinoma. Barium swallow study shows a large fundal carcinoma. (Courtesy of Dr H. Shawdon.)

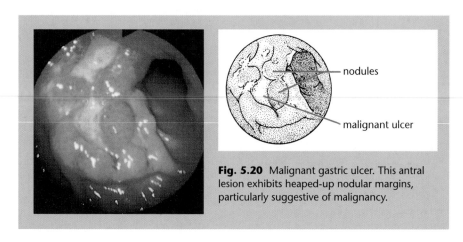

Fig. 5.20 Malignant gastric ulcer. This antral lesion exhibits heaped-up nodular margins, particularly suggestive of malignancy.

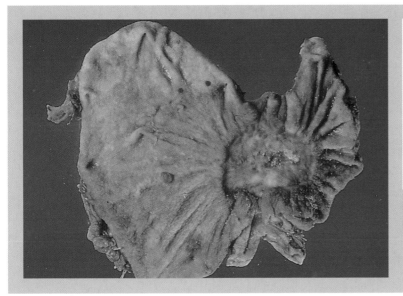

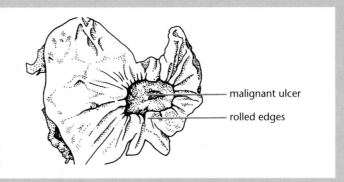

Fig. 5.21 Malignant gastric ulcer. Partial gastrectomy specimen shows a large malignant ulcer of the lesser curvature, with raised, rolled margins.

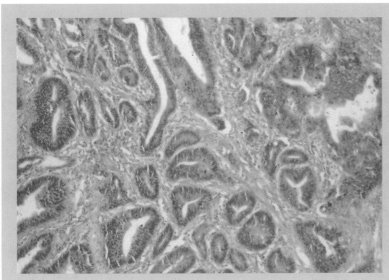

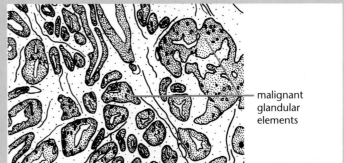

Fig. 5.22 Adenocarcinoma. This intestinal-type tumor exhibits well-formed malignant glandular elements.

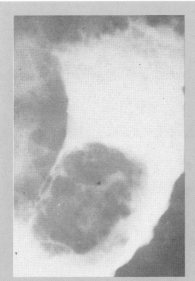

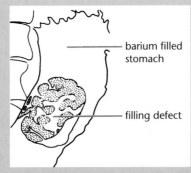

Fig. 5.23 Adenocarcinoma (polypoid type). Barium swallow study reveals a large polypoid lesion in the body of the stomach, causing a filling defect.

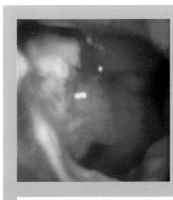

Fig. 5.24 Adenocarcinoma (fungating type). Endoscopic view reveals a hemorrhagic tumor near the lesser curvature, with ulceration and necrosis.

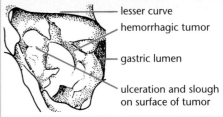

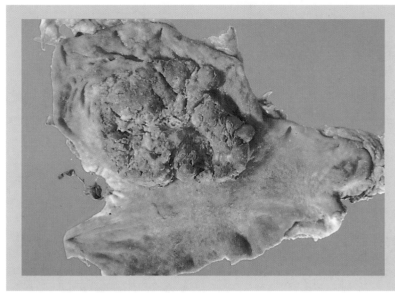

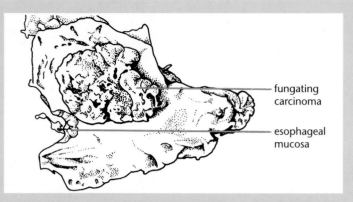

fungating carcinoma

esophageal mucosa

Fig. 5.25 Adenocarcinoma (fungating type). This specimen, opened along the greater curvature of the stomach, exhibits a large, fungating tumor occupying the lesser curvature.

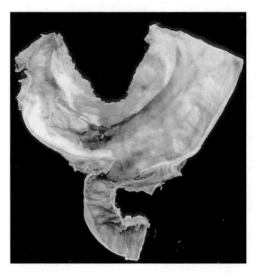

Fig. 5.26 Stenosing pyloric carcinoma. This postmortem specimen, showing the distal stomach and pylorus, is from an 84-year-old woman who presented with severe anemia and a 3-month history of weight loss. Palliative gastroenterostomy was performed 4 days before death. A localized, nodular, stenosing tumor, measuring 6 cm in diameter, can be seen in the pyloric canal. There is obvious deep mural invasion, but the proximal duodenum is completely unaffected. The gastroenterostomy, 2 cm proximal to the tumor, is patent.

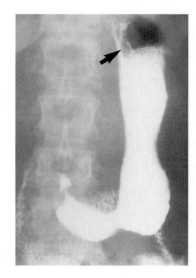

Fig. 5.27 Diffuse adenocarcinoma (linitis plastica). Barium study (erect view) shows the typical appearance of an extensive linitis plastica involving the entire stomach, which appears fixed and narrowed. No peristalsis was observed and barium flowed out of the stomach quickly. The mucosal edge is only slightly irregular; ulceration of the mucosa may be minimal or absent in this type of carcinoma. (Arrow indicates the gastric fundus.)

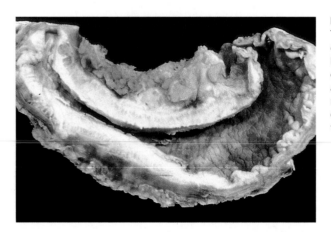

Fig. 5.28 Diffuse adenocarcinoma (linitis plastica). This gastrectomy specimen, opened anteriorly, is from a 64-year-old man who had a 3-year history of dyspepsia. Barium swallow and endoscopy revealed a gastric carcinoma. There is diffuse infiltration of the pylorus and body of the stomach by pale tumor, as well as marked luminal narrowing, although the tumor has no exophytic component. Note the irregular infiltration of the muscle coat.

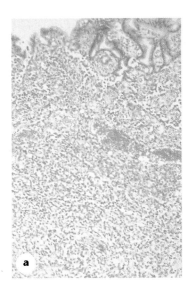

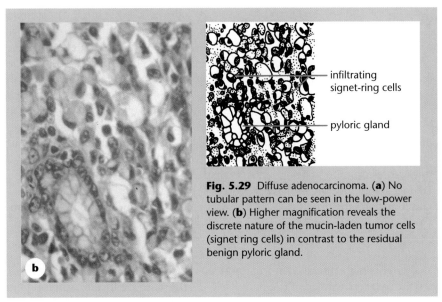

Fig. 5.29 Diffuse adenocarcinoma. (**a**) No tubular pattern can be seen in the low-power view. (**b**) Higher magnification reveals the discrete nature of the mucin-laden tumor cells (signet ring cells) in contrast to the residual benign pyloric gland.

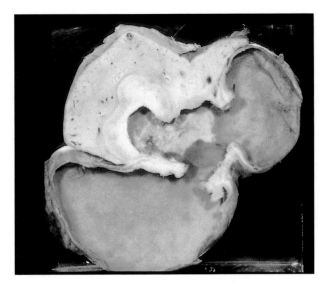

Fig. 5.30 Liver invasion. This specimen, showing the stomach opened anteriorly, is from a 62-year-old man who presented with a 6-month history of epigastric pain, vomiting and weight loss, as well as a palpable epigastric mass. Total gastrectomy with partial hepatic lobectomy was performed. An ulcerating neoplasm of the lesser curvature has spread extensively into the adherent hepatic parenchyma. Extensive local invasion by gastric cancer is common.

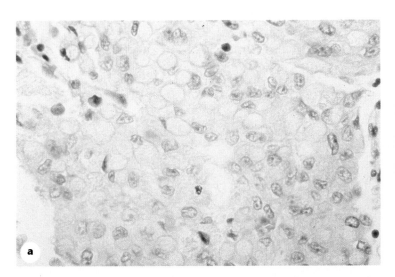

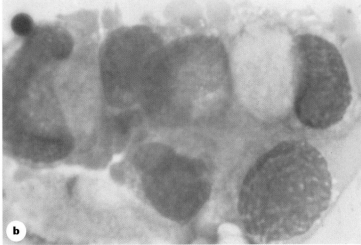

Fig. 5.31 Bone marrow metastases. A 60-year-old man presented with microangiopathic hemolytic anemia (MAHA). (**a**) Bone marrow biopsy shows metastatic mucin-producing adenocarcinoma. (**b**) High-power view of a bone marrow aspirate demonstrates a clump of malignant cells. Further evaluation revealed a primary gastric cancer. Chemotherapy led to a complete clinical remission lasting 9 months. Cancer-related MAHA is most commonly seen with gastric carcinoma. Fragmentation of red blood cells is due to many factors, including the shearing effect of fibrin strands secondary to disseminated intravascular coagulation (DIC) (associated with mucin-producing adenocarcinomas) or shearing by direct contact with intravascular tumor cells or with secondary proliferation of pulmonary arterioles.

PANCREATIC CANCERS

The increasing incidence of exocrine pancreatic cancers in the US reflects the aging of the population. About 30 000 new cases are diagnosed each year, with 25 000 deaths. It is the fourth most common cause of cancer-related mortality in adults in the US. The median age of patients with these tumors is approximately 70 years, with one-third of cases occurring in persons aged 75 years or older. About one-quarter of patients are under 60 years. The etiology remains obscure, except for a known association with cigarette smoking; pancreatic cancer is 2–4 times more common in heavy smokers than in non-smokers. Other risk factors include alcohol abuse, chronic pancreatitis and juvenile-onset diabetes mellitus.

HISTOLOGY

About 75% of pancreatic malignancies are ductal adenocarcinomas, of which approximately 70% occur in the head of the pancreas. A variety of uncommon types of pancreatic carcinoma have been described, including acinar, adenosquamous, anaplastic, papillary, mucous and microadenocarcinomas, each of which comprises less than 5% of the total. All of these have similarly poor prognoses and are treated in a similar fashion. Also uncommon are mucinous cystic neoplasms (cystadenoma/cystadenocarcinoma) of the pancreas, which occur most frequently in middle-aged women. These are typically located in the tail of the pancreas. Clinical behavior can be difficult to predict pathologically, leading some to conclude that all mucinous cystic neoplasms of the pancreas have malignant potential. Complete surgical resection results in cure rates of 30–60%. The remaining 5–10% of pancreatic neoplasms are predominantly islet cell derived (*see* Chapter 7). Other rare neoplasms include pancreatoblastomas, most of which occur in children, and the solid and cystic neoplasms. The latter occurs most frequently in young women and carries an excellent prognosis following resection.

STAGING OF PANCREATIC CANCERS

Pancreatic cancer most commonly presents at an advanced stage. Early or local disease (stage I), with cancer confined to the pancreas, is unusual. Regional disease (stage II or III) is more common and includes tumor invasion into the bile duct, duodenum, adjacent peripancreatic tissue or adjacent lymph nodes. Extensive disease (stage IV) signifies either invasion of tumor into the stomach, colon, spleen or blood vessels, or the presence of distant metastases. The overall prognosis of pancreatic carcinoma (excluding mucinous cystic neoplasms) is dismal, with a median survival time of 3–5 months and a 5-year survival rate of 1%.

Staging procedures include ultrasonography, CT scanning and magnetic resonance imaging. A diagnostic laparoscopy may also be performed to detect peritoneal disease that is not visible radiologically. Regardless of these studies, an accurate histologic diagnosis is necessary to distinguish benign disease from carcinoma, islet cell tumors and retroperitoneal lymphomas, owing to the major therapeutic and prognostic differences between these disease entities. When liver metastases are present, fine-needle aspiration biopsy is often successful in establishing a diagnosis of metastatic disease. In the case of locally unresectable disease, endoscopic retrograde cholangiopancreatography (ERCP) or fine-needle aspiration may be used. In the setting of a resectable pancreatic mass, biopsy may be deferred in favor of proceeding directly with surgical resection.

CLINICAL MANIFESTATIONS

Carcinoma of the head of the pancreas leads to jaundice caused by biliary obstruction. The gallbladder is usually distended (Courvoisier's sign). Carcinomas of the body and tail are accompanied by severe pain resulting from retroperitoneal invasion and infiltration of the celiac ganglia and splanchnic nerves. About 75% of patients present with pain and progressive weight loss. Splenomegaly, due to encasement and obstruction of the splenic vein, may also occur. Other features include depression, diabetes mellitus (5–10% of cases), alterations in bowel function (particularly obstipation) and venous thrombosis with migratory thrombophlebitis (Trousseau's sign; *see* section on Hepatobiliary Cancers).

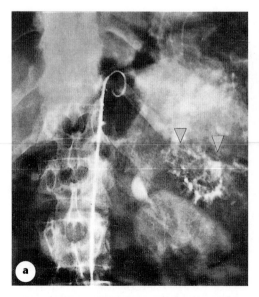
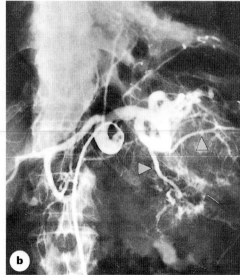
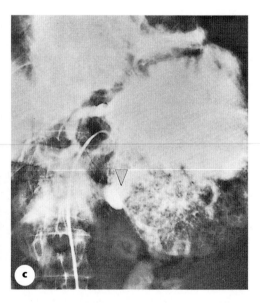

Fig. 5.32 Cystadenoma-cystadenocarcinoma. Cystadenomas and cystadenocarcinomas are often quite large at the time of clinical detection. (**a**) As their names imply, both tumors contain cystic elements and both frequently show internal calcification, often in a stellate pattern (arrows).

(**b,c**) The tumor is typically hypervascular, angiography demonstrates hypertrophied pancreatic branches (arrows) of the splenic artery feeding the lesion in the tail of the pancreas.

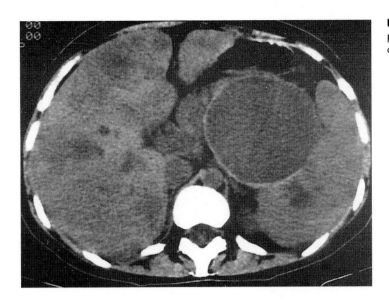

Fig. 5.33 Cystadenocarcinoma. CT scan of a 33-year-old woman who presented with metastatic disease shows one of several large pancreatic cysts and many liver metastases.

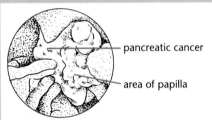

pancreatic cancer

area of papilla

Fig. 5.34 Pancreatic carcinoma. Endoscopic view shows a tumor invading the duodenal wall just above the papilla of the pancreatic duct. The folds are irregular and nodular.

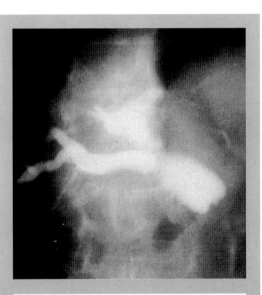

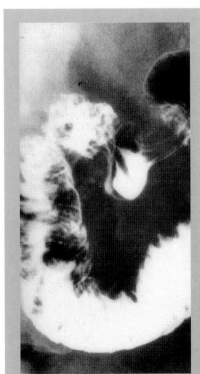

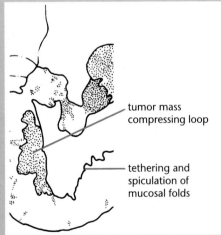

tumor mass compressing loop

tethering and spiculation of mucosal folds

Fig. 5.35 Pancreatic carcinoma. Barium study shows a tumor mass in the head of the pancreas invading the duodenal loop and producing changes in the fold pattern.

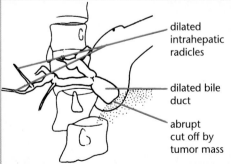

dilated intrahepatic radicles

dilated bile duct

abrupt cut off by tumor mass

Fig. 5.36 Pancreatic carcinoma. Percutaneous transhepatic cholangiogram demonstrates obstruction of the common bile duct by tumor, which produced jaundice in this patient.

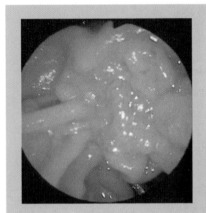

127

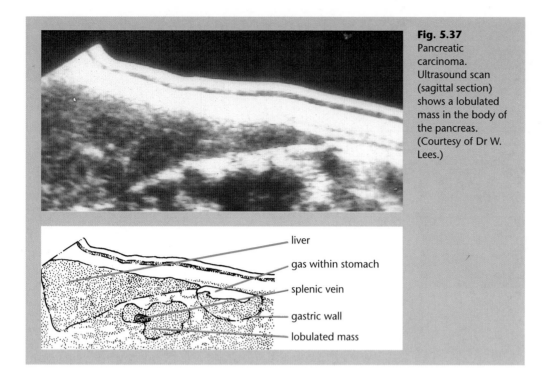

Fig. 5.37 Pancreatic carcinoma. Ultrasound scan (sagittal section) shows a lobulated mass in the body of the pancreas. (Courtesy of Dr W. Lees.)

liver

gas within stomach

splenic vein

gastric wall

lobulated mass

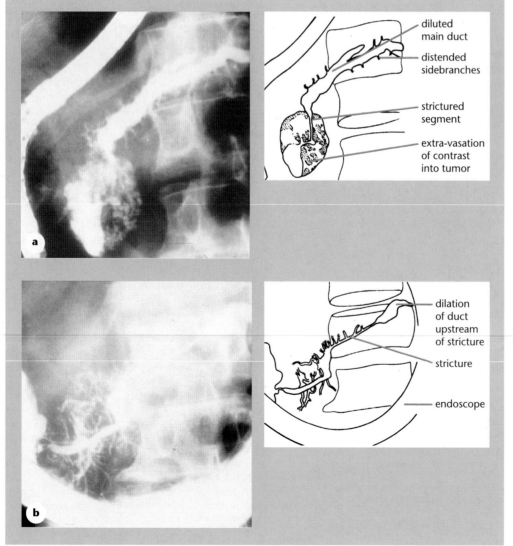

diluted main duct

distended sidebranches

strictured segment

extra-vasation of contrast into tumor

dilation of duct upstream of stricture

stricture

endoscope

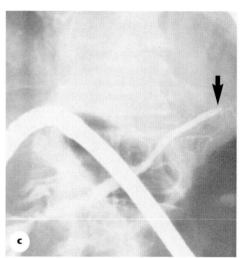

Fig. 5.38 Pancreatic carcinoma. Endoscopic retrograde cholangiopancreatography (ERCP) shows stricture of the pancreatic duct with dilatation upstream due to carcinoma. Shown are examples of carcinoma of the head (**a**), body (**b**) and tail (**c**) of the pancreas producing obstruction of the pancreatic duct (arrow).

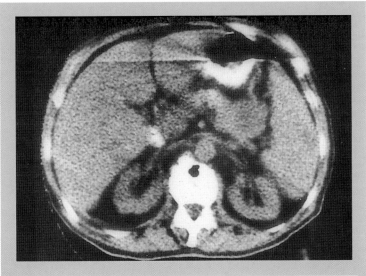

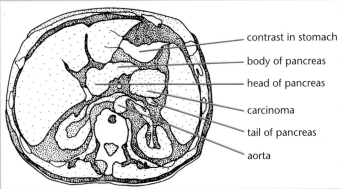

contrast in stomach

body of pancreas

head of pancreas

carcinoma

tail of pancreas

aorta

Fig. 5.39 Pancreatic carcinoma. Abdominal CT scan shows a large focal mass in the tail of the pancreas.

Definition of TNM

Primary Tumor (T)

TX	Primary tumor cannot be assessed
T0	No evidence of primary tumor
Tis	In situ carcinoma
T1	Tumor limited to the pancreas 2 cm or less in greatest dimension
T2	Tumor limited to the pancreas more than 2 cm in greatest dimension
T3	Tumor extends directly into any of the following: duodenum, bile duct, peripancreatic tissues
T4	Tumor extends directly into any of the following: stomach, spleen, colon, £ Adjacent large vessels

Regional Lymph Nodes (N)

NX	Regional lymph nodes cannot be assessed
N0	No regional lymph node metastasis
N1	Regional lymph node metastasis
	pN1a Metastasis in a single regional lymph node
	pN1a Metastasis in multiple regional lymph nodes

Distant Metastasis (M)

MX	Distant metastasis cannot be assessed
M0	No distant metastasis
M1	Distant metastasis

Stage grouping

Stage	Tis	N0	M0
Stage I	T1	N0	M0
	T2	N0	M0
Stage II	T3	N0	N0
Stage III	T1	N1	M0
	T2	N1	M0
	T3	N1	M0
Stage IVA	T4	Any N	M0
Stage IVB	Any T	Any N	M1

Fig. 5.40 Staging of pancreatic carcinoma (from Flemming *et al.*, 1997).

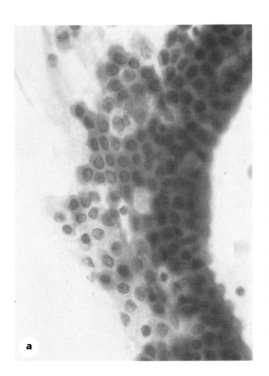

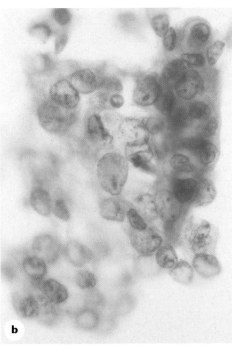

a

b

Fig. 5.41 Benign vs. malignant pancreatic cytology. In contrast to (**a**) a sheet of benign ductal cells, (**b**) malignant cells exhibit the usual characteristics of malignancy: an increased nucleus to cytoplasm ratio, hyperchromatic nuclei and irregular nuclear contours. Note the uniform distribution of the benign, compared to the malignant, cells.

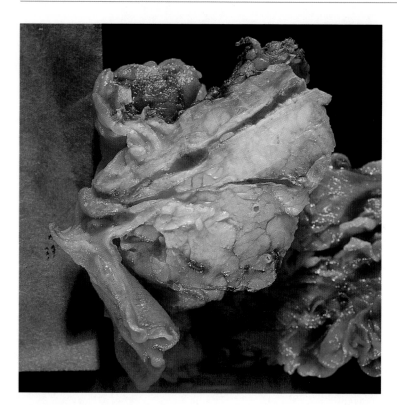

Fig. 5.42
Adenocarcinoma of the pancreas often appears as a diffuse infiltrative, tan/white fibrotic lesion effacing the normal lobular architecture of the pancreatic parenchyma, as shown here in the head of the pancreas (between the pancreatic and common bile ducts) in a Whipple resection specimen. Note: (1) ampulla, (2) common bile duct, (3) cancer, (4) pancreatic duct, (5) duodenal wall.

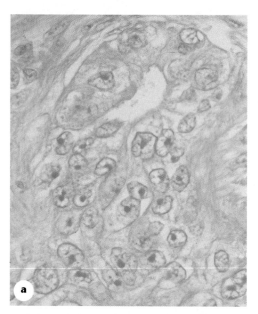

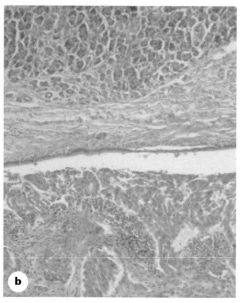

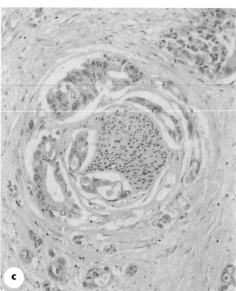

Fig. 5.43 Pancreatic carcinoma. Three histologic patterns may be found in pancreatic carcinoma. (**a**) Well-differentiated tumors are marked by well-formed glands of tumor cells. (**b**) In this moderately differentiated lesion, nests of tumor cells produce a squamoid configuration. (**c**) Pancreatic carcinomas typically induce an intense desmoplastic response. Perineural tumor invasion is also a frequent finding. In some cases, diagnosis of malignancy from a needle biopsy which samples only the desmoplastic stroma may be difficult to distinguish from dense fibrosis in chronic pancreatitis.

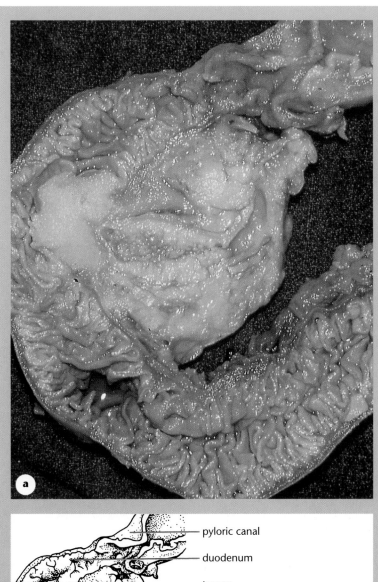

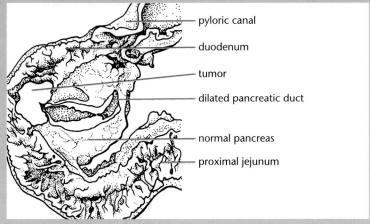

- pyloric canal
- duodenum
- tumor
- dilated pancreatic duct
- normal pancreas
- proximal jejunum

Fig. 5.44 Pancreatic carcinoma. These autopsy specimens demonstrate (**a**) a carcinoma invading the head of the pancreas, infiltrating the duodenum and destroying the pancreatic duct, and tumors (**b**) of the body (arrows) and (**c**) tail. Note the well-demarcated masses and areas of necrosis. (**a**: Courtesy of Mr M. Knight; **b**: courtesy of Dr J. Newman.)

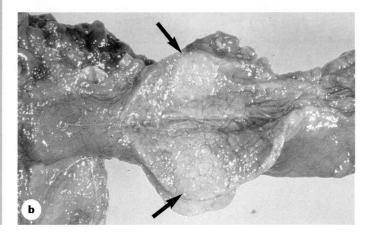

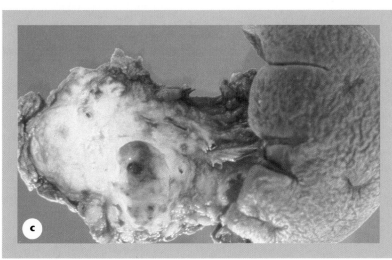

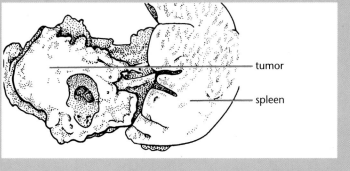

- tumor
- spleen

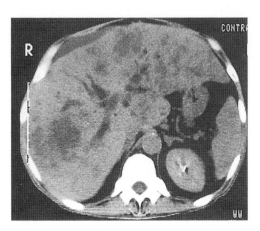

Fig. 5.45 Liver metastases. Abdominal CT scan in a patient with pancreatic carcinoma shows an enlarged, abnormal-looking liver, with dilated bile ducts centrally (to which the patient's jaundice can be ascribed) and widespread metastases more peripherally. Other CT sections showed a mass in the head of the pancreas.

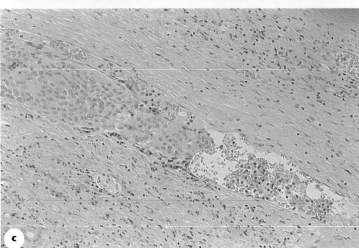

a

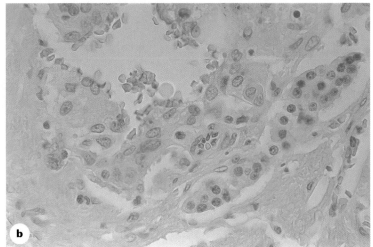

b

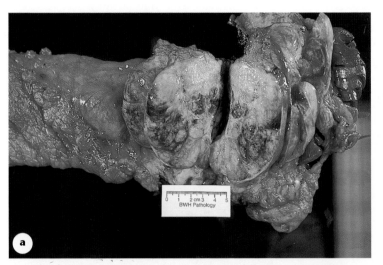

c

Fig. 5.46 (**a**) Solid pseudopapillary tumor of the pancreas, as shown here in the tail of the pancreas (P) abutting the spleen (S), typically has hemorrhagic/necrotic foci on gross examination; occasionally such foci impart a pseudocystic appearance (not shown). The tumor is classically encountered as an incidental finding or as a cause of abdominal pain in young adult females. The cytologic appearance on direct smears prepared from fine-needle aspirates is characteristic: loosely cohesive tumor cells appear to show off a 'pseudopapilla', that is, a core of myxoid stroma containing a central capillary. Although more than 95% of patients are cured by excision alone, this case showed cytologic atypia (**b**), vascular invasion (**c**) and frequent mitoses (not shown), warranting designation as the malignant variant of solid pseudopapillary tumor. An isolated metastasis in the lesser sac was identified at the time of resection (not shown).

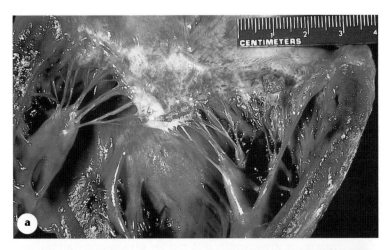

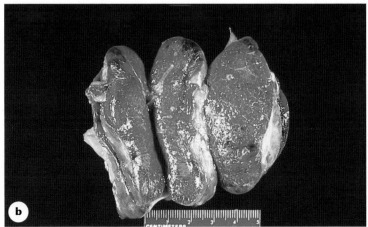

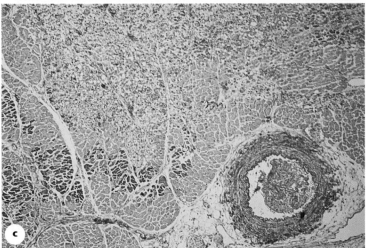

Fig. 5.47 (**a**) Non-bacterial thrombotic endocarditis (NBTE). A 70-year-old man with pancreatic cancer developed fatal pulmonary and cerebral emboli. Autopsy findings included classic features of NBTE, characterized by sterile thrombi without inflammation at the lines of closure of cardiac valve leaflets (arrows). This complication is associated with the hypercoaguable state classically referred to as the Trousseau syndrome in patients with mucinous adenocarcinoma. The thrombi may embolize or disseminated intravascular coagulation may supervene, leading to vascular occlusion in end organs such as the spleen, which displays wedge-shaped hemorrhagic infarcts (**b**, arrows), or the heart, where microscopy reveals a thrombus in a small muscular artery supplying an organizing, infarcted zone of myocardium (**c**).

HEPATOBILIARY CANCERS

LIVER CANCERS

Hepatocellular carcinoma is relatively rare in the US although in parts of Africa and Asia it is one of the most common forms of malignant disease – a difference probably attributable to environmental influences (including diet and the increased incidence of hepatitis B). In the US hepatocellular carcinoma is the cause of 3000–4000 deaths per year, mainly in elderly patients. About 60–80% of these cases are preceded by and associated with hepatic cirrhosis. In contrast to the US, in areas of high incidence, hepatocellular carcinoma often occurs without cirrhosis in middle-aged patients. Risk factors include hereditary hemochromatosis, hepatitis B infection and possibly hepatitis C viral infection and other causes of cirrhosis, including alcohol abuse, schistosome infestation and homozygous α1-antitrypsin deficiency. Non-cirrhotic causes include chronic ingestion of food containing aflatoxins (metabolites of the mold *Aspergillus flavus*), plant derivatives found in 'bush tea' (cycasin and pyrrolizidine) and possibly long-term use of androgens or oral contraceptives.

Hepatocellular carcinomas (hepatomas) have a wide range of histologic appearances, from well-differentiated tumors (which may be difficult to distinguish from regenerative nodules) to anaplastic malignancies. Diagnostic studies include CT-guided needle core biopsy and fine-needle aspiration biopsy, radionuclide scanning, ultrasonography, liver CT scanning and determination of α-fetoprotein (AFP) level. The AFP is elevated in about 70% of cases, usually above 400 ng/ml (normal 20–40 ng/ml). Unfortunately, AFP is also increased in certain benign diseases (e.g. hepatitis) and in other malignancies (germ cell tumors and gastric, pancreatic and pulmonary cancers). Hepatic angiography can be informative, showing a hypervascular tumor, and can also delineate the anatomic distribution for evaluating the possibility of successful resection.

The AJCC staging system for hepatocellular carcinoma is based on tumor size, number of tumor nodules, involvement of one or more liver lobes, vascular invasion, nodal metastases and presence or absence of distant metastases. In Africa one proposed clinical staging system is based on risk factors, the presence or absence of ascites, weight loss, portal hypertension and jaundice. In general, surgical resectability is the most important factor, as hepatocellular carcinomas are highly resistant to chemotherapy. The ability to resect the tumor completely while leaving adequate liver to support life is critical. The highest success rates have been in patients with incidental hepatocellular carcinomas discovered at transplantation for chronic liver disease. Survival in unresectable tumors varies from less than 2 months for advanced disease to 3 or more months for early hepatoma. Selected patients with resectable tumors may do significantly better, with some series reporting 10-year survival rates of nearly 20%.

Clinical manifestations depend on the presence or absence of underlying cirrhosis. In the latter case, the presence of hepatoma may be heralded by sudden deterioration of hepatic function, leading rapidly to death. The most frequent presenting symptom, however, is weight loss associated with a painful mass in the epigastrium or right upper quadrant. The sudden development of ascites may be due to a Budd–Chiari syndrome (hepatic vein obstruction or thrombosis). Clinically evident metastases are not common and occur mainly to the lung and bones. Hepatic cancer may be accompanied by any of several paraneoplastic syndromes, including erythrocytosis, hypercalcemia, hypoglycemia, dysfibrinogenemia and thrombocytosis.

BILIARY TRACT CANCERS

Carcinoma of the gallbladder is uncommon, causing about 3000 deaths per year in the United States. The malignancy is most often an incidental pathologic finding at the time of cholecystectomy for cholelithiasis and is present in 0.2–5% of patients who undergo cholecystectomy; there is a female predominance. The presence of gallstones is strongly associated with gallbladder cancer, particularly gallstones of large size. However, the incidence of gallbladder carcinoma in patients with gallstones is only 1%.

Over half the malignancies discovered at an early stage originate in the fundus of the gallbladder. These early cases have an increased chance of long-term survival. Unfortunately, the majority of patients present with involvement of the entire gallbladder and the 5-year survival rate is only 5%. Histologically, 85–95% of cases are adenocarcinomas, with the remainder comprising squamous cell carcinomas and other rare malignancies. Most patients die as the result of direct invasion of the liver, although metastases to other sites, particularly regional lymph nodes, may occur.

Cholangiocarcinomas, which are more commonly extra- than intrahepatic in origin, are primary carcinomas of the bile ducts. They may be located in the common duct (40% of cases), the confluence of the cystic, common and hepatic ducts (24%), hepatic ducts and bifurcation (19%), common hepatic duct (10%) and cystic duct (7%). This tumor typically arises in late adult life, in either sex, and, unlike carcinoma of the gallbladder, shows no association with cholelithiasis. In some Asians, biliary infestation with the fluke *Clonorchis sinensis* is a predisposing factor. In other cases, an association with choledochal cysts or ulcerative colitis and associated primary sclerosing cholangitis may be present. Virtually all cases are adenocarcinomas, with variable degrees of mucus production, fibroblastic reaction and in some cases anaplasia. Jaundice is present in most patients, associated with severe pruritus and pain. Cure is rare but is occasionally achieved by radical surgery.

Carcinomas of the ampulla of Vater are uncommon but unique: they have a high potential for cure because cases can sometimes be diagnosed at an early stage, owing to their tendency to cause obstructive jaundice early in the course of the disease. Most tumors are papillary and histologically are moderately to well-differentiated adenocarcinomas. The presenting symptoms include jaundice, pain, pruritus, fever and weakness due to blood loss. A characteristic sign is caused by incorporation of blood into the acholic and fat-laden stool, which produces the 'silver stool' sign of Thomas.

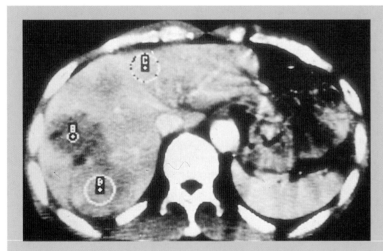

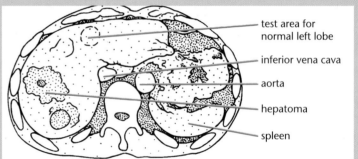

test area for normal left lobe

inferior vena cava

aorta

hepatoma

spleen

Fig. 5.48 Hepatoma. CT scan shows a diffuse lesion in the right lobe of an otherwise normal liver.

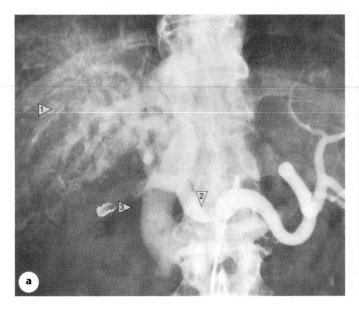

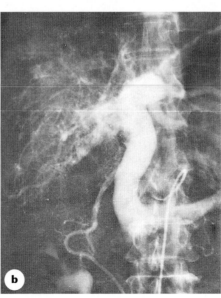

Fig. 5.49 Hepatocellular carcinoma with esophageal varices. A 72-year-old man presented with massive upper GI bleeding. (**a**) Celiac arteriogram shows a hypervascular mass in the liver (arrow 1). There is massive shunting from the hepatic artery (arrow 2) to the main portal vein (arrow 3). (**b**) Later-phase film shows further filling of the portal vein and hepatofungal flow, causing the variceal bleeding.

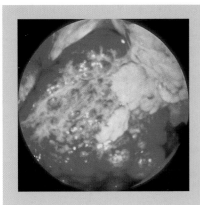

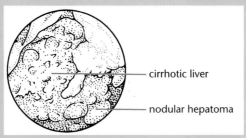

cirrhotic liver

nodular hepatoma

Fig. 5.50 Hepatocellular carcinoma. Laparoscopic view shows a cirrhotic liver with a nodular hepatoma.

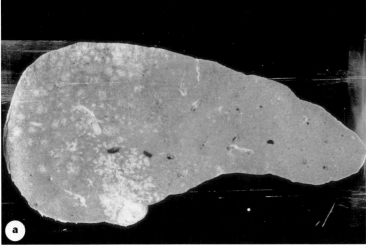

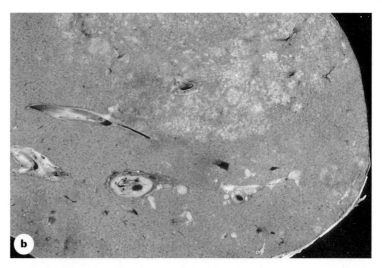

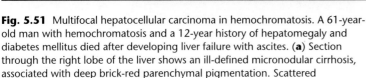

Fig. 5.51 Multifocal hepatocellular carcinoma in hemochromatosis. A 61-year-old man with hemochromatosis and a 12-year history of hepatomegaly and diabetes mellitus died after developing liver failure with ascites. (**a**) Section through the right lobe of the liver shows an ill-defined micronodular cirrhosis, associated with deep brick-red parenchymal pigmentation. Scattered throughout the posterior region are many pale nodules of carcinoma. (**b**) The right main portal vein and its branches are occluded by similar pale neoplastic tissue. Multifocal hepatocellular carcinoma is the most common type of malignancy (about two-thirds of cases) arising in cases of long-standing hemochromatosis.

Definition of TNM

Primary Tumor (T)
TX Primary tumor cannot be assessed
T0 No evidence of primary tumor
T1 Solitary tumor 2 cm or less in greatest dimension without vascular invasion
T2 Solitary tumor 2 cm or less n greatest dimension with vascular invasion, or multiple tumors limited to one lobe, none more than 2 cm in greatest dimension without vascular invasion, or solitary tumor more than 2 cm in greatest dimension without vascular invasion
T3 Solitary tumor more than 2 cm in greatest dimension with vascular invasion, or multiple tumors limited to one lobe, none more than 2 cm in greatest dimension, with vascular invasion, or multiple tumors limited to one lobe, any more than 2 cm in greatest dimension, with or without vascular invasion.
T4 Multiple tumors in more than one lobe or tumor(s) involve(s) a major branch of the portal or hepatic vein(s) or invasion of adjacent organs other than the gallbladder or perforation of the visceral peritoneum

Regional Lymph Nodes (N)
NX Regional lymph nodes cannot be assessed
N0 No regional lymph node metastasis
N1 Regional lymph node metastasis

Distant Metastasis (M)
MX Distant metastasis cannot be assessed
M0 No distant metastasis
M1 Distant metastasis

Stage grouping

Stage	T	N	M
Stage I	T1	N0	M0
Stage II	T1	N0	M0
Stage IIIA	T3	N0	M0
Stage IIIB	T1	N1	M0
	T2	N1	M0
	T3	M1	M0
Stage IVA	T4	Any N	M0
Stage IVB	Any T	Any N	M1

Fig. 5.52 Staging of hepatocellular carcinoma (including intrahepatic bile ducts) (from Flemming *et al.*, 1997).

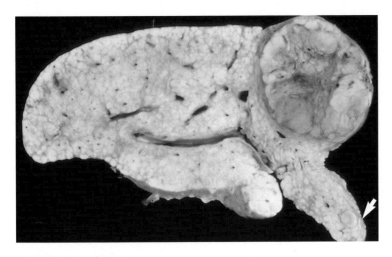

Fig. 5.53 Uninodular hepatocellular carcinoma. Autopsy of a 77-year-old man who collapsed and died while undergoing treatment in a psychiatric hospital revealed rupture of a hepatic tumor through the visceral peritoneum; death resulted from exsanguination with hemoperitoneum. The cut surface of the liver shows fine, uniform, micronodular cirrhosis. A rounded, apparently well-circumscribed, partly bile-stained tumor (6.5 cm in diameter) arises near the diaphragmatic surface. A smaller nodule of similar tumor is apparent at the bottom right (arrow). The uninodular type of hepatocellular carcinoma represents about 30% of cases. An encapsulated type, which is rare in the US but common in Japan, has a slightly better prognosis.

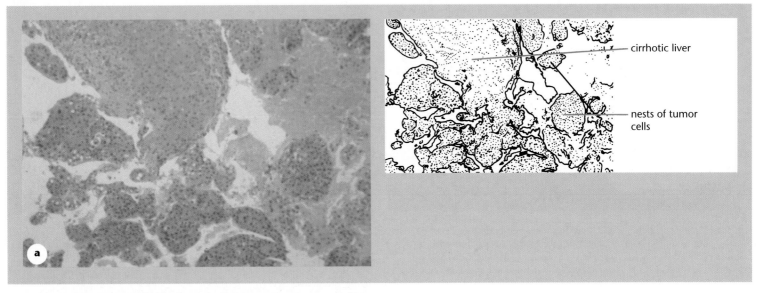

cirrhotic liver

nests of tumor cells

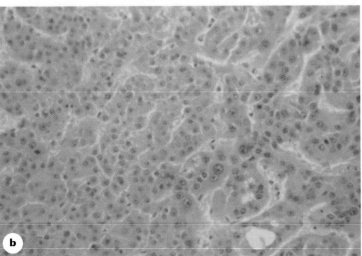

Fig. 5.54 Hepatocellular carcinoma. (**a**) Low-power photomicrograph shows a typical fragmented biopsy specimen, with nests of tumor cells and a fragment of cirrhotic liver. The malignant cells resemble normal liver cells and may be well differentiated. (**b**) At higher magnification, however, the cells are often pleomorphic, with prominent nucleoli. Immunoperoxidase stains for AFP, α1-antitrypsin, carcinoembryonic antigen and cytokeratins are useful in distinguishing hepatocellular carcinoma from metastatic tumors.

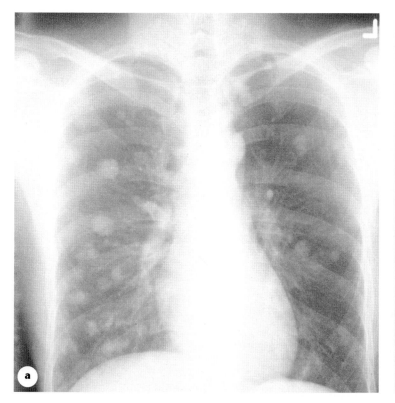

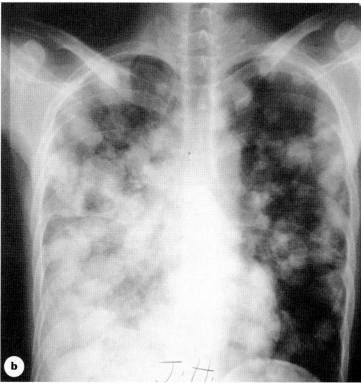

Fig. 5.55 Lung metastases. (**a**) Chest film of a 19-year-old Asian man who presented with hepatocellular carcinoma shows the well-defined pulmonary nodules characteristic of metastatic deposits. (**b**) Rapid disease progression occurred within 2 months. Metastases are unusual with hepatoma but do occur to the bones, lung and brain.

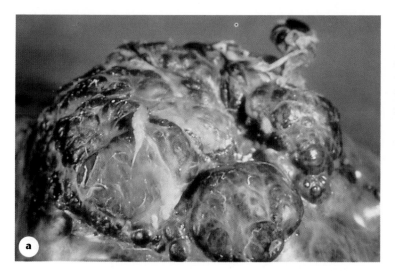

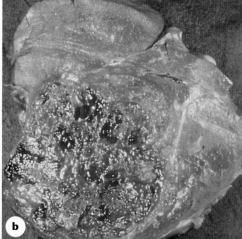

Fig. 5.56 Primary hepatic angiosarcoma. Typically, these tumors may appear as (**a**) a surface vascular tumor or (**b**) a hemorrhagic tumor mass. They are associated with industrial exposure to vinyl chloride and the radiographic contrast agent Thorotrast and usually comprise multicentric hemorrhagic nodules. (Courtesy of Prof. K. Weinbren.).

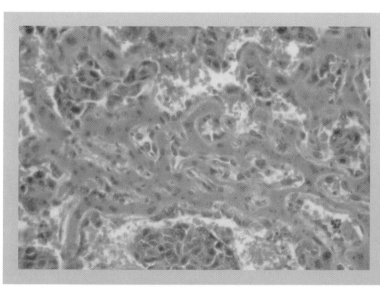

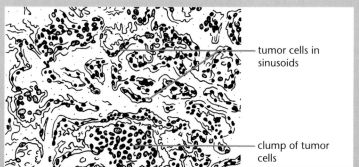

tumor cells in sinusoids

clump of tumor cells

Fig. 5.57 Primary hepatic angiosarcoma. Its characteristic pattern is marked by growth of tumor cells along the sinusoids.

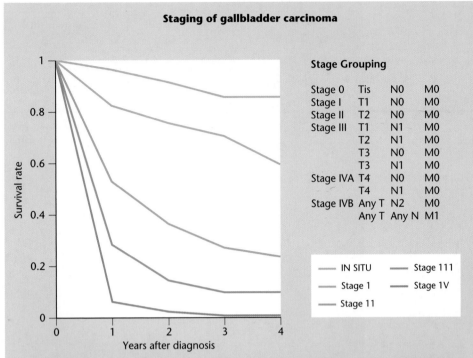

Staging of gallbladder carcinoma

Survival rate vs Years after diagnosis

Stage Grouping

Stage 0	Tis	N0	M0
Stage I	T1	N0	M0
Stage II	T2	N0	M0
Stage III	T1	N1	M0
	T2	N1	M0
	T3	N0	M0
	T3	N1	M0
Stage IVA	T4	N0	M0
	T4	N1	M0
Stage IVB	Any T	N2	M0
	Any T	Any N	M1

Legend: IN SITU, Stage 1, Stage 11, Stage 111, Stage 1V

Relative survival rates for 877 patients with gallbladder cancer. Data taken from the Surveillance, Epidemiology, and End Results Program of the National Cancer Institute for the years 1983–1987. Stage 0 includes 40 patients; stage I, 105; Stage II, 101; Stage III, 132; and Stage IV, 499.

Fig. 5.58 Staging of gallbladder carcinoma (from Flemming *et al.*, 1997).

Definition of TNM

Primary Tumor (T)

TX Primary tumor cannot be assessed
T0 No evidence of primary tumor
Tis Carcinoma *in situ*
T1 Tumor invades mucosa or muscle layer
   T1a Tumor invades the mucosa
   T1b Tumor invades the muscle layer
T2 Tumor invades the perimuscular connective tissue; no extension beyond the serosa or into the liver
T3 Tumor perforates the serosa (visceral peritoneum) or directly invades into one adjacent organ, or both (extension 2 cm or less into the liver)
T4 Tumor extends more than 2 cm into the liver and/or into two or more adjacent organs (stomach, duodenum, colon, pancreas, omentum, extrahepatic bile ducts, any involvement of liver)

Regional Lymph Nodes (N)

NX Regional lymph nodes cannot be assessed
N0 No regional lymph node metastasis
N1 Metastasis in cystic duct, pericholedochal, and/or hilar lymph nodes (i.e., in the hepatoduodenal ligament)
N2 Metastasis in peripancreatic (head only), periduodenal, periportal, celiac, and/or superior mesenteric lymph nodes

Distant Metastasis (M)

MX Presence of distant metastasis cannot be assessed
M0 No distant metastasis
M1 Distant metastasis

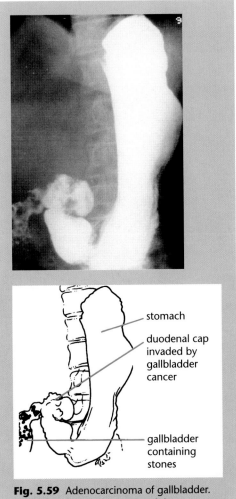

Fig. 5.59 Adenocarcinoma of gallbladder. Barium study shows invasion of the duodenum by a gallbladder tumor, accompanied by a fistula.

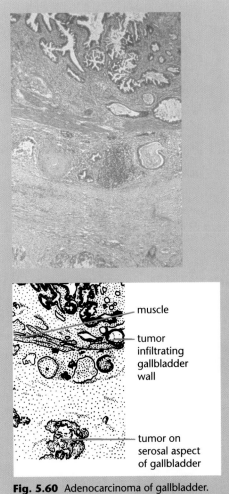

Fig. 5.60 Adenocarcinoma of gallbladder. Nests of tumor cells can be seen invading the gallbladder wall.

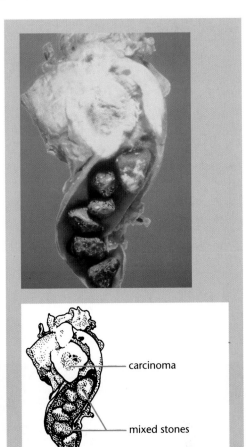

Fig. 5.61 Adenocarcinoma of neck of gallbladder. These tumors are frequently associated with gallstones, as shown here. Most cases of gallbladder malignancy are associated with a long-standing history of cholelithiasis and cholecystitis.

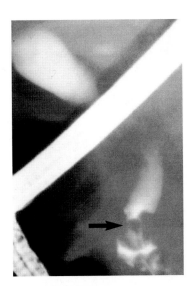

Fig. 5.62 Cholangiocarcinoma. Endoscopic retrograde cholangiogram shows a lesion obstructing the common bile duct (arrow).

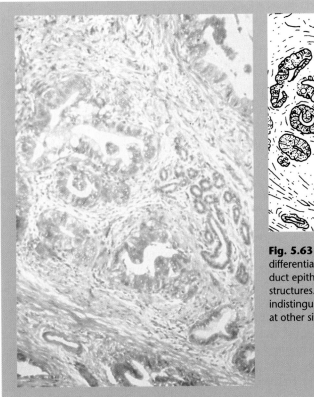

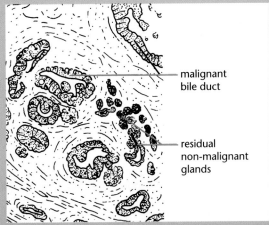

Fig. 5.63 Cholangiocarcinoma. In this moderately differentiated adenocarcinoma, glands of malignant bile duct epithelium can be seen adjacent to benign structures. When intrahepatic, such tumors may be indistinguishable from metastatic adenocarcinoma arising at other sites. (Courtesy of Prof. K. Weinbren.)

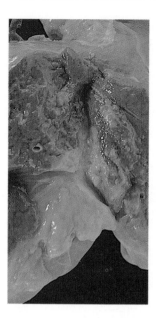

Fig. 5.64 Cholangiocarcinoma arising at the confluence of the right and left main hepatic ducts is a pale, locally infiltrative tumor. Each of the ducts is markedly dilated.

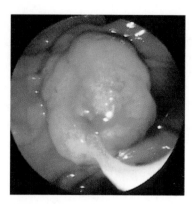

Fig. 5.65 Adenocarcinoma of ampulla of Vater. Endoscopic view shows a periampullary lesion with an area of minimal bleeding in the center. The tumor is cannulated for ERCP to determine the extent of obstruction.

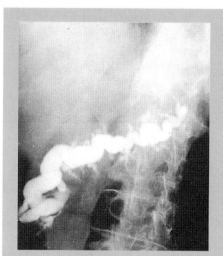

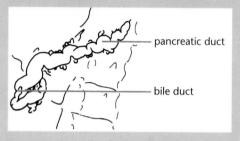

— pancreatic duct

— bile duct

Fig. 5.66 Adenocarcinoma of ampulla of Vater. The pancreatic duct is dilated secondary to obstruction by tumor. The partially filled and dilated bile duct can also be seen. The gallbladder is palpable in 30% of such cases, with painless jaundice.

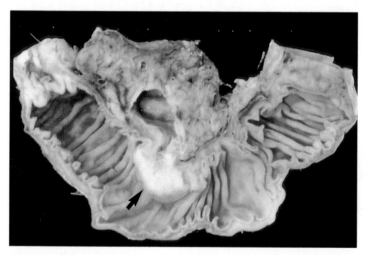

Fig. 5.67 Adenocarcinoma of ampulla of Vater. This specimen is from a 56-year-old man who presented with a 3-week history of jaundice, itching and slight fever. Radiologic studies were normal, but at laparotomy the gallbladder and common bile duct were found to be distended owing to distal obstruction. Pancreaticoduodenectomy and cholecystojejunostomy were performed. The head of the pancreas, the duodenum and the distal common bile duct are dissected to reveal a small, nodular, pale neoplasm arising in the ampulla of Vater beneath the duodenal mucosa (arrow). The tumor (1.5 cm in diameter) has obstructed the orifice of the ampulla, leading to marked dilatation of the common bile duct (middle right).

CANCERS OF THE SMALL INTESTINE

Primary malignant neoplasms of the small bowel develop in 1200 to 1500 individuals in the US each year. Typically, patients are in their fifth or sixth decade of life. There is a significant association with pre-existing Crohn's disease or celiac disease (sprue, gluten enteropathy). The most common malignancies are carcinoid tumors and adenocarcinomas, each of which constitutes 30–35% of cases. Lymphomas comprise about 20% of cases and 10–15% are malignant gastrointestinal stromal tumors (leiomyosarcomas). An equal number of benign tumors occur, but most of these are incidental findings.

Carcinoid tumors occur most commonly in the appendix, followed in frequency by the distal small bowel. In the latter site they are often multicentric and may be clinically aggressive. Adenocarcinomas occur most frequently in the proximal small bowel; about half involve the duodenum. Symptoms include bleeding, obstruction and pain. Both regional and distant metastases occur, as in cancers of the colon.

Lymphomas may be localized or diffuse and may occur throughout the gastrointestinal tract. They are most common in the stomach (up to 60%) and nearly 35% occur in the small intestine. The frequency is lowest in the duodenum, moderate in the jejunum and highest in the ileum. Primary small intestinal lymphomas are most often solitary lesions, with multiple separate lesions present in up to 20% of cases. The lymphomas are typically large at time of discovery, averaging 8 cm. Histologically, primary small intestinal lymphomas are similar to lymphomas of mucosal associated lymphoid tissue (MALTomas) in the remainder of the gastrointestinal tract and the respiratory system. In children, most GI lymphomas are histiocytic (large cell) or Burkitt's (undifferentiated) types, with a predilection for the terminal ileum and the ileocecal valve. Although systemic lymphomas may involve the small intestine, involvement by Hodgkin's disease is quite rare.

Malignant gastrointestinal stromal tumors constitute about 15% of small bowel malignancies; they appear to have a slight predilec-

tion for the duodenum and jejunum. They often reach large sizes (20 cm or greater) before diagnosis and the tumor mass may be predominantly extraluminal. Perforation with abscess formation, peritonitis or fistula formation is an unusual but dramatic event. Most patients present with abdominal pain, with or without gastrointestinal bleeding. Regional lymph node involvement is rare but hematogenous metastases, directly related to the histologic aggressiveness of the tumor, develop in many patients.

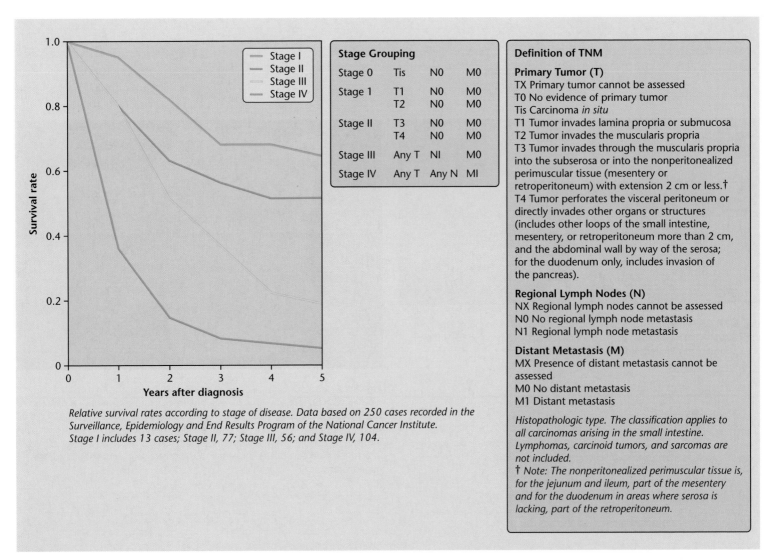

Stage Grouping			
Stage 0	Tis	N0	M0
Stage 1	T1	N0	M0
	T2	N0	M0
Stage II	T3	N0	M0
	T4	N0	M0
Stage III	Any T	N1	M0
Stage IV	Any T	Any N	M1

Definition of TNM

Primary Tumor (T)
TX Primary tumor cannot be assessed
T0 No evidence of primary tumor
Tis Carcinoma *in situ*
T1 Tumor invades lamina propria or submucosa
T2 Tumor invades the muscularis propria
T3 Tumor invades through the muscularis propria into the subserosa or into the nonperitonealized perimuscular tissue (mesentery or retroperitoneum) with extension 2 cm or less.†
T4 Tumor perforates the visceral peritoneum or directly invades other organs or structures (includes other loops of the small intestine, mesentery, or retroperitoneum more than 2 cm, and the abdominal wall by way of the serosa; for the duodenum only, includes invasion of the pancreas).

Regional Lymph Nodes (N)
NX Regional lymph nodes cannot be assessed
N0 No regional lymph node metastasis
N1 Regional lymph node metastasis

Distant Metastasis (M)
MX Presence of distant metastasis cannot be assessed
M0 No distant metastasis
M1 Distant metastasis

Histopathologic type. The classification applies to all carcinomas arising in the small intestine. Lymphomas, carcinoid tumors, and sarcomas are not included.
† Note: The nonperitonealized perimuscular tissue is, for the jejunum and ileum, part of the mesentery and for the duodenum in areas where serosa is lacking, part of the retroperitoneum.

Relative survival rates according to stage of disease. Data based on 250 cases recorded in the Surveillance, Epidemiology and End Results Program of the National Cancer Institute. Stage I includes 13 cases; Stage II, 77; Stage III, 56; and Stage IV, 104.

Fig. 5.68 Staging of cancers of the small intestine. Histopathologic type: the classification applies to all carcinomas arising in the small intestine. Lymphomas, carcinoid tumors and sarcomas are not included (from Flemming *et al.*, 1997).

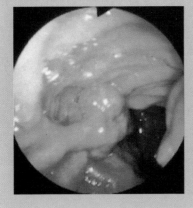

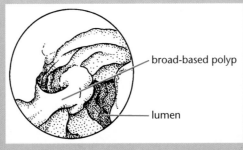

broad-based polyp

lumen

Fig. 5.69 Hamartomatous polyp in Peutz–Jeghers syndrome. Endoscopic view shows a broad-based polyp in the duodenum in a patient with Peutz–Jeghers syndrome. These small intestinal polyps only rarely become malignant. This syndrome is an autosomal dominant condition that is also marked by deposits of melanin on the buccal mucosa, lips and digits. Ovarian neoplasms arise in almost 5% of women with this syndrome.

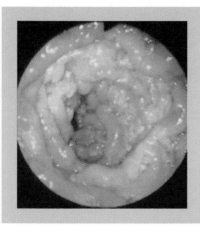
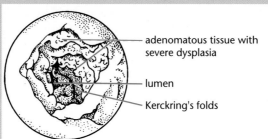

adenomatous tissue with
severe dysplasia

lumen

Kerckring's folds

Fig. 5.70 Diffuse adenomatosis in familial adenomatous polyposis. The proximal small intestine has been almost entirely affected by adenomatous (dysplastic) changes. Note the difference in color between adenomatous tissue and uninvolved Kerckring's folds.

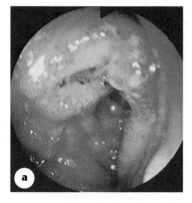
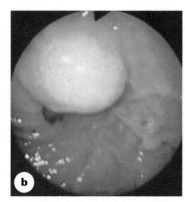

Fig. 5.71 Malignant gastrointestinal stromal tumor of duodenum. Endoscopy demonstrates (**a**) destruction of the duodenal wall by tumor and (**b**) a tumor mass compressing the antrum.

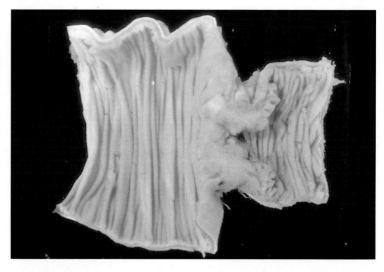

Fig. 5.72 Adenocarcinoma of jejunum. This specimen is from a 75-year-old woman who presented with a 6-week history of profuse vomiting. A barium study was not diagnostic and laparatomy was performed. A segment of jejunum has been opened to show an annular, stenosing tumor, extending over a length of 1.5 cm: it has infiltrated the full thickness of the bowel wall. The intestine is markedly dilated proximal to the obstruction and exhibits muscle hypertrophy.

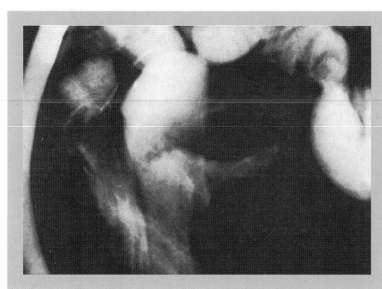
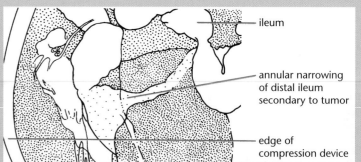

ileum

annular narrowing
of distal ileum
secondary to tumor

edge of
compression device

Fig. 5.73 Adenocarcinoma of ileum. Barium study shows an annular constricting lesion. (Courtesy of Dr D. Nolan.)

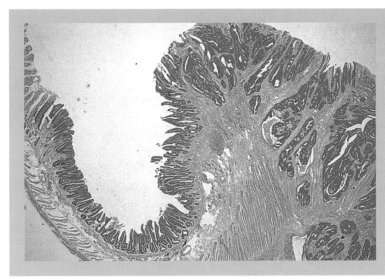

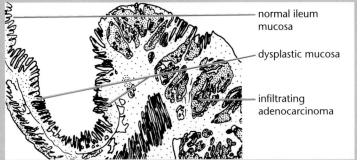

normal ileum mucosa

dysplastic mucosa

infiltrating adenocarcinoma

Fig. 5.74 Adenocarcinoma of ileum. Low-power photomicrograph demonstrates a gradual transition from normal mucosa through dysplasia to invasive adenocarcinoma.

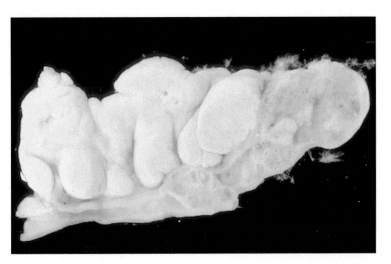

Fig. 5.75 Mucinous cystadenocarcinoma of appendix. This specimen is from an 83-year-old man who died of peritoneal carcinomatosis; the primary tumor site was not identified before death. The appendix is diffusely expanded by a multilocular cystic tumor largely composed of pale, mucinous material. Adenocarcinoma of the appendix is extremely rare and is usually of the mucinous type. The elderly are typically affected and may present with symptoms of acute appendicitis. The clinical behavior and prognostic features are the same as those of cecal adenocarcinoma. These tumors occasionally give rise to pseudomyxoma peritonei, a condition marked by progressive accumulation of intra-abdominal pearly, gelatinous, mucoid material grossly indistinguishable from ruptured benign mucocele. (Courtesy of the Gordon Museum, Guy's Hospital Medical School, London, UK.)

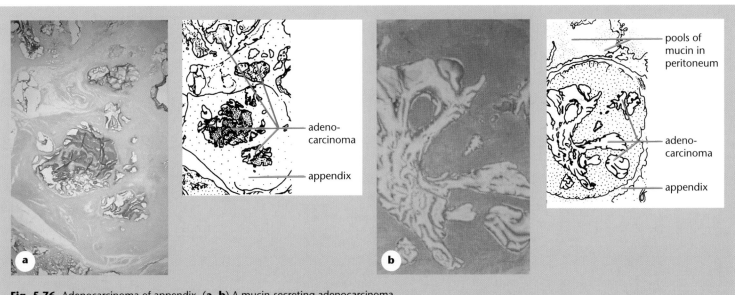

pools of mucin in peritoneum

adeno-carcinoma

appendix

adeno-carcinoma

appendix

Fig. 5.76 Adenocarcinoma of appendix. (**a, b**) A mucin-secreting adenocarcinoma has penetrated the full thickness of the appendiceal wall (**a** Alcian blue; **b** H&E).

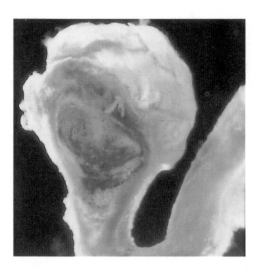

Fig. 5.77 Carcinoid tumor of appendix. This tumor was found incidentally during cholecystectomy in a 59-year-old woman. The appendix has been mounted to show a pear-shaped, yellow-brown tumor (2.5 cm in length) at the distal end. The appendix is the single most common primary site of GI carcinoid tumors, the ileum being second in frequency. Appendiceal lesions are typically seen in young adults and usually follow a benign course, in contrast to those arising in the small bowel. As a consequence, the carcinoid syndrome is a rare complication of appendiceal lesions.

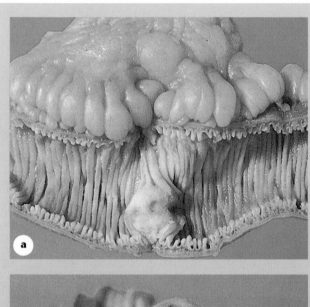

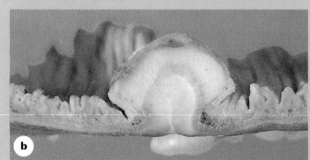

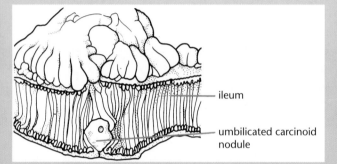

ileum

umbilicated carcinoid nodule

Fig. 5.78 Carcinoid tumor of ileum. (**a**) A small, umbilicated carcinoid nodule from a patient with carcinoid syndrome arises from the submucosa, as seen on sectioning (**b**). The yellow color of the tumor is the result of formalin fixation. Such tumors may not be detectable on barium examination. Carcinoid tumors of the ileum show a predilection for men, typically between the ages of 50 and 70. An indolent clinical course is common, but the majority of these tumors eventually metastasize to lymph nodes or the liver. These lesions secrete 5-hydroxytryptamine, which is normally metabolized in the liver and, therefore, has no systemic effects. However, the development of liver metastases circumvents this metabolic process and the carcinoid syndrome may then ensue. Thus, the clinical development of the carcinoid syndrome in a patient with a history of small intestinal carcinoid tumor should suggest the likelihood of extraintestinal metastases.

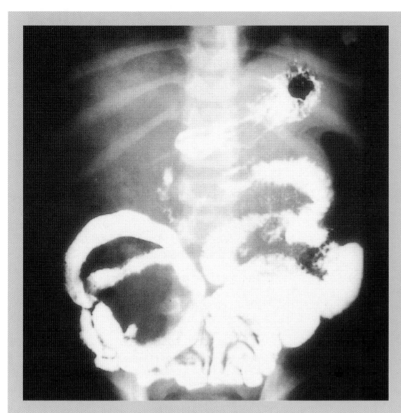

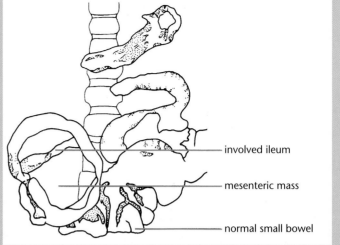

involved ileum

mesenteric mass

normal small bowel

Fig. 5.79 Lymphoma. Barium film in a patient with celiac disease shows a small bowel lymphoma giving rise to a large mesenteric mass in the right lower quadrant. The tumor displaces and compresses several ileal loops, which show effacement of the fold pattern, as well as nodular irregularity indicating mucosal invasion. (Courtesy of Dr R. Dick.)

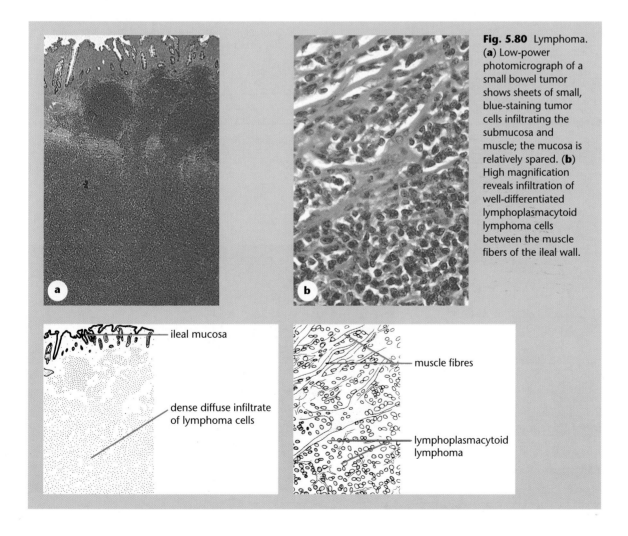

Fig. 5.80 Lymphoma. (**a**) Low-power photomicrograph of a small bowel tumor shows sheets of small, blue-staining tumor cells infiltrating the submucosa and muscle; the mucosa is relatively spared. (**b**) High magnification reveals infiltration of well-differentiated lymphoplasmacytoid lymphoma cells between the muscle fibers of the ileal wall.

ileal mucosa

dense diffuse infiltrate of lymphoma cells

muscle fibres

lymphoplasmacytoid lymphoma

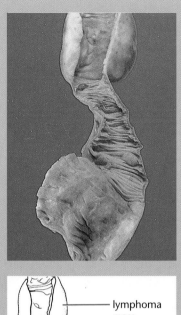

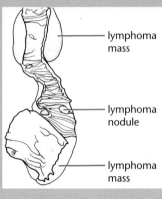

Fig. 5.81 Lymphoma. Plaque-like growths of a large cell lymphoma have infiltrated the ileal wall; note the smaller intervening nodule. In such instances, intestinal obstruction is the most common presentation.

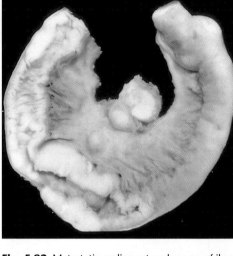

Fig. 5.82 Metastatic malignant melanoma of ileum. This specimen is from a 60-year-old man who presented with a change in bowel habits, weight loss and frequent vomiting. The case was initially believed to represent a multicentric lymphoma. However, the source of his primary tumor was not detected before signs of intestinal obstruction developed and laparotomy was performed. This partly opened loop of small bowel shows three separate pale amelanotic infiltrative deposits of tumor, along with several enlarged mesenteric nodes, which are replaced by further metastases. The propensity of malignant melanoma to metastasize to almost any site is well known. Such lesions, when amelanotic, may be misdiagnosed both clinically and pathologically. In general, metastasis of any tumor to the small bowel is uncommon.

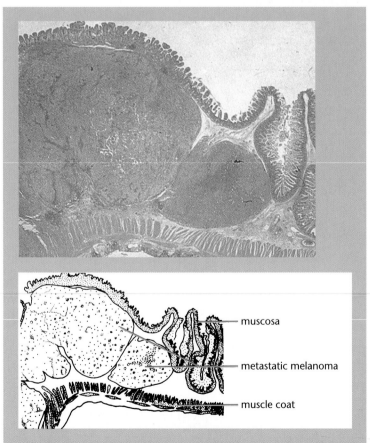

Fig. 5.83 Metastatic malignant melanoma of jejunum. Metastatic deposits of tumor can be seen in the submucosa of the jejunum. The lesion is predominantly amelanotic. Radiographic studies in such instances may reveal 'target' or 'bull's eye' lesions.

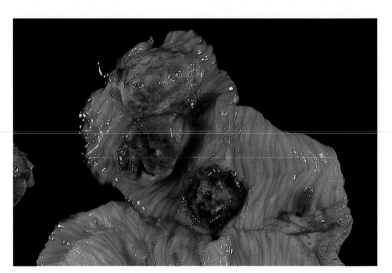

Fig. 5.84 The small bowel is a favored site for metastases from melanoma. This jejunal resection specimen shows the typical appearance of multiple pigmented nodules; some show surface ulceration and associated central necrosis. These appear as 'target' lesions on radiographic contrast studies.

COLORECTAL CANCERS

Over 140 000 cases of colorectal cancer are diagnosed in the United States annually. Carcinomas of the large bowel and rectum are the second most common cause of cancer-related deaths, falling just behind lung cancer. The incidence of colon cancer is highest in industrialized regions such as the United States and Europe. Several proposed etiologic hypotheses implicate dietary risk factors. Diets high in red meat and animal fats have been associated with an increased risk of colorectal cancer. Fiber intake, on the other hand, was once thought to play a major role in the development of colorectal cancer but has recently been shown to have little or no effect on colorectal cancer risk. Another risk factor for colorectal cancer is inflammatory bowel disease; individuals with ulcerative colitis for more than 10 years are at particularly high risk.

Up to 25% of all patients with colorectal cancer have a family history of the disease. Several hereditary syndromes are associated with an increased risk for colon cancer. Familial adenomatous polyposis (FAP) is a rare autosomal dominant condition that is characterized by the development of numerous polyps throughout the colon. Virtually all patients with FAP will develop colon cancer by age 40 unless prophylactic colectomy is performed. FAP is caused by germline mutations in the tumor suppressor gene APC. The identity of the involved gene in FAP and Gardner's syndrome kindreds suggests that the separation of Gardner's syndrome from FAP may be artificial. The importance of APC is emphasized by the observation that it is mutated in colon tumors (but not the germ line) of some patients with sporadic (i.e. non-hereditary) colon cancer.

Heriditary non-polyposis colon cancer (HNPCC), another inherited syndrome, is characterized by the early onset of colon cancer, often involving the right side of the colon, and typically occurring in the absence of numerous colonic polyps. Several germline defects responsible for HNPCC have been identified; the most common of these are mutations in hMLH1 and hMSH2. These genes are essential components of a nucleotide mismatch repair system. HNPCC is also associated with the development of extracolonic tumors, including malignancies of the endometrium, ovary, stomach and small bowel. Genetic screening for individuals at risk for HNPCC is now available.

HISTOLOGY

Over 98% of cancers of the large bowel are adenocarcinomas. Characteristic subgroups include mucinous or colloid tumors and signet ring cell tumors. Adenocarcinomas are classified as well, moderately or poorly differentiated, each category having a distinct prognostic implication. Most colorectal carcinomas originate from adenomatous polyps. Pathologically, progression from early adenomatous proliferations through adenomatous polyp, high-grade dysplasia and, ultimately, invasive carcinoma occurs as a continuum. This progression coincides with the accumulation of genetic alterations within the neoplasm. These alterations include mutations of tumor suppressor genes, e.g. p53, DCC and APC, as well as activation and/or overexpression of oncogenes, e.g. c-*myc* and k-*ras*. While the order of occurrence of these genetic changes may vary, the quantitative accumulation of defects correlates with biologic and histologic parameters of neoplastic progression, suggesting a multistep model of tumorigenesis. The majority of bowel cancers arise in the rectum and sigmoid colon; however, recent studies show that, for unknown reasons, the proportion of cancers arising in the rectum is decreasing, whereas the percentage of those originating in the cecum and ascending colon is increasing. The remaining 2% of colorectal cancers consist of lymphomas, leiomyosarcomas and miscellaneous tumors.

STAGING OF COLORECTAL CANCERS

Colorectal cancers are generally staged at the time of surgery. CT scans of the abdomen and pelvis and chest radiographs are usually also performed to evaluate for metastatic disease. Bone scans are not routinely carried out in the absence of bone pain, due to a low incidence of bone metastases. Extension of primary rectal cancers into adjacent soft tissues can often be assessed by endorectal MRI or ultrasound.

Several systems have been employed in staging colorectal cancer. The AJCC recently revised the TNM staging classification (*see* Fig. 5.103); new subcategories are included to differentiate tumors based on the number of involved lymph nodes (1–3 vs >4). A practical and frequently used system was introduced by Dukes and subsequently modified by Kirklin and colleagues, Astler and Coller, and others (*see* Fig. 5.102). This classification is based on three prognostic variables: depth of tumor invasion through the bowel wall, regional lymph node involvement and distant metastases. Unlike other cancers, the size of the primary colon carcinoma does not in itself affect prognosis. As recent studies have shown, the 5-year survival rate for each stage of disease, except for Dukes stage D, has improved. The reasons for this trend may not necessarily be related to improvements in early detection and in surgical technique but rather to more thorough and accurate staging.

Colorectal cancers spread by direct invasion, through lymphatic channels, along hematogenous routes and by implantation. Spread of colon cancers through the portal venous circulation leads to liver metastases, which are present in about two-thirds of patients at autopsy. Cancers that originate within 12 cm of the anal verge are considered rectal cancers. The location of these lesions and the lymphatic drainage of this area necessitate special management decisions. Rectal cancers situated below the peritoneal reflection have a high rate of local recurrence. Cancers of the lower rectum may metastasize via the paravertebral plexus to supraclavicular nodes, lungs, bone and brain, without liver involvement.

CLINICAL MANIFESTATIONS

Patients with cancer of the cecum and ascending colon usually present with anemia caused by intermittent GI bleeding. Obstruction is rare, because the bowel wall is more distensible and has a greater circumference than the descending colon. These cancers are often large and may be fungating or friable. Carcinomas of the transverse colon and either the hepatic or the splenic flexure, which account for about 10% of total cases, are somewhat less common than cecal neoplasms and much less common than rectosigmoid tumors. They frequently cause cramping pain, bleeding and sometimes obstruction or perforation. Large bowel obstruction is the most common complication of colon carcinoma and may lead to proximal ulceration or perforation. Obstruction is the principal reason why up to 30% of cases present as surgical emergencies. Other complications include iron deficiency anemia, hypokalemia (particularly associated with large villous rectal lesions) and intussusception in adults. Tumors of the sigmoid colon and rectum cancers usually cause changes in normal bowel habits, with tenesmus, decrease in stool caliber and hematochezia.

Colorectal cancer is usually initially diagnosed with colonoscopy. A full colonoscopy should be performed in all patients with colorectal cancer to rule out the possibility of second occult primary colon cancers, which occur in about 5% of patients. Surgical resection of the primary colorectal cancer is generally performed either with curative intent or, in patients with metastatic disease, as a palliative procedure to reduce the risk of obstruction and bleeding.

MOLECULAR BIOLOGY AND PROGNOSTIC FACTORS

The use of molecular prognostic factors in colorectal cancer remains an area of intense investigation. Numerous molecular markers have been examined for potential prognostic significance. These include but are not limited to allelic loss of chromosome 18 q, mutation in the *k-ras* oncogene, hypermethylation of p16, the presence of microsatellite instability, and overexpression of thymidylate synthase, vascular endothelial growth factor, p53, p27 and COX-2. The clinical utility of these markers has not yet been formally tested in prospective trials.

ANAL CANCERS

There are over 3000 new cases of anal carcinoma in the United States annually. Due to the transitional (columnar to squamous) nature of the epithelium of the anorectal junction and the presence of glandular epithelium, endocrine cells and melanocytes, several different histologies may develop. These include squamous cell carcinomas (>50%), basaloid carcinoma, colonic-type adenocarcinoma and, rarely, mucinous carcinoma, melanoma and small cell carcinoma. The incidence of anal cancer and its precursor lesions (such as anal intraepithelia neoplasia) is increasing, particularly in HIV-positive men and women (*see* Chapter 17). The development of anal carcinoma is also strongly associated with human papilloma virus infection. Patients with Crohn's disease and chronic perianal fistulae are also at increased risk. Screening in high-risk persons includes physical exam, an anal Pap smear and anoscopy if the Pap smear is abnormal.

Squamous cell carcinomas can be divided into tumors arising in the anal canal, most often above the dentate line, and those arising in the skin at the anal margin. Tumors of the anal canal, which are three times as common as those at the anal margin, tend to spread proximally and to disseminate predominantly to intrapelvic lymph nodes; the 5-year survival rate is about 50%. In contrast, squamous cell cancers arising at the anal margin tend to be more indolent, metastasize to inguinal lymph nodes and have a favorable prognosis.

Anal malignant melanoma, like squamous carcinoma, can be divided into two types: tumors arising in the anal canal and those arising from anal skin. The latter group is entirely comparable to conventional cutaneous malignant melanomas. Malignant melanoma of the anal canal is fairly rare and tends to present in late adulthood in either sex. It shows a predilection for extensive local invasion and early lymph node metastases and is associated with a poor prognosis.

Table 5.2 Classification of colonic polyps.

Type	Histopathology	Associated Diseases
Neoplastic	Adenoma	None (sporadic)
	tubular adenoma	Familial adenomatous polyposis
	tubulovillous adenoma	Gardner's syndrome
	villous adenoma	Turcot syndrome
Non-neoplastic	Hyperplastic polyp	None (sporadic)
		Hyperplastic polyposis
	Hamartomatous polyp	None (sporadic)
		Peutz–Jeghers syndrome
	Inflammatory fibroid polyp	None (sporadic)
	Inflammatory pseudopolyp	Ulcerative colitis, Crohn's disease
		Ischemic colitis
		Infection (amebiasis, schistosomiasis)
		Ulceration
	Juvenile polyp	None (sporadic)
		Juvenile polyposis syndrome
		Cronkhite–Canada syndrome
	Lymphoid polyp	None (incidental, reactive)
		Lymphoid polyposis

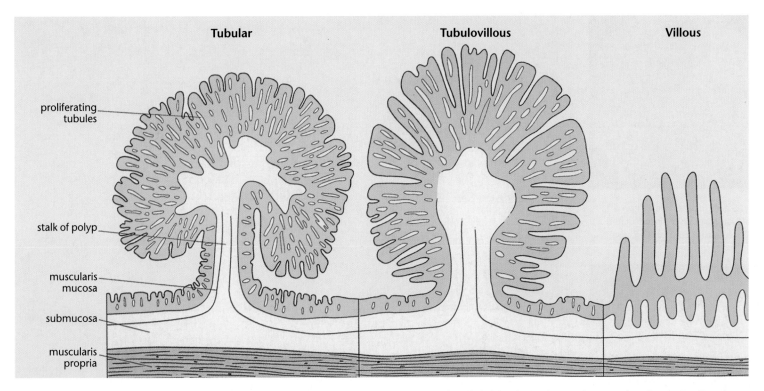

Tubular **Tubulovillous** **Villous**

proliferating tubules

stalk of polyp

muscularis mucosa

submucosa

muscularis propria

Fig. 5.85 Patterns of adenomatous colonic polyps. Polyps may be pedunculated (left, middle) or sessile (right). The surface epithelium of the stalk may be non-neoplastic (left) or adenomatous (middle). Polyps may be solitary or multiple; the presence of more than approximately 100 polyps suggests the diagnosis of familial adenomatous polyposis. Although they can arise at any site in the large bowel, the largest and more often symptomatic lesions tend to be situated in the left side of the colon. The diagnosis of adenoma requires the presence of epithelial dysplasia. These polyps are, therefore, premalignant neoplastic tissue. Factors believed to increase the risk of malignant change include large polyp size (particularly > 2 cm in diameter), severe epithelial dysplasia and villous architecture. Penetration of the muscularis mucosa by dysplastic epithelium, with invasion of submucosa, is the distinguishing sign of invasive carcinoma.

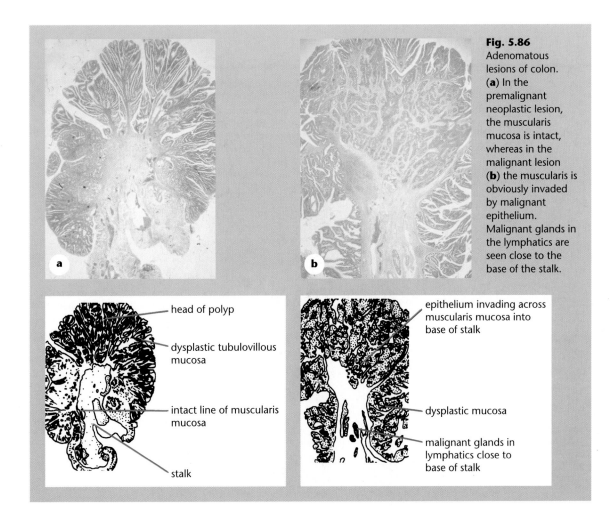

Fig. 5.86 Adenomatous lesions of colon. (**a**) In the premalignant neoplastic lesion, the muscularis mucosa is intact, whereas in the malignant lesion (**b**) the muscularis is obviously invaded by malignant epithelium. Malignant glands in the lymphatics are seen close to the base of the stalk.

head of polyp

dysplastic tubulovillous mucosa

intact line of muscularis mucosa

stalk

epithelium invading across muscularis mucosa into base of stalk

dysplastic mucosa

malignant glands in lymphatics close to base of stalk

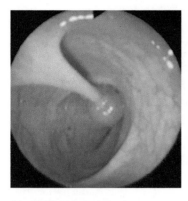

Fig. 5.87 Tubular adenoma. Endoscopy shows a pedunculated adenomatous polyp of the colon.

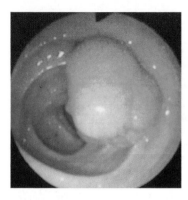

Fig. 5.89 Tubulovillous adenoma. Endoscopic view shows a moderate-sized sessile polyp. Several lobules are evident.

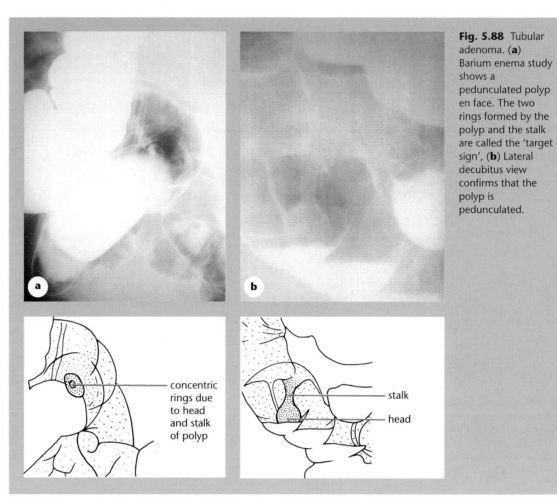

Fig. 5.88 Tubular adenoma. (**a**) Barium enema study shows a pedunculated polyp en face. The two rings formed by the polyp and the stalk are called the 'target sign'. (**b**) Lateral decubitus view confirms that the polyp is pedunculated.

concentric rings due to head and stalk of polyp

stalk

head

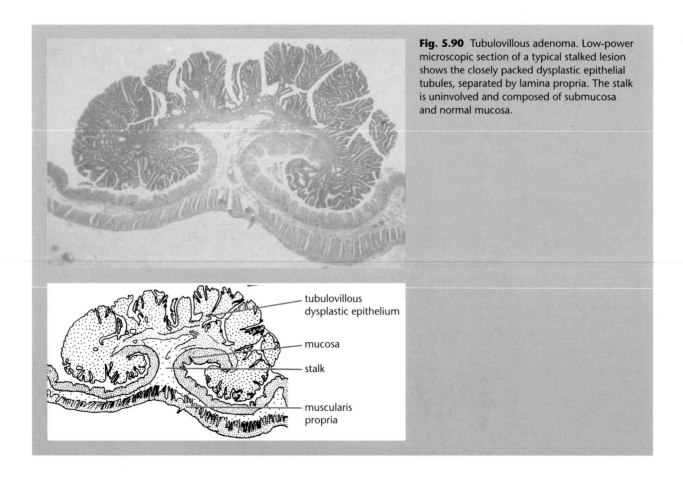

Fig. 5.90 Tubulovillous adenoma. Low-power microscopic section of a typical stalked lesion shows the closely packed dysplastic epithelial tubules, separated by lamina propria. The stalk is uninvolved and composed of submucosa and normal mucosa.

tubulovillous dysplastic epithelium

mucosa

stalk

muscularis propria

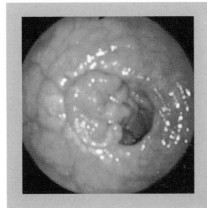
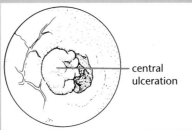

Fig. 5.91 Villous adenoma. Malignant rectal villous polyp. Endoscopy shows superficial central ulceration in this rectal polyp, suggestive of malignancy.

central ulceration

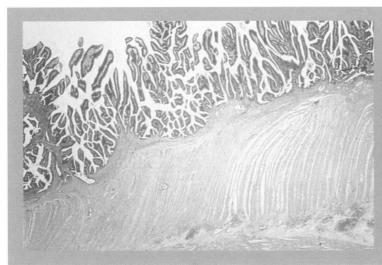

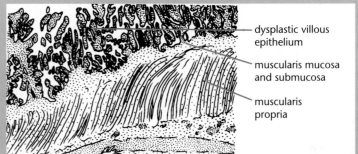

dysplastic villous epithelium

muscularis mucosa and submucosa

muscularis propria

Fig. 5.92 Sessile villous adenoma. Histologic section of a villous polyp demonstrates its sessile nature. Note the numerous finger-like villi, with dysplastic epithelium over a core of lamina propria, resting directly on the muscularis mucosa. No invasion is present.

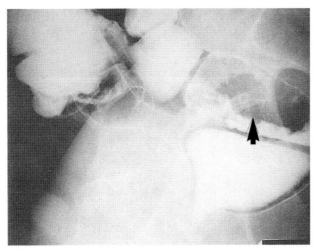

Fig. 5.93 Villous adenoma. A broad rectal lesion can be seen rising posteriorly (arrow). Histologic examination revealed a villous adenoma. Tumors of this size have a high probability of malignancy and are too large and broad-based for endoscopic removal. Typical symptoms include copious, watery, mucus-containing diarrhea, rectal bleeding and tenesmus.

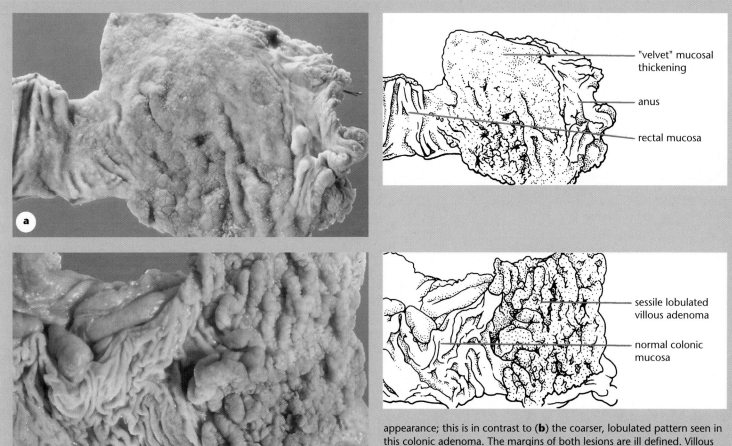

appearance; this is in contrast to (**b**) the coarser, lobulated pattern seen in this colonic adenoma. The margins of both lesions are ill defined. Villous adenomas are most common in the rectum, where they tend to be larger and to show more severe dysplasia than tubular adenomas; they therefore more commonly progress to adenocarcinoma. Villous adenomas of the rectum sometimes secrete large amounts of potassium or albumin, giving rise to hypokalemia or hypoalbuminemia.

Fig. 5.94 Villous adenoma. These two large, broad-based, sessile, colorectal lesions demonstrate common macroscopic patterns of large villous adenomas. (**a**) A fine villous pattern gives the mucosa of this rectal lesion a velvety

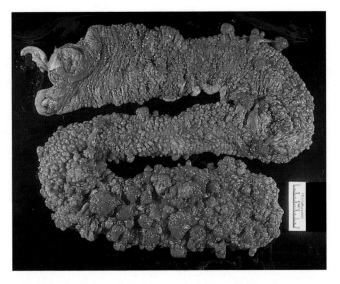

Fig. 5.96 Familial adenomatous polyposis, with innumerable adenomatous polyps, increasing in size and density from proximal (upper left) to distal (lower right). Microscopic section of one of the largest polyps (left) demonstrates a focal area of invasive adenocarcinoma (right) characterized by irregular, infiltrative gland architecture and an associated desmoplastic stroma.

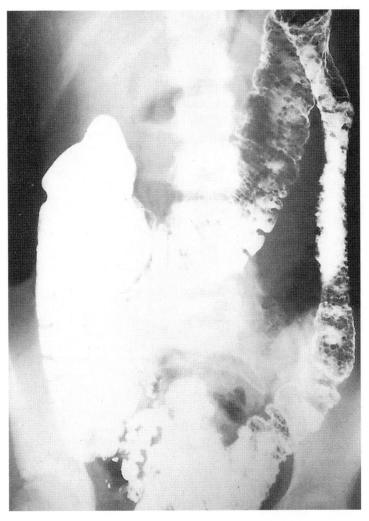

Fig. 5.95 Familial adenomatous polyposis. Barium enema study demonstrates multiple, small polyps throughout the colon.

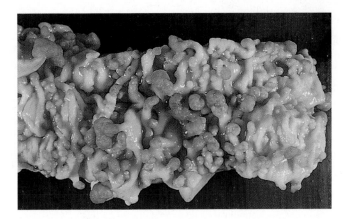

Fig. 5.97 Familial adenomatous polyposis. This disorder is marked by the development of hundreds of large bowel adenomas, as seen in this segment of large bowel, which is covered with adenomas of various sizes. It usually arises in the second and third decades.

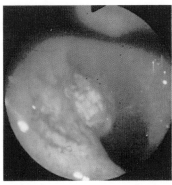

Fig. 5.99 Polypoid epithelial dysplasia in ulcerative colitis. Endoscopy reveals epithelial dysplasia with surrounding chronic active colitis in a patient who had ulcerative colitis for nearly 20 years. Histologic examination showed high-grade mucosal dysplasia. The dysplasia is histologically identical to that seen in adenomatous polyps. However, in the setting of ulcerative colitis of >10 years duration, high-grade dysplasia is strongly associated with the development of invasive cancer and should prompt serious consideration of colectomy.

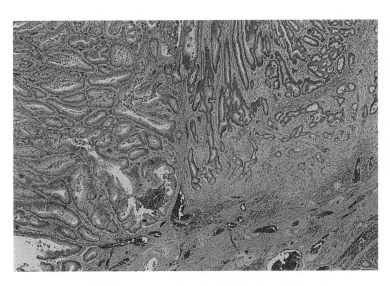

Fig. 5.98 Familial adenomatous polyposis (FAP). Section of colon shows immumerable polyps characteristic of FAP. If left untreated, the risk of colon cancer in such patients approaches 100% by the age of 40.

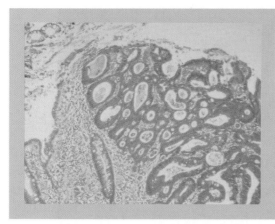
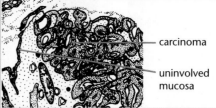

Fig. 5.100 Intramucosal carcinoma in ulcerative colitis. Frank intramucosal carcinoma is evident in this colon biopsy specimen from a patient with ulcerative colitis. The lesion infiltrates the lamina propria but does not extend beyond the muscularis mucosa. The tumor evolves through ascending grades of dysplasia in non-polypoid mucosa, as evidenced by the uninvolved mucosa at the left margin.

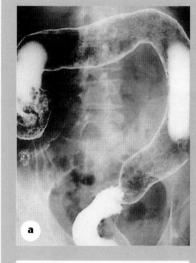
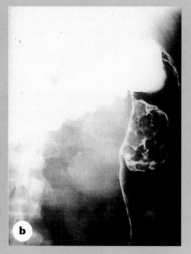
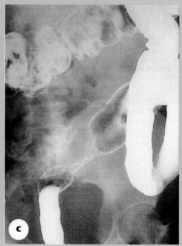
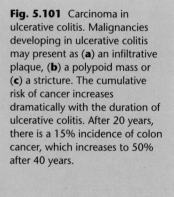
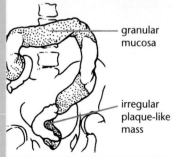
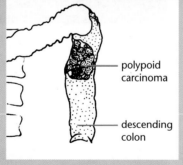
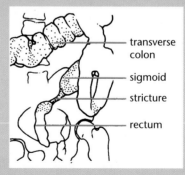

Fig. 5.101 Carcinoma in ulcerative colitis. Malignancies developing in ulcerative colitis may present as (**a**) an infiltrative plaque, (**b**) a polypoid mass or (**c**) a stricture. The cumulative risk of cancer increases dramatically with the duration of ulcerative colitis. After 20 years, there is a 15% incidence of colon cancer, which increases to 50% after 40 years.

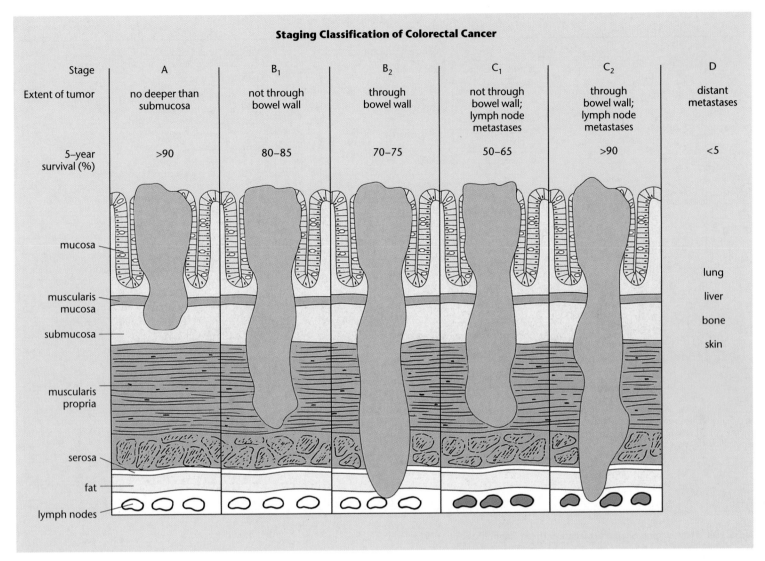

Staging Classification of Colorectal Cancer

Stage	A	B₁	B₂	C₁	C₂	D
Extent of tumor	no deeper than submucosa	not through bowel wall	through bowel wall	not through bowel wall; lymph node metastases	through bowel wall; lymph node metastases	distant metastases
5-year survival (%)	>90	80–85	70–75	50–65	>90	<5

mucosa

muscularis mucosa

submucosa

muscularis propria

serosa

fat

lymph nodes

lung

liver

bone

skin

Fig. 5.102 Modified Dukes' staging classification of colorectal cancer. Stages B3 and C3 (not shown) signify perforation or invasion of contiguous organs or structures (T4). The TNM classification provides a more accurate staging system: Dukes B is a composite of better (T2N0) and worse (T3N0, T4N0) prognostic groups as is Dukes C (T×N1 or T×N2).

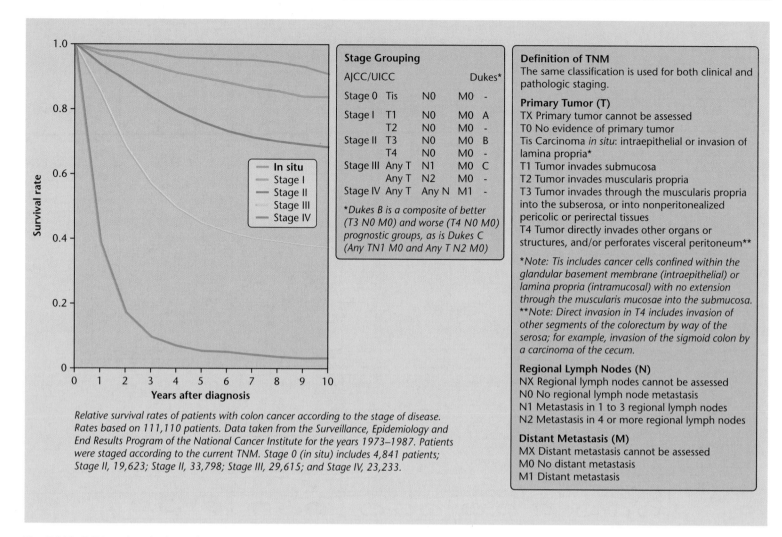

Stage Grouping

AJCC/UICC				Dukes*
Stage 0	Tis	N0	M0	-
Stage I	T1	N0	M0	A
	T2	N0	M0	-
Stage II	T3	N0	M0	B
	T4	N0	M0	-
Stage III	Any T	N1	M0	C
	Any T	N2	M0	-
Stage IV	Any T	Any N	M1	-

Dukes B is a composite of better (T3 N0 M0) and worse (T4 N0 M0) prognostic groups, as is Dukes C (Any TN1 M0 and Any T N2 M0)

Definition of TNM
The same classification is used for both clinical and pathologic staging.

Primary Tumor (T)
TX Primary tumor cannot be assessed
T0 No evidence of primary tumor
Tis Carcinoma *in situ*: intraepithelial or invasion of lamina propria*
T1 Tumor invades submucosa
T2 Tumor invades muscularis propria
T3 Tumor invades through the muscularis propria into the subserosa, or into nonperitonealized pericolic or perirectal tissues
T4 Tumor directly invades other organs or structures, and/or perforates visceral peritoneum**

*Note: Tis includes cancer cells confined within the glandular basement membrane (intraepithelial) or lamina propria (intramucosal) with no extension through the muscularis mucosae into the submucosa.
**Note: Direct invasion in T4 includes invasion of other segments of the colorectum by way of the serosa; for example, invasion of the sigmoid colon by a carcinoma of the cecum.*

Regional Lymph Nodes (N)
NX Regional lymph nodes cannot be assessed
N0 No regional lymph node metastasis
N1 Metastasis in 1 to 3 regional lymph nodes
N2 Metastasis in 4 or more regional lymph nodes

Distant Metastasis (M)
MX Distant metastasis cannot be assessed
M0 No distant metastasis
M1 Distant metastasis

Relative survival rates of patients with colon cancer according to the stage of disease. Rates based on 111,110 patients. Data taken from the Surveillance, Epidemiology and End Results Program of the National Cancer Institute for the years 1973–1987. Patients were staged according to the current TNM. Stage 0 (in situ) includes 4,841 patients; Stage II, 19,623; Stage II, 33,798; Stage III, 29,615; and Stage IV, 23,233.

Fig. 5.103 TNM staging of colorectal cancer (from Flemming *et al.*, 1997).

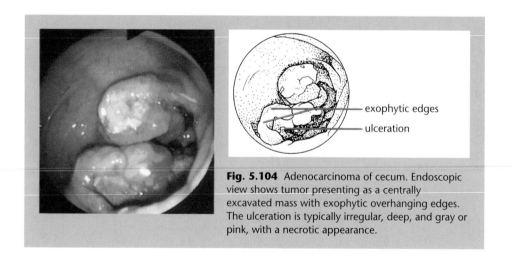

Fig. 5.104 Adenocarcinoma of cecum. Endoscopic view shows tumor presenting as a centrally excavated mass with exophytic overhanging edges. The ulceration is typically irregular, deep, and gray or pink, with a necrotic appearance.

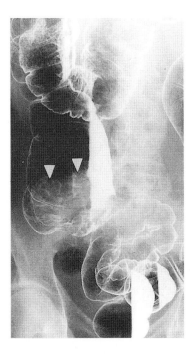

Fig. 5.105 Adenocarcinoma of cecum. Intestinal obstruction occurs late in the course of the disease. Although this lesion (arrows) is relatively large, there was no obstruction to retrograde filling of the ileum and no dilatation of the small intestine. Symptoms may include anemia or dyspepsia and weight loss reminiscent of a benign or malignant gastric ulcer.

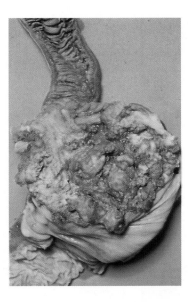

Fig. 5.106 Adenocarcinoma of cecum. Large, fungating tumors, as seen here, are a less common presentation of colorectal tumors; they predominate in the cecum.

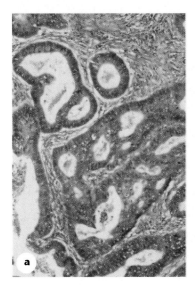
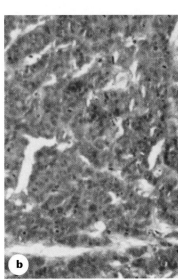
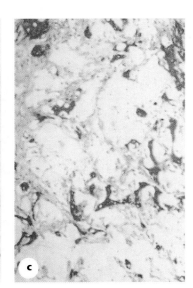

Fig. 5.107 Adenocarcinoma. (**a**) Moderately differentiated tumors are marked by gland (acinar) formation by malignant epithelium; there is considerable nuclear pleomorphism within individual cells. (**b**) In poorly differentiated lesions, sheets of malignant epithelial cells can be seen with little acinar formation. (**c**) The mucinous (colloid) variant exhibits nests of malignant epithelium in pools of mucin.

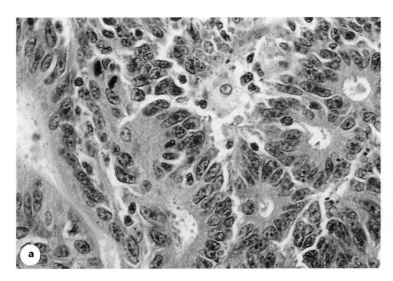
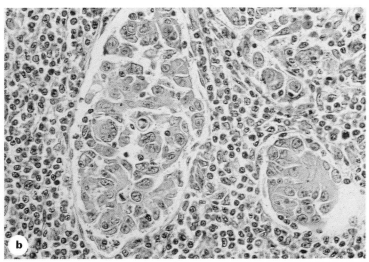

Fig. 5.108 Adenocarcinoma. (**a**) High-power view of a moderately differentiated tumor shows irregular and hyperchromatic nuclei, prominent nucleoli and several mitoses. (**b**) Metastases are evident in this lymph node biopsy.

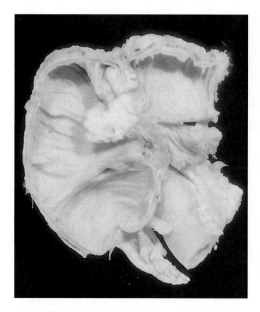

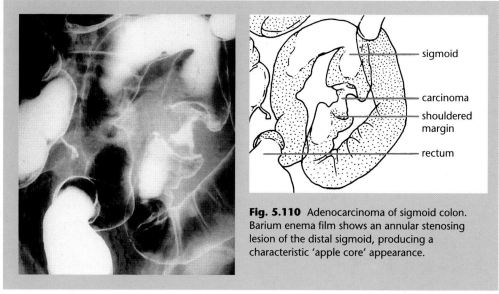

Fig. 5.110 Adenocarcinoma of sigmoid colon. Barium enema film shows an annular stenosing lesion of the distal sigmoid, producing a characteristic 'apple core' appearance.

Fig. 5.109 Adenocarcinoma of ascending colon. This specimen is from a 57-year-old man who presented with a 1- year history of right upper quadrant abdominal pain. Examination revealed a tender mass beneath the right costal margin and barium enema film showed a tumor just proximal to the hepatic flexure. A right hemicolectomy was performed. The distal ileum, cecum and ascending colon have been opened to show an annular, stenosing neoplasm at the hepatic flexure; the bowel lumen has been reduced to a narrow cleft. Proximally, there is obvious dilatation of the intestine, with some associated muscle hypertrophy.

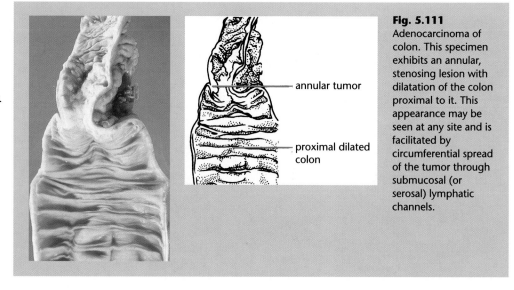

Fig. 5.111 Adenocarcinoma of colon. This specimen exhibits an annular, stenosing lesion with dilatation of the colon proximal to it. This appearance may be seen at any site and is facilitated by circumferential spread of the tumor through submucosal (or serosal) lymphatic channels.

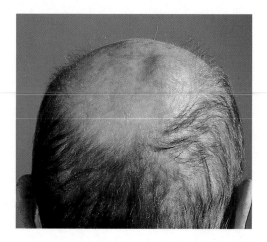

Fig. 5.112 Metastatic colon cancer. A 60-year-old man with previous colectomy for stage III colon cancer 4 years earlier developed a nodule on his posterior scalp. Biopsy was positive for poorly differentiated adenocarcinoma, similar to the original cancer. CEA was elevated at 50 ng/ml. Subsequent studies showed multiple liver metastases. Skin metastases are not common, but have been reported in colon, pancreatic, breast and lung cancers as well as miscellaneous other malignancies.

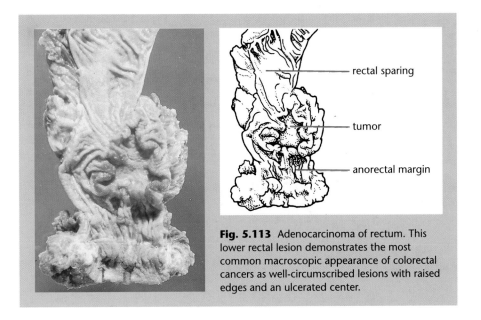

Fig. 5.113 Adenocarcinoma of rectum. This lower rectal lesion demonstrates the most common macroscopic appearance of colorectal cancers as well-circumscribed lesions with raised edges and an ulcerated center.

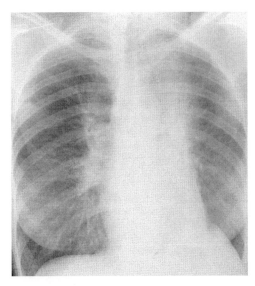

Fig. 5.114 Metastatic colorectal cancer. A 34-year-old woman with prior anterior-posterior resection for a stage II rectal cancer 3 years earlier presented with clinical features of SVC syndrome. Chest radiograph showed mediastinal adenopathy and atelactatic changes in the left upper lobe. Chest CT scan and nuclide flow studies (not shown) revealed tumor obstruction of the SVC. Mediastinoscopy was positive for adenocarcinoma with features similar to the original rectal carcinoma. Bronchoscopy showed no intrinsic lesions. Radiotherapy resulted in a partial remission. Liver metastases eventually occurred. Metastatic colorectal carcinoma may spread to the lungs and mediastinum and bypass the liver due to lymphatic spread via the paravertebral vascular channels of Batson as well as lower pelvic collaterals.

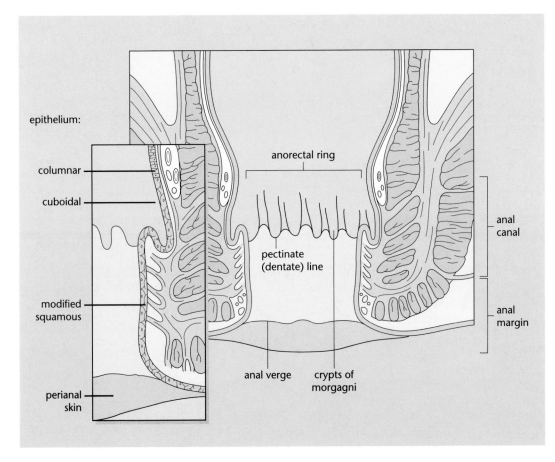

Fig. 5.115 Anatomy of the lower rectum and anal canal. The anal canal extends from the anorectal ring to an area about halfway between the dentate (pectinate) line and the anal verge. The anal margin consists of the area distal to the anal canal, including the perianal skin.

Definition of TNM	Stage grouping			
Primary Tumor (T)				
TX Primary tumor cannot be assessed	Stage 0	Tis	N0	M0
T0 No evidence of primary tumor	Stage I	T1	N0	M0
Tis Carcinoma in situ	Stage II	T2	N0	M0
T1 Tumor 2cm or less in greatest dimension		T3	N0	M0
T2 Tumor more than 2cm, but not more than 5cm in greatest dimension	Stage IIIA	T1	N1	M0
T3 Tumor more than 5cm in greatest dimension		T2	N1	M0
T4 Tumor of any size invades adjacent organ(s), e.g. vagina, urethra,		T3	N1	M0
bladder (involvement of sphincter muscle(s) alone is not classified as		T4	N0	M0
T4)	Stage IIIB	T4	N1	M0
		Any T	N2	M0
Regional Lymph Nodes (N)		Any T	N3	M0
NX Regional lymph nodes cannot be assessed	Stage IV	Any T	Any N	M1
N0 No regional lymph node metastasis				
N1 Metastasis in perirectal lymph node(s)				
N2 Metastasis in unilateral iliac and/or inguinal lymph node(s)				
N3 Metastasis in perirectal and inguinal lymph nodes and/or bilateral internal iliac and/or inguinal lymph nodes				
Distant Metastasis (M)				
MX Presence of distant metastasis cannot be assessed				
M0 No distant metastasis				
M1 Distant metastasis				

Fig. 5.116 Staging of cancer of the anal canal. The staging system applies to all carcinomas arising in the anal canal, including carcinomas that arise within anorectal fistulae. The classification also includes cloacogenic carcinomas. Melanomas are excluded (From Flemming *et al.*, 1997).

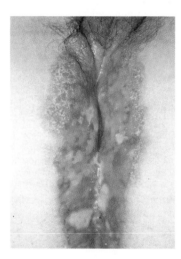

Fig. 5.117 Paget's disease of perianal skin. Extramammary Paget's disease is an intraepithelial adenocarcinoma, whereas Bowen's disease is an intraepithelial squamous cell carcinoma. Any abnormal skin in the perianal area should be biopsied to establish the diagnosis and should not be assumed to represent eczema or psoriasis.

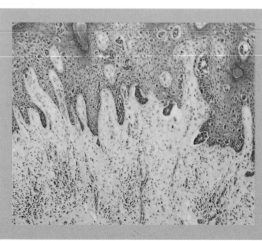
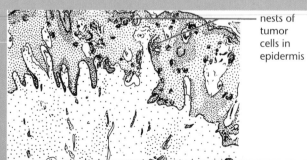

nests of tumor cells in epidermis

Fig. 5.118 Extramammary Paget's disease. Histologic section of anal tissue shows nests of malignant cells within the epidermis.

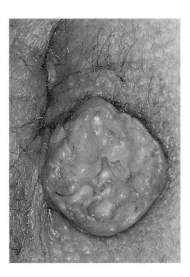

Fig. 5.119 Squamous cell carcinoma of anal margin. Squamous cancers of the anus are divided into tumors arising in the anal canal (most often above the dentate line) and those arising in the skin at the anal margin, as shown here. This lesion measures 1 cm across. Neoplasms at this site tend to be slow growing and metastasize to inguinal lymph nodes. They have a 5-year survival rate of approximately 70%.

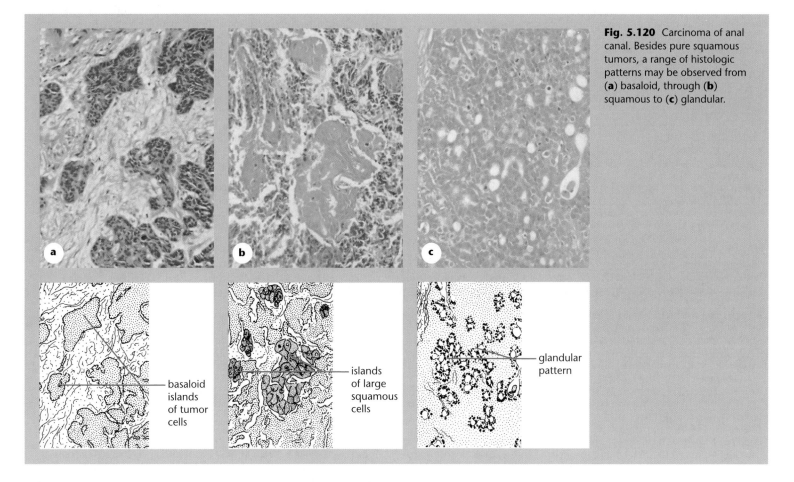

Fig. 5.120 Carcinoma of anal canal. Besides pure squamous tumors, a range of histologic patterns may be observed from (**a**) basaloid, through (**b**) squamous to (**c**) glandular.

basaloid islands of tumor cells

islands of large squamous cells

glandular pattern

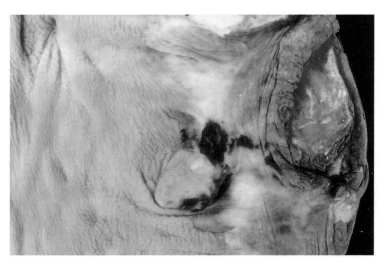

Fig. 5.121 Malignant melanoma of anal canal. This specimen is from a 74-year-old woman who presented with a brief history of episodic rectal bleeding. A hard mass was palpable in the lateral wall of the anal canal and an abdominoperineal resection was performed. The anal canal has been opened to show a flattened, ovoid nodule (2 cm in diameter) arising at about the level of the dentate line. The edge of the tumor shows obvious melanotic pigmentation and an irregular streak of pigment extends from the nodule to the anal margin. Anorectal melanoma is rare, accounting for about 1% of anal cancers.

REFERENCES

Aaltonen LA, Salovaara R, Kristo P, *et al.*: Incidence of hereditary nonpolyposis colorectal cancer and the feasibility of molecular screening for the disease. N Engl J Med 1998; 338 : 1481–1487.

Asaka M, Kimura T, Kato M, *et al.*: Possible role of *Helicobacter pylori* infection in early gastric cancer development. Cancer 1994; 73 : 2691–2694.

Ashley SW, Wells SA: Tumors of the small intestine. Semin Oncol 1988; 15 : 116–128.

Beahrs OH, Henson DE, Hutter RVP, Myers MH (American Joint Committee on Cancer): Manual for Staging of Cancer, 4th edn. Lippincott, Philadelphia, 1993.

Blot WJ: Esophageal cancer trends and risk factors. Semin Oncol 1004; 21 : 403–410.

Bossari S, Viale G, Bossi P, *et al.*: Cytoplasmic accumulation of p53 protein: an independent prognostic indicator in colorectal adenocarcinomas. J Natl Cancer Inst 1994; 86 : 681–687.

Bronner CE, Baker SM, Morrison PT, *et al.*: Mutation in the DNA mismatch repair gene homologue hMLH1 is associated with hereditary non-polyposis colon cancer, Nature 1994; 368 : 258–261.

Cho KR, Vogelstein B: Genetic alterations in the adenoma-carcinoma sequence. Cancer 1992; 70(6 suppl):1727–1731.

Correa P: Clinical implications of recent developments in gastric cancer pathology and epidemiology. Semin Oncol 1985; 12 : 2–10.

Davessar K, Pezzullo JC, Kessimian N, *et al.*: Gastric adenocarcinoma: prognostic significance of several pathologic parameters and histologic classifications. Hum Pathol 1990; 21 : 325–332.

Devesa SS, Blot WJ, Frangioni JF: Changing patterns in the incidence of esophageal and gastric carcinoma in the United States. Cancer 1998; 83 : 2049–2053.

Di Bisceglie AM, Rustgi VK, Hoofnagle JH: Hepatocellular carcinoma. Ann Intern Med 1988; 108 : 390–401.

Edwards JM, Hillier VF, Lawson RAM, *et al.*: Squamous carcinoma of the oesophagus: histological criteria and their prognostic significance. Br J Cancer 1989; 59 : 429–433.

Falkson G, Cnaan A, Schutt AJ: Prognostic factors for survival in heptocellular carcinoma. Cancer Res 1988; 48 : 7314–7318.

Flavia Di Renzo M, Olivero M, Giacomini A, *et al.*: Overexpression and amplification of the Met/HGF receptor gene during the progression of colorectal cancer. Clin Ca Res 1995; 1 : 147–154.

Flemming I, Cooper J, Henson D, *et al.*: (eds) for the AJCC: AJCC Cancer Staging Manual, 5th edn. Lippincott-Raven, Philadelphia, 1997.

Fuchs C, Giovannucci E, Colditz G, *et al.*: A prospective study of family history and the risk of colorectal cancer. N Engl J Med 1994; 331 : 1669–1674.

Fuchs C, Giovannucci E, Colditz G, *et al.*: Dietary fiber and the risk of colorectal cancer and adenoma in women. N Engl J Med 1999; 340 : 169–176.

Fuchs C, Mayer RJ: Gastric carcinoma. N Engl J Med 1995; 333 : 32–41.

Gibby DG, Hanks JB, Wanebo HJ: Bile duct carcinoma. Ann Surg 1985; 202 : 139–144.

Greenlee RT, Hill-Harmon MB, Murray T, Thun M. Cancer statistics 2001. CA Cancer J Clin 2001; 51 : 15–36.

Groden J, Thliveris A, Samowitz W, *et al.*: Identification and characterization of the familial adenomatous polyposis coli gene. Cell 1991; 66(3):589–600.

Haber DA, Mayer RJ: Primary gastrointestinal lymphoma. Semin Oncol 1988; 15 : 154–169.

Harris NL: Low-grade B-cell lymphoma of mucosa-associated lymphoid tissue and monocytoid B-cell lymphoma. Related entities that are distinct from other low-grade B-cell lymphomas [editorial; comment]. Arch Pathol Lab Med 1993; 117(8):771–775.

Iizuka T, Isono K, Kakegawa T, Watanabe H: Parameters linked to ten-year survival in Japan of resected esophageal carcinoma. Japanese Committee for Registration of Esophageal. Carcinoma Cases [see comments]. Chest 1989; 96(5):1005–1011.

Jen J, Kim H, Piantadosi S, *et al.*: Allelic loss of chromosome 18 q and prognosis in colorectal cancer. N Engl J Med 1994; 331 : 213–221.

Kalser MH, Barkin J, MacIntyre JM: Gastrointestinal sarcomas. Semin Oncol 1988; 15 : 181–188.

Karpe M, Leon L, Klinistra D, Brennan M: Lymph node staging in gastric cancer: is location more important than number? Ann Surg 2000; 232(3):362–371.

Kinzler KW, Nilbert MC, Su LK, *et al.*: Identification of FAP locus genes from chromosome 5q21. Science 1991; 253(5020):661–665.

Lagergren J, Bergstrom R, Lindgren A, Nyren O: Symptomatic gastroesophageal reflux as a risk factor for esophageal adenocarcinoma. N Engl J Med 1999; 340 : 825–831.

Leach FS, Nicolaides NC, Papadopoulos N, *et al.*: Mutations of a mutS homolog in hereditary nonpolyposis colorectal cancer. Cell 1993; 75 : 1215–1225.

Licht JD, Weissman LB, Antman K: Gastrointestinal sarcomas. Semin Oncol 1988; 15 : 181–188.

Manabe T, Myashita T, Ohshio G, *et al.*: Small cell carcinoma of the pancreas. Cancer 1988; 62 : 135–141.

Markowitz A, Saleemi MS, Freeman LM: Role of In-111 labeled CYT-103 immunoscintigraphy in the evaluation of patients with recurrent colorectal carcinoma. Clin Nucl Med 1993; 18 : 685–700.

Mitchell EP: Carcinoma of the anal region. Semin Oncol 1988; 15 : 146–153.

Nagasue N, Kohno H, Chang YC, *et al.*: Liver resection for hepatocellular carcinoma. Results of 229 consecutive patients during 11 years. Ann Surg 1993; 217(4):375–384.

Nagorney DM, McPerson GAD: Carcinoma of the gallbladder and extrahepatic bile ducts. Semin Oncol 1988; 15 : 106–115.

Nakamura T, Nekarda H, Hoelscher AH, *et al.*: Prognostic value of DNA ploidy and c-*erb*B-2 oncoprotein overexpression in adenocarcinoma of Barrett's esophagus. Cancer 1994; 73 : 1784–1794.

Palefsky JM: Anal human papillomavirus infection and anal cancer in HIV-positive individuals: an emerging problem. AIDS 1994; 8 : 283–295.

Papadopoulos N, Nicolaides NC, Wei Y-F, *et al.*: Mutations of a mutL homolog in hereditary colon cancer. Science 1994; 263 : 1625–1629.

Parsons R, Li GM, Longley MJ, *et al.*: Hypermutability and mismatch repair deficiency in RER+ tumor cells. Cell 1993; 75(6):1227–1236.

Powell SM, Petersen GM, Krush AJ, *et al.*: Molecular diagnosis of familial adenomatous polyposis. N Engl J Med 1993; 329 : 1982–1987.

Rubinfield B, Souza B, Albert I, *et al.*: Association of the APC gene product with beta-catenin. Science 1993; 262(5140):1731–1734.

Ryan DP, Compton CC, Mayer RJ: Carcinoma of the anal canal. N Engl J Med 2000; 342 : 792–800.

Sinicrope F, Ruan S, Cleary K, *et al.*: bcl-2 and p53 oncoprotein expression during colorectal tumorigenesis. Cancer Res 1995; 55 : 237–241.

Su LK, Vogelstein B, Kinzler KW: Association of the APC tumor suppressor protein with catenins. Science 1993; 262(5140):1734–1737.

Toribara N, Sleisenger M: Screening for colorectal cancer. N Engl J Med 1995; 332 : 861–867.

Wanebo HJ, Kennedy BJ, Chmiel JS, Steele GD, Winchester DP: Cancer of the stomach. A patient care study by the American College of Surgeons. Ann Surg 1993; 218 : 583–592.

Willson JKV: Biology of large bowel cancer. Hematol Oncol Clin North Am 1989; 3 : 19–34.

Winawer SJ, Zauber AG, Nah M, *et al.*: Prevention of colorectal cancer by colonoscopic polypectomy. N Engl J Med 1993; 329 : 1977–1981.

Cancer of the genitourinary tract

William K. Oh, Marc B. Garnick, Christopher L. Corless, Philip W. Kantoff

6

PROSTATE CANCER

Prostate cancer is the most commonly diagnosed non-cutaneous malignancy in men in the United States. In 2001, over 198 000 cases will be diagnosed and over 30 000 men will die of the disease. The incidence of prostate cancer increased rapidly in the early 1990s because of the widespread use of the prostate-specific antigen (PSA) test, but subsequently leveled off in the late 1990s. Mortality from prostate cancer has also appeared to begin to decline recently, though the cause for this drop is not known.

The incidence of prostate cancer increases rapidly with age, particularly after the age of 50, although the presence of pathologic prostate cancer in men less than 50 years of age has been demonstrated in autopsy series. There are strong ethnic and racial differences in the incidence of prostate cancer. Scandinavians and Americans, particularly African Americans, have a very high incidence of prostate cancer compared to Asian men. The results of studies including men who migrate from areas of low incidence to areas of high incidence and acquire intermediate probabilities of developing prostate cancer suggest that environmental factors contribute to these differences. One such factor may be the high-fat diet of the Western developed world. Serum androgen levels may also contribute to the development of prostate cancer. This has been suggested on the basis of epidemiologic studies wherein higher serum testosterone levels or higher tissue levels of 5-α reductase (the enzyme that converts testosterone to dihydrotestosterone) may be associated with a higher likelihood of the development of prostate cancer.

A subset of patients who develop prostate cancer probably do so on the basis of genetic predisposition. Familial prostate cancer may be an important factor among patients who develop prostate cancer at a young age.

HISTOLOGY

The vast majority of prostate cancers are adenocarcinomas. Most exhibit acinar-type differentiation, but some also have features of ductal differentiation; pure large duct prostatic adenocarcinomas are uncommon. Typical prostatic adenocarcinomas may contain foci of mucinous differentiation or neuroendocrine differentiation but the prognostic significance of these features remains uncertain. Small cell undifferentiated carcinoma of the prostate is rare but when present, is often associated with areas of adenocarcinoma. Whether presenting in pure form or intermixed with adenocarcinoma, small cell undifferentiated carcinoma in the prostate carries a grave prognosis. Other tumors occurring in the prostate include transitional cell carcinoma (most often by invasion from the urethra), sarcomas of stromal origin and metastases from other organs.

The putative precursor of invasive adenocarcinoma is prostatic intraepithelial neoplasia (PIN), in which cytologically dysplastic cells are found lining normal ducts and acini. PIN is divided into low and high grades; however, only the latter is geographically associated with invasive adenocarcinoma. Although the natural history of PIN is unknown, many foci of high-grade PIN demonstrate partial loss of the basal cell layer and a transition to small invasive glands is occasionally observed. A diagnosis of high-grade PIN on needle biopsy should prompt additional studies to rule out invasive tumor.

Small foci of adenocarcinoma are found incidentally at autopsy in more than 30% of men over the age of 50 who die of unrelated causes. Thus, there is a large pool of these so-called latent or 'autopsy' prostate cancers present in the older male population. Whether clinical cancers arise from latent tumors or develop by an independent pathway is unknown.

Although a variety of grading schemes for prostate cancer have been developed, the most widely used in the United States is the Gleason grading system, which is based strictly upon architectural rather than cytologic features of the cancer. According to this scheme, the pattern of infiltrating tumor glands is assigned a grade from 1 (well differentiated) to 5 (poorly differentiated). Since many adenocarcinomas exhibit more than one pattern, the grades for the two most common patterns present in a tumor are added together to give a Gleason sum or Gleason score. The prognostic utility of the Gleason grading system has been validated in numerous studies wherein patients diagnosed with low Gleason score cancers have an excellent prognosis, while those with high Gleason score cancers have a poor prognosis. The main shortcoming of the Gleason grading system is that the majority of cancers are intermediate in grade. Less than 30% of cancers in most studies are within the Gleason score 2–4 or 8–10 groups. As a result, the Gleason score provides little prognostic information in most cases.

Tissue staining for PSA has become an important adjunct to confirming the diagnosis of prostate cancer. This is particularly useful in poorly differentiated cancers or those cancers that manifest themselves initially at metastatic sites as poorly differentiated carcinoma.

DIAGNOSIS AND STAGING OF PROSTATE CANCER

The detection of prostate cancer has been greatly enhanced by the introduction of the PSA. Optimal detection of prostate cancer is now achieved through the combination of the digital rectal examination (DRE) and PSA. Biopsies are facilitated by the concurrent use of transrectal ultrasound, which enables the physician to locate the areas of abnormality. The morbidity from biopsy is now minimal with the use of spring-loaded biopsy guns. Optimal information is acquired when multiple specially co-ordinated biopsies are performed. With such biopsies, the grade of the cancer, the number of cores positive for cancer and percentage of cancer per core should be determined.

A bone scan should be performed after the diagnosis of prostate cancer is made, particularly in men with a PSA in excess of 10 ng/ml. Although the incidence of radiographically detected regional lymph nodes is quite low, scanning by CT or MRI should be considered, particularly in patients with high-grade, high-stage cancers or those patients with high PSA serum levels. Endorectal coil MRI should be performed in patients being considered for radical prostatectomy in whom the extent of local disease needs to be assessed. With the widespread use of PSA, the proportion of localized prostate cancers has increased.

Approximately 80% of cancers arising in the prostate gland arise in the peripheral zones and 20% arise in the periureteral or transition zone. Cancers arising in the transition zone traditionally had been diagnosed by transurethral resection of the prostate. However, with increasing use of PSA and of medical therapies for benign prostatic hyperplasia (BPH), the frequency of stage A (T1a) cancers has diminished. Transrectal biopsies of the transition zone are possible if a transition zone cancer is suspected. A distinction between A1 and A2 cancers is made on the basis of grade and volume of cancer. A1 cancers are low-grade, low-volume cancers.

The majority of cancers that are currently diagnosed are picked up as a result of an abnormal PSA, an abnormal DRE or both. Organ-confined, palpable cancers are T2 or B cancers (*see* Fig. 6.11). Cancers diagnosed strictly on the basis of an abnormal PSA with no associated palpable abnormality are currently classified as T1C or B0 cancers. Cancers which on physical exam extend into the seminal vesicles or palpably exceed beyond the prostate are categorized as T3 or stage C cancers. Stage D cancers are those that have metastasized either to regional lymph nodes – stage D1 – or distant lymph nodes, bone or viscera – stage D2 (*see* Fig. 6.11).

Careful examination of the prostate following its removal at the time of radical prostatectomy provides critical prognostic information. There is good correlation between the grade of cancer found at the time of biopsy and that found at the time of radical prostatectomy. With careful examination of the prostate, the volume of cancer can be ascertained. Similarly, vascular or perineural invasion can be ascertained as can the degree of local extension. Cancers that are confined within the capsule are less likely to recur than those that invade through the capsule or into the seminal vesicle or demonstrate positive margins. Clinically localized tumors are frequently upstaged into stage C cancers pathologically. The frequency of lymph node involvement at the time of radical prostatectomy has apparently decreased in recent years, perhaps in part due to the more careful selection of surgical patients afforded by the use of the PSA.

CLINICAL MANIFESTATIONS

Most patients diagnosed with prostate cancer are asymptomatic and the diagnosis is made as a result of an abnormal PSA or DRE. Since the prevalence of BPH in the population of men susceptible to prostate cancer is high, many men will manifest mild degrees of prostatism. With locally advanced prostate cancer, urinary obstruction may occur, as may hematospermia. Carcinoma should be considered when obstructive urinary symptomatology develops over a short period of time. Some patients initially present with symptoms of metastatic disease either from painful bony metastasis or from lymphadenopathy. In such patients, immunostaining for PSA may be of particular value in distinguishing a carcinoma of prostatic origin.

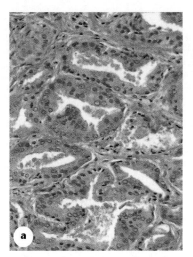
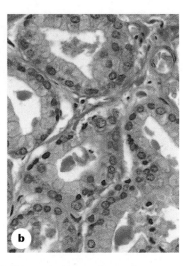

Fig. 6.1 Adenomatous hyperplasia. (**a**) In this atypical example, small, irregular, closely packed glands form a circumscribed nodule. (**b**) At higher power, the epithelial cells lack the prominent nucleoli of adenocarcinoma. A two-cell layer is present focally. Distinction of atypical adenomatous hyperplasia from well-differentiated adenocarcinoma may be difficult.

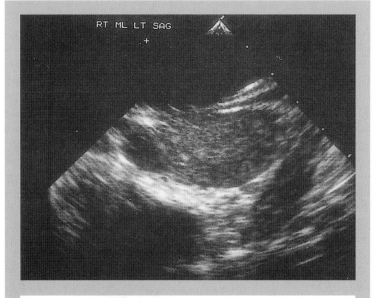

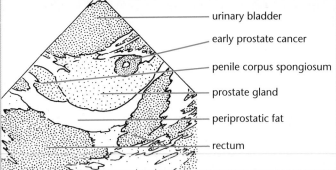

Fig. 6.2 Prostate cancer. Sagittal ultrasonogram demonstrates hypoechoic areas, which are the most common abnormalities seen with prostate cancer. Needle biopsy of hypoechoic lesions can be performed directly under ultrasonographic guidance.

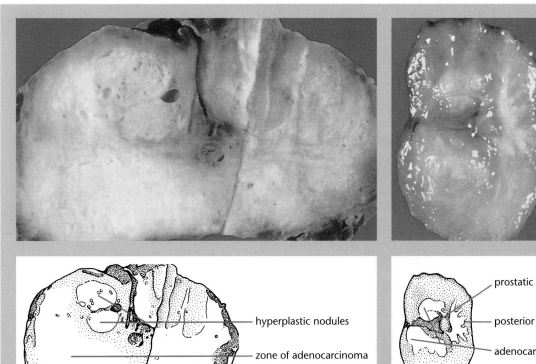

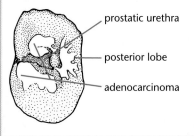

Fig. 6.3 Adenocarcinoma. (**a**) Many prostatic carcinomas arise in the posterior portion of the gland. Cystic areas in this specimen represent zones of nodular hyperplasia unrelated to the carcinoma. This site of origin is not invariably the case, however. (**b**) A yellow zone of coloration in the periurethral region in this specimen corresponds to a lesion involving both lateral lobes.

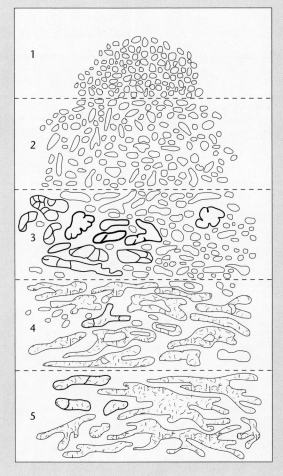

Fig. 6.4 Gleason pattern scores. This is one of the standard grading systems for prostate adenocarcinomas. Five histologic patterns are identified. Patterns 1 and 2 correspond to well-differentiated cancers. Pattern 3 marks a moderately differentiated cancer and patterns 4 and 5 correspond to poorly differentiated or anaplastic lesions.

Histological grading of prostatic adenocarcinoma

1
- Sharply circumscribed aggregate of small, closely packed, uniform glands

2
- Greater variation in glandular size
- More stroma between glands
- More infiltrative margins

3
- Further variation in glandular size
- Glands more widely dispersed in stroma
- Distinctly infiltrative margins, with loss of circumscription

4
- "Fused gland" pattern – irregular masses of neoplastic glands coalescing and branching
- Infiltration of prostatic stroma

5
- Diffusely infiltrating tumor cells with only occasional gland formation

Adapted from Gleason, 1977

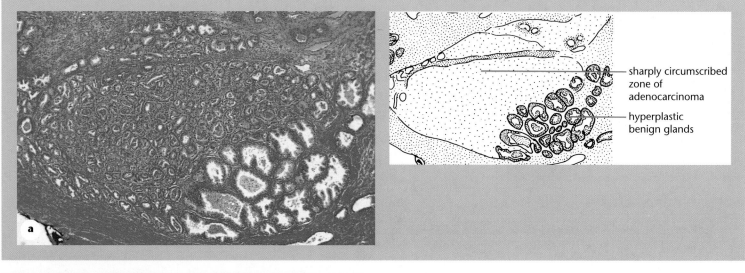

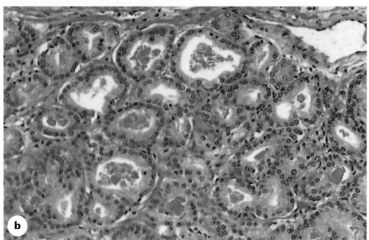

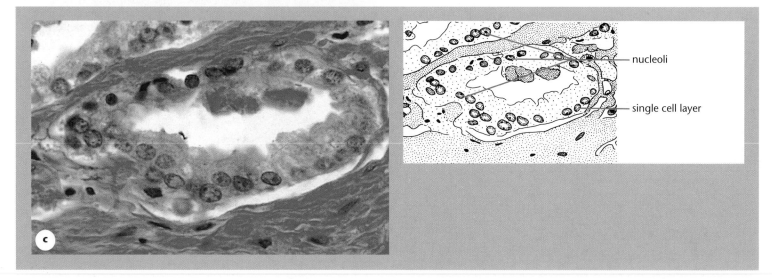

Fig. 6.5 Adenocarcinoma (Gleason grade 1). (**a**) This lesion forms a sharply circumscribed aggregate of small, uniform glands. At this magnification, distinction from atypical adenomatous hyperplasia is not possible. The larger surrounding glands are hyperplastic. (**b**) Small, uniform, closely spaced glands are the hallmark of this low-grade malignancy. Note the sharply circumscribed border, with the surrounding storma at the top left of the field. Intraluminal crystalloids are also present. (**c**) The presence of large nucleoli in the glandular cells has been used to distinguish low-grade carcinoma from atypical adenomatous hyperplasia. This admittedly arbitrary distinction has little if any biologic importance.

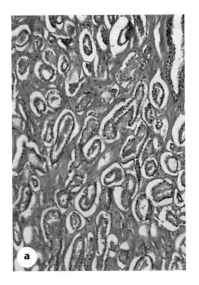

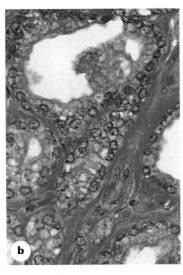

Fig. 6.6 Adenocarcinoma (Gleason grade 2). (**a**) This grade exhibits greater variation in glandular size, more stroma between glands and a more infiltrative margin than the much less common grade 1 pattern. Distinction of grade 2 lesions from grade 3 is somewhat subjective. (**b**) Carcinomatous glands are composed of a single layer of cells. The nuclei are enlarged and have prominent nucleoli.

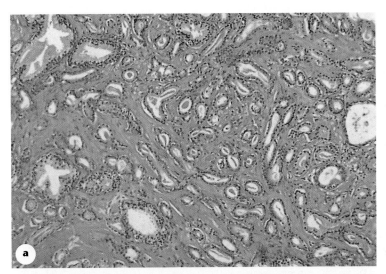

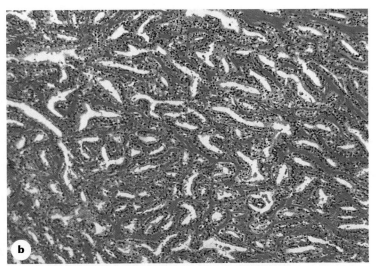

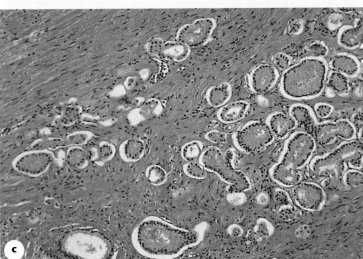

Fig. 6.7 Adenocarcinoma (Gleason grade 3). (**a**) The features of this lesion represent an extension of the changes seen in the grade 2 pattern. The glands are even more irregular in size and shape. The tumor is distinctly infiltrative, without any of the circumscription characterizing grade 1 and 2 lesions. (**b**) Glandular size and shape in this example are markedly irregular. (**c**) Diffuse infiltration of single, irregular glands is evident. Small foci such as these are commonly encountered in needle biopsy specimens.

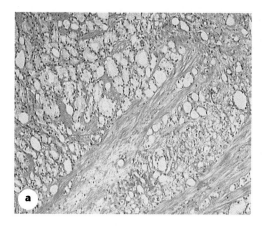
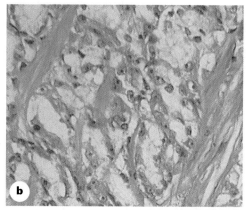
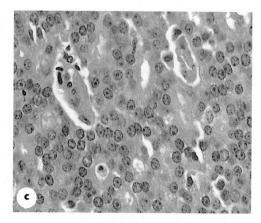

Fig. 6.8 Adenocarcinoma (Gleason grade 4). (**a**) The most common grade 4 variant of prostatic adenocarcinoma is the fused-gland pattern seen here. Back-to-back glands without intervening stroma infiltrate the prostate. (**b**) Higher-power view shows back-to-back glands infiltrating the stroma. (**c**) In another example of the fused-gland pattern, the carcinoma grows as an infiltrating sheet of cells containing scattered lumina.

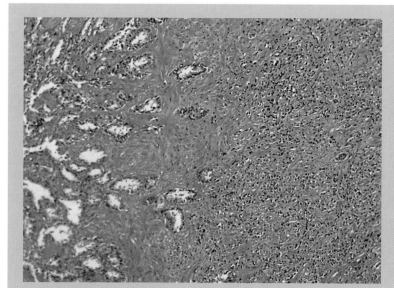

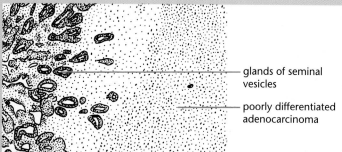

Fig. 6.9 Adenocarcinoma (Gleason grade 5). A seminal vesicle has been invaded by single tumor cells of a high-grade lesion.

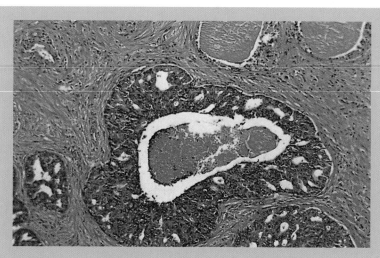

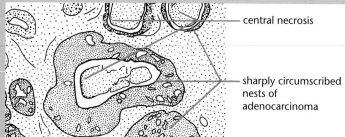

Fig. 6.10 Adenocarcinoma (Gleason grade 5). This lesion exhibits a comedocarcinomatous pattern. Circumscribed nests of tumor cells are similar to those seen at low power in the cribriform variant of Gleason grade 3. The presence of a central area of necrosis distinguishes this pattern from grade 3. The cells of this variant have pleomorphic, vesicular nuclei.

Staging of Prostate Cancer

AJCC TNM	Stage		Whitmore-Jewett	
T1a	I	Microscopic tumor in ≤5% of prostatic chips	A1	Microscopic tumor in ≤5% of prostatic chips
T1b	II	Microscopic tumor in >5% of Prostatic chips. Tumor is not well differentiated	A2	Microscopic tumor in >5% of prostatic chips. Tumor is not well differentiated
T1c		Non-palpable tumor identified By needle biopsy	B0	Non-palpable tumor identified by needle biopsy
T2a		Tumor confined within prostate, involves one lobe	B1	Palpable <1.5 cm organ confined
			B2	Palpable >1.5 cm organ confined
T2b		Tumor confined within prostate, Prostate, involves both lobes	B3	Nodule involving both lobes
T3a	III	Tumor extends through the Prostate capsule (unilateral or bilateral)		
T3b		Tumor invades seminal vesicle	C1	Unilateral seminal vesicle involvement
			C2	Bilateral seminal vesicle involvement
T4	IV	Tumor is fixed or invades bladder, External sphincter, rectum, levator Muscles and/or pelvic wall	C3	Extension to pelvic wall
N1		Metastases in regional lymph nodes	D1	Metastases to 3 or fewer pelvic lymph nodes
			D2	Metastases to >3 lymph nodes or above aortic bifurcation
M1		Distant metastases	D2	Distant metastases

Fig. 6.11 Clinical staging of prostate cancer. The 1997 AJCC TNM classification is compared with the Whitmore–Jewett system which is still used in North America. Note that for patients with non-palpable cancer detected by biopsy performed because of an elevated PSA level, there is a new stage assignment in the Whitmore–Jewett system, stage BO. The AJCC system assigns these cancers to stage TIC, if the malignancy is not detected by imaging.

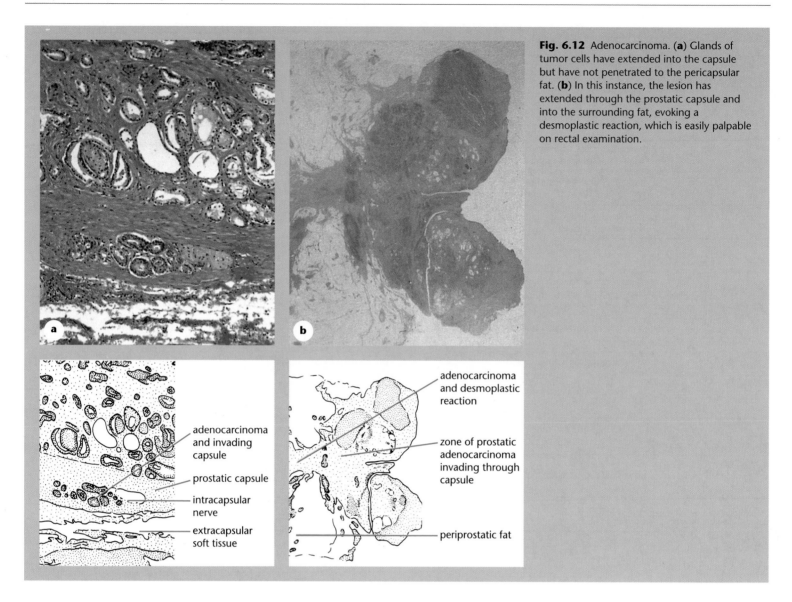

Fig. 6.12 Adenocarcinoma. (**a**) Glands of tumor cells have extended into the capsule but have not penetrated to the pericapsular fat. (**b**) In this instance, the lesion has extended through the prostatic capsule and into the surrounding fat, evoking a desmoplastic reaction, which is easily palpable on rectal examination.

adenocarcinoma
and desmoplastic
reaction

adenocarcinoma
and invading
capsule

prostatic capsule

intracapsular
nerve

extracapsular
soft tissue

zone of prostatic
adenocarcinoma
invading through
capsule

periprostatic fat

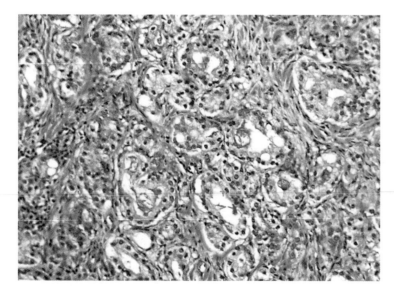

Fig. 6.13 Adenocarcinoma. Even histologically typical lesions like the one shown here often stain positively (red) with the mucicarmine technique, in contrast to normal or hyperplastic prostatic tissue. This stain, therefore, may be valuable as an adjunct to diagnosis.

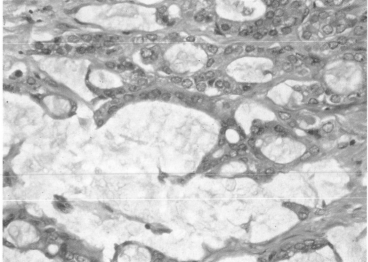

Fig. 6.14 Adenocarcinoma. Some prostatic adenocarcinomas produce abundant extracellular mucin which forms large pools in the stroma, separating tumor cells. Such carcinomas are not readily amenable to Gleason grading and may be confused with metastases from a primary gastrointestinal tumor.

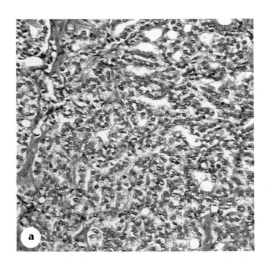

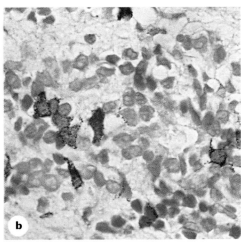

Fig. 6.15 Carcinoid-like tumor. (**a**) Nests of cells with uniform nuclei show a glandular-trabecular growth pattern resembling gastrointestinal carcinoid tumors. (**b**) Argyrophil stain demonstrates many positive (brown) cells in a prostatic carcinoid-like tumor, confirming its neuroendocrine differentiation (Churukian–Schenk stain).

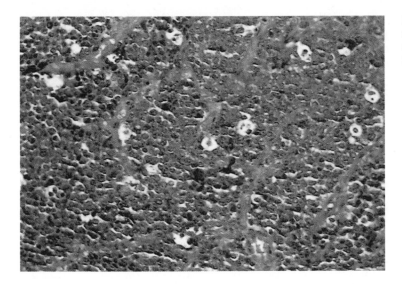

Fig. 6.16 Small cell carcinoma. Carcinomas indistinguishable by light microscopy from pulmonary small cell (oat cell) carcinoma occasionally arise in the prostate. They are usually seen in association with areas of more conventional adenocarcinoma.

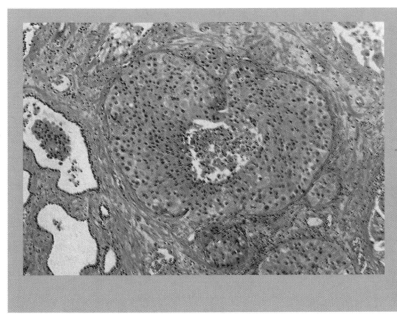

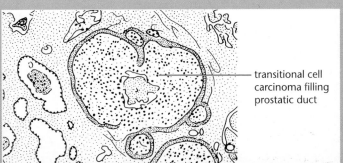

transitional cell carcinoma filling prostatic duct

Fig. 6.17 Transitional cell carcinoma. This tumor may arise in the prostatic ducts or may extend into the ducts from an initial focus in the prostatic urethra. Cytologically identical to analogous lesions of the bladder and urethra, it is characteristically composed of highly plemorphic cells without any evidence of squamous or glandular differentiation. The closely packed, irregular contour of the tumor nests and the surrounding fibroplastic stromal reaction suggest that this is an invasive lesion rather than an *in situ* change in normal ducts.

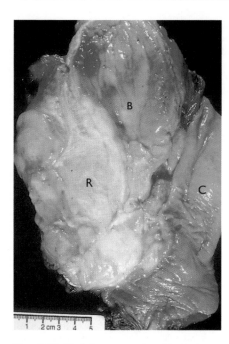

Fig. 6.18 Rhabdomyosarcoma. The tumor forms a large, fleshy mass that replaces the prostate gland and invades the bladder and signmoid colon. R = rhabdomyosarcoma replacing prostate gland; B= urinary bladder; C = distal sigmoid colon.

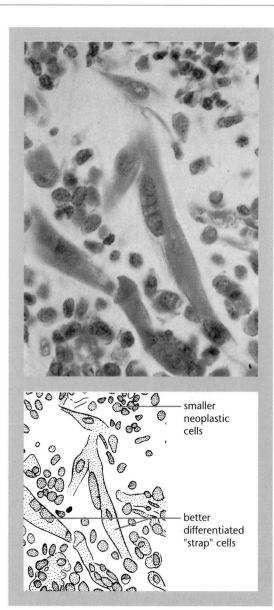

smaller neoplastic cells

better differentiated "strap" cells

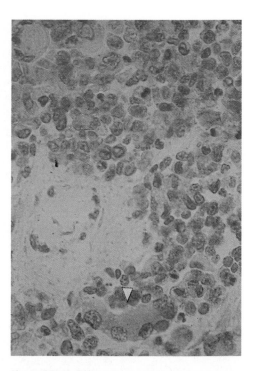

Fig. 6.19 Rhabdomyosarcoma. (**a**) Prostatic rhabdomyosarcomas are usually of the embryonal type and are predominantly composed of small cells with little evidence of differentiation. Rare 'strap' cells may be found in some tumors with more obvious skeletal muscle features. (**b**) In questionable cases, staining for skeletal muscle markers such as myoglobin may be helpful. The large, brown-staining cell (arrow) is positive in this tumor.

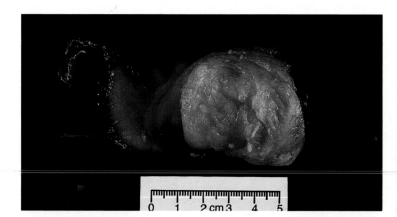

Fig. 6.20 Leiomyosarcoma of prostate. Leiomyosarcoma of prostate, although rare (comprising less than 0.1% of primary prostatic neoplasms), is the single most common prostatic sarcoma typically occurring in older adults (26% of cases). The tumor is characterized by fascicular arrangements of spindle-shaped cells with brightly eosinophilic cytoplasm and strong immunohistochemical positivity for smooth muscle actin and weaker positivity for desmin. Precise criteria for distinction from (benign) leiomyoma have not been proven reliable. Reactive myofibroblastic/fibroblastic proliferations such as postoperative spindle cell nodule should also be considered in the differential diagnosis.

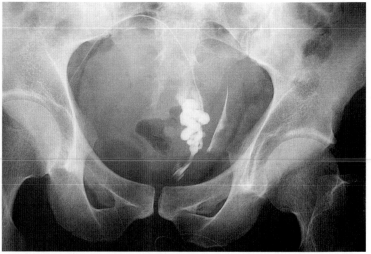

Fig. 6.21 Prostate sarcoma. 35-year-old man with an unusual sarcoma of the prostate. Vasogram shows dilated seminal vesicle due to obstruction from the tumor.

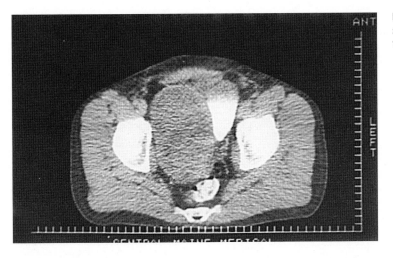

Fig. 6.22 Prostate sarcoma. Same patient. CT scan shows large sarcoma of the prostate (S) displacing the urinary bladder (B) and rectum (R).

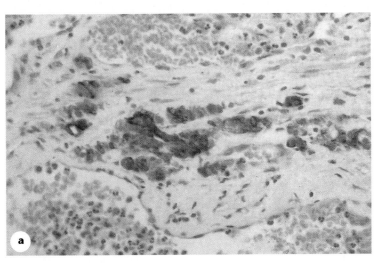

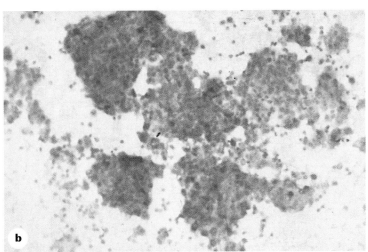

Fig. 6.23 Metastatic adenocarcinoma of prostate. (**a**) This biopsy specimen containing a high-grade adenocarcinoma stains positively for anti-PSA, strongly supporting a prostatic origin. (**b**) Antibodies directed against PSA and prostatic acid phosphatase in this needle aspiration cytology specimen of lung tissue react positively for the latter, indicating a prostatic origin.

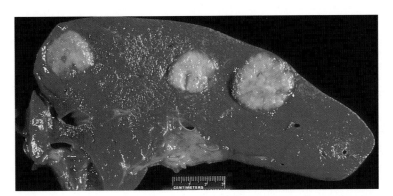

Fig. 6.24 Liver metastases. In unusual instances, prostate cancer can metastasize to the liver. Discrete nodularity is the most common pattern. (Courtesy of Pathology Department, Brigham and Women's Hospital, Boston, MA.)

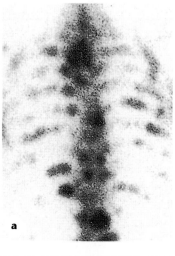

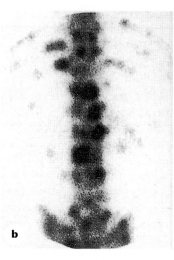

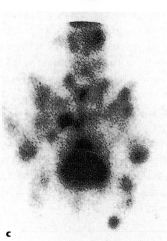

a

b

c

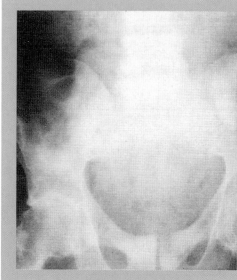

Fig. 6.26 Bone metastases. Radiograph of the lumbar spine and pelvis in a patient presenting with back pain shows multiple sclerotic deposits from a previously undiagnosed primary prostatic carcinoma.

Fig. 6.25 Bone metastases. (**a, b**) Typically, bone scans in metastatic prostate cancer exhibit a 'Christmas tree' pattern of radionuclide uptake, with multiple rib, vertebral and long bone metastases. Osteoblastic metastases in the pelvis and ribs may be confused with metastases from another site. An immunohistochemical PSA determination on tumor tissue (or a serum level) can confirm the diagnosis.

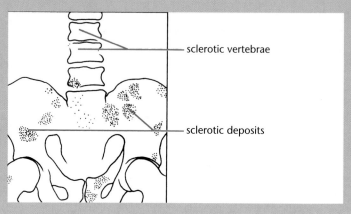

sclerotic vertebrae

sclerotic deposits

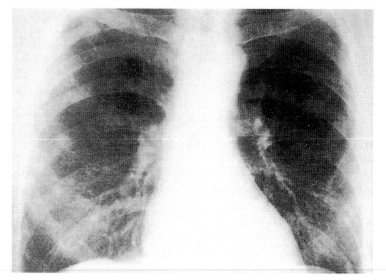

Fig. 6.27 Bone metastases. Plain film of the chest shows multiple dense sclerotic rib lesions which were initially misinterpreted as pulmonary metastases.

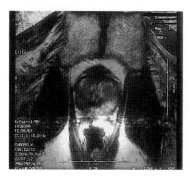

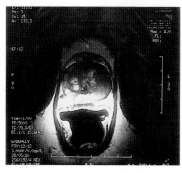

Fig. 6.28 Endorectal magnetic resonance imaging (MRI). Use of endorectal MRI may improve the sensitivity and specificity of detecting cancer that is extracapsular or involving the seminal vesicles.

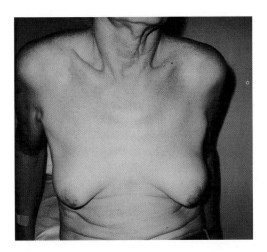

Fig. 6.29 Gynecomastia in a man treated with diethylstilbestrol (DES) for advanced prostate cancer. As estrogenic therapies (including the herbal therapy PC-SPES) are now being increasingly used for androgen-independent prostate cancer, recognition of this complication is important. In addition, antiandrogen monotherapy can also lead to significant gynecomastia. A short course of prophylactic breast irradiation may inhibit growth of breast tissue.

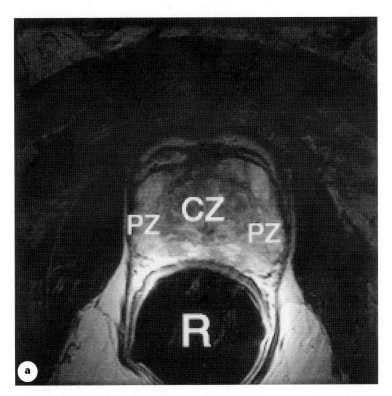

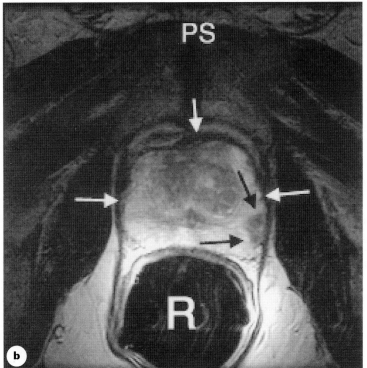

Fig. 6.30 Two axial T$_2$-weighted images from a prostate MR using an endorectal coil. (**a**) At a relatively superior level in the prostate, the normal differentiation between the lower signal central zone (CZ) and the higher signal peripheral zone (PZ) is evident. The rectum (R) is distended by the coil. (**b**) At a lower position in the prostate, a focal area of low signal in the left peripheral zone is seen (black arrows) indicating an area of infiltration with tumor. The margins of the prostate capsule (white arrows) appear intact. The rectum (R) and pubic symphysis (PS) are marked for orientation.

BLADDER CANCER

Over 50 000 new cases of bladder cancer are diagnosed in the United States each year, with over twice as many men affected as women. Bladder cancer generally arises as a result of exposure to environmental carcinogens. In the US, the most important carcinogen is cigarette smoke, contributing to at least 50% of cases. On a worldwide basis, environmental toxins and *Schistosoma haematobium* play a more significant role. Specific genetic abnormalities have been delineated in association with bladder cancer. Monosomy 9 is frequently associated with superficial papillary transitional cell carcinomas. Tumors associated with a higher malignant potential frequently contain abnormalities on chromosome 17p, including p53 abnormalities.

HISTOLOGY

Ninety percent of bladder cancers are transitional cell carcinomas. These are designated grade 1 (well differentiated) to grade 3 (poorly differentiated). They often exhibit a papillary architecture when presenting as superficial lesions. High-grade tumors may be localized within the bladder, but are sometimes associated with widespread transitional cell carcinoma *in situ*. Alternatively, patients may present with carcinoma *in situ* in the absence of grossly recognizable tumor. Both high-grade papillary lesions and carcinoma *in situ* are associated with a substantial risk for developing muscularis invasion. Some transitional cell carcinomas exhibit areas of squamous or adenocarcinomatous differentiation, the significance of which is uncertain. Pure squamous cell carcinomas and adenocarcinomas of the bladder are much less common than transitional cell carcinomas, but are less responsive to therapy.

STAGING OF BLADDER CANCER

Because bladder cancer can metastasize rapidly, sometimes even before symptoms become apparent, staging studies in a patient with this diagnosis are imperative. Chest films, radionuclide bone scanning, tests of liver and renal function and CT scans are all valuable.

Standard staging systems have been based on intravenous urography, bimanual examination, and transurethral resection. At present, two systems are used: the Jewett–Strong–Marshall (JSM) system and the American Joint Committee on Cancer (AJCC) system (*see* Fig. 6.31). Both classify bladder cancers as superficial, invasive or metastatic. Superficial disease is limited to the mucosa or submucosa (JSM stages O and A or AJCC stages Ta and T1); this is the most common form of bladder cancer. Lesions that extend through the submucosa and into the muscularis are classified as invasive bladder cancer. These include lesions that involve superficial or deep muscles (JSM stages B1 and B2 or AJCC T2a and T2b). Although it was formerly believed that the depth of muscle invasion (superficial vs deep) was most important, it now appears that the presence of any muscle involvement is prognostically significant. Almost 50% of patients with muscle invasion eventually die of disease, usually associated with distant metastases. Stages C (T3, T4) and D (N+) denote lesions invading the perivesical fat and extending beyond it, respectively.

CLINICAL MANIFESTATIONS

The most common symptom of bladder cancer is painless hematuria. Carcinoma *in situ* can cause symptoms of urinary tract irritation. Endoscopically, the bladder mucosa may appear normal; a definitive diagnosis can be established only after a urinary cytologic specimen or a mucosal biopsy is obtained and examined. Urinary obstruction caused by urethral blockage and pain secondary to metastatic disease occur occasionally but are relatively uncommon initial manifestations. Sites of metastases include the liver, lung, lymphatic system and bones.

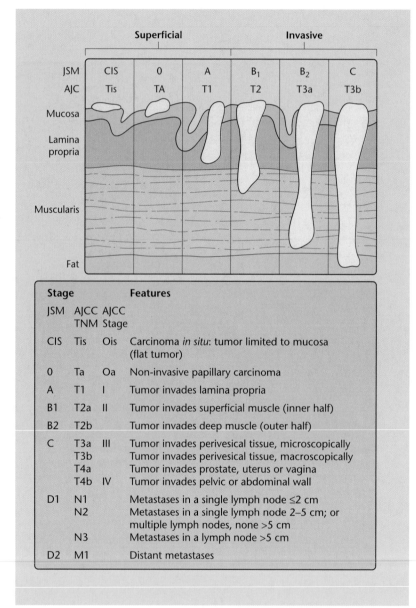

Fig. 6.31 The Jewett–Strong–Marshall (JSM) and AJCC staging systems for bladder cancer.

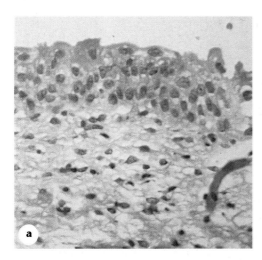 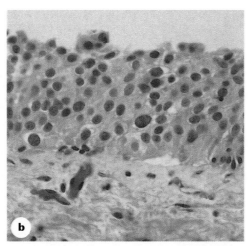 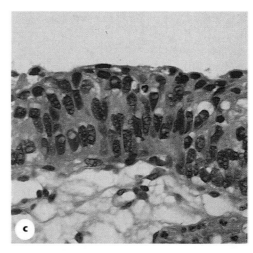

Fig. 6.32 Urothelial dysplasia. (**a**) In mild urothelial dysplasia, cell polarity is altered and there is irregular crowding of nuclei, which are enlarged and focally notched. (**b**) Moderate urothelial dysplasia is marked by more evident loss of cytoplasmic clearing and there are greater numbers of enlarged, slightly irregular, hyperchromatic nuclei. (**c**) Although polarity is not totally lost and there is maturation to superficial cells, the degree of pleomorphism present in this severely dysplastic urothelium approaches carcinoma *in situ*. It should be considered neoplastic and carries a high risk for invasion.

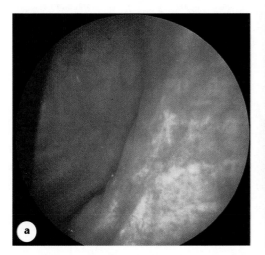 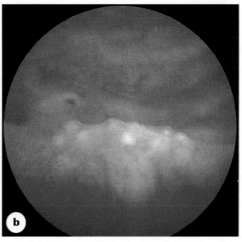 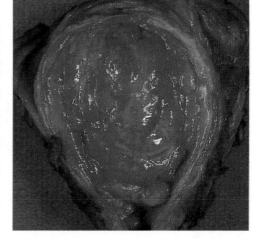

Fig. 6.33 Carcinoma *in situ*. (**a**) Diffuse mucosal erythema with redness not confined within blood vessels is seen in the foreground of this cystoscopic view. This is one appearance of a diffuse *in situ* lesion. (**b**) This raised, sessile *in situ* lesion at the bladder neck exhibits many round, whitish, submucosal aggregates of cystitis follicularis. The background bladder wall has patches of reddened mucosa and other areas consistent with multifocal carcinoma *in situ*. (Courtesy of B. Bracken MD, Cincinnati, OH.)

Fig. 6.34 Carcinoma *in situ*. This cystectomy specimen has a granular and erythematous mucosa, with hemorrhagic areas marking sites of extensive denudation. Numerous poorly defined areas have a cobblestone appearance.

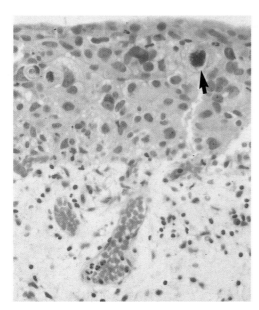

Fig. 6.35 Transitional cell carcinoma *in situ*. The cells exhibit loss of polarity with respect to the surface and contain large, irregular nuclei. An atypical mitosis is evident on the right (arrow), suggesting possible aneuploidy.

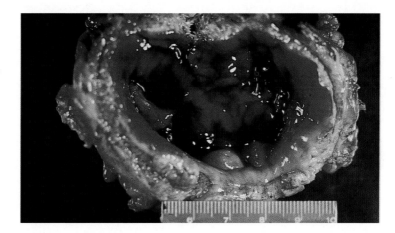

Fig. 6.36 Hemorrhagic cystitis. This 70-year-old woman had recurrent episodes of hemorrhagic cystitis over many years related to chronic use of cyclophosphamide. Cystectomy was required for control of symptoms. Note markedly thickened bladder wall. In some cases, the metabolites (especially acrolein) of cyclophosphamide can result in bladder carcinoma.

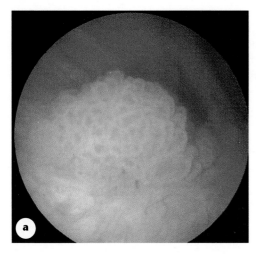

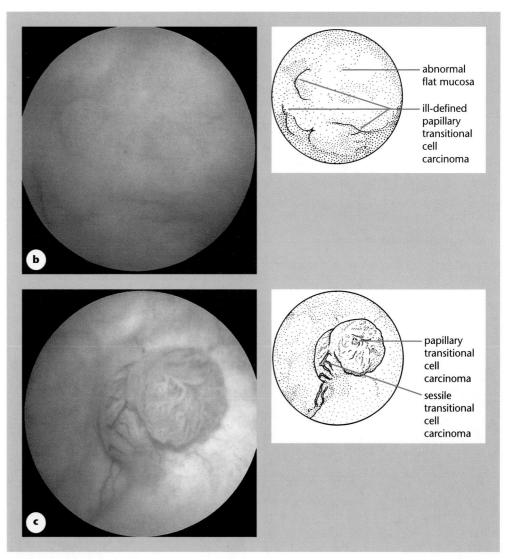

Fig. 6.37 Transitional cell carcinoma. Cystoscopic findings are frequently predictive of the histologic grade of tumor and are useful in assessing adjacent urothelium. (**a**) This discrete grade II papillary lesion (TA or T1) is surrounded by normal mucosa. (**b**) Multiple grade II papillary lesions (TA or T1) are poorly defined because of the surrounding mucosal abnormalities. This lack of definition between malignant and benign mucosa makes definitive transurethral resection uncertain. (**c**) A grade II papillary transitional cell carcinoma (TA or T1) is associated with a sessile invasive tumor (T2 or greater), thus forming a 'collision tumor'. (Courtesy of B. Bracken MD, Cincinnati, OH.)

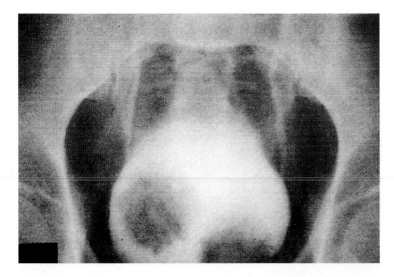

Fig. 6.38 Transitional cell carcinoma. The two large, round masses evident in this cystogram represent papillary tumors. The contrast material enters the crypts, causing a fuzzy, ill-defined appearance at the edges of the masses.

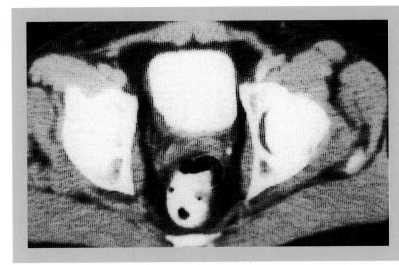

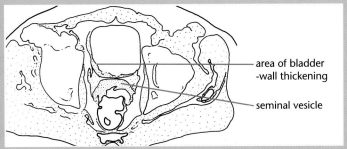

Fig. 6.39 Transitional cell carcinoma. Abdominopelvic CT scanning is helpful in staging bladder cancers. In this example, the neoplasm has thickened the bladder wall without definite extension into the surrounding fat.

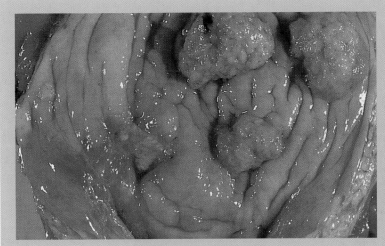

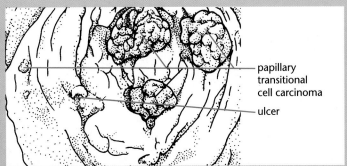

Fig. 6.40 Transitional cell carcinoma. This cystectomy specimen exhibits three large and two small papillary tumors. Transurethral resection of an additional papillary tumor, which documented muscle invasion, has left an ulcerated area in the right posterolateral wall.

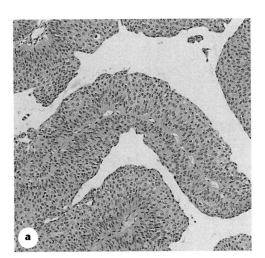

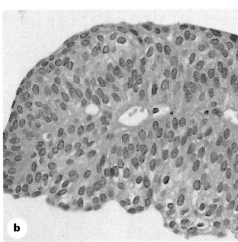

Fig. 6.41 Transitional cell carcinoma. (**a**) This grade I papillary tumor exhibits well-formed papillae that are covered by hyperplastic urothelium. (**b**) Urothelium shows orderly maturation to superficial cells. The slightly hyperchromatic nuclei are crowded together secondary to mild to moderate enlargement.

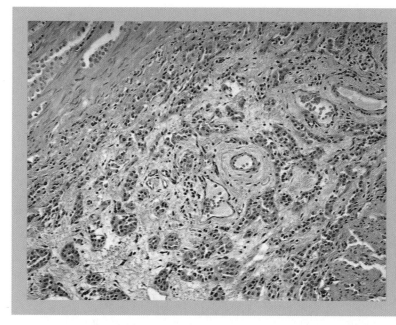

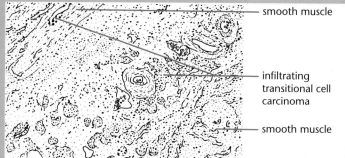

Fig. 6.42 Transitional cell carcinoma. Nests and cords of an infiltrating grade II lesion are present between and within smooth muscle bundles of the bladder wall.

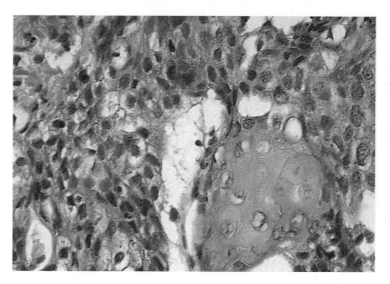

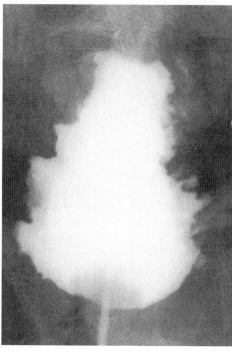

Fig. 6.44 Squamous cell carcinoma. An earlier cystogram in this patient demonstrated a typical 'Christmas tree' bladder with round diverticula. Six years later the flattening and irregularity of the side walls of the bladder strongly suggest tumor infiltration.

Fig. 6.43 Transitional cell carcinoma. This high-grade tumor exhibits focal squamous differentiation (center). It should not be misdiagnosed as a squamous cell carcinoma, which usually shows intercellular bridging and keratin pearls.

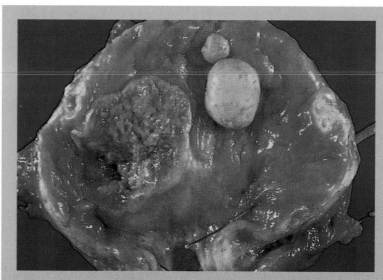

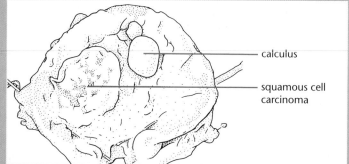

Fig. 6.45 Squamous cell carcinoma. The ulcerated, necrotic tumor in this cystectomy specimen has raised edges that appear sharply demarcated from the surrounding mucosa. Several bladder calculi are present.

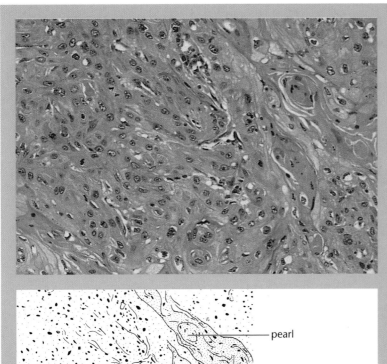

Fig. 6.46 Squamous cell carcinoma. In this well-differentiated tumor, sheets of polygonal keratinizing cells with intercellular bridges produce extracellular keratin and form pearls.

— pearl

— keratin

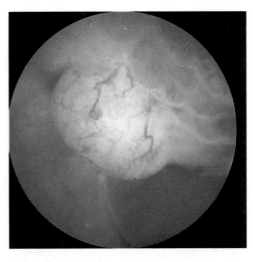

Fig. 6.47 Adenocarcinoma of urachus. A tumor in the bladder dome stretches the intact normal mucosa and appears to be invading the bladder from an intramural or extravesical source. These cystoscopic findings are characteristic of an urachal adenocarcinoma.

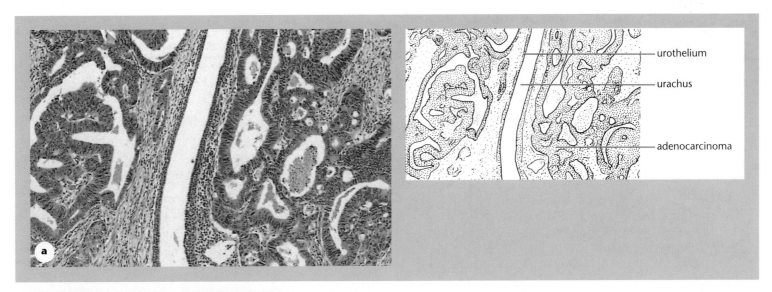

— urothelium

— urachus

— adenocarcinoma

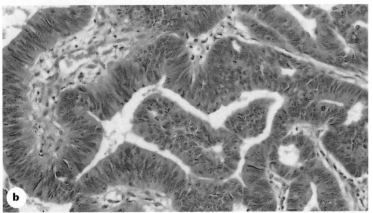

Fig. 6.48 Adenocarcinoma of urachus. (**a**) Low-power photomicrograph of a tumor that arose in the wall of the bladder dome shows that the urachus, lined by a thin layer of urothelium, is microscopically patent. (**b**) Papillae and glands are lined by stratified columnar epithelium. (**a**: Courtesy of B. Bracken MD, Cincinnati, OH.)

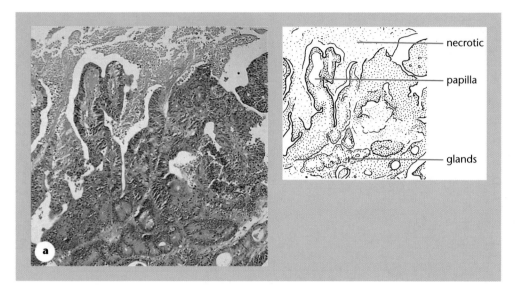

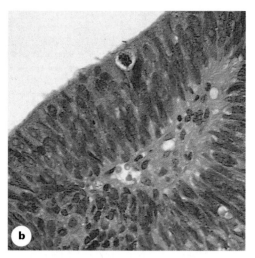

Fig. 6.49 Adenocarcinoma. (**a**) These tumors are commonly papillary and glandular, resembling intestinal neoplasms. The luminal surface in this example is covered with necrotic cellular debris and mucin. (**b**) Like urachal adenocarcinoma, papillae and glands contain stratified columnar epithelium. Intracytoplasmic mucin may be absent.

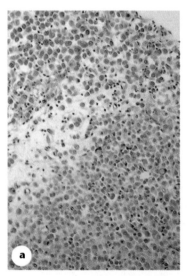

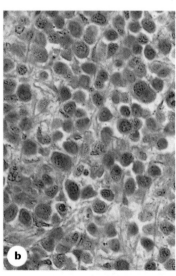

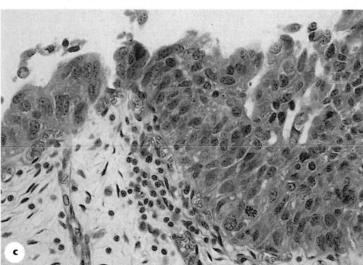

Fig. 6.50 Signet ring cell carcinoma. (**a**) The lamina propria contains a dense infiltrate of neoplastic cells. Overlying urothelium is denuded. (**b**) Many cells contain mucin vacuoles. Cells with displaced nuclei have a signet ring cell appearance. (**c**) The presence of carcinoma *in situ* (on the left) supports a bladder origin for this cancer.

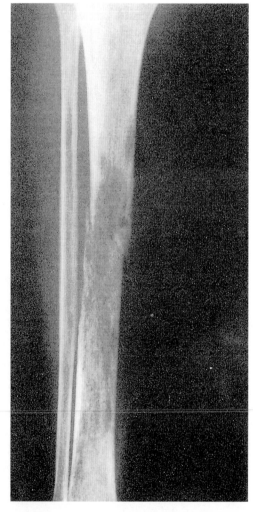

Fig. 6.51 Bone metastases. Plain film of the tibia shows osteolytic metastases in the midshaft in a patient with advanced transitional cell carcinoma of the bladder. Surprisingly, these lesions can undergo healing with intensive combination chemotherapy. If the lesion is isolated and small, it can be surgically resected.

KIDNEY CANCER

Over 30 000 new cases of renal cell carcinoma are diagnosed on an annual basis. In the past, renal cell carcinoma was frequently diagnosed when symptoms arose from local extension of disease, metastases or a variety of paraneoplastic phenomena. However, an increasing proportion of patients are currently diagnosed as a result of an incidental finding on non-invasive radiologic examination performed for other reasons.

HISTOLOGY

Most renal cancers are adenocarcinomas. They are subclassified according to architectural and cytologic features as follows (including relative incidences): clear cell (70%) granular (10%), papillary (10%), chromophobic (5%), sarcomatoid (2%), collecting duct carcinoma (<1%). Cytogenetic studies support the distinction of these histologic variants. Whereas almost all clear cell tumors have a deletion in the short arm of chromosome 3, papillary tumors are characterized by trisomy 7 and 17. Low-grade clear cell tumors may be entirely cystic. Papillary tumors are significantly associated with cortical adenomas and are relatively more common in the setting of end-stage renal disease. The sarcomatoid variant of renal cell carcinoma is associated with a worse prognosis.

Most renal cell carcinomas exhibit features suggesting proximal tubule differentiation; however, markers of distal tubule differentiation are sometimes observed. The old term hypernephroma should be abandoned. When investigated in detail, many so-called sarcomas of the kidney have turned out to be sarcomatoid carcinomas; true renal sarcomas are very rare. Angiomyolipomas and oncocytomas of the kidney are more common tumors, each associated with an essentially benign prognosis. In pediatric patients, Wilms' tumor is the most common renal neoplasm.

STAGING OF KIDNEY CANCER

Renal cancer can be classified into stage I through IV (*see* Fig. 6.56). Staging is usually determined at surgery. The stage of disease, which reflects the sites of invasion, is an important predictor of outcome; however, the prognosis does not necessarily become worse with increasingly higher stages. At one time it was believed that all patients with stage III disease could anticipate a similar outcome. Now it is known that individuals with renal vein involvement may actually have a better prognosis; some investigators, in fact, classify renal vein involvement as stage II.

CLINICAL MANIFESTATIONS

The classic triad of symptoms – hematuria, flank pain and abdominal mass – is observed in only about 10% of patients. However, individual symptoms occur in almost half of patients with kidney cancer. A variety of paraneoplastic phenomena can be associated with renal adenocarcinoma, including hypertension and hepatosplenomegaly not caused by metastases.

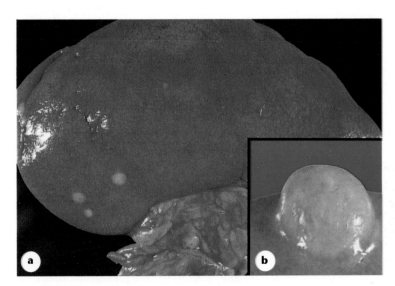

Fig. 6.52 Cortical adenoma. This benign lesion is a common incidental finding at autopsy; it may be multiple. (**a**) The three adenomas in this kidney are each less than 5 mm in diameter, slightly raised, sharply demarcated, gray-white, subcapsular nodules. (**b**) An adenoma protrudes from the cortical surface. Although predominantly gray-white, it has multiple yellow areas, indicating that it is composed of both granular and clear cells.

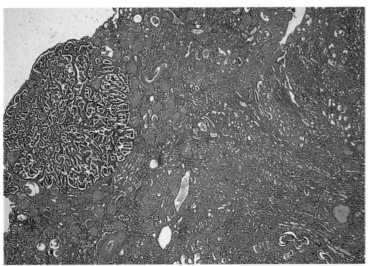

Fig. 6.53 Cortical adenoma. An unencapsulated tubular epithelial neoplasm in the subcapsular cortex merges imperceptibly with the surrounding parenchyma. It has a uniform papillary growth pattern and lacks hemorrhage and necrosis.

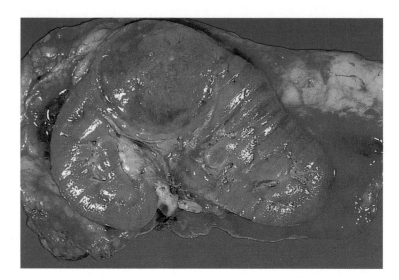

Fig. 6.54 Oncocytoma. Apparently arising from epithelial cells of the proximal renal tubule, these tumors have a low malignant potential when they are less than 5 cm in diameter and are well circumscribed. They have a characteristic mahogany-brown color. Uncommon focal hemorrhage is also present.

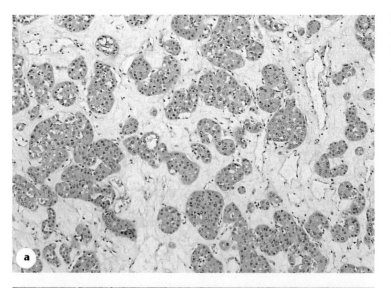

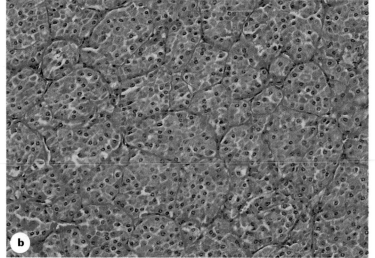

Fig. 6.55 Oncocytoma. (**a**) The central scar is composed of loose, relatively acellular, fibrous tissue. Organoid packeting of oncocytes is prominent. (**b**) Compact peripheral nests are separated by a delicate fibrovascular stroma. Oncocytomas comprise a uniform population of tubular cells with abundant eosinophilic, granular cytoplasm and minimal nuclear atypia.

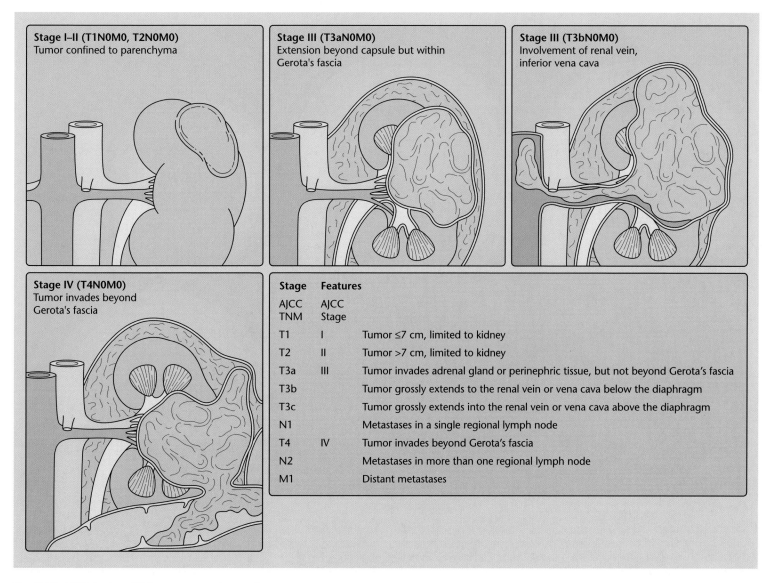

Stage I–II (T1N0M0, T2N0M0)
Tumor confined to parenchyma

Stage III (T3aN0M0)
Extension beyond capsule but within Gerota's fascia

Stage III (T3bN0M0)
Involvement of renal vein, inferior vena cava

Stage IV (T4N0M0)
Tumor invades beyond Gerota's fascia

Stage	Features	
AJCC TNM	AJCC Stage	
T1	I	Tumor ≤7 cm, limited to kidney
T2	II	Tumor >7 cm, limited to kidney
T3a	III	Tumor invades adrenal gland or perinephric tissue, but not beyond Gerota's fascia
T3b		Tumor grossly extends to the renal vein or vena cava below the diaphragm
T3c		Tumor grossly extends into the renal vein or vena cava above the diaphragm
N1		Metastases in a single regional lymph node
T4	IV	Tumor invades beyond Gerota's fascia
N2		Metastases in more than one regional lymph node
M1		Distant metastases

Fig. 6.56 AJCC staging of kidney cancer and examples.

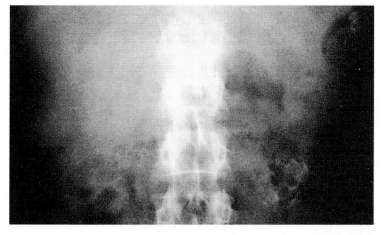

Fig. 6.57 Renal cell carcinoma. Calcifications in both renal beds are suggestive of renal carcinoma, especially in this patient with von Hippel–Lindau disease.

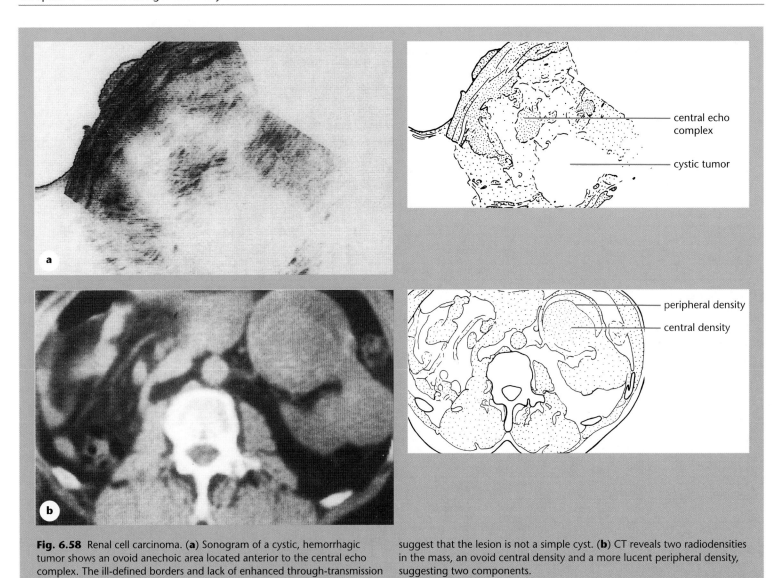

central echo
complex

cystic tumor

peripheral density

central density

Fig. 6.58 Renal cell carcinoma. (**a**) Sonogram of a cystic, hemorrhagic tumor shows an ovoid anechoic area located anterior to the central echo complex. The ill-defined borders and lack of enhanced through-transmission suggest that the lesion is not a simple cyst. (**b**) CT reveals two radiodensities in the mass, an ovoid central density and a more lucent peripheral density, suggesting two components.

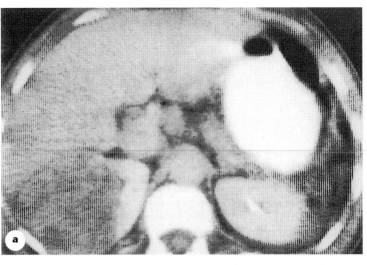

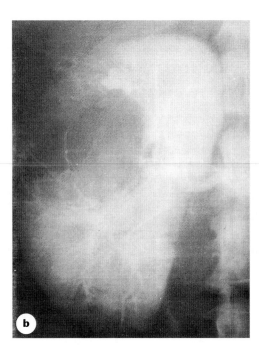

Fig. 6.59 Renal cell carcinoma. (**a**) A solid tumor with areas of hemorrhage or necrosis, which appeared echogenic on sonography, shows mixed density on CT scan. (**b**) Arteriography reveals a hypovascular mass.

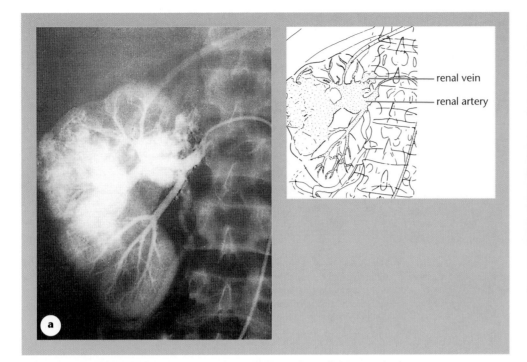

renal vein

renal artery

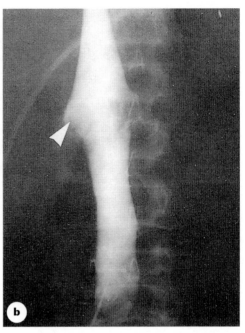

Fig. 6.60 Renal cell carcinoma. (**a**) In addition to renal vein invasion, this arteriogram shows neovascularity in the tumor, as well as in the course of the renal vein. (**b**) On the inferior vena cavagram, the contrast column defines the tumor thrombus on the right (arrow). There is wash-in from the normal left renal vein flow.

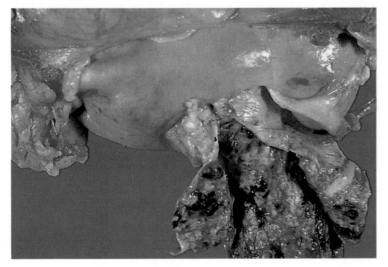

Fig. 6.61 Renal cell carcinoma. With massive invasion by tumor, the renal vein may become occluded by adherent tumor thrombus.

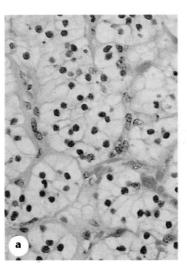
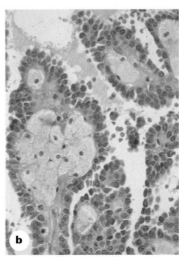
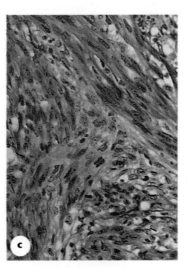

Fig. 6.62 Renal cell carcinoma histology. (**a**) The classic clear cell variant of renal cell carcinoma is composed of cells with abundant cytoplasm containing lipid and glycogen. (**b**) Tumor cells in the papillary variant are arranged around fibrovascular cores that frequently contain clusters of foamy macrophages. (**c**) Intersecting fascicles of anaplastic spindle cells are present in this sarcomatoid variant.

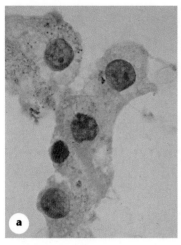
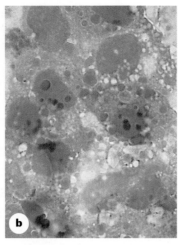
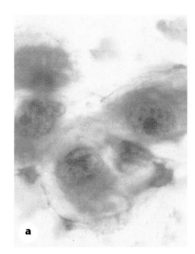
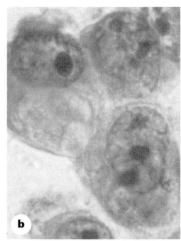

Fig. 6.63 Renal cell carcinoma. (**a, b**) Fine-needle aspiration biopsy of a well-differentiated tumor shows small sheets and groups of cells with slight nuclear enlargement and hyperchromatism, small nucleoli and abundant cytoplasm containing hemosiderin granules and lipid vacuoles.

Fig. 6.64 Renal cell carcinoma. (**a, b**) Fine-needle aspiration biopsy of a poorly differentiated tumor shows cells that have prominent nuclear pleomorphism with chromatin clearing and single or multiple macronucleoli. Nucleus to cytoplasm ratios are high. In the section on the left, perinuclear cytoplasm is distinctly granular. Urine cytology may reveal similar cells.

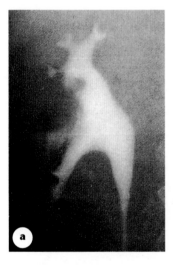
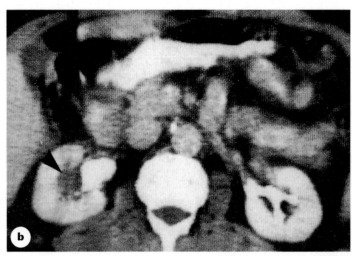
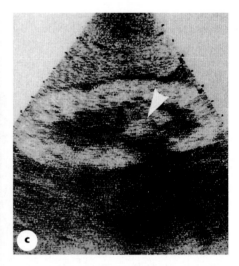

Fig. 6.65 Transitional cell carcinoma. (**a**) The urogram reveals a mass with ill-defined margins either arising in or impinging on the lateral portion of the renal pelvis. (**b**) CT shows a minimally enhancing mass in the renal sinus/pelvis displacing the contrast in the pelvis medially (arrow). (**c**) Because the mass (arrow) is echogenic on the sonogram, it is solid rather than cystic.

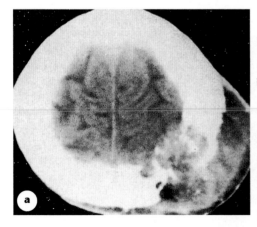
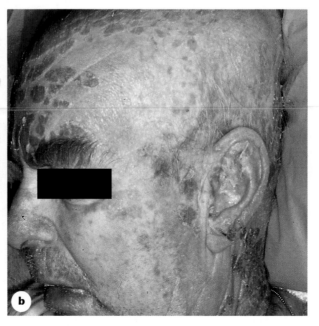

Fig. 6.66 Skull metastases. (**a, b**) This 74-year-old man developed metastatic renal cell cancer to the skull with marked protuberance of the temporal bone. Cranial radiotherapy, administered because of the brain metastases (not seen on this CT scan), was followed by radiation dermatitis.

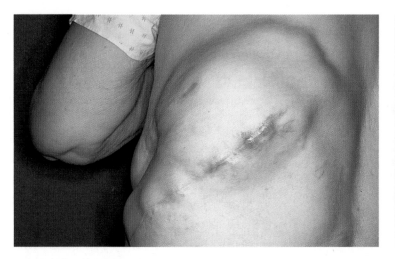

Fig. 6.67 Renal cell carcinoma. Soft tissue metastases in the lower chest and flank developed in this 57-year-old woman, 1 year after nephrectomy.

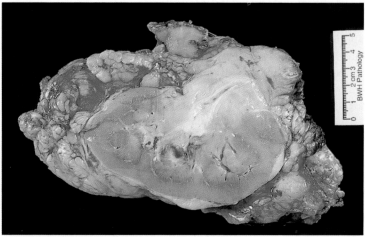

Fig. 6.68 Renal lymphoma. The kidney and perirenal lymph nodes were secondarily involved by non-Hodgkin's lymphoma, predominantly diffuse (focally nodular), large B-cell type, with focal CD10 positivity in nodular areas, consistent with transformation from lower grade follicular lymphoma (as demonstrated in the separately submitted right retroperitoneal nodes).

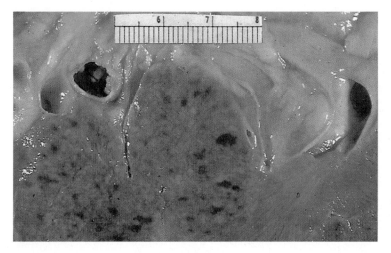

Fig. 6.69 Metastatic malignant melanoma. The urinary tract is a common site of metastases. If not amelanotic, the metastatic nodules are brown-black. Urine may also be black.

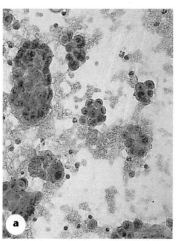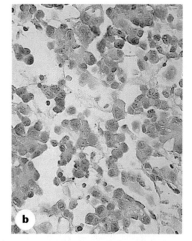

Fig. 6.70 Metastatic adenocarcinoma. (**a, b**) Fine-needle aspiration kidney biopsy from a patient with pulmonary and renal masses contains papillary and glandular epithelial fragments. The presence of intracytoplasmic mucin (right, center) excludes renal cell carcinoma and is consistent with metastatic adenocarcinoma, in this case originating in the lung.

TESTICULAR CANCER

Testicular cancer, which in the United States is diagnosed in over 7000 patients each year, serves as a model of a curable neoplasm. Most patients are young, in their third or fourth decade of life. In patients over the age of 50, testicular neoplasms are usually due to a malignant lymphoma.

HISTOLOGY

Germ cell cancers of the testis can be divided into seminomas and non-seminomas. This distinction is based on the fact that seminomas are extremely radioresponsive and tend toward localized tissue invasion, whereas non-seminomas are more radioresistant and metastasize via hematogenous routes to the lung or liver. Histologic variants of non-seminoma include embryonal carcinoma, teratoma, choriocarcinoma (and mixtures of these such as teratocarcinoma, a histologic combination of teratoma and embryonal cell cancer), and yolk sac tumor (also known as endodermal sinus tumor).

Less than 5% of testicular malignancies originate from the gonadal stroma; these are mainly Leydig cell tumors, which can occur at any age and secrete both testosterone and estradiol, causing sexual precocity in prepubertal boys and gynecomastia in adults. About 10% of Leydig cell tumors metastasize; these demonstrate histologic features of aggressive behavior, such as blood vessel invasion and poor cell differentiation. Sertoli cell tumors are rare (only about 100 cases have been reported) and are also found in all age groups. They may secrete estrogens and thus cause gynecomastia. Metastases occur in 10–20% of cases.

Lymphomas, usually of the diffuse large cell type, represent 5% or less of testicular malignancies. They tend to be bilateral and often disseminate, particularly to the central nervous system. Involvement of the testes may occur in systemic lymphomas (about 10% of cases) and in some patients may herald an underlying malignant lymphoma.

STAGING OF TESTICULAR CANCER

The staging evaluation of testicular cancers usually includes an abdominal-pelvic CT scan and chest radiography; sometimes suspicious abnormalities on a chest film prompt CT scanning of the chest as well. In certain high-risk patients (usually those with signs suggestive of choriocarcinoma), a bone scan and CT scan of the head are performed. Stage I non-seminomas are often surgically staged by retroperitoneal lymph node dissection. Circulating biologic markers, such as human chorionic gonadotropin (HCG) and α-fetoprotein (AFP), are prognostically important and are useful in following the clinical course.

Cancer confined to the testis, with no clinical or radiologic evidence of distant metastases, constitutes stage I disease (*see* Fig. 6.71). If there is no disease above the diaphragm but evidence of retroperitoneal adenopathy is demonstrated on CT scan or lymphangiogram, the cancer is classified as stage II disease. Stage III disease is marked by persistence of positive biologic markers after orchidectomy or by subdiaphragmatic visceral involvement (e.g. of the liver, spleen or inferior vena cava) or supradiaphragmatic metastases to the lung parenchyma or central nervous system. Prognosis can be determined by criteria established by the International Germ Cell Consensus Criteria (Table 6.1).

CLINICAL MANIFESTATIONS

The manifestations of testicular cancer are protean, ranging from detection of an asymptomatic nodule or swelling on self-examination of the testes to the development of symptoms secondary to metastatic disease. Patients who present with a painful lesion in the scrotum are often initially diagnosed and treated for epididymitis before the true diagnosis of cancer is established. Epididymitis often occurs concomitantly in patients with testicular cancer and may explain the associated pain. The sudden, acute appearance of a rapidly enlarging testis, particularly characteristic of choriocarcinoma, is usually associated with hemorrhage into neoplastic tissue. Back or abdominal pain secondary to retroperitoneal adenopathy, dyspnea caused by pulmonary metastases, weight loss, gynecomastia, supraclavicular lymphadenopathy and urinary obstruction may also be evident at the time of presentation.

Table 6.1 International Germ Cell Consensus Criteria for testicular cancer

Non-seminoma	Seminoma
Good prognosis	
Testis/retroperitoneal primary *and* No non-pulmonary visceral metastases *and* Good markers – all of • AFP <1000 ng/ml and • hCG <5000 iu/l (1000 ng/ml) and • LDH <1.5 × upper limit of normal	Any primary site *and* No non-pulmonary visceral metastases *and* Normal AFP, any hCG, any LDH
58% of non-seminomas 5-year PFS 89% 5-year survival 92%	90% of seminomas 5-year PFS 82% 5-year survival 86%
Intermediate prognosis	
Testis/retroperitoneal primary *and* No non-pulmonary visceral metastases *and* Intermediate markers – any of • AFP ≥1000 and ≤10 000 ng/ml or • hCG ≥5000 iu/l and ≤50 000 iu/l or • LDH ≥1.5 × N and ≤10 × N	Any primary site *and* Non-pulmonary visceral metastases *and* Normal AFP, any hCG, any LDH
28% of non-seminomas 5-year PFS 75% 5-year survival 80%	10% of seminomas 5-year PFS 67% 5-year survival 72%
Poor prognosis	
Mediastinal primary *or* Non-pulmonary visceral metastases *or* Poor markers – any of • AFP > 10 000 ng/ml or • hCG > 50 000 iu/l (10 000 ng/ml) or • LDH > 10 × upper limit of normal	No patients classified as poor prognosis
16% of non-seminomas 5-year PFS 41% 5-year survival 48%	

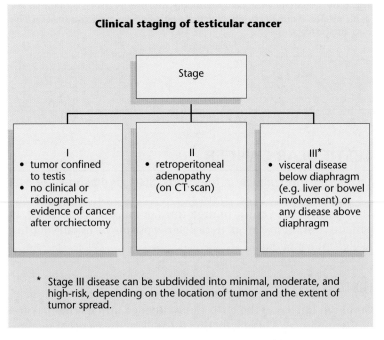

Clinical staging of testicular cancer

Stage

I
• tumor confined to testis
• no clinical or radiographic evidence of cancer after orchiectomy

II
• retroperitoneal adenopathy (on CT scan)

III*
• visceral disease below diaphragm (e.g. liver or bowel involvement) or any disease above diaphragm

* Stage III disease can be subdivided into minimal, moderate, and high-risk, depending on the location of tumor and the extent of tumor spread.

Fig. 6.71 Clinical staging of testicular cancer. The AJCC TNM staging system is less commonly used since it is based upon histologic evaluation of the orchidectomy specimen and retroperitoneal peri-aortic lymph node dissection. Since the latter may not be performed in every patient, the clinical staging system is generally more practical.

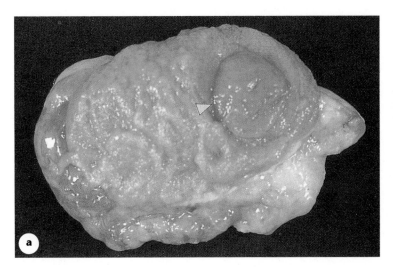

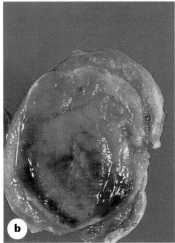

Fig. 6.72 Leydig cell tumor. (**a**) This tumor forms a small, circumscribed, yellow nodule (arrow) within the testis. (**b**) An encapsulated, focally hemorrhagic tumor has replaced most of the testicular parenchyma.

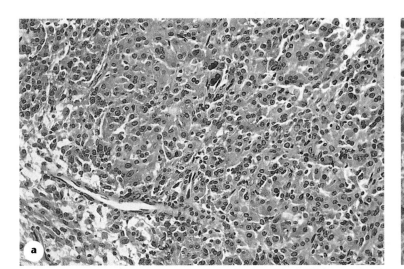

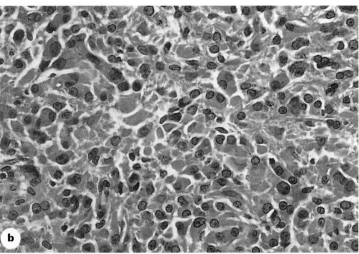

Fig. 6.73 Leydig cell tumor. (**a**) Sheets of tumor cells with prominent, eosinophilic cytoplasm infiltrate the testicular stroma. (**b**) High-power view reveals that the tumor is composed of polygonal, ovoid and spindled cells with dense eosinophilic cytoplasm and round to ovoid nuclei. There is moderate nuclear pleomorphism.

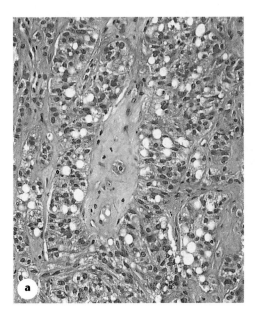

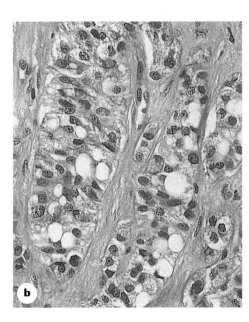

Fig. 6.74 Sertoli cell tumor. (**a**) Low- and (**b**) high-power photomicrographs reveal irregular cords of tumor cells with vacuolated cytoplasm infiltrating the testicular stroma.

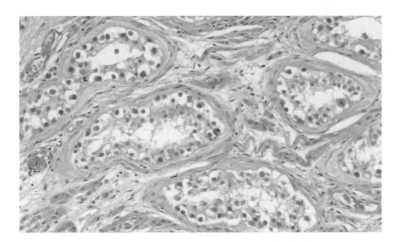

Fig. 6.75 Germ cell neoplasia *in situ*. Neoplastic germ cells with abundant, clear cytoplasm line the seminiferous tubules. The nuclei are larger and more hyperchromatic than normal germ cells. Spermatogenesis is decreased or absent.

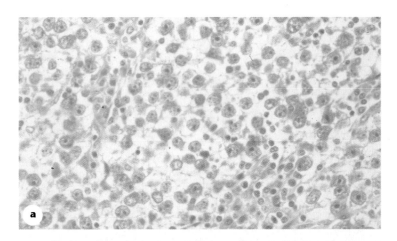

Fig. 6.76 Seminoma. (**a**) A lymphatic infiltrate is typical in seminomas. (**b**) Multinucleate histiocytes (giant cells) may be seen in seminomas and should not be confused with syncytiotrophoblastic cells. The nuclei of the giant cells have a uniform vesicular appearance identical to that of mononuclear histiocytes. (**c**) The large, irregular giant cells in this seminoma are syncytiotrophoblastic cells resembling placental syncytial cells and producing the β-subunit of human chorionic gonadotrophin (β-hCG). In the absence of a mixture of cytotrophoblastic and syncytiotrophoblastic elements, choriocarcinoma should not be diagnosed.

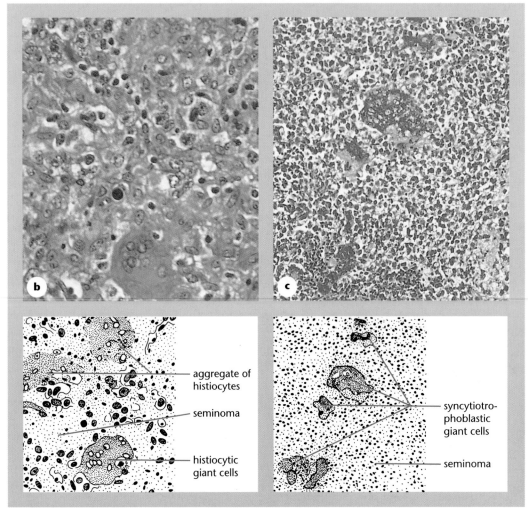

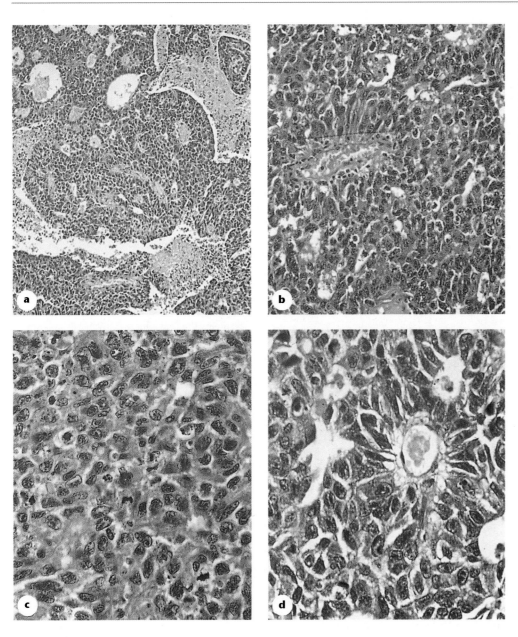

Fig. 6.77 Embryonal carcinoma. (**a**) Nests and cords of neoplastic cells are surrounded by zones of necrosis. (**b**) Medium-power view demonstrates highly pleomorphic tumor cells clustering around small blood vessels. (**c**) The degree of nuclear pleomorphism, a high mitotic rate and eosinophilic cytoplasm distinguish this tumor from seminoma. However, it may be difficult to distinguish it from anaplastic seminoma. (**d**) Perivascular rosettes and irregular lumen-like structures are common. Many of the luminal structures probably form when central cells become necrotic and disappear.

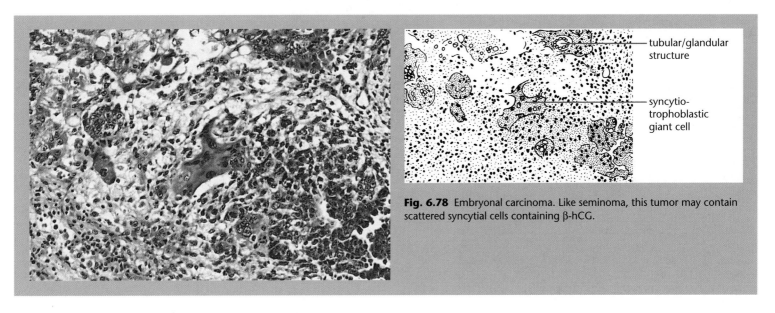

Fig. 6.78 Embryonal carcinoma. Like seminoma, this tumor may contain scattered syncytial cells containing β-hCG.

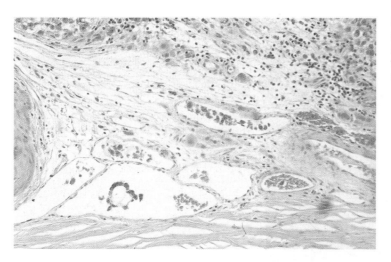

Fig. 6.79 Embryonal carcinoma. Lymphatic invasion, as demonstrated here, is a very important prognostic feature for the subsequent development of retroperitoneal metastases. The possibility should be considered in all patients with primary testicular tumors, especially if retroperitoneal lymph node dissection is contemplated.

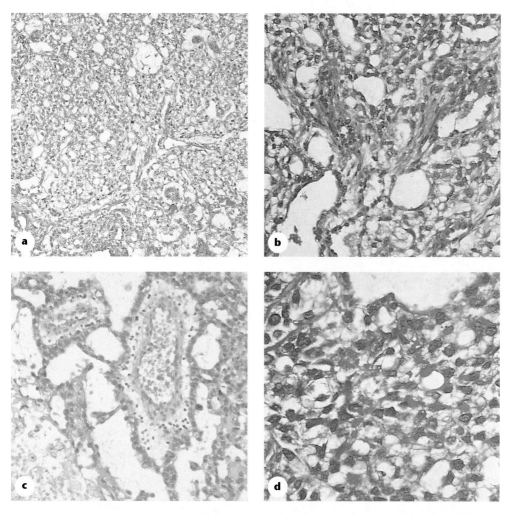

Fig. 6.80 Yolk sac (endodermal sinus) tumor. (**a**) Low- and (**b**) medium-power photomicrographs show irregular cystic spaces alternating with more solid areas. The cells appear cytologically uniform. (**c**) Diagnostic Schiller–Duval bodies are papillary structures containing a vascular core invested by loose connective tissue and surrounded by a layer of tumor cells. (**d**) Eosinophilic globules are frequently seen in yolk sac tumors. The globules have been shown to contain AFP and α1-antitrypsin.

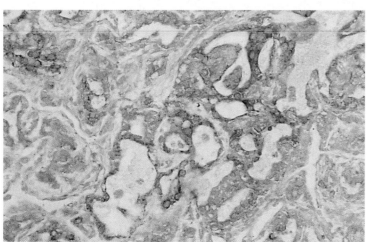

Fig. 6.81 Yolk sac (endoderma sinus) tumor. The brown staining corresponds to deposits of AFP localized by immunocytochemistry.

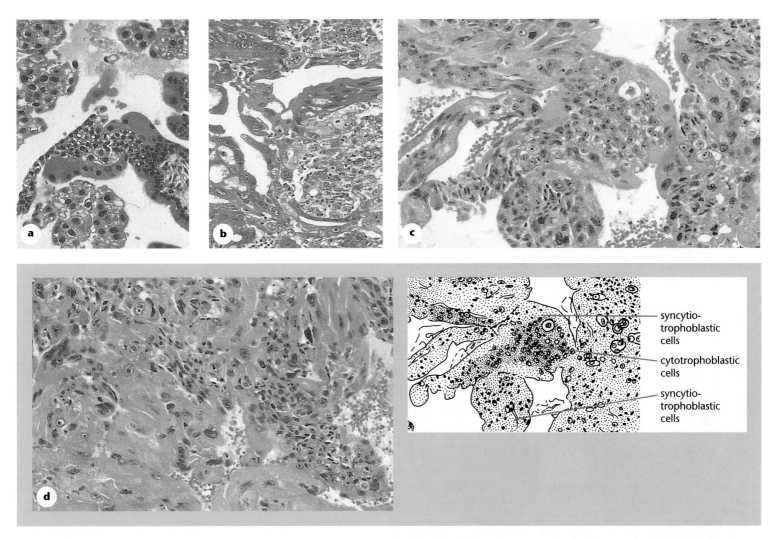

Fig. 6.82 Choriocarcinoma. Microscopically, developing placental tissue (**a**) closely resembles choriocarcinoma (**b**). The intimate mixture of neoplastic cytotrophoblastic and syncytiotrophoblastic cells is diagnostic.

(**c**) Syncytiotrophoblastic cells with abundant eosinophilic cytoplasm surround central aggregates of cytotrophoblastic cells. (**d**) Aggregates of syncytial and cytotrophoblastic cells are associated with stromal hemorrhage.

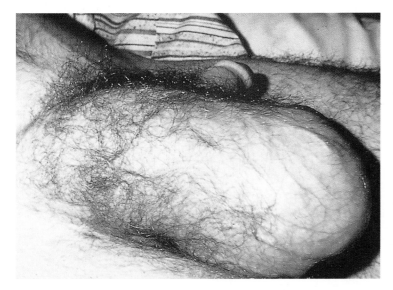

Fig. 6.83 Teratoma. Testicular teratomas may reach enormous size. (Courtesy of JE Fowler Jr MD, Chicago, IL.)

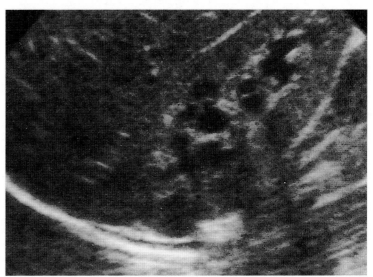

Fig. 6.84 Teratoma. The multicystic structure in the center of this ultrasonogram is a small teratoma containing several cystic spaces. (Courtesy of TL Pope Jr MD, Charlottesville, VA.)

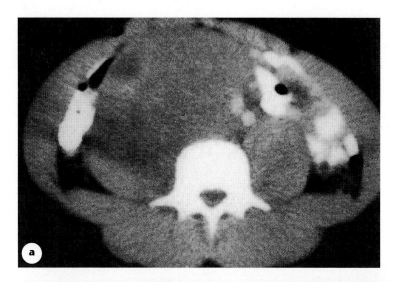

Fig. 6.85 Mature teratoma. A 24-year-old patient with metastatic mixed embryonal cell carcinoma and teratoma (often called teratocarcinoma) and a persistent mass in the abdomen (**a**) and lung (**b**). Biopsy of the large mass after chemotherapy showed pure teratoma without evidence of embryonal cell carcinoma. Although histologically benign, teratomas may increase in size. Surgical resection is indicated because they are unresponsive to chemotherapy. (Courtesy of TL Pope Jr MD, Charlottesville, VA.)

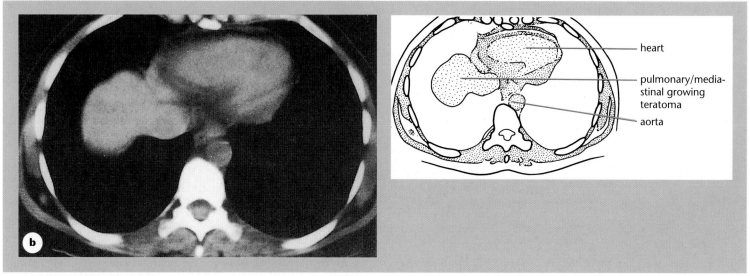

Fig. 6.86 Metastatic teratoma. Microscopic section of a resected pulmonary nodule shows a mature teratoma. The large, fibrous nodule contains blunt papillary projections lined by columnar epithelial cells surrounding a central lumen. A stromal lymphocytic infiltrate (blue cells) underlies the papillary mucosa (enteric derived). Mature teratomas recapitulate endodermal, mesodermal and entodermal structures, typically showing adult tissue from more than one germ cell line.

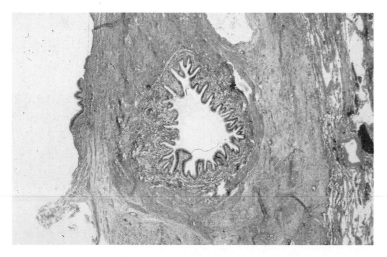

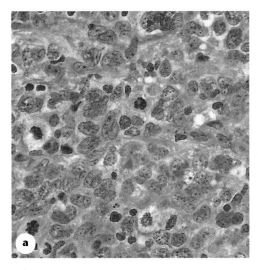
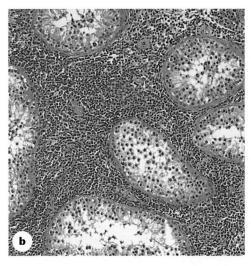
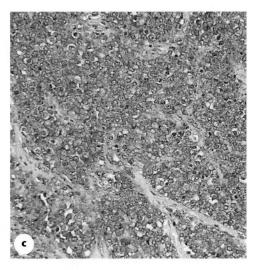

Fig. 6.87 Primary lymphoma of testis. (**a**) Most testicular lymphomas are of the diffuse large cell type, characterized by large cells with pleomorphic nuclei and a high mitotic rate. (**b**) The growth of testicular lymphoma around normal seminiferous tubules may be helpful in distinguishing it from seminoma.

(**c**) Immunocytochemical localization of leukocyte common antigen (brown pigment) is extremely helpful in identifying lymphoma when the distinction from seminoma is difficult.

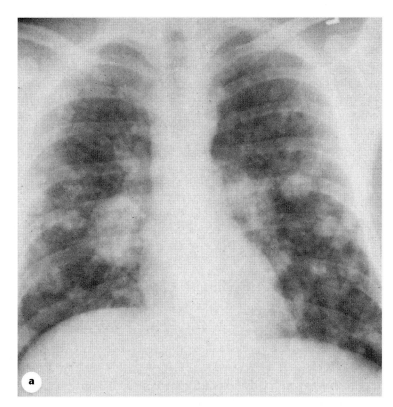
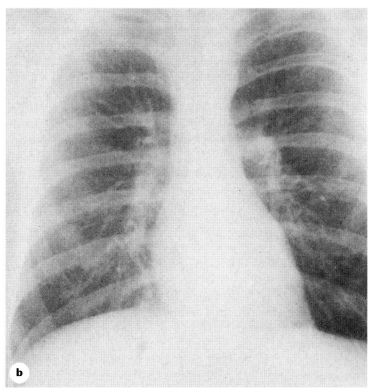

Fig. 6.88 Pulmonary metastases. (**a**) Chest film shows numerous metastatic deposits of testicular embryonal cell carcinoma. (**b**) A dramatic response can be seen following combination chemotherapy containing cisplatin. This chemotherapeutic protocol achieves over a 90% cure rate for metastatic disease.

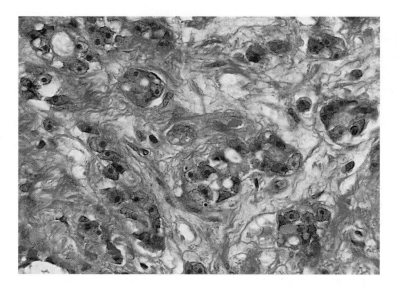

Fig. 6.89 Metastatic adenocarcinoma of prostate. Small, glandular clusters of tumor cells can be seen in the testicular interstitium. This is a rare site for metastases.

PENILE CANCER

Cancer of the penis, which occurs almost exclusively in uncircumcised men, is exceedingly uncommon in the United States, representing less than 2% of malignancies of the male genitourinary tract. The highest rate of incidence is seen in men over 45 years of age, with a predominance of Afro-Americans over whites in a ratio of 3 : 1. A higher incidence of penile cancer is observed in those Eastern nations where circumcision is not routinely practiced.

Although the precise etiology of penile cancer is unknown, a clear link to poor hygiene in the uncircumcised male has been established, implicating the growth of possibly carcinogenic micro-organisms in smegma retained beneath the prepuce. Approximately 20% of patients have a history of past or present venereal disease. An etiologic role for Herpes simplex infection has been postulated but not proven.

HISTOLOGY

The vast majority of penile cancers are squamous cell carcinomas. Rare cases of adenocarcinoma, melanocarcinoma and sarcoma have been reported, the latter being in some instances associated with Kaposi's sarcoma. Metastatic disease of the penis originating from primary tumors of the rectum, prostate or bladder also occurs but is quite uncommon.

Approximately 50% of penile cancers metastasize via lymphatic vessels to the deep and superficial inguinal nodes. Most of these

malignancies are relatively unresponsive to radiotherapy and a consistently effective chemotherapeutic protocol has yet to be developed. Treatment of penile cancer is therefore heavily reliant on surgery. Depending on the extent of disease, this may involve partial, complete or radical penectomy, with inguinal lymphadenectomy when necessary to remove affected nodes. In cases of penile cancer detected at an early stage, cure is sometimes achieved by a partial penectomy that preserves a penile stump adequate for sexual activity and urination. The overall 5-year survival for cancer of the penis is approximately 50%.

CLINICAL MANIFESTATIONS

At the time of presentation, the penile lesion, invariably located in the preputial area, may appear either as a flat ulcer with raised edges, usually extending into the underlying tissues, or as a clustered papillomatous growth resembling the much more common, sexually transmitted condyloma acuminatum. All such penile lesions are suspect and should be biopsied to confirm the histologic diagnosis. Because of overlying psychological factors associated with any abnormality of the penis, patients may delay seeking medical attention until the malignancy is well established. However, most of these lesions are slow to grow and metastasize and therefore the prognosis even for fairly well-advanced cases remains relatively good unless extensive involvement of the inguinal lymph nodes is already present.

Fig. 6.90 AJCC staging of penile cancer.

Definition of TNM

Primary tumor (T)

TX	Primary tumor cannot be assessed
T0	No evidence of primary tumor
Tis	Carcinoma in situ
Ta	Noninvasive verrucous carcinoma
T1	Tumor invades subepithelial connective tissue
T2	Tumor invades the corpus spongiosum or cavernosum
T3	Tumor invades the urethra or prostate
T4	Tumor invades the adjacent structures

Regional lymph nodes (N)

NX	Regional lymph nodes cannot be assessed
N0	No regional lymph node metastasis
N1	Metastasis in a single superficial inguinal lymph node
N2	Metastasis in multiple or bilateral superficial inguinal lymph nodes
N3	Metastasis in deep inguinal or pelvic lymph node(s), unilateral or bilateral

Distant metastasis (M)

MX	Presence of distant metastasis cannot be assessed
M0	No distant metastasis
M1	Distant metastasis

Stage grouping

Stage 0	Tis	N0	M0
	Ta	N0	M0
Stage I	T1	N0	M0
Stage II	T1	N1	M0
	T2	N0	M0
	T2	N1	M0
Stage III	T1	N2	M0
	T2	N2	M0
	T3	N0	M0
	T3	N1	M0
	T3	N2	M0
Stage VI	T4	Any N	M0
	Any T	N3	M0
	Any T	Any N	M1

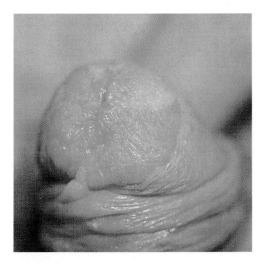

Fig. 6.91 Carcinoma *in situ*. This lesion presents clinically as a well-demarcated, slightly elevated erythematous plaque. (Courtesy of KR Greer MD, Charlottesville, VA.)

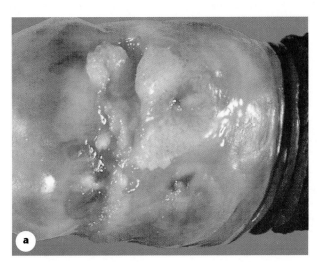
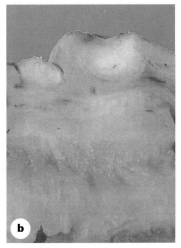

Fig. 6.92 Squamous cell carcinoma. (**a**) This resection specimen shows a small lesion arising in the coronal sulcus. (**b**) Cut section from the specimen demonstrates two small nodules of invasive tumor.

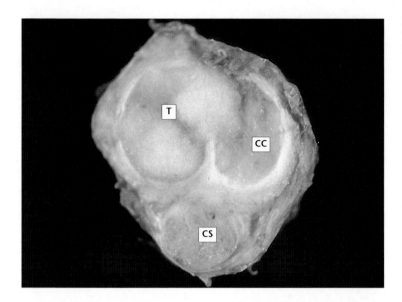

Fig. 6.93 Squamous cell carcinoma. A cross-section of the penile shaft illustrating replacement of the corpus cavernosum (CC) by tumor (T). CS = corpus spongiosum.

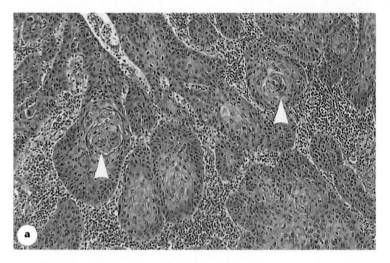

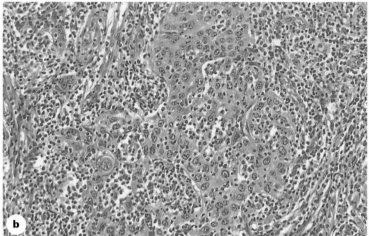

Fig. 6.94 Squamous cell carcinoma. (**a**) Irregular nests of neoplastic cells invade the underlying tissue. Note the foci of keratinization (arrows). (**b**) At the point of deepest invasion, the squamous carcinoma cells are non-keratinizing and exhibit considerable pleomorphism, with large vesicular nuclei. Note the associated intense inflammation often seen in invasive carcinoma.

REFERENCES

Abrahamsson PA: Neuroendocrine differentiation in prostatic carcinoma. Prostate 1999; 39(2):135–148.

Albertsen PC, Hanley JA, Gleason DF, Barry MJ: Competing risk analysis of men aged 55 to 74 years at diagnosis managed conservatively for clinically localized prostate cancer. JAMA 1998; 280(11):975–980.

Bosl GJ, Motzer RJ: Testicular germ-cell cancer. N Engl J Med 1997; 337(4):242–253.

Bostwick DG, Grignon DJ, Hammond ME, et al.: Prognostic factors in prostate cancer. College of American Pathologists Consensus Statement 1999. Arch Pathol Lab Med 2000; 124(7):995–1000.

Carlin BI, Andriole GL: The natural history, skeletal complications, and management of bone metastases in patients with prostate carcinoma. Cancer 2000; 88(12 suppl):2989–2994.

Catalona WJ, Southwick PC, Slawin KM, et al.: Comparison of percent free PSA, PSA density, and age-specific PSA cutoffs for prostate cancer detection and staging. Urology 2000; 56(2):255–260.

Comiter CV, Kibel AS, Richie JP, Nucci MR, Renshaw AA: Prognostic features of teratomas with malignant transformation: a clinicopathological study of 21 cases. J Urol 1998; 159(3):859–863.

D'Amico AV, Schnall M, Whittington R, et al.: Endorectal coil magnetic resonance imaging identifies locally advanced prostate cancer in select patients with clinically localized disease. Urology 1998; 51(3):449–454.

D'Amico AV, Whittington R, Malkowicz SB, et al.: Clinical utility of the percentage of positive prostate biopsies in defining biochemical outcome after radical prostatectomy for patients with clinically localized prostate cancer. J Clin Oncol 2000; 18(6):1164–1172.

Elgamal AA, Troychak MJ, Murphy GP: ProstaScint scan may enhance identification of prostate cancer recurrences after prostatectomy, radiation, or hormone therapy: analysis of 136 scans of 100 patients. Prostate 1998; 37(4):261–269.

Epstein JI: Gleason score 2–4 adenocarcinoma of the prostate on needle biopsy: a diagnosis that should not be made. Am J Surg Pathol 2000; 24(4):477–478.

Fleming S, O'Donnell M: Surgical pathology of renal epithelial neoplasms: recent advances and current status. Histopathology 2000; 36(3):195–202.

George DJ, Kantoff PW: Prognostic indicators in hormone refractory prostate cancer. Urol Clin North Am 1999; 26(2):303–310, viii.

Gleason DF: Histologic grading of prostate cancer: a perspective. Hum Pathol 1992; 23(3):273–279.

Greenlee RT, Hill-Harmon MB, Murray T, Thun M: Cancer statistics, 2001. CA Cancer J Clin 2001; 51(1):15–36.

Guinan P, Sobin LH, Algaba F, et al.: TNM staging of renal cell carcinoma: Workgroup No. 3. Union International Contre le Cancer (UICC) and the American Joint Committee on Cancer (AJCC). Cancer 1997; 80(5):992–993.

Han M, Walsh PC, Partin AW, Rodriguez R: Ability of the 1992 and 1997 American Joint Committee on Cancer staging systems for prostate cancer to predict progression-free survival after radical prostatectomy for stage T2 disease. J Urol 2000; 164(1):89–92.

International Germ Cell Cancer Collaborative Group: International Germ Cell Consensus Classification: a prognostic factor-based staging system for metastatic germ cell cancers. J Clin Oncol 1997; 15:594–603.

Krieg R, Hoffman R: Current management of unusual genitourinary cancers. Part 1: Penile cancer. Oncology (Huntingt) 1999; 13(10):1347–1352.

Motzer RJ, Bander NH, Nanus DM: Renal-cell carcinoma. N Engl J Med 1996; 335(12):865–875.

Motzer RJ, Russo P: Systemic therapy for renal cell carcinoma. J Urol 2000; 163(2):408–417.

Oh WK, Kantoff PW: Management of hormone refractory prostate cancer: current standards and future prospects. J Urol 1998; 160(4):1220–1229.

Oh WK, Hurwitz M, D'Amico AV, Richie JP, Kantoff PW: Prostate cancer. In: Bast R, Kufe D, Pollock R, et al., eds: Cancer Medicine, 5th edn. BC Decker, Hamilton, Ontario, 2000.

Olumi AF: A critical analysis of the use of p53 as a marker for management of bladder cancer. Urol Clin North Am 2000; 27(1):75–82, ix.

Shuin T, Kondo K, Ashida S, et al.: Germline and somatic mutations in von Hippel–Lindau disease gene and its significance in the development of kidney cancer. Contrib Nephrol 1999; 128:1–10.

Smith JA, Labasky RF, Cockett AT, Fracchia JA, Montie JE, Rowland RG: Bladder cancer clinical guidelines panel summary report on the management of nonmuscle invasive bladder cancer (stages Ta, T1 and TIS). The American Urological Association. J Urol 1999; 162(5):1697–1701.

Steele GS, Richie JP: Management of low-stage nonseminomatous germ cell tumors of the testis. Compr Ther 2000; 26(3):210–219.

Stein JP, Lieskovsky G, Cote R, et al.: Radical cystectomy in the treatment of invasive bladder cancer: long-term results in 1,054 patients. J Clin Oncol 2001; 19(3):666–675.

Truong LD, Caraway N, Ngo T, et al.: The diagnostic and therapeutic roles of fine-needle aspiration. Am J Clin Pathol 2001; 115:18–31.

Varghese SL, Grossfeld GD: The prostatic gland: malignancies other than adenocarcinomas. Radiol Clin North Am 2000; 38(1):179–202.

FIGURE CREDITS

The following books published by Gower Medical Publishing are sources of figures in the present chapter. The figure numbers given in the listing are those of the figures in the present chapter. The page numbers given in parentheses are those of the original publication.

Dieppe PA, Bacon PA, Bamji AN, et al.: Atlas of Clinical Rheumatology. Lea and Febiger/Gower Medical Publishing, Philadelphia/London, 1986: Fig. 6.26 (p. 21.5).

Weiss MA, Mills SE: Atlas of Genitourinary Tract Disorders. JB Lippincott/Gower Medical Publishing Philadelphia/New York. 1988: Figs 6.1 (p. 13.15), 6.4 (p. 14.8), 6.5 (p. 14.12), 6.6 (p. 14.13), 6.7 (p. 14.13), 6.8 (p. 14.14), 6.9 (p. 14.11), 6.10 (p. 14.16), 6.12 (p. 14.10), 6.13 (p. 14.18), 6.15 (p. 14.20), 6.16 (p. 14.20), 6.17 (p. 14.21), 6.19 (4.24), 6.23 (p. 14.17), 6.32 a, b (p. 12.14), 6.32c (p. 12.14), 6.33 (p. 12.9), 6.34 (p. 12.9), 6.37 (p. 12.16), 6.38 (p. 12.6), 6.39 (p. 12.8), 6.40 (p. 12.16), 6.41 (p. 12.17), 6.42 (p. 12.19), 6.43 (p. 12.21), 6.44 (p. 12.7), 6.45 (p. 12.27), 6.46 (p. 12.28), 6.47, (p. 12.31), 6.48 (p. 12.31), 6.49 (p. 12.32), 6.50 (p. 12.33), 6.52 (p. 11.2), 6.53 (p. 11.3), 6.54 (p. 11.5), 6.55 (p. 11.7), 6.57 (p. 11.9), 6.58 (p. 11.12), 6.59 (p. 11.13), 6.60 (p. 11.10), 6.61 (p. 11.21), 6.62 (p. 11.17), 6.63 (p. 11.8), 6.64 (p. 11.9), 6.65 (p. 11.49), 6.69 (p. 11.55), 6.70 (p. 11.57), 6.72 (p. 16.24), 6.73 (p. 16.24), 6.74 (p. 16.25), 6.76 (p. 16.9), 6.77 (p. 16.13), 6.78 (p. 16.14), 6.80 (p. 16.15), 6.81 (p. 16.16), 6.82 c, d (p. 16.17), 6.83 (p. 16.18), 6.84 (p. 16.19), 6.85 (p. 16.22), 6.87 (p. 16.31), 6.89 (p. 16.31), 6.91 (p. 19.2), 6.92 (p. 19.8), 6.94 (p. 19.7).

7

Gynecologic tumors and malignancies

Ursula Matulonis, Karen J. Krag, David R. Genest

OVARIAN CARCINOMA

Although not the most common, epithelial ovarian cancer is the most lethal, affecting approximately 26 000 women per year and causing 14 500 deaths in the United States. Ovarian cancer is the fourth most frequent cause of cancer death in women. The median age of diagnosis is 63 and close to 50% of patients are 65 years of age or older. The risk factors for epithelial ovarian cancer include nulliparity, while protective factors include multiple births and use of oral contraceptives. Family history of ovarian cancer is an important risk factor and compared to the general population whose lifetime risk is 1.6%, a woman with a single relative affected by ovarian cancer has a 4–5% risk. Genes implicated in increased susceptibility if germline inheritance occurs in an autosomal dominant pattern include BRCA1, BRCA2 (heriditary breast-ovarian cancer) and mismatch repair genes such as hMSH2 and hMLSH1 (hereditary non-polyposis colorectal syndrome). For women carrying a mutated high-risk gene, parity lowers risk but protective use of oral contraception remains controversial.

HISTOLOGY

The majority of malignant ovarian tumors are of epithelial origin (*see* Table 7.1). Papillary serous cystadenocarcinomas, which constitute the majority of these tumors, are characterized by papillary fronds and psammoma bodies with cells reminiscent of fallopian tube mucosa. The contralateral ovary is involved either grossly or microscopically in up to half of cases. Endometrioid tumors are second in frequency and are less commonly bilateral. The remaining epithelial malignancies – mucinous, clear cell and undifferentiated carcinomas and malignant Brenner tumors – are all less common. Multiple histologies may occur in the same patient and squamous differentiation may be present, especially within endometrioid tumors.

With the exception of the poor prognosis associated with clear cell tumors, multivariate analyses have generally not shown histologic subtype to influence survival. The grade of tumor contributes more significantly to prognosis, with shorter survival times associated with high-grade tumors. Poorly differentiated carcinomas usually have a more virulent course; survival without treatment may be measured in months rather than years. Borderline epithelial tumors contain individual malignant appearing cells, but show no evidence of invasion. Approximately 90% of borderline tumors are serous and 10% are mucinous; rarely, endometrioid and clear cell varieties are encountered. Borderline tumors have a very long natural history, although they can metastasize and cause death.

Germ cell tumors constitute approximately 20% of benign ovarian neoplasms but represent only about 5% of ovarian malignancies. They are most common in young women and children, in whom cure and preservation of fertility are frequently achieved. Dysgerminoma accounts for nearly half of all malignant germ cell tumors, with a median age at diagnosis of 22 years. Other types include immature teratoma, endodermal sinus tumor, embryonal carcinoma and non-gestational choriocarcinoma. They are all rare, but interesting because of their similarity to male testicular cancers in both natural history and responsiveness to chemotherapy.

Other non-epithelial ovarian tumors may be divided into sex cord-stromal tumors, metastatic malignancies and sarcomas. Of the sex cord tumors, granulosa cell tumors are the most common and constitute 2% of all ovarian malignancies. Composed of granulosa cells with or without theca cells, they may be hormonally active, causing resumption of menses in older women or precocious pseudopuberty in the rare young person developing this malignancy. Sertoli–Leydig cell tumors (androblastomas) are sex cord-stromal tumors marked by some testicular differentiation and often by androgen production; they are rarely malignant. Metastatic tumors, which represent 10% of ovarian malignancies, most commonly originate from primary sites in the endometrium, gastrointestinal tract and breast. They include Krukenberg tumors of gastric origin, which exhibit a classic mucus-secreting, 'signet ring' cell histology. Primary colon and pancreatic carcinomas are also known to metastasize to the ovary. Primary ovarian sarcomas are very rare and may be classified in a manner similar to that used for uterine sarcomas. Mixed tumors marked by the presence of both sarcomatous and epithelial elements also occur, and are termed malignant mixed Müllerian tumors (MMMT) or carcinosarcomas.

Small cell tumors can arise in the ovary and typically are very aggressive and have a poor prognosis.

STAGING OF OVARIAN CARCINOMA

Early stage ovarian carcinoma is confined to the ovary (stage I) or the pelvic organs (stage II) (*see* Fig. 7.1). However, because of the vague nature of symptoms and the lack of effective screening programs, most women present with spread throughout the peritoneal cavity (stage III). Ovarian carcinomas usually disseminate intraperitoneally and careful exploration even in stage I cases discloses intra-abdominal metastases in approximately 25% of patients. Extraperitoneal dissemination (stage IV) is uncommon and usually occurs late in the course of the disease. Pleural effusions are the most common manifestation of extra-abdominal disease. Although the mechanism for this tendency is unclear, the right hemidiaphragm is commonly involved in stage IV disease, and there are connections between the lymphatic systems above and below the diaphragm. Parenchymal lung involvement is unusual. Nodal spread may also occur to Virchow's node (supraclavicular), the inguinal nodes or Sister Mary-Joseph's node in the paraumbilical region. The FIGO staging system requires assessment of the ovarian capsule, lymph node dissection and multiple biopsies for accurate staging. Without careful surgical evaluation, up to 30% of women may be understaged.

CLINICAL MANIFESTATIONS

Early stage epithelial ovarian carcinoma rarely causes symptoms, although large masses may cause pelvic pain, constipation, tenesmus and urinary frequency or dysuria. Abdominal cramping, flatulence, bloating and gas pains are more common presenting symptoms, usually due to tumor dissemination throughout the peritoneal cavity. These symptoms unfortunately are often poorly defined and occasionally mild; they may be attributed to benign gastrointestinal pathology, until the woman has obvious abdominal distension, most often related to increasing ascites or intestinal obstruction. The importance of a pelvic examination in the initial evaluation of any woman with gastrointestinal complaints cannot be overemphasized. Late in the course of the disease, shortness of breath from pleural effusions may occur. Hematogenous dissemination to the liver, lungs and left supraclavicular or axillary nodes is a less common occurrence, and bone, brain or meningeal metastases are rare. However, unusual metastases may occur, especially in patients with a prolonged natural history.

In the postmenopausal woman with an ovarian mass, useful diagnostic tests include a transvaginal ultrasound and CT scan. The CA125 blood test has not been shown to be a useful screening tool, but is important in monitoring the results of therapy once a diagnosis has been established.

Non-epithelial tumors often present in a fashion similar to epithelial malignancies. Granulosa cell tumors and other stromal neoplasms are usually detected when a woman presents with pelvic discomfort or vague abdominal symptoms; these tumors also may secrete estrogen and cause resumption of menses in the postmenopausal woman. This hyperestrogenic effect may lead to the simultaneous development of endometrial carcinoma. Germ cell tumors are seen almost exclusively in premenopausal women. They are occasionally detected as an asymptomatic pelvic mass, but more commonly they present acutely with symptoms of rapid tumor growth or as abdominal emergencies secondary to hemorrhage, rupture or torsion. (Text on 'Endometrial Carcinoma' appears on page 217.)

Table 7.1 Classification of malignant ovarian tumors

	Tumor	Frequency (%)
Epithelial	Papillary serous cystadenocarcinoma	38
	Mucinous cystadenocarcinoma	11
	Endometrioid carcinoma	13
	Clear cell carcinoma	5
	Malignant Brenner tumor	< 0.5
	Undifferentiated carcinoma	15
Sex cord-stromal	Granulosa cell tumor	2
	Sertoli–Leydig tumor	< 1
	Mixed tumors	< 0.5
Germ cell	Immature teratoma	< 0.5
	Embryonal carcinoma	< 0.5
	Endodermal sinus tumor	< 1
	Choriocarcinoma	< 0.5
	Mixed	< 1
	Dysgerminoma	2
Stromal	Sarcomas	< 0.5
Miscellaneous	Metastatic carcinoma	10
	Lymphoma	< 0.5

FIGO staging system of the ovary

Stage I **Growth limited to ovaries**

Stage IA
Growth limited to one ovary. No ascites; no tumor on external surface; capsule intact.

Stage IB
Growth limited to both ovaries. No ascites; no tumor on external surface; capsule intact.

Stage IC
Tumor either stage IA or IB, but with tumor on the surface of one or both ovaries; or with capsule rupture; or with ascites containing malignant cells; or with positive peritoneal washings.

Stage II **Growth involving one or both ovaries with pelvic extension**

Stage IIA
Extension and/or metastases to uterus and/or tubes.

Stage IIB
Extension to other pelvic tissues.

Stage IIC
Tumor either stage IIA or IIB, but with tumor on the surface of one or both ovaries; or with capsule rupture; or with ascites containing malignant cells; or with positive peritoneal washings.

Stage III **Tumor involving one or both ovaries with peritoneal implants outside the pelvis and/or retroperitoneal or inguinal nodes. Superficial liver metastases equals stage III. Tumor is limited to the true pelvis, but with histologically verified malignant extension to small bowel or omentum.**

Stage IIIA
Tumor grossly limited to true pelvis with negative nodes but with histologically confirmed microscopic seeding of abdominal peritoneal surface.

Stage IIIB
Tumor of one or both ovaries with histologically confirmed implants on abdominal peritoneal surfaces, none > 2 cm in diameter. Nodes negative.

Stage IIIC
Abdominal implants > 2 cm in diameter and/or positive retroperitoneal or inguinal nodes.

Stage IV **Growth involving one or both ovaries with distant metastases. If pleural effusion is present, there must be positive cytologic test results to assign a case to stage IV. Parenchymal liver metastases equals stage IV.**

Fig. 7.1 FIGO staging system for carcinoma of the ovary (1989).

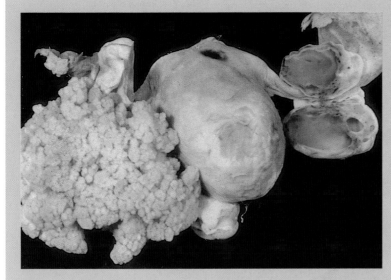

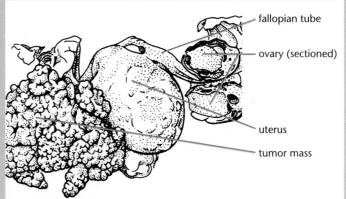

by sessile papillae. At its upper pole, a small mature (benign) teratoma is also visible. The uterus is distorted by leiomyomas, and the right ovary contains a follicular cyst and corpus luteum. Both serous and mucinous tumors of borderline malignancy are now well defined histologically and clearly recognized clinically. The median age at presentation is 5–10 years younger than patients with invasive cancer, and borderline malignancies are not unusual in premenopausal women.

Fig. 7.2 Papillary serous borderline malignancy. This specimen, from a 29-year-old woman who presented with menorrhagia, consists of the uterus with both tubes and ovaries. The left ovary is largely replaced by a tumor covered

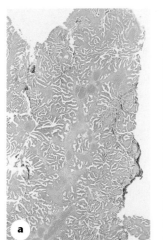

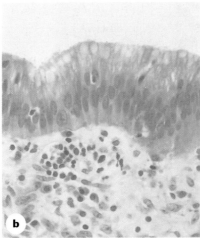

Fig. 7.3 Papillary serous borderline malignancy. (**a**) Complex papillary structure. (**b**) Histologic examination at higher magnification reveals mitotic activity and nuclear atypia, together with multilayering and cell proliferation, but the absence of stromal invasion marks the neoplasm as borderline malignant. These tumors may spread throughout the peritoneum and implant on serosal surfaces, although invasive implants are rare. The 5-year survival rate is around 95%, but 10-year survival falls to 75%. A small percentage of tumors are aggressive, and chemotherapy appears to be ineffective.

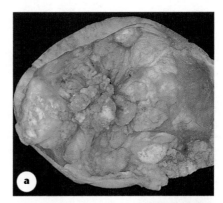

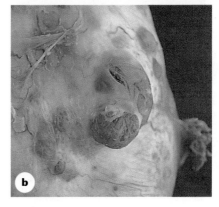

Fig. 7.4 Papillary serous cystadenocarcinoma. (**a**) The ovary is replaced by a large, unilocular tumor, the lining of which is composed of solid, papillary tumor exhibiting hemorrhage and focal necrosis. (**b**) In a different specimen, tumor can be seen extending through the serosal surface. Capsule excrescences, dense adherence of tumor to peritoneum, the presence of cytologically positive peritoneal fluid, and a high histologic grade are all poor prognostic signs in stage I patients and suggest the necessity for further therapy.

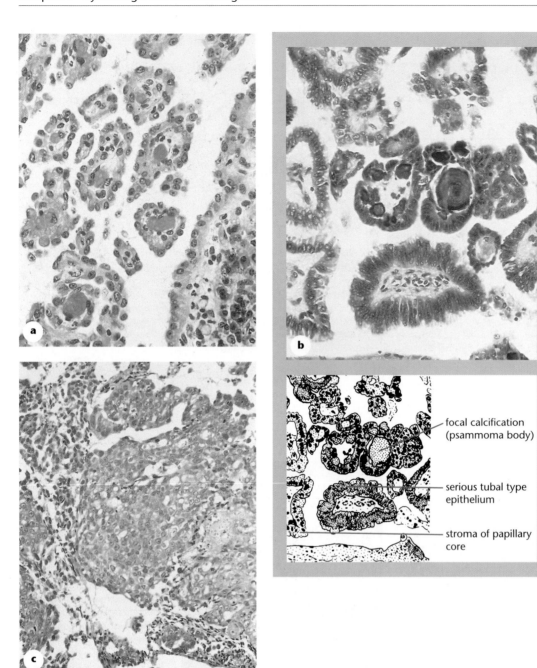

Fig. 7.5 Papillary serous cystadenocarcinoma. Histologically, these tumors range from (**a**) well-differentiated neoplasms with obvious papillae and minimal atypia, to (**b**) moderate differentiation with more proliferative epithelium, and to (**c**) poorly differentiated solid nests of cells. Psammoma bodies (see **b**) can occur in all grades but are more frequent in well-differentiated tumors.

focal calcification (psammoma body)

serious tubal type epithelium

stroma of papillary core

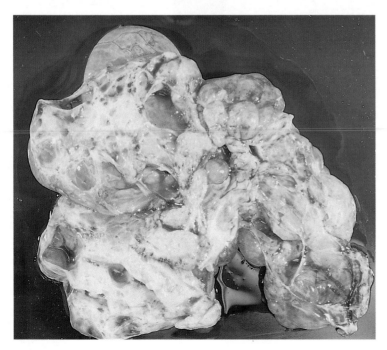

Fig. 7.6 Mucinous cystadenocarcinoma. The ovary is replaced by a multiloculated, partly cystic, partly solid mass. Cystic spaces contain viscid fluid. This tumor is common, arising largely in middle-aged or elderly women. Like its benign counterpart, mucinous cystadenoma, it may attain great size.

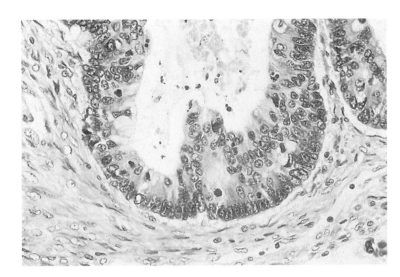

Fig. 7.7 Mucinous cystadenocarcinoma. This epithelium is barely recognizable as mucinous. It is papillary, piled up, and exhibits both nuclear atypia and multiple mitotic figures.

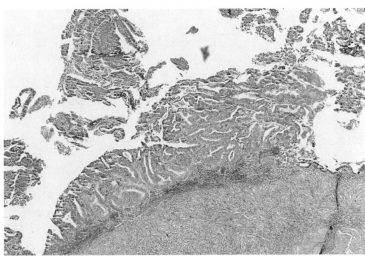

Fig. 7.8 Endometrioid carcinoma. A 44-year-old woman presented with intermenstrual bleeding and underwent surgery for presumed endometriosis. A 2 mm focus of endometrioid carcinoma was discovered inside one endometriotic cyst. There was no disease elsewhere in the abdomen. Endometrioid carcinoma occurs in approximately 0.5% of cases of ovarian endometriosis and is the most common pathologic subtype associated with this condition. The tumor is usually semicystic and may be filled with a chocolate-brown fluid. Microscopically, the glands resemble endometrial carcinoma, and an associated uterine carcinoma may be seen in 20% of patients.

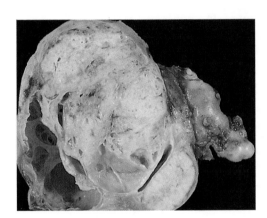

Fig. 7.9 Clear cell adenocarcinoma. Arising in the ovary is a large, predominantly solid, yellowish neoplasm that shows focal cystic change and necrosis. Cystic changes are common in these tumors.

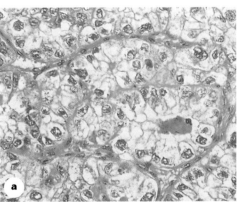

Fig. 7.10 Clear cell adenocarcinoma. Histology is typically variable, usually including solid sheets or tubular arrangement of cells with abundant clear cytoplasm (**a**), and cystic spaces lined by hobnail cells, with nuclei projecting apically (**b**). In more than 60% of patients, the tumors are confined to the ovary at presentation, but stage for stage, the prognosis is worse than for papillary serous adenocarcinomas. Hematogenous metastases are more frequent, and some patients have a fulminant course.

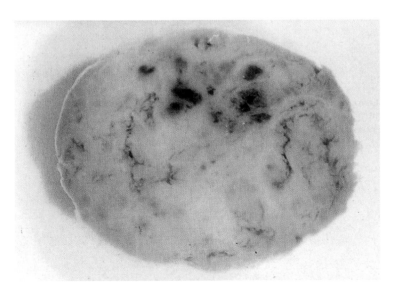

Fig. 7.11 Granulosa cell tumor. This specimen is from a 46-year-old woman. The yellowish tumor is well circumscribed and largely solid, measuring 4 cm in diameter. Small foci of poorly defined cystic change are also visible. This appearance is typical of this sex cord-stromal tumor, which can occur at any age, including childhood, but most frequently secretes excessive amounts of estrogen, leading to menstrual irregularity or postmenopausal bleeding. All granulosa cell tumors should be regarded as malignant, but the clinical course is often indolent.

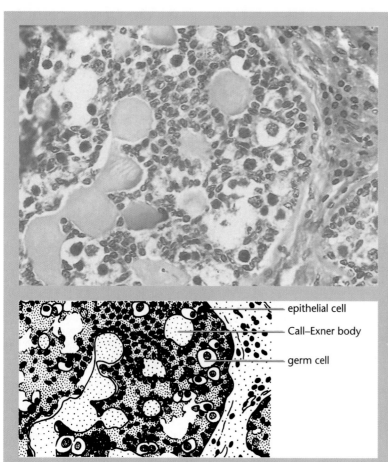

Fig. 7.12 Granulosa cell tumor. This tumor is composed of nests of cells with inconspicuous cytoplasm; bland, oval nuclei with little cytologic atypia; and occasional longitudinal nuclear grooves ('coffee bean appearance'). Germ cells and epithelial cells are intermixed; epithelial cells may form Call–Exner bodies, consisting of pink, inspissated material.

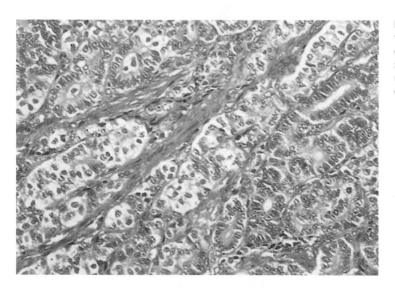

Fig. 7.13 Sertoli–Leydig cell tumor. Tubules containing well-developed Sertoli-type cells are seen at lower left, whereas at right the epithelium is less well differentiated.

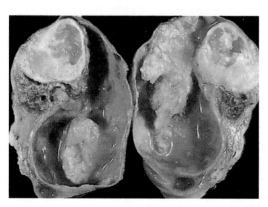

Fig. 7.14 Mature cystic teratoma. The bisected ovary reveals replacement by a multicystic tumor within which sebaceous material and matted hair can be seen.

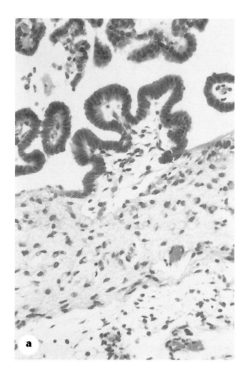
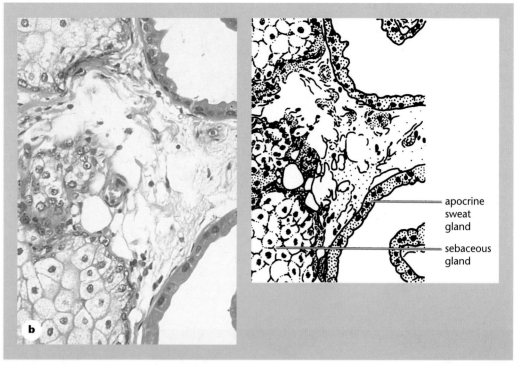

apocrine
sweat
gland

sebaceous
gland

Fig. 7.15 Mature cystic teratoma. (**a**) A small focus of mature choroid plexus lies above equally mature-appearing brain tissue. (**b**) Normal sebaceous glands below are adjacent to well-developed apocrine sweat glands above. Stroma ovarii is an uncommon variant of this germ cell tumor, composed predominantly of thyroid tissue.

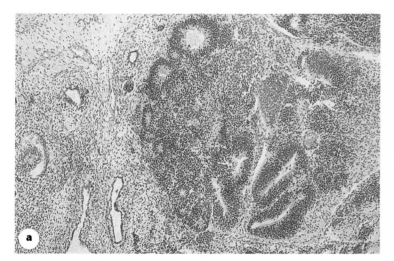
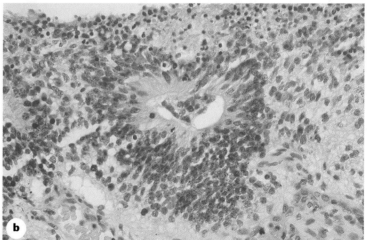

Fig. 7.16 Immature teratoma. (**a**) A large region of immature neuroepithelium is present.
(**b**) Neuroepithelial rosettes, indicative of embryonic differentiation, are characteristic of immature teratomas.

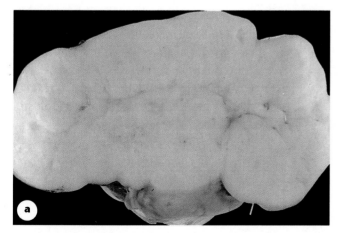
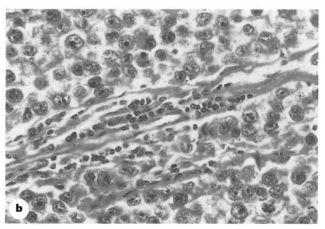

Fig. 7.17 Dysgerminoma. (**a**) This large, uniform, well-circumscribed whitish tumor arising in the ovary is analogous to testicular seminoma; it usually secretes neither human chorionic gonadotrophin (HCG) nor α-fetoprotein (AF). Dysgerminomas are extremely sensitive to radiation and chemotherapy and carry an excellent prognosis, with many patients retaining their fertility. (**b**) Histologically, nests of large, uniform cells with pale to clear cytoplasm and prominent nucleoli are separated by stroma infiltrated by lymphocytes and plasma cells.

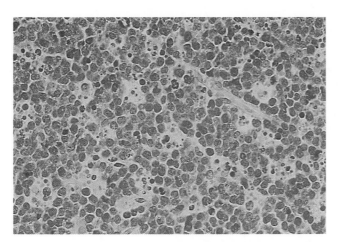

Fig. 7.18 Burkitt's lymphoma. Occasionally, the ovary is the primary site for an extranodal lymphoma. This tumor, which may occur in children, is characterized by the classic starry-sky pattern marked by large, light-staining benign histiocytes. Malignant cells are small, blue staining, and undifferentiated.

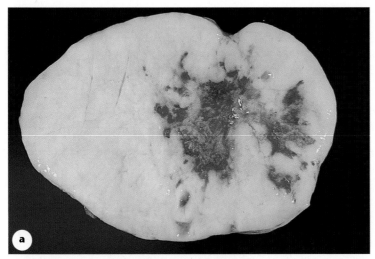

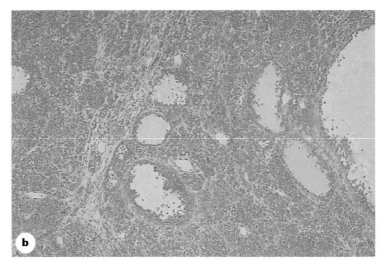

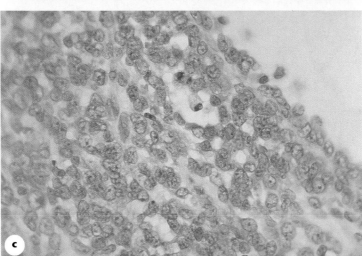

Fig. 7.19 Small cell carcinoma of the ovary of the hypercalcemic type. (**a**) The ovary is entirely replaced by a solid, tan tumor with central area of hemorrhage. (**b**) Histologically, there are solid sheets of closely packed, undifferentiated, small cells, with occasional microfollicles. (**c**) Tumor cells have scant cytoplasm, round vesicular nuclei and numerous mitoses.

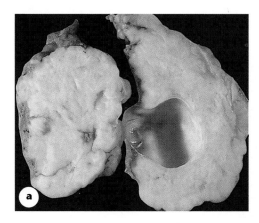

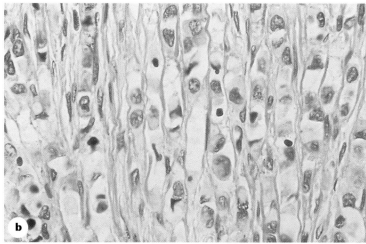

Fig. 7.20 Metastatic breast cancer. (**a**) Both ovaries are diffusely replaced by pale, rather nodular tumor; a follicular cyst is also present on the right. Bilateral involvement by metastases is common. (**b**) Metastatic breast cancer cells are arranged in long lines perpendicular to the surface of the ovarian cortex.

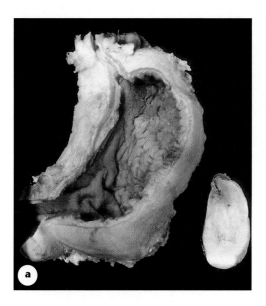

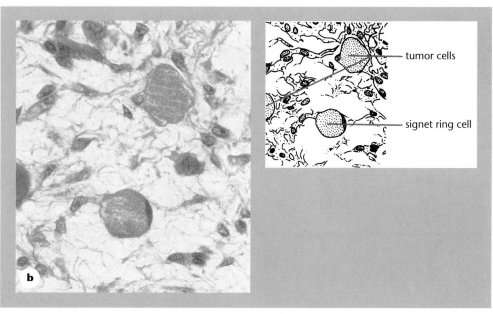

tumor cells

signet ring cell

Fig. 7.21 Gastric adenocarcinoma with ovarian metastasis (Krukenberg tumor). (**a**) These specimens are from a 65-year-old woman who had a four-month history of dysphagia. A barium meal revealed a tumor of the gastric fundus, and esophagogastrectomy with resection of a right ovarian tumor was performed. The sectioned ovary at the right shows total replacement by pale tumor. (**b**) When the gastric tumor is a mucus-secreting signet ring cell adenocarcinoma, the ovarian moiety is known as a Krukenberg tumor. Ovarian involvement may be bilateral. Other primary sources of signet ring histology are carcinomas of the breast and colon.

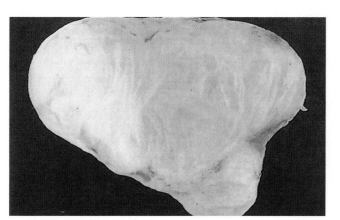

Fig. 7.22 Fibroma. The ovary is replaced by a pale, lobulated tumor, the cut surface of which is fibrous and whorled. Ovarian fibromas, derived from stromal mesenchyme, usually arise in the fifth or sixth decade, and are almost invariably benign. They are sometimes accompanied by ascites or pleural effusions (Meigs' syndrome).

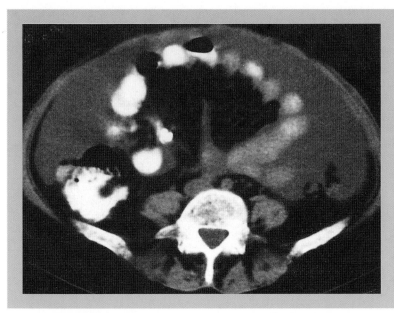

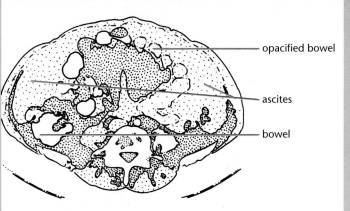

Fig. 7.23 Stage III ovarian cancer (ascites). CT scan in a 57-year-old woman with recurrent ovarian cancer who presented with ascites shows peritoneal fluid surrounding loops of small bowel.

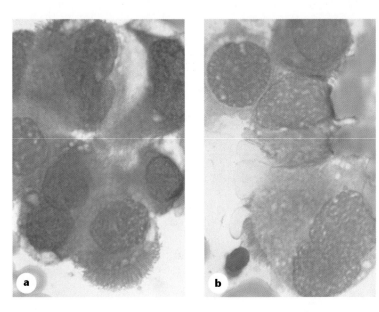

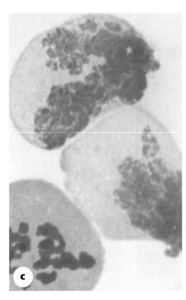

Fig. 7.24 Stage III ovarian cancer (ascites). (**a, b**) Malignant cells in ascitic fluid exhibit characteristic brush borders. (**c**) Mitotic figures can also be seen, as well as (**d**) a large, immature binucleate cell with prominent nucleoli.

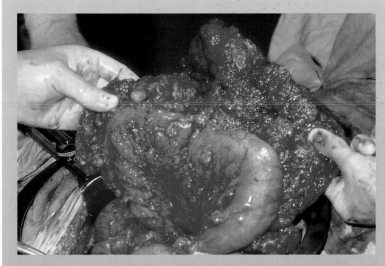

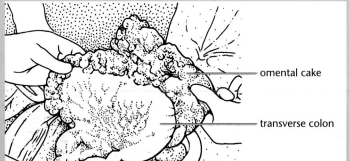

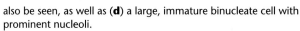

this 55-year-old woman had few symptoms: vague abdominal bloating, increased gas, and a feeling of fullness. Histologic examination showed a moderately differentiated papillary serous cystadenocarcinoma. (Courtesy of Howard Goodman MD, Department of Gynecologic Oncology, Brigham and Women's Hospital, Boston, MA.)

Fig. 7.25 Stage III ovarian cancer (peritoneal implants). Despite extensive tumor with mesenteric studding, together with a large omental cake of tumor,

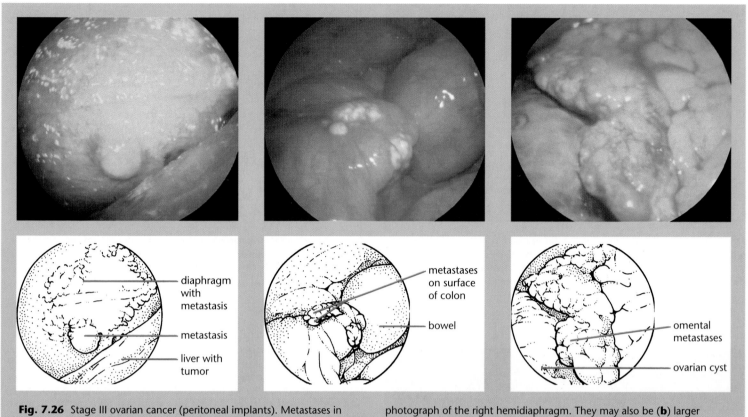

Fig. 7.26 Stage III ovarian cancer (peritoneal implants). Metastases in patients in this stage may be tiny seedlings, as (**a**) in this laparoscopic photograph of the right hemidiaphragm. They may also be (**b**) larger nodules on bowel serosa or (**c**) extensive omental cakes.

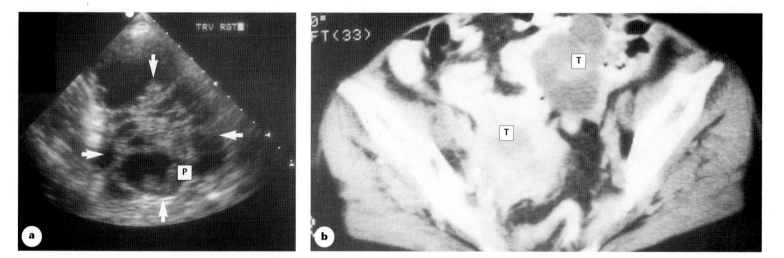

Fig. 7.27 Stage III ovarian cancer. This 72-year-old woman had a 2-month history of diarrhea, a 5-pound weight loss and abdominal bloating. The pelvic ultrasound (**a**) shows a complex multicystic mass (arrows). Solid and cystic components are seen, as well as an irregular wall and papillary projections (P) within the cystic structures. The most common adnexal mass in the premenopausal woman is a functional cyst which should resolve over a few weeks; in the postmenopausal patient, any cyst over 5 cm or with internal septations must be fully evaluated. This pelvic CT scan (**b**) confirms the large multicystic mass (T). At surgery she had diffuse peritoneal studding, extensive retroperitoneal adenopathy, and an unresectable pelvic mass. She responded well to chemotherapy, with normalization of markers and total regression of her symptoms.

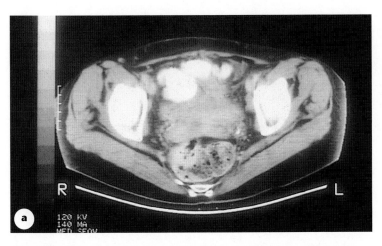

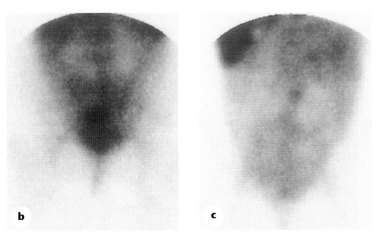

Fig. 7.28 Recurrent ovarian cancer. This 54-year-old woman was 9 months out from her diagnosis of ovarian cancer when her CA125 began to rise. CT scan (**a**) showed a pelvic mass, and OncoScint confirmed extensive pelvic disease (**b**), but also showed diffuse peritoneal involvement and para-aortic disease (**c**). At surgery she had disease documented in all three areas. OncoScint is an In^{111} labeled monoclonal antibody to TAG-72, an antigen present on the majority of ovarian carcinoma cells.

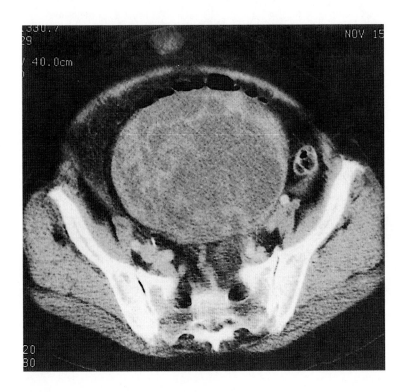

Fig. 7.29 Ovarian granulosa cell tumor. This CAT scan was taken of a 72-year-old woman who presented with a several month history of abdominal pressure. It shows a large pelvic mass, which was resectable at surgery. Pathology demonstrated a granulosa cell tumor, and she had some bloody although cytologically negative ascites. These tumors are usually cystic, filled with serous fluid and blood, and 15% of women present with hemoperitoneum due to partial or complete cyst rupture.

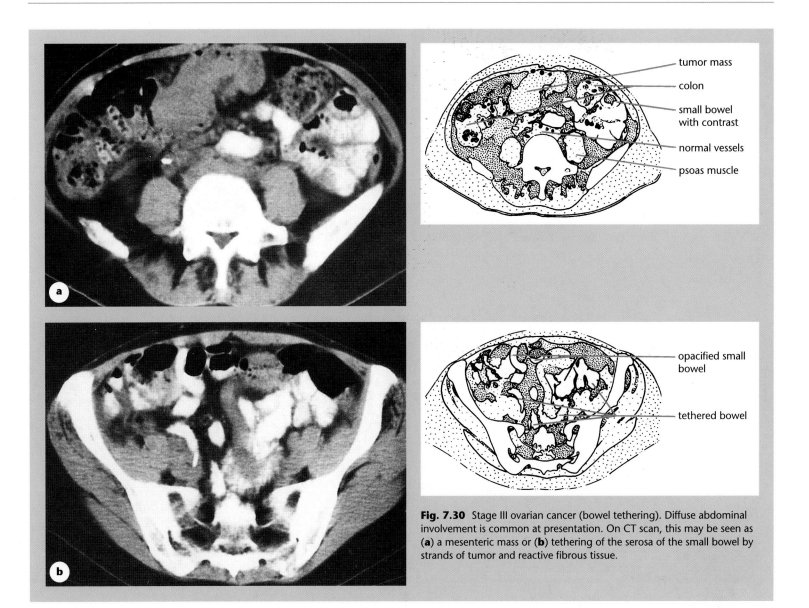

tumor mass
colon
small bowel with contrast
normal vessels
psoas muscle

opacified small bowel
tethered bowel

Fig. 7.30 Stage III ovarian cancer (bowel tethering). Diffuse abdominal involvement is common at presentation. On CT scan, this may be seen as (**a**) a mesenteric mass or (**b**) tethering of the serosa of the small bowel by strands of tumor and reactive fibrous tissue.

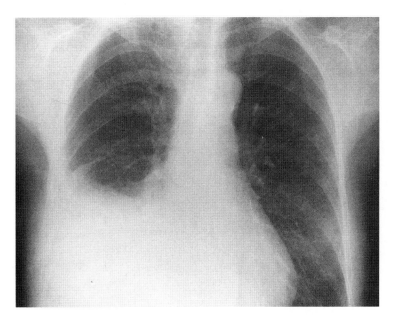

Fig. 7.31 Stage IV ovarian cancer (pleural effusion). A 54-year-old non-smoker presented with shortness of breath; she had no abdominal symptoms. Plain film of the chest demonstrates a large pleural effusion which was cytologically positive for carcinoma. Pelvic examination revealed a large left ovarian mass. Her CA125 level was 2000. After six cycles of chemotherapy, there was complete resolution of the effusion, the pelvic mass, and the elevated CA125. She remains without evidence of disease 24 months later.

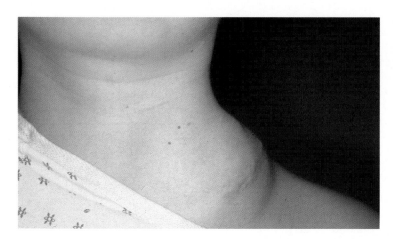

Fig. 7.32 Stage IV ovarian cancer. This 35-year-old woman presented with a large supraclavicular mass 10 years after surgery and adjuvant chemotherapy for stage III ovarian carcinoma. Pathologic examination showed papillary serous adenocarcinoma identical to her initial tumor. Although such nodal involvement is occasionally seen at presentation, spread to the left supraclavicular (Virchow's) node or left axillary (Irish's) node, as well as to the liver, lung or brain, is usually a late occurrence. Even at autopsy, liver or lung metastases are present in only 15% of cases.

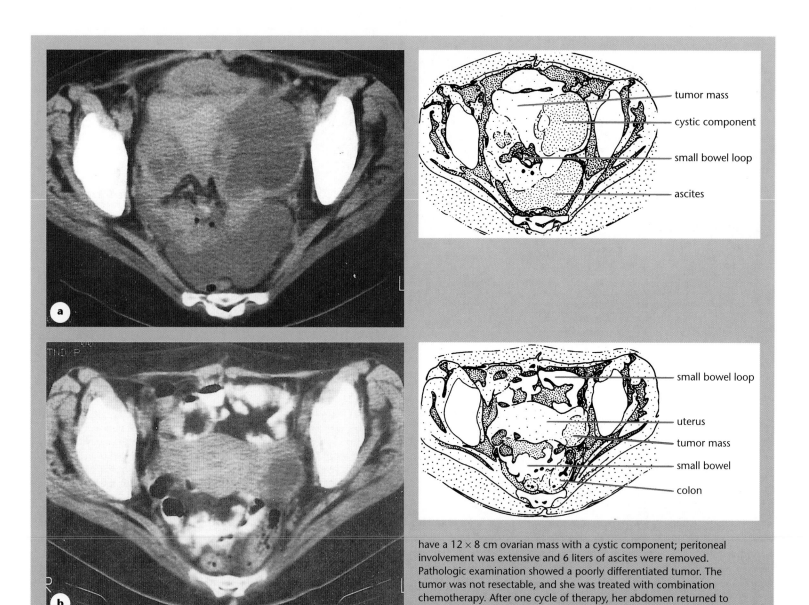

Fig. 7.33 Response to chemotherapy. A 51-year-old woman presented with a rapid increase in abdominal girth. (**a**) On CT scan, she was found to have a 12 × 8 cm ovarian mass with a cystic component; peritoneal involvement was extensive and 6 liters of ascites were removed. Pathologic examination showed a poorly differentiated tumor. The tumor was not resectable, and she was treated with combination chemotherapy. After one cycle of therapy, her abdomen returned to normal size. (**b**) A CT scan reveals only a small residual ovarian mass. Surgery after four cycles of chemotherapy showed no gross or microscopic tumor. She received four more cycles of chemotherapy but relapsed 1 year later with abdominal metastases.

ENDOMETRIAL CARCINOMA

Endometrial carcinoma is the most common malignancy of the female genital tract, with 37 000 cases a year. Despite its prevalence, there are only 3000 deaths per year. Most likely because of patient and physician education, cases are diagnosed at an earlier stage than in the past, and death rates are continuing to decrease. Its incidence peaks late in the sixth decade. Proven associations include obesity (50 pounds overweight increases the risk 10-fold), diabetes mellitus, late menopause, and probably hypertension, as well as other factors such as nulliparity and infertility, which increase estrogenic stimulation to the endometrium. Exogenous estrogens clearly increase the risk for carcinoma, but this can be reversed by cycling estrogens with progestins, which may actually decrease the risk. Polycystic ovarian disease and other illnesses that cause chronic anovulation increase the risk for this malignancy and women with these problems may develop endometrial carcinoma while in the reproductive age group.

There is no effective screening method for detecting endometrial carcinoma. However, on occasion an endometrial cancer may be revealed by Papanicolaou smear either as malignant cells or as normal endometrial cells, which are not usually seen in cervical smear. The presence of normal endometrial cells may indicate a carcinoma in approximately 10% of postmenopausal women. Evaluation in these women, as well as in women with postmenopausal bleeding, requires endometrial sampling or dilatation and curettage. The majority of women with well-differentiated stage I cancers are cured by surgery alone. Radiotherapy is used for significant myometrial invasion and higher grade tumors.

HISTOLOGY

Adenocarcinoma constitutes more than 90% of endometrial cancers. In their gross appearance, these tumors are often polypoid or exophytic. Their microscopic appearance is marked by multiple glands crowding out supporting stroma; individual cells may vary from mildly atypical to totally bizarre. Tumor grade, which takes into account cell type, nuclear atypia and glandular architecture, appears to be an important prognostic feature; lymphatic and vascular space involvement may also be significant for prognosis. Squamous elements may be present and may be either benign (adenocanthoma) or malignant (adenosquamous carcinoma). However, prognosis in these mixed tumors is determined by the grade of the glandular element only. Papillary serous adenocarcinoma is a rare, highly aggressive type of endometrial cancer which is histologically identical to its ovarian counterpart, exhibiting extensive papillary fronds and often psammoma bodies.

Sarcomas, of which leiomyosarcoma is the most common, represent approximately 5% of uterine malignancies. Believed to arise *de novo* and not from leiomyomas, leiomyosarcomas usually occur in the fifth and sixth decades. They are homologous tumors, containing elements derived from uterine smooth muscle, and are usually intramural in location. Microscopically, they are composed of spindle cells with 10 or more mitoses per 10 high-power fields (HPF). A variant exhibiting 5–10 mitoses per 10 HPF is of uncertain malignant potential and possesses a very long natural history. It may

spread to the lungs, in which case it is termed benign metastasizing leiomyoma. Endometrial stromal sarcoma is also a homologous tumor, derived from uterine mesenchyme, but it differs from normal endometrial stroma by the presence of cellular atypia and invasion through the myometrium. Low-grade tumors, also called endolymphatic stromal myosis, resemble proliferative endometrial stroma, with little cytologic atypia, often with prominent vessels, and up to 10 mitoses per 10 HPF. High-grade malignancies, on the other hand, have more than 10, and frequently as many as 20, mitoses per 10 HPF, together with a greater degree of nuclear atypia and pleomorphism. Heterologous tumors, which are extremely rare, contain foreign elements, such as bone or cartilage; they may also contain an epithelial component.

Malignant mixed Müllerian tumors (MMMT) or carcinosarcomas are derived from Müllerian mesenchyme and therefore contain both epithelial (carcinoma) and connective tissue (sarcoma) elements. The epithelial component is most commonly endometrioid, whereas the sarcomatous portion may be homologous or heterologous.

STAGING OF ENDOMETRIAL CARCINOMA

Most endometrial malignancies are confined to the uterus at the time of diagnosis (stage I) (*see* Fig. 7.34). Spread to the cervix marks stage II tumors. Microscopic cervical involvement does not worsen prognosis. More advanced stages – spread to pelvic organs or retroperitoneal lymph nodes (stage III) or hematogenous spread to distant sites (stage IV), usually to the lungs – are occasionally seen; they have a poor prognosis.

Chest radiography is useful in all patients and selected patients should have a cystoscopy and proctoscopy. Depth of invasion of the myometrium as assessed at surgery, as well as evaluation of pelvic and para-aortic lymph nodes, is also essential for staging. These factors provide useful information for determining prognosis and aid in the choice of adjuvant therapy.

CLINICAL MANIFESTATIONS

More than 90% of women with endometrial carcinoma present with abnormal vaginal bleeding. Although atrophic vaginitis is the most common cause of vaginal bleeding in low-risk postmenopausal women, patients presenting with this complaint require an endometrial biopsy for proper evaluation. With increasing age, abnormal postmenopausal bleeding is more often associated with carcinoma; overall, about 20% of such women will be found to have a malignancy. Carcinoma in perimenopausal women or anovulatory women may present with heavy or prolonged bleeding; these women may ignore changes in their bleeding pattern, considering them to be signs of approaching menopause. If the tumor spreads outside the uterus, adjacent organs are most commonly involved. Vaginal or suburethral metastases may cause pain, bleeding, or discharge; abdominal distension and bowel or urinary dysfunction may develop from involvement of the bladder or rectum. Back pain may result from para-aortic nodal involvement. Pulmonary metastases may occur late in the course of disease due to hematogenous spread and brain metastases may occur.

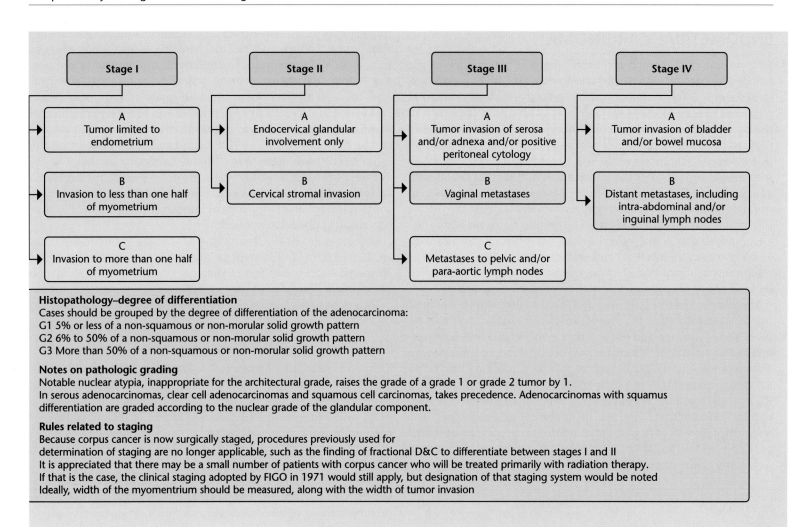

Histopathology–degree of differentiation
Cases should be grouped by the degree of differentiation of the adenocarcinoma:
G1 5% or less of a non-squamous or non-morular solid growth pattern
G2 6% to 50% of a non-squamous or non-morular solid growth pattern
G3 More than 50% of a non-squamous or non-morular solid growth pattern

Notes on pathologic grading
Notable nuclear atypia, inappropriate for the architectural grade, raises the grade of a grade 1 or grade 2 tumor by 1.
In serous adenocarcinomas, clear cell adenocarcinomas and squamous cell carcinomas, takes precedence. Adenocarcinomas with squamus differentiation are graded according to the nuclear grade of the glandular component.

Rules related to staging
Because corpus cancer is now surgically staged, procedures previously used for
determination of staging are no longer applicable, such as the finding of fractional D&C to differentiate between stages I and II
It is appreciated that there may be a small number of patients with corpus cancer who will be treated primarily with radiation therapy.
If that is the case, the clinical staging adopted by FIGO in 1971 would still apply, but designation of that staging system would be noted
Ideally, width of the myomentrium should be measured, along with the width of tumor invasion

Fig. 7.34 FIGO staging system for endometrial carcinoma (1990).

TNM staging compared to the FIGO system

Definition of TNM

Primary tumor (T)*

TNM	FIGO	Definition
TX	–	Primary tumor cannot be assessed
T0	–	No evidence of primary tumor
Tis	–	Carcinoma in situ
T1	1	Tumor confined to the corpus uteri
T1a	IA	Tumor limited to the endometrium
T1b	IB	Tumor invades up to or less than one-half of the myometrium
T1c	IC	Tumor invades more than one-half of the myometrium
T2	II	Tumor invades the cervix but not extending beyond the uterus
T2a	IIA	Endocervical glandular involvement only
T2b	IIB	Cervical stromal invasion
T3 and/or N1	III	Local and/or regional spread as specified in T3a, b, NI and FIGO IIIA, B, and C below
T3a	IIIA	Tumor involves the serosa and/or adnexa (direct extension or metastasis) and/or cancer cells in ascites or peritoneal washings
T3b	IIIB	Vaginal involvement (direct extension or metastasis)
N1	IIIC	Metastasis to the pelvic and/or para-aortic lymph nodes
T4†	IVA	Tumor invades the bladder mucosa or the rectum and/or the bowel mucosa
M1	IVB	Distant metastasis (excluding metastasis to the vagina, pelvic serosa, or adnexa; including metastasis to intra-abdominal lymph nodes other than para-aortic, and/or inguinal lymph nodes.)

Regional lymph nodes (N)

NX Regional lymph nodes cannot be assessed
NO No regional lymph node metastasis
NI Regional lymph node metastasis

Distant metastasis (M)

TNM	FIGO	Definition
MX	–	Presence of distant metastasis cannot be assessed
MO	–	No distant metastasis
M1	IVB	Distant metastasis

Stage grouping

AJCC/UICC				FIGO
Stage 0	Tis	N0	M0	
Stage IA	T1a	N0	M0	Stage IA
Stage IB	T1b	N0	M0	Stage IB
Stage IC	T1c	N0	M0	Stage IC
Stage IIA	T2a	N0	M0	Stage IIA
Stage IIB	T2b	N0	M0	Stage IIB
Stage IIIA	T3a	N0	M0	Stage IIIA
Stage IIIB	T3b	N0	M0	Stage IIIB
Stage IIIC	T1	N1	M0	Stage IIIC
	T2	N1	M0	
	T3a	N1	M0	
	T3b	N1	M0	
Stage IVA	T4	Any N	M0	Stage IVA
Stage IVB	Any T	Any N	M1	Stage IVB

* The predominant lesion is adenocarcinoma, but all histologic types should be reported. However, choriocarcinomas, sarcomas, mixed mesodermal tumors, and carcinosarcomas should be presented separately.

† Note: The presence of bullous edema is not sufficient evidence to classify a tumor as T4.

Fig. 7.35 TNM staging compared to the FIGO system. (AJCC: Manual for Staging of Cancer, 4th edn. Lippincott, Philadelphia, 1993)

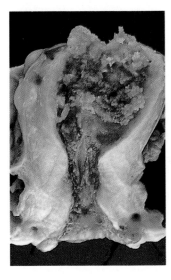

Fig. 7.36 Endometrial adenocarcinoma. Arising from the endometrium in the body of the uterus is a large, polypoid, focally necrotic neoplasm.

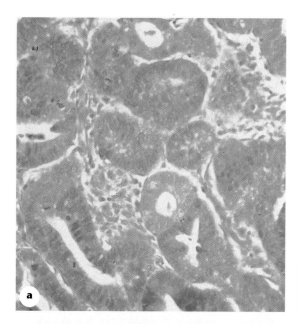

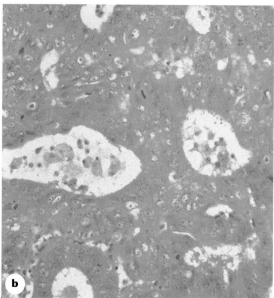

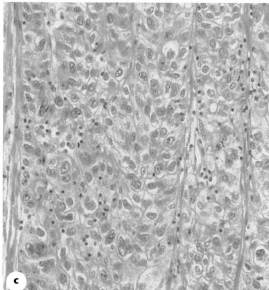

Fig. 7.37 Endometrial adenocarcinoma. (**a**) In a grade I tumor, the glands are well preserved, indicating continuing differentiation; supporting stroma, however, has been crowded out. (**b**) Grade II lesions are marked by piling up and bridging of malignant epithelium within gland spaces. This results in a cribriform pattern and focally solid areas. (**c**) All organization is lost in grade III tumors, which show solid sheets of cancer cells. Grade is associated with depth of invasion, probability of pelvic nodal involvement, likelihood of response to hormonal therapy, and survival.

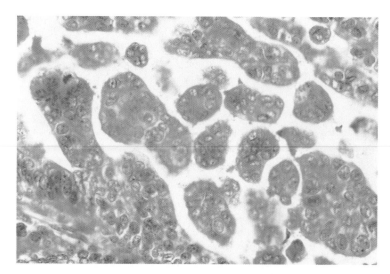

Fig. 7.38 Papillary serous adenocarcinoma. Histologically and clinically, this rare and virulent form of endometrial cancer resembles its ovarian counterpart; its pattern of transperitoneal spread is also similar.

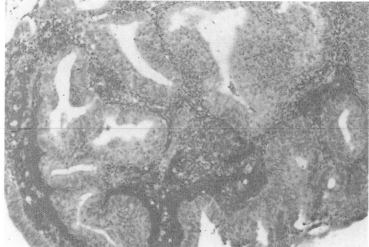

Fig. 7.39 Atypical endometrial hyperplasia. Crowded, irregular endometrial glands with pronounced cytologic atypia, characterized by epithelial disorganization, nuclear stratification, variation in nuclear size and shape, and prominent nucleoli. Atypical hyperplasias are considered at high risk for malignant change.

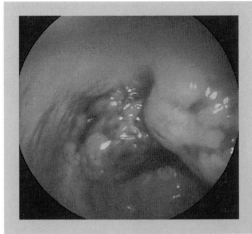

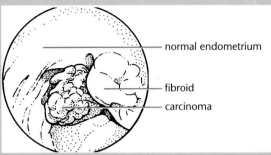

Fig. 7.40 Stage I endometrial carcinoma. A small carcinoma can be seen adjacent to a uterine fibroid in this hysteroscopy photograph. Occasionally, a tumor this small may be missed on curettage.

normal endometrium

fibroid

carcinoma

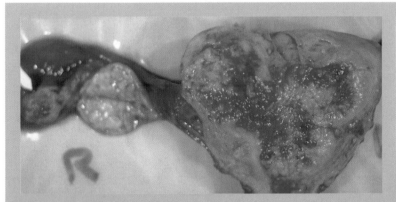

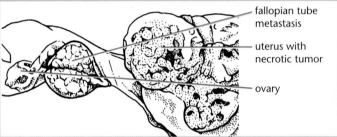

fallopian tube metastasis

uterus with necrotic tumor

ovary

Fig. 7.41 Stage III endometrial carcinoma. This specimen is from a 64-year-old woman with a 1-year history of postmenopausal bleeding. The

tumor is ulcerative, deeply invasive, and has spread to the fallopian tube. Pathologic examination showed a poorly differentiated adenocarcinoma. (Courtesy of Howard Goodman MD, Department of Gynecologic Oncology, Brigham and Women's Hospital, Boston, MA.)

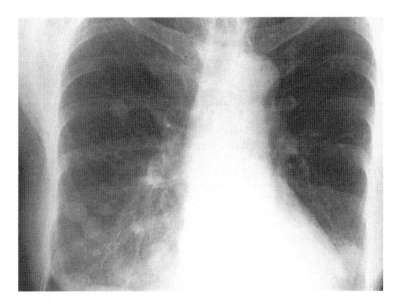

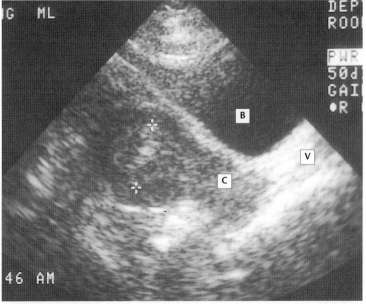

Fig. 7.42 Stage IV endometrial carcinoma (pulmonary metastases). This 74-year-old woman presented with vaginal bleeding and was found to have a stage IB poorly differentiated adenosquamous carcinoma of the endometrium, which was invasive to one third of the myometrium. One year after surgery the disease recurred with pulmonary nodules. A significant number of patients at recurrence have only distant metastases, the pulmonary parenchyma being the most common site.

Fig. 7.43 Endometrial cancer. Sagittal midline real-time ultrasound image of the pelvis, transabdominal in a patient with abnormal vaginal bleeding. No normal endometrium is visible in the fundus, with a heterogeneous central mass present (between asterisks). B = bladder; C = cervix; V = vagina.

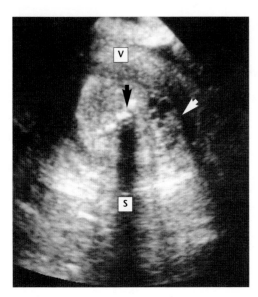

Fig. 7.44 Endometrial cancer. Coronal real-time ultrasound image through the uterine fundus in the patient in Fig. 7.43, using an endovaginal transducer. Note more detailed image of internal structure of the mass, with small areas of calcification (arrow) showing acoustic shadow (S), as well as small cystic areas (arrowhead). V = vaginal wall.

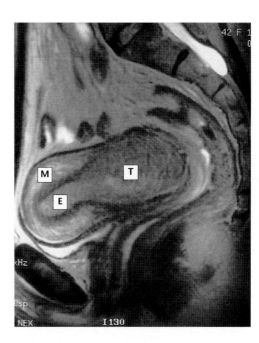

Fig. 7.45 Endometrial cancer. This MRI clearly defines normal myometrium (M), endometrium (E), and a large tumor (T) arising posteriorly from the uterus. While MRI gives excellent definition to pelvic tissues, CT scans are better able to differentiate between contrast-filled bowel and nodal disease.

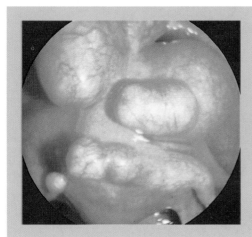
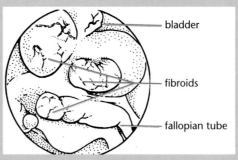

Fig. 7.46 Leiomyoma. This laparascopic photograph shows multiple large intramural fibroids.

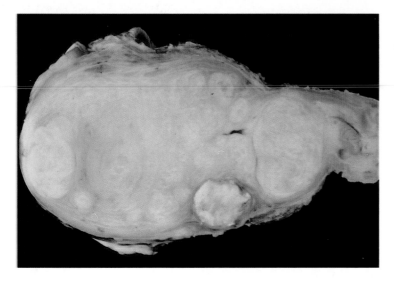

Fig. 7.47 Leiomyoma. This grossly enlarged and distorted uterus has been sectioned to show multiple, well-circumscribed intramural and submucosal tumors displacing and compressing the uterine cavity. The lesions have a typical whorled appearance except for one (bottom right), which has undergone degeneration and dystrophic calcification. These benign neoplasms of uterine smooth muscle, also known as 'fibroids', are very common and arise only during the reproductive years. They are usually multiple and are thought to be caused by excessive estrogen stimulation; they tend to atrophy after menopause. Various forms of degenerative changes are common, but malignant transformation in a leiomyoma is very rare.

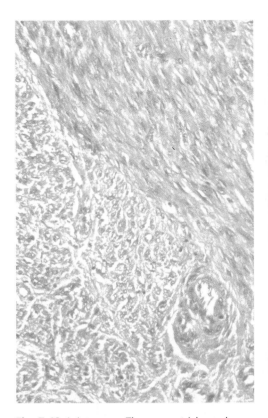

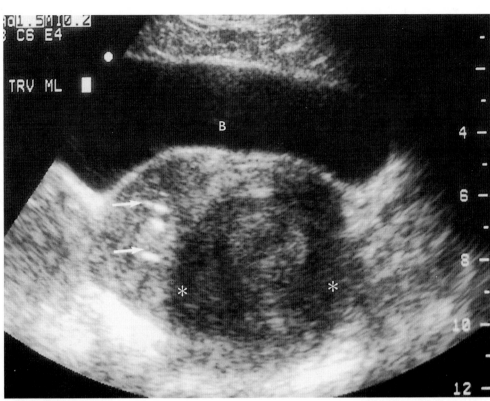

Fig. 7.48 Leiomyoma. The myometrial muscle bundles above and to the right in this photomicrograph run parallel to the plane of the section. Below and to the left, the plane of the section cuts across the muscle bundle. These are characteristic features of smooth muscle tumors.

Fig. 7.49 Transverse real-time ultrasound image through the uterine fundus in a patient with abdominal pain. A large hypoechoic mass is seen to the left of the midline (asterisks) compatible with a uterine fibroid. Note several portions of an IUD (arrows) within the plane of the scan. B = bladder.

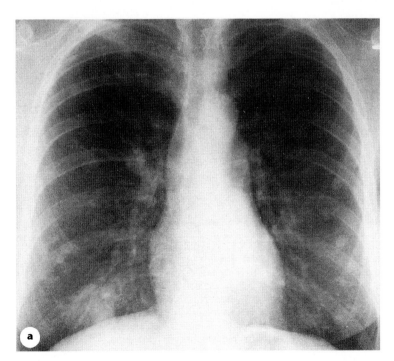

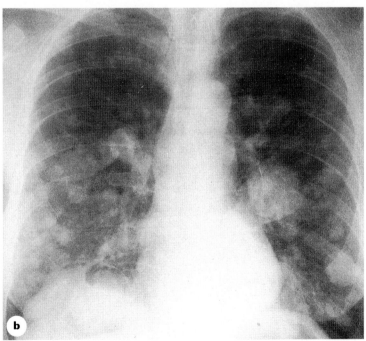

Fig. 7.50 Metastatic leiomyoma. This 39-year-old woman had a hysterectomy for menorrhagia due to uterine leiomyomas. (**a**) Five years later bilateral asymptomatic pulmonary nodules developed. Biopsy showed histologic findings similar to the tumor seen at hysterectomy. (**b**) Over a 6-year interval, the size of the lesions slowly increased, still with no major symptoms. This entity has been termed 'benign metastasizing leiomyoma' but it undoubtedly represents a very low-grade malignancy (leiomoysarcoma).

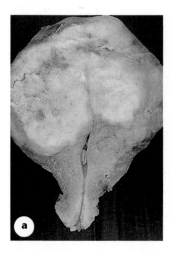

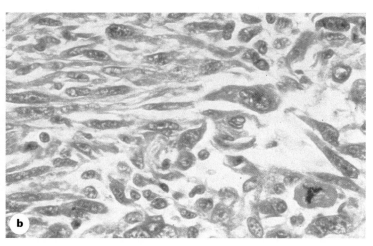

Fig. 7.51 Leiomyosarcoma. (**a**) In the myometrium of the fundus and body of this uterine specimen is an irregular pale neoplasm showing focal hemorrhage and necrosis, with serosal invasion. (**b**) Pleomorphism and a brisk mitotic rate clearly identify the malignant nature of this tumor. Prognosis is related to stage, number of mitotic figures, depth of invasion, and perhaps to extent of pleomorphism; the 5-year survival rate is about 30%.

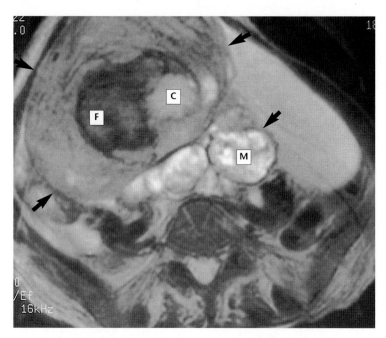

Fig. 7.52 Unresectable leiomyosarcoma. This MRI is from a 50-year-old woman who presented with abdominal swelling. The MRI shows a heterogeneous tumor (arrows) with areas of solid and cystic (C) tumor, mucin production (M) and fibrosis (F). While CT scan can define a mass, MRI can differentiate some tissue types within a tumor.

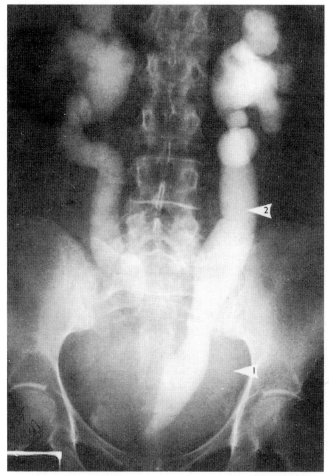

Fig. 7.53 Leiomyosarcoma. A 51-year-old woman had recurrent low-grade uterine leiomyosarcoma. She first presented with a large pelvic mass and was treated surgically. Disease recurred 6 years later and again 3 years afterward, when radiologic evaluation showed a large pelvic mass (arrow 1) with bilateral hydronephrosis and hydroureters (arrow 2). Renal function was normal and the pelvic mass was resected. Chest CT scan showed a single pulmonary nodule, which on resection proved to be a primary, well-differentiated lymphocytic lymphoma.

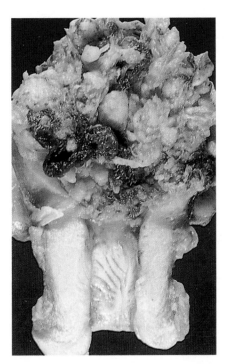

Fig. 7.54 Malignant mixed Müllerian tumor. Arising in the uterine fundus is a large, polypoid, hemorrhagic mass with extensive myometrial invasion. These tumors arise most often in the elderly and carry a poor prognosis.

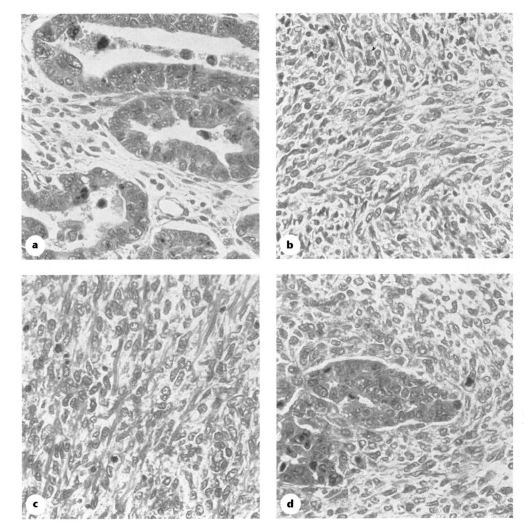

Fig. 7.55 Malignant mixed Müllerian tumor. These four photomicrographs are all from the same tumor. (**a**) In this portion of the tumor, the apparent diagnosis is adenocarcinoma, but (**b**) in another section, the tissue organization suggests the whorls of a muscle tumor; the impression is that of a leiomysarcoma. (**c**) The tissue organization in this instance is more consistent with a stromal sarcoma. (**d**) Both epithelium and stroma are malignant and malignant mixed Müllerian tumor (carcinosarcoma) is present.

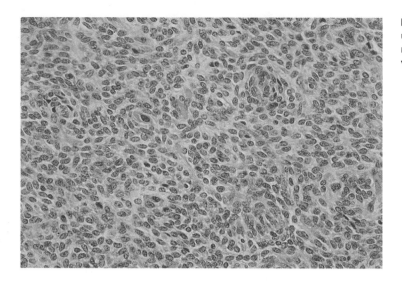

Fig. 7.56 Endometrial stromal sarcoma. This homologous tumor arises from uterine mesenchyme. The high-grade type seen in this photomicrograph is marked by greater nuclear atypia and pleomorphism than the low-grade variant, together with more than 10 mitoses per 10 HPF.

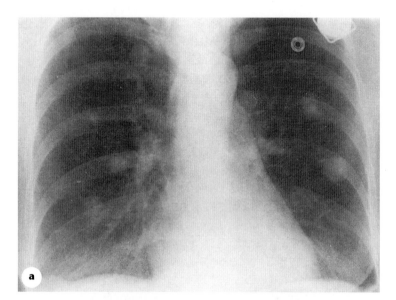

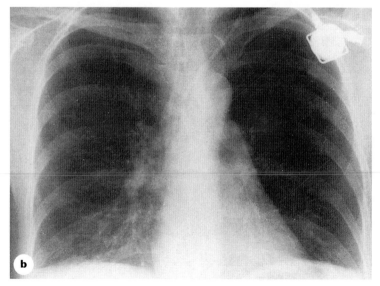

Fig. 7.57 Endometrial stroma sarcoma. A 37-year-old woman presented with menometrorrhagia and was found at surgery to have a high-grade malignant uterine tumor and a benign Brenner tumor of the ovary. Disease recurred in the abdomen 2 months after surgery, and she was treated with whole-abdominal radiotherapy. **(a)** Pulmonary metastases developed 3 months after completion of radiotherapy, and she was treated with chemotherapy, which resulted **(b)** in complete remission within 2 months. Endometrial stromal sarcoma appears to be the most chemoresponsive form of uterine sarcoma.

CERVICAL CANCER

Cancer of the cervix once accounted for half of the cancer-related deaths in the United States. Although its incidence has decreased, it still accounts for 12 900 cases per year and 4400 deaths per year. This cancer occurs most frequently in the fifth and sixth decades. Risk factors include early age of first intercourse, multiple sexual partners, lower socio-economic status and history of sexually transmitted diseases. Cervical cancer is thought to arise in pre-existing areas of intraepithelial neoplasia over the period of 10–20 years. Human papilloma virus (HPV) is the virus implicated in most cases of cervical cancer. There are over 80 types of HPV but only 25 infect the genital tract; certain types (HPV 16 and 18) are high risk for development of cervical cancer.

HISTOLOGY

Cervical squamous intraepithelial lesion (SIL) is divided into low-grade SIL (koilocytosis, mild dysplasia, CIN I) and high-grade SIL (severe dysplasia, carcinoma *in situ*, CIN III); it is a precursor lesion of invasive cervical cancer. It takes years for this orderly progression to occur and diagnosis by Papanicolaou smear and subsequent treatment of these preinvasive lesions have markedly decreased the mortality from invasive cancer.

Squamous cell carcinomas, including small cell variants, constitute 80% of cervical malignancies. Microscopically, the tumors are marked by disorder in the progression of squamous epithelium from flattened surface cells to cuboidal cells at the basement membrane. Moreover, nests of neoplastic epithelial cells invade through the basement membrane; microinvasive cancers infiltrate less than 3–5 mm into the cervical stroma. Keratin pearls may be seen, especially in well-differentiated tumors, but they are absent in poorly differentiated lesions. Poorly differentiated squamous cell carcinomas have dense, hyperchromatic nuclei and frequent mitoses. Lymphatic and vascular invasion is more frequent than in well-differentiated tumors and is associated with nodal involvement and a poorer prognosis. More often the small cell variant represents a poorly differentiated squamous cell tumor and less commonly a neuroendocrine tumor. The distinction may need to be made by electron microscope or immunoperoxidase staining.

Adenocarcinomas are less common than squamous cell tumors, constituting 5–20% of cervical neoplasia; however, there appears to be an increase in incidence of these malignancies among younger women. They are more difficult to diagnose by Papanicolaou smear or clinical examination because they are often confined to the endocervix. Grossly, cervical adenocarcinomas may present as a fungating, polypoid mass, but they may also exhibit an endophytic growth pattern that may internally expand the cervix, leading to its having a barrel shape; thus, the lower uterine segment may show no external lesion. Arising from endocervical glands, the tumors are marked by glands lined by high-columnar, mucin-secreting cells. Squamous differentiation, which may be malignant (adenosquamous carcinoma) or benign (adenoacanthoma), may also be present within adenocarcinomas and some researchers report a worse prognosis with adenosquamous variants. Tumors of other cell types are occasionally seen in the cervix, among them clear cell carcinoma, adenoid cystic carcinoma, botryoid sarcoma and melanoma.

STAGING OF CERVICAL CARCINOMA

In the majority of cases, cervical cancers are diagnosed while they are still confined to the cervix either as occult tumors discovered by Papanicolaou smear screening (stage IA) or as larger lesions (stage IB). More advanced tumors have spread either to the vagina or to the parametrium (stages II and III); stage IV tumors are defined as involving the bladder or rectum or as having spread to distant sites.

Clinical staging is completed with a pelvic examination under anesthesia, during which cystoscopy and proctoscopy are performed to rule out adjacent organ involvement. Lymphatic spread is not uncommon, as the cervix is rich in lymphatics; however, the clinical staging system does not include abdominal CT scan or MRI to assess pelvic and para-aortic nodes. Hematogenous spread to the liver, lung, and bone can occur but is usually associated with massive pelvic disease. Whereas the disease is clinically staged, patients may be found at surgery to have more advanced disease. Nodal involvement is common and affects both prognosis and the need for further therapy. Information gained at surgery and from CT or MR scans may not be used to alter the assigned stage, although such information is of course useful for treatment planning.

CLINICAL MANIFESTATIONS

As these tumors are usually asymptomatic, in most instances they are discovered at routine pelvic examination and by Papanicolau smear. The Pap test may pick up an entirely unsuspected lesion, in which case colposcopy is performed to view the entire cervix under magnification in the search for changes indicating intraepithelial or invasive neoplasia: white epithelium with vascular punctation or mosaicism or atypical vessels. In addition to obtaining biopsies of abnormal areas, an endocervical curettage is performed.

When cervical tumors progress in size and become symptomatic, the most common complaints are abnormal vaginal bleeding, which may be postcoital, postmenopausal or intermenstrual, or vaginal discharge, which is often yellow, serosanguineous and malodorous. Advanced or recurrent disease may present with pelvic pain, tenesmus, bladder irritation, lower extremity edema, renal obstruction or back pain from retroperitoneal lymph node involvement. Pulmonary or bone metastases may occur late in the course of disease.

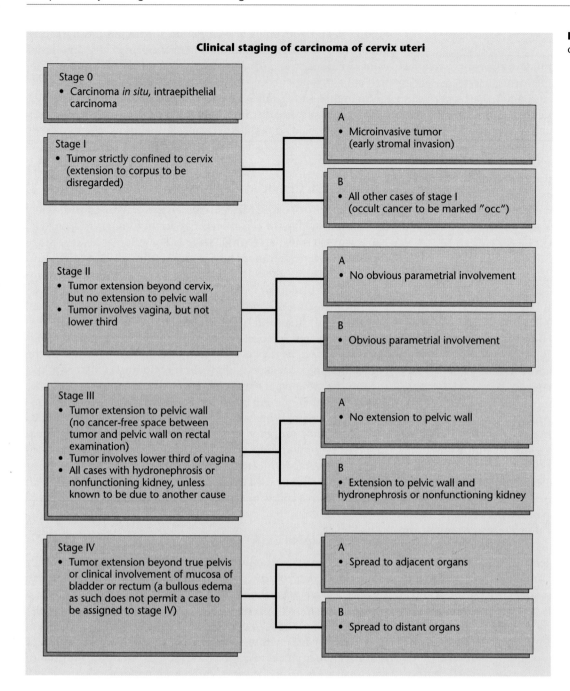

Clinical staging of carcinoma of cervix uteri

Stage 0
- Carcinoma *in situ*, intraepithelial carcinoma

Stage I
- Tumor strictly confined to cervix (extension to corpus to be disregarded)

A
- Microinvasive tumor (early stromal invasion)

B
- All other cases of stage I (occult cancer to be marked "occ")

Stage II
- Tumor extension beyond cervix, but no extension to pelvic wall
- Tumor involves vagina, but not lower third

A
- No obvious parametrial involvement

B
- Obvious parametrial involvement

Stage III
- Tumor extension to pelvic wall (no cancer-free space between tumor and pelvic wall on rectal examination)
- Tumor involves lower third of vagina
- All cases with hydronephrosis or nonfunctioning kidney, unless known to be due to another cause

A
- No extension to pelvic wall

B
- Extension to pelvic wall and hydronephrosis or nonfunctioning kidney

Stage IV
- Tumor extension beyond true pelvis or clinical involvement of mucosa of bladder or rectum (a bullous edema as such does not permit a case to be assigned to stage IV)

A
- Spread to adjacent organs

B
- Spread to distant organs

Fig. 7.58 Staging for carcinoma of the cervix uteri (FIGO 1984).

AJCC primary	FIGO tumor (T)	
TX	-	Primary tumor cannot be assessed
T0	-	No evidence of primary tumor
Tis	0	Carcinoma in situ
T1	I	Cervical carcinoma confined to uterus (extension to corpus should be disregarded)
T1a	IA	Invasive carcinoma, diagnosed only by microscopy. All macroscopically visible lesions even with superficial invasion are T1b/Ib. Stromal invasion with a maximum depth of 5 mm measured from the base of the epithelium and horizontal spread of 7 mm or less. Vascular space involvement, venous or lymphatic, does not affect classification.
T1a1	IA1	Measured stromal invasion 3 mm or less and 7 mm or less in Horizontal spread
T1a2	IA2	Measured stromal invasion more than 3 mm and not more than 5 mm with a horizontal spread of 7 mm or less
T1b	IB	Clearly visible lesion confined to the cervix or microscopic lesion greater than T1a2/IA2
T1b1	IB1	Clearly visible lesion 4 cm or less in greatest dimension
T1b2	IB2	Clearly visible lesion more than 4 cm in greatest dimension
T2	II	Cervical carcinoma invades beyond uterus but not to pelvic wall or to the lower third of vagina
T2a	IIA	Tumor without parametrial invasion
T2b	IIB	Tumor with parametrial invasion
T3	III	Cervical carcinoma extends to the pelvic wall and/or involves lower third of vagina or causes hydronephrosis or non functioning kidney
T3a	IIIA	Tumor involves lower third of the vagina, no extension to the pelvic wall
T3b	IIIB	Tumor extends to pelvic wall or causes hydronephrosis or non functioning kidney
T4*	IVA	Tumor invades mucosa of bladder or rectum and/or extends beyond true pelvis
M1	IVB	Distant metastasis

Regional lymph nodes (N)
Regional lymph nodes include paracervical, parametrial, hypogastric (obturator), common, internal and external iliac, presacral an sacral.

NX	-	Regional lymph nodes cannot be assessed
N0	-	No regional lymph node metastasis
N1	-	Regional lymph node metastasis

Distant metastasis (M)

MX	-	Presence of distant metastasis connot be assessed
M0	-	No distant metastasis
M1	IVB	Distant metastasis

AJCC, American Joint Committee on Cancer; FIGO, International Federation of Gynecology and Obstetrics. *Presence of bulleous edema is not sufficient evidence to classify a tumor T4.

Stage grouping

Stage	Primary tumor	Regional lymph nodes	Distant metastases
0	Tis	N0	M0
IA1	T1a1	N0	M0
IA2	T1a2	N0	M0
IB1	T1b1	N0	M0
IB2	T1b2	N0	M0
IIA	T2a	N0	M0
IIB	T2b	N0	M0
IIIA	T3a	N0	M0
IIIB	T1	N1	M0
	T2	N1	M0
	T3a	N1	M0
	T3b	Any N	M0
IVA	T4	Any N	M0
IVB	Any T	Any N	M1

Fig. 7.59 Staging of cervical cancer (from Flemming *et al.*, 1997).

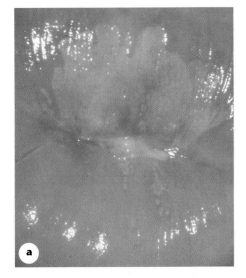
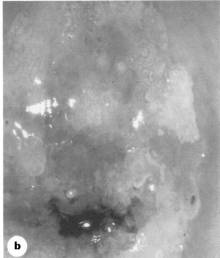
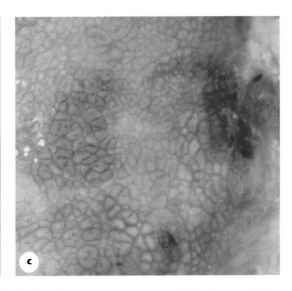

Fig. 7.60 Cervical squamous intraepithelial lesion (SIL, CIN). This sequence of photographs, taken through the colposcope, shows progressively more severe examples of SIL. (**a**) Low-grade SIL is marked by mild dysplasia, appearing as a whitened area of epithelium emanating from the transformation zone. (**b**) Early high-grade SIL (moderate dysplasia, CIN II) shows early vascular mosaicism and vessel punctuation findings that are more pronounced (**c**) in advanced high-grade SIL (CIN III severe dysplasia). Any of these findings on colposcopic examination requires biopsy. (Courtesy of Howard Goodman MD, Department of Gynecologic Oncology, Brigham and Women's Hospital, Boston, MA.)

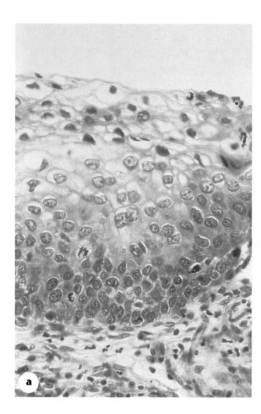
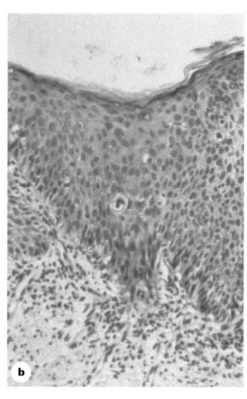

Fig. 7.61 Cervical squamous intraepithelial lesion (SIL). (**a**) Koilocytosis, multinucleation, hyperchromasia and nuclear enlargement are present in the upper layers of the epithelium, consistent with a low-grade lesion (LSIL). (**b**) Full-thickness atypia with absence of normal maturation is indicative of a high-grade lesion (HSIL).

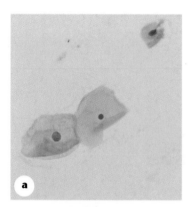
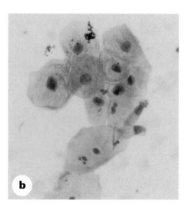
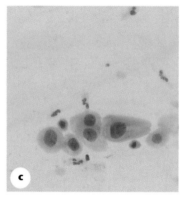
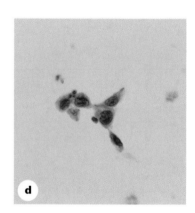

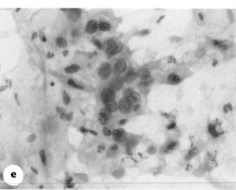

Fig. 7.62 Cervical squamous intraepithelial lesion (SIL). This series of Papanicolaou smears shows progression from normal through invasive carcinoma. (**a**) Two normal squamous cells with small pyknotic nuclei are visible. (**b**) Low grade SIL (CIN I) is characterized by a slightly higher nucleus to cytoplasm ratio. The presence of columnar cells signifies that this is an adequate smear sampling of the endocervix. In high-grade SIL, the nucleus to cytoplasm ratio is higher than in low-grade SIL. Both moderate dysplasia/CIN II (**c**) and severe dysplasia/CINIII/carcinoma *in situ* (**d**) are now categorized as high-grade SIL. (**e**) Invasive carcinoma is marked by spindle cells, prominent nucleoli in large nuclei, and extensive acellular necrotic debris in the background. (Courtesy of Edmund Cibas MD, Department of Pathology, Brigham and Women's Hospital, Boston, MA.)

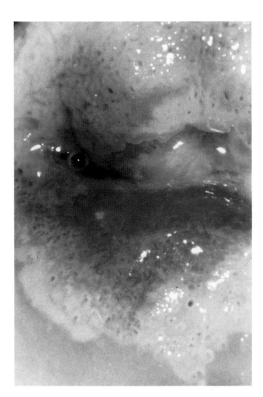

Fig. 7.63 High-grade squamous intraepithelial lesion. This colposcopic photograph shows extensive areas of white epithelium and punctation. Biopsy revealed an *in situ* lesion.

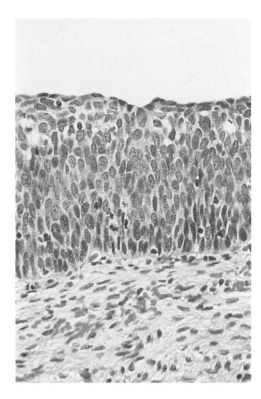

Fig. 7.64 High-grade squamous intraepithelial lesion. No squamous cytoplasmic maturation is present except that the topmost cell layer may be flattened, as shown here.

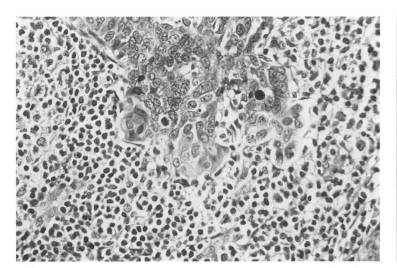

Fig. 7.65 Microinvasive squamous cell carcinoma. Three tongues of cells with relative cytoplasmic eosinophilia extend from the overlying basophilic epithelium into the underlying stroma. An intense inflammatory reaction is present. The exact definition of microinvasive carcinoma is controversial, but the inclusion in this category of a tumor such as this, showing less than I mm of invasion, no lymphatic or vascular invasion, and no confluence of invasive tongues, cannot be questioned. The risk of nodal involvement in this case is negligible.

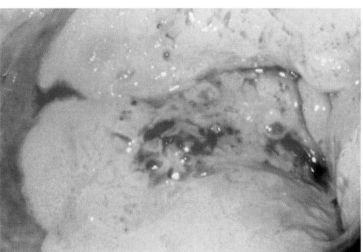

Fig. 7.66 Squamous cell carcinoma. This colposcopic photograph shows the white epithelium and the grossly atypical vessels and hemorrhage that are characteristic of invasive lesions. (Courtesy of Howard Goodman MD, Department of Gynecologic Oncology, Brigham and Women's Hospital, Boston MA.)

Fig. 7.67 Squamous cell carcinoma. Arising from the ectocervix is an irregular, fungating, pale neoplasm.

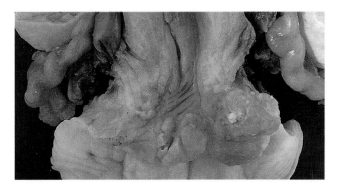

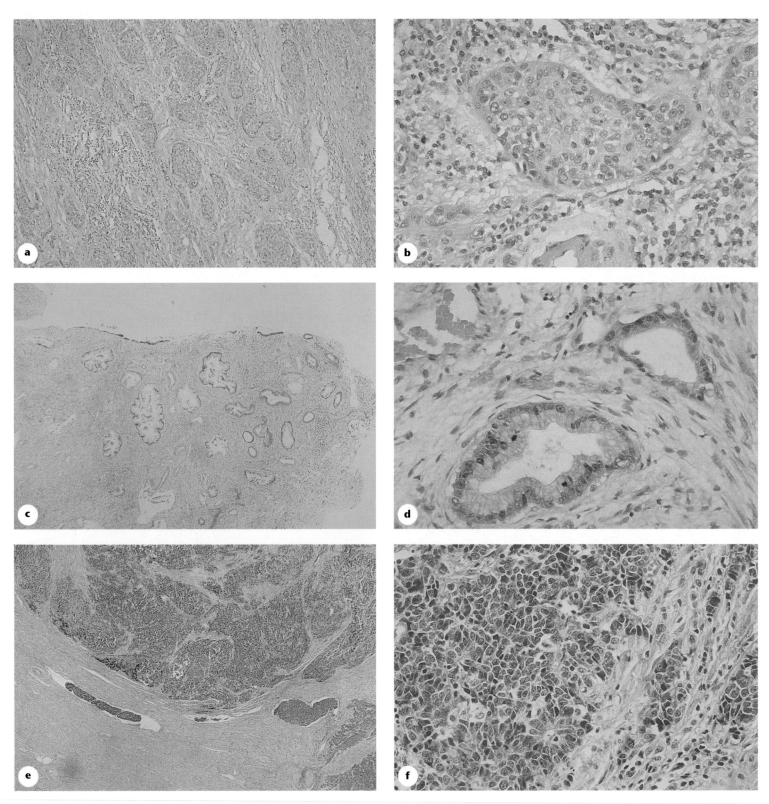

Fig. 7.68 *Squamous cell carcinoma.* (**a**) Tumor widely infiltrates the cervical stroma. (**b**) This tumor is composed of nests of moderately differentiated squamous epithelium. *Adenocarcinoma.* (**c**) The superficial and deep endocervical stroma is widely infiltrated by malignant glands. (**d**) Irregular glands with mucinous epithelium and occasional mitoses infiltrate the stroma. *Small cell neuroendocrine carcinoma.* (**e**) Solid nests of hyperchromatic tumor cells infiltrate stroma, involving lymphatic and vascular channels. (**f**) Tumor cells have scant cytoplasm and hyperchromatic, molded nuclei.

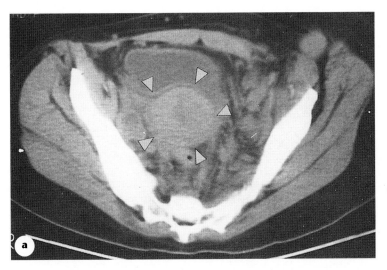
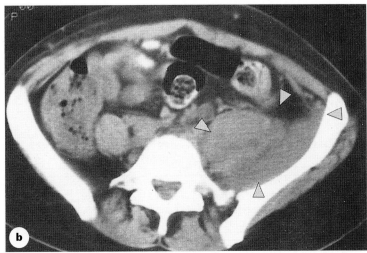

Fig. 7.69 Stage IIIB cervical carcinoma. A 27-year-old woman presented with increased vaginal bleeding, left leg swelling and abdominal pain. Examination revealed a large fixed pelvic mass. CT scan evaluation (**a**) confirms the mass (arrows) and (**b**) shows extension into the left psoas and iliacus muscles (arrows). She also had hydronephrosis. Pathologic examination showed an adenosquamous carcinoma.

OTHER GYNECOLOGIC MALIGNANCIES

VULVAR CARCINOMA

Vulvar carcinoma accounts for approximately 4% of gynecologic malignancies. Whereas preinvasive disease occurs primarily in the premenopausal woman, the median age for invasive vulvar cancer is 60 years. The etiology is unclear, but the tumor may be related to sexually transmitted diseases, especially HPV, cigarette smoking, vulvar trauma and immunosuppression: however, it does not appear to be endocrinologically mediated. Vulvar cancer is more common in diabetics and in women with a history of breast, endometrial or cervical cancer.

Carcinoma *in situ* may represent a preinvasive lesion, especially in the elderly and immunosuppressed. The significance of chronic vulvar dystrophy is unknown, as it represents a heterogenous group of disorders, but in the absence of cellular atypia, most cases of chronic vulvar dystrophy will not progress to invasive carcinoma. Invasive carcinoma is usually well differentiated, keratinizing, and squamous, but other histologic types such as melanoma, adenocarcinoma or basal cell carcinoma may occur. The staging system for vulvar carcinoma is shown in Figure 7.70.

VAGINAL CARCINOMA

Vaginal carcinoma is usually metastatic from primary tumors of the endometrium, ovary, cervix, breast or gastrointestinal tract. Primary tumors of the vagina are rare, but they may occur in infants (endodermal sinus tumor, embryonal rhabdomyosarcoma), adolescents (clear cell carcinoma) or adults (carcinomas, sarcomas, melanomas). Squamous cell carcinomas, the most common type of malignancy, usually present late in life with abnormal vaginal discharge or bleeding. Clear cell carcinomas are rare, but may occur in approximately 0.1% of women exposed *in utero* to diethylstilbestrol; the risk for devel-

opment of these tumors is greatest between the ages of 15 and 25 years. The staging system for vaginal carcinoma is shown in Figure 7.77.

FALLOPIAN TUBE CARCINOMA

Primary fallopian tube carcinoma is very rare. It parallels ovarian carcinoma in natural history, pathology, staging, and treatment. Although frequently asymptomatic, it may present with vaginal bleeding or in the same manner as ovarian cancer, with increasing abdominal girth and vague gastrointestinal complaints. Like ovarian carcinoma, spread is most often peritoneal, but hematogenous dissemination to lung, brain or pericardium may occur.

GESTATIONAL TROPHOBLASTIC NEOPLASIA

This category of gynecologic tumors includes the hydatidiform mole (complete and partial), the invasive mole, choriocarcinoma and placental site trophoblastic tumor (PSTT). Molar pregnancies occur with a frequency of 1 in 1500 live births in the US; in other areas of the world, the frequency may be as high as 1 in 120. Although dietary factors have been implicated, the etiology is unknown. Invasive moles or choriocarcinoma develop in 15% of women with complete molar pregnancies; it can usually be cured with a few courses of single agent chemotherapy, thus preserving fertility. Simple hysterectomy and chemotherapy may be used in women who have completed their child-bearing. Choriocarcinoma most commonly follows molar pregnancy but may also complicate an abortion, ectopic pregnancy, or normal delivery. The lung, gastrointestinal tract, oral cavity, liver and central nervous system may be sites of metastatic disease. The latter two sites are poor prognostic features, but the majority of these patients may be cured with chemotherapy. The staging system for gestational trophoblastic neoplasms is shown in Figure 7.85.

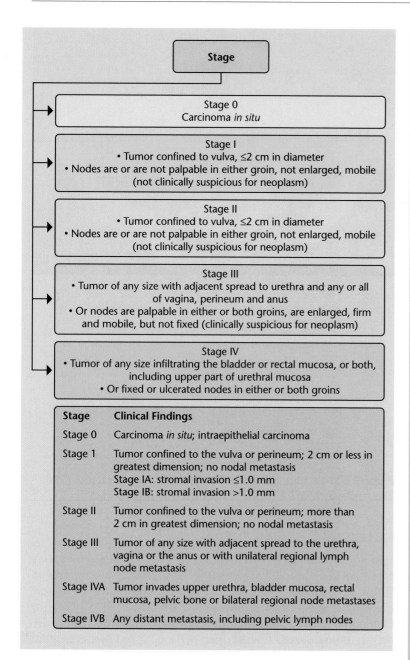

Stage

Stage 0
Carcinoma *in situ*

Stage I
• Tumor confined to vulva, ≤2 cm in diameter
• Nodes are or are not palpable in either groin, not enlarged, mobile (not clinically suspicious for neoplasm)

Stage II
• Tumor confined to vulva, ≤2 cm in diameter
• Nodes are or are not palpable in either groin, not enlarged, mobile (not clinically suspicious for neoplasm)

Stage III
• Tumor of any size with adjacent spread to urethra and any or all of vagina, perineum and anus
• Or nodes are palpable in either or both groins, are enlarged, firm and mobile, but not fixed (clinically suspicious for neoplasm)

Stage IV
• Tumor of any size infiltrating the bladder or rectal mucosa, or both, including upper part of urethral mucosa
• Or fixed or ulcerated nodes in either or both groins

Stage	Clinical Findings
Stage 0	Carcinoma *in situ*; intraepithelial carcinoma
Stage 1	Tumor confined to the vulva or perineum; 2 cm or less in greatest dimension; no nodal metastasis Stage IA: stromal invasion ≤1.0 mm Stage IB: stromal invasion >1.0 mm
Stage II	Tumor confined to the vulva or perineum; more than 2 cm in greatest dimension; no nodal metastasis
Stage III	Tumor of any size with adjacent spread to the urethra, vagina or the anus or with unilateral regional lymph node metastasis
Stage IVA	Tumor invades upper urethra, bladder mucosa, rectal mucosa, pelvic bone or bilateral regional node metastases
Stage IVB	Any distant metastasis, including pelvic lymph nodes

Fig. 7.70 FIGO staging system for carcinoma of the vulva (1990).

TNM staging vs FIGO staging

Definition of TNM

Primary tumor (T)*

TNM	FIGO	Definition
TX	–	Primary tumor cannot be assessed
T0	–	No evidence of primary tumor
T1	I	Carcinoma *in situ*
T2	II	Tumor confined to the vagina
T3	III	Tumor invades paravaginal tissues but not to the pelvic wall
T4†	IVA	Tumor extends to the pelvic wall Tumor invades the mucosa of the bladder or rectum
and/or		
		extends beyond the true pelvis
M1	IVB	Distant metastasis

Regional lymph nodes (N)

NX	Regional lymph nodes cannot be assessed
N0	No regional lymph node metastasis

Upper two-thirds of the vagina

N1	Pelvic lymph node metastasis

Lower one-third of the vagina

N1	Unilateral inguinal lymph node metastasis
N2	Bilateral inguinal lymph node metastasis

Distant metastasis (M)

TNM	FIGO	Definition
MX	–	Presence of distant metastasis cannot be assessed
M0	–	No distant metastasis
M1	IVB	Distant metastasis

Stage grouping

AJCC/UICC				FIGO
Stage 0	Tis	N0	M0	Stage 0
Stage I	T1	N0	M0	Stage I
Stage II	T2	N0	M0	Stage II
Stage III	T1	N1	M0	Stage III
	T2	N1	M0	
	T3	N0	M0	
	T3	N1	M0	
Stage IVA	T1	N2	M0	Stage IVA
	T2	N2	M0	
	T3	N2	M0	
	T4	Any N	M0	
Stage IVB	Any T	Any N	M1	Stage IVB

* Squamous cell carcinoma is the most common type of cancer occurring in the vagina but infrequently an adenocarcinoma may occur in the upper one-third.

† Note: The presence of bullous edema is not sufficient evidence to classify a tumor as T4. If the mucosa is not involved, the tumor is Stage III.

Fig. 7.71 TNM staging compared to the FIGO staging system. (AJCC: Manual for Staging of Cancer, 4th edn. Lippincott, Philadelphia, 1993)

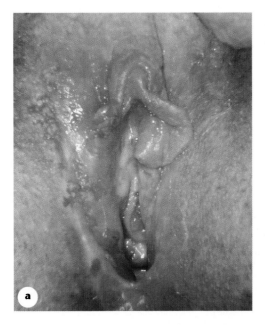

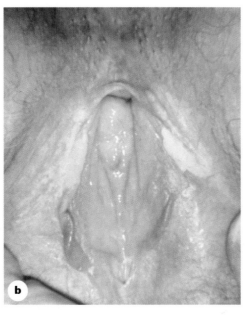

Fig. 7.72 Carcinoma *in situ*. Clinically, this lesion may present variously. (**a**) In this instance, an erythematous patch extends across the midline, whereas in another example (**b**) there is marked whitening of non-contiguous patches of tumor due to hyperkeratosis.

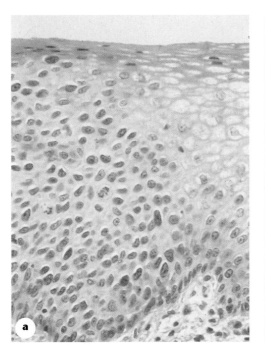

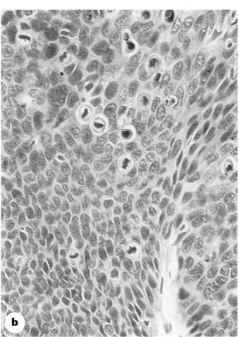

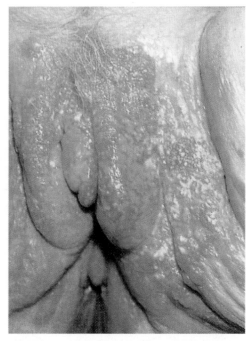

Fig. 7.73 Carcinoma *in situ*. (**a**) On the right side of the field, there is normal stratified squamous epithelium, whereas the left side is marked by loss of normal cytoplasmic maturation and by cells with enlarged atypical nuclei. (**b**) Multiple atypical mitotic figures, as well as atypical nuclei without degenerative features, are characteristic.

Fig. 7.74 Paget's disease. Involvement of the vulva is clinically identical to the far less common penile counterpart of this lesion. Raised erythematous plaques with crusting to excoriation are typical. The clinical circumscription is deceptive, however, because grossly uninvolved margins often contain neoplastic cells. Paget's disease may be associated with invasive adenocarcinoma of the apocrine glands of the vulva or with carcinoma of other organs, most notably the cervix, uterus, breast and colon.

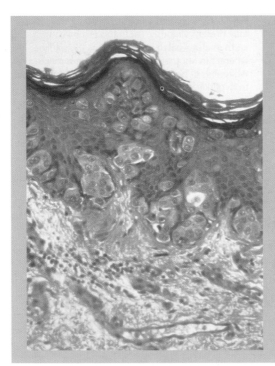
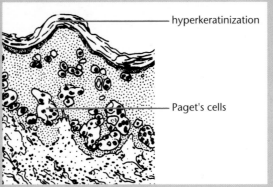

Fig. 7.75 Paget's disease. Basal nests of large, pale cells are found along the basement membrane of the epithelium; between them are less well-differentiated basal cells. Hyperkeratinization also is present. Paget's cells are often seen in rete pegs pushing deep into the dermis. Because of this, a more extensive vulvectomy, including epidermis and dermis, is required for treatment.

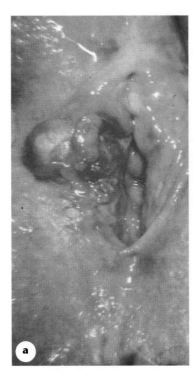

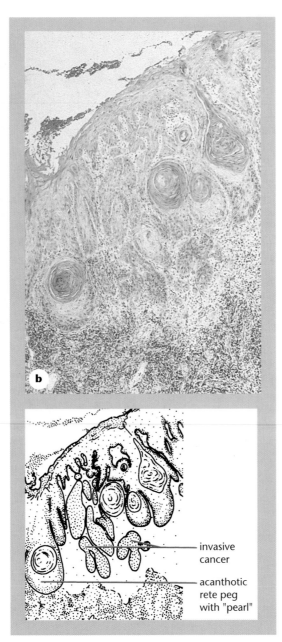

Fig. 7.76 Squamous cell carcinoma (**a**) The ulcerative lesion seen here affects a vulva in which many surface structures are inapparent owing to atrophic dystrophy. The labia and clitoris are no longer well defined. (**b**) The left side of this field shows acanthotic rete pegs that contain prematurely keratinized pearls, but there is no subepithelial infiltration. This is atypical hyperplastic dystrophy. In the right side of the field, there is infiltration by invasive cancer.

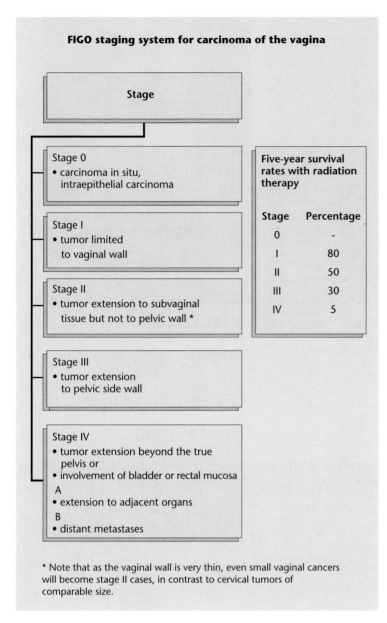

FIGO staging system for carcinoma of the vagina

Stage

Stage 0
• carcinoma in situ, intraepithelial carcinoma

Stage I
• tumor limited to vaginal wall

Stage II
• tumor extension to subvaginal tissue but not to pelvic wall *

Stage III
• tumor extension to pelvic side wall

Stage IV
• tumor extension beyond the true pelvis or
• involvement of bladder or rectal mucosa
A
• extension to adjacent organs
B
• distant metastases

Five-year survival rates with radiation therapy	
Stage	**Percentage**
0	-
I	80
II	50
III	30
IV	5

* Note that as the vaginal wall is very thin, even small vaginal cancers will become stage II cases, in contrast to cervical tumors of comparable size.

Fig. 7.77 FIGO staging system for carcinoma of the vagina.

Definition of TNM

Primary tumor (T)*

TNM	FIGO	Definition
TX	–	Primary tumor cannot be assessed
T0	–	No evidence of primary tumor
T1	I	Carcinoma in situ
T2	II	Tumor confined to the vagina
T3	III	Tumor invades paravaginal tissues but not to the pelvic wall
T4†	IVA	Tumor extends to the pelvic wall
		Tumor invades the mucosa of the bladder or rectum and/or extends beyond the true pelvis
M1	IVB	Distant metastasis

Regional lymph nodes (N)

NX   Regional lymph nodes cannot be assessed
N0   No regional lymph node metastasis

Upper two-thirds of the vagina
N1   Pelvic lymph node metastasis

Lower one-third of the vagina
N1   Unilateral inguinal lymph node metastasis
N2   Bilateral inguinal lymph node metastasis

Distant metastasis (M)

TNM	FIGO	Definition
MX	–	Presence of distant metastasis cannot be assessed
M0	–	No distant metastasis
M1	IVB	Distant metastasis

Stage grouping

AJCC/UICC			FIGO	
Stage 0	Tis	N0	M0	Stage 0
Stage I	T1	N0	M0	Stage I
Stage II	T2	N0	M0	Stage II
Stage III	T1	N1	M0	Stage III
	T2	N1	M0	
	T3	N0	M0	
	T3	N1	M0	
Stage IVA	T1	N1	M0	Stage VIA
	T2	N2	M0	
	T3	N2	M0	
	T4	Any N	M0	
Stage IVB	Any T	Any N	M1	Stage IVB

* Squamous cell carcinoma is the most common type of cancer occurring in the vagina, but infrequently an adenocarcinoma may occur in the upper one-third.

† Note: the presence of bullous edema is not sufficient evidence to classify a tumor as T4. If the mucosa is not involved, the tumor is stage III.

Fig. 7.78 TNM staging compared to the FIGO staging system. (AJCC: Manual for Staging of Cancer, 4th edn. Lippincott, Philadelphia, 1993)

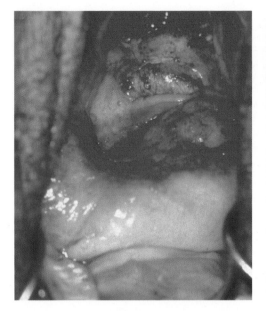

Fig. 7.79 Vaginal carcinoma. The ulceration in the posterior wall of the vagina is an invasive vaginal cancer. Its endophytic growth pattern has resulted in significant penetration of the vaginal wall, although the tumor mass is still small. The cervix is everted and appears inflamed but is univolved.

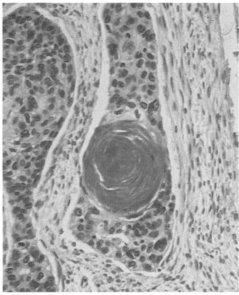

Fig. 7.80 Squamous cell carcinoma. As is usual with these tumors, keratin pearls are often formed. The degree of histologic differentiation is not a prognostic factor.

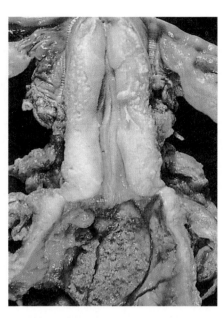

Fig. 7.81 Squamous cell carcinoma. Arising in the posterior vaginal wall is a raised, irregular neoplasm.

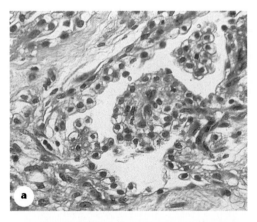

Fig. 7.82 Clear cell adenocarcinoma. (**a**) Clear cells line the glandular spaces and papillae. (**b**) In the other specimen, clear cells with large atypical nuclei form a solid sheet of tumor.

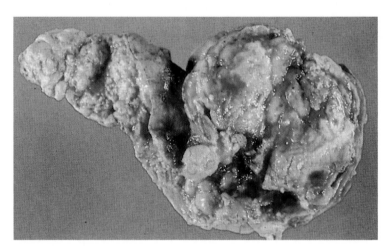

Fig. 7.83 Fallopian tube carcinoma. A typical tubal cancer has dilated and filled the tubal lumen without destroying the tubal wall.

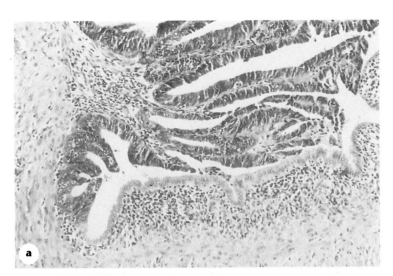

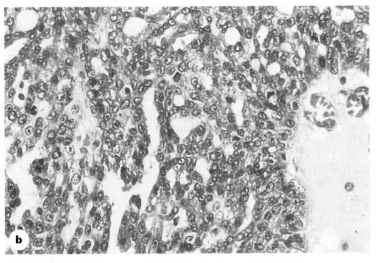

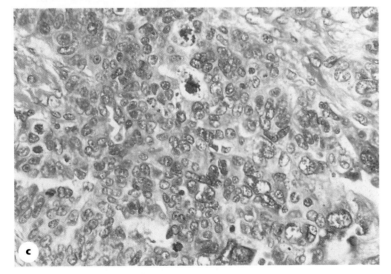

Fig. 7.84 Fallopian tube carcinoma. (**a**) Normal tubal epithelium is seen in the lower portion of this field, but tubal carcinoma forms the papillary structures above. (**b**) Papillary-alveolar patterns are formed by this relatively aggressive tubal cancer. (**c**) A solid pattern can be seen in more aggressive tumors.

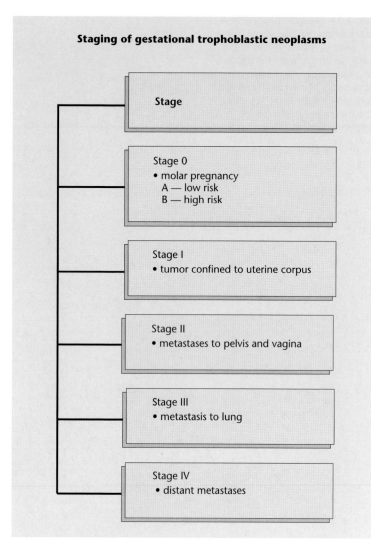

Staging of gestational trophoblastic neoplasms

Stage

Stage 0
- molar pregnancy
  A — low risk
  B — high risk

Stage I
- tumor confined to uterine corpus

Stage II
- metastases to pelvis and vagina

Stage III
- metastasis to lung

Stage IV
- distant metastases

Fig. 7.85 Staging of gestational trophoblastic neoplasms. (Adapted from Goldstein and Berkowitz, 1980)

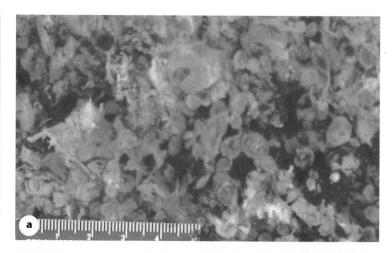

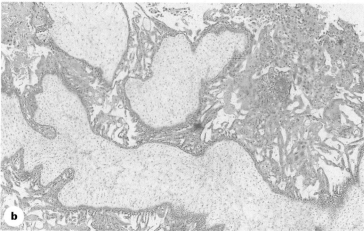

Fig. 7.86 Complete hydatidiform mole. (**a**) Numerous grape-like swellings ('vesicles', molar villi) in placental tissue are characteristic of complete moles; no fetal tissues are present. (**b**) Molar villi are enlarged and edematous and are covered by a thick covering of proliferating, markedly atypical trophoblast.

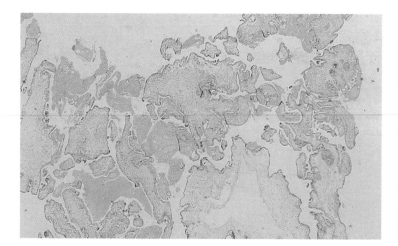

Fig. 7.87 Partial hydatidiform mole. The placenta is a mixture of small, normal-appearing villi and large, edematous 'molar' villi, the latter with irregular shapes ('scalloping') and minimal trophoblast hyperplasia.

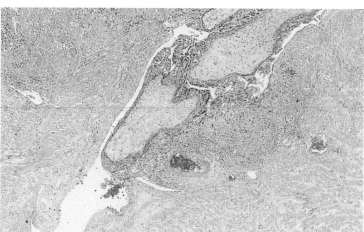

Fig. 7.88 Invasive mole. Two villi from a complete mole (covered by a thick layer of hyperplastic trophoblast) are present deep within the myometrium in this hysterectomy specimen.

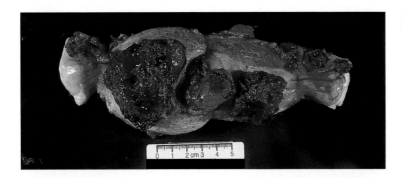

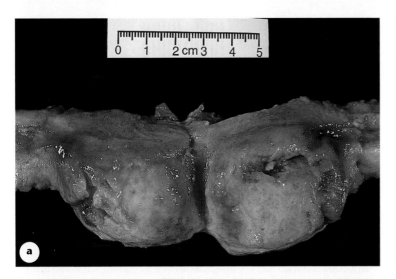

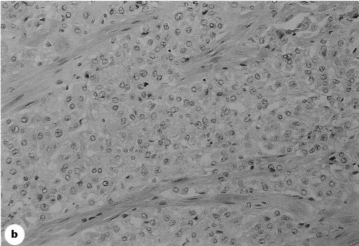

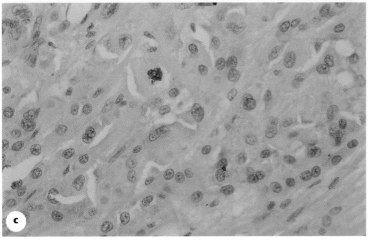

Fig. 7.90 Placental site trophoblastic tumor. (**a**) Myometrium is transmurally replaced by solid tan tumor. (**b**) Histologically, sheets of monomorphic, single, spindled and epithelioid cells infiltrate between myometrial fibers. (**c**) Tumor cells have abundant trophoblastic cells found normally in the placental bed.

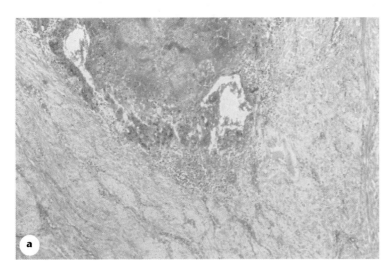

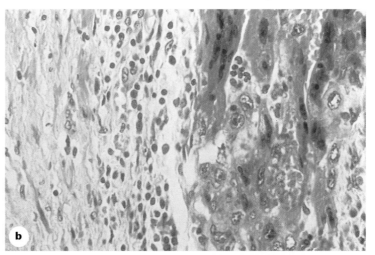

Fig. 7.91 Choriocarcinoma of fundus. (**a**) The typical invasive cancer seen here is marked by a large amount of hemorrhage and very little tumor tissue.

(**b**) Myometrium on the left of this field is being destroyed by a mixture of malignant cytophoblasts and syncytiotrophoblasts on the right.

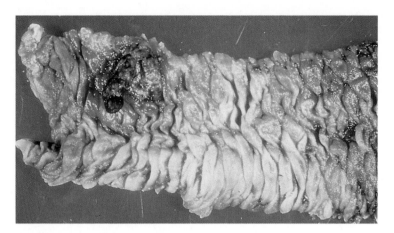

Fig. 7.92 Intestinal metastases. Bowel metastases from choriocarcinoma are a bad prognostic sign and indicate stage IV disease. They may cause life-threatening hemorrhage and are often treated surgically. (Courtesy of Ross Berkowitz MD, Department of Gynecologic Oncology, Brigham and Women's Hospital, Boston MA.)

REFERENCES

Averette AE, Donato M, Lovecchio JL, Sevin BU: Surgical staging of gynecologic malignancies. Cancer 1987; 60 : 2010–2020.

Averette HE, Donato DM: Ovarian carcinoma: advances in diagnosis, staging and treatment. Cancer 1990; 65 : 703–708.

Boronow RC: Advances in diagnosis, staging and management of cervical and endometrial cancer, stages I and II. Cancer 1990; 65 : 648–659.

Crum C: Contemporary theories in cervical carcinogenesis: the virus, the host and the stem cell. Mod Pathol 2000; 13 : 2451–2459.

Daly M, Obrams GI: Epidemiology and risk assessment for ovarian cancer. Semin Oncol 1998; 25 : 255.

DiSaia PJ: Conservative management of the patient with early gynecologic cancer. CA 1989; 39 : 135–154.

Flemming I, Cooper J, Henson D, *et al.*: AJCC Cancer Staging Manual, 5th edn. Lippincott, Philadelphia, 1997.

Frank TS: Testing for hereditary risk of ovarian cancer. Cancer Control 1999; 6(4):327.

Goldstein D, Zantern-Przybysz I, Bernstein M, Berkowitz R: Revised FIGO staging system for gestational trophoblastic tumors: recommendations regarding therapy. J Reprod Med 1998; 43 : 37–43.

Goldstein DP, Berkowitz RS: The management of gestational trophoblastic neoplasms. Curr Probl Obstet Gynecol 1980; 4 : 20.

Greenlee RT, Hill-Harmon MB, Murray T, *et al*: Cancer statistics, 2001. CA Cancer J Clin 2001; 50 : 7.

Hall W: Ovarian cancer, screening, treatment, and follow-up. NIH Consensus Development Panel. JAMA 1995; 273 : 491–497.

Hoskins W, Perez C, Young R: Principles and Practice of Gynecologic Oncology, 3rd edn. Lippincott, Williams and Wilkins, Philadelphia, 2000.

Janicek MF, Averette HE: Cervical cancer: prevention, diagnosis, and therapeutics. CA Cancer J Clin 2001; 51 : 92.

Lynch HT, Bewtra C, Lynch JF: Familial ovarian cancer clinical nuances. Am J Med 1983; 81 : 1073.

Lynch HT, Casey MJ, Lynch J, *et al.*: Genetics and ovarian cancer. Semin Oncol 1998; 25(3):265.

Mackey SE, Creaseman WT: Ovarian cancer screening. J Clin Oncol 1995; 13 : 783.

Moore TD, Phillips PH, Nerenstone SR, Cheson BD: Systemic treatment of advanced and recurrent endometrial carcinoma: current status and future directions. J Clin Oncol 1991; 9 : 1071–1088.

National Institutes of Health Consensus Development Conference Statement: Ovarian cancer: screening, treatment, and follow-up. Gynecol Oncol 1994; 55(3):S4.

Nelson J, Averette H, Richart R: Dysplasia, carcinoma in situ and early invasive cervical carcinoma. CA 1984; 34 : 306–327.

Ozols RF, Young RC: Chemotherapy of ovarian cancer. Semin Oncol 1984; 11 : 251–263.

Ries LAG, Kosary CL, Hankey BF, *et al.*: SEER cancer statistics review 1973–1994, National Cancer Institute. National Institute for Health, Bethesda, MD, 1997.

Seidman J, Kurman R: Ovarian serous borderline tumors: a critical view of the literature with emphasis on prognostic indicators. Human Pathol 2000; 31 : 539–557.

Surwit EA, Childers JM, Krag DM, *et al.*: Clinical assessment of CYT-103 immunoscintigraphy in ovarian cancer. Gyn Oncol 1993; 48 : 285.

Yancik R, Ries LG, Yates JW: Ovarian cancer in the elderly: an analysis of surveillance. Am J Obstet Gynecol 1986; 154 : 639.

Zaioudek C: Ovarian neoplasms. In: Gompel C, Silverberg SG, eds: Pathology in Gynecology and Obstetrics, 4th edn. Lippincott, Philadelphia, 1994; 330–413.

FIGURE CREDITS

The following books published by Gower Medical Publishing are sources of figures in the present chapter. The figure numbers given in the listing are those of the figures in the present chapter. The page numbers (or slide numbers) given in parentheses are those of the original publication.

Fletcher CDM, McKee PH: An Atlas of Gross Pathology. Edward Arnold/Gower Medical Publishing, London, 1987: Figs 7.4 (p 74), 7.6 (p 75), 7.9 (p 75) 7.14 (p 76), 7.17 (p 76), 7.20A (p 77), 7.22 (p 76), 7.36 (p 80), 7.51A (p 80), 7.54 (p 80), 7.67 (p 82), 7.81 (p 82).

Fox H. McKee PH, Pugh RCB, eds: Reproductive system. In: Turk JL, Fletcher CDM, eds: RCSI Slide Atlas of Pathology. Gower Medical Publishing, London, 1986: Figs 7.2 (slide 9), 7.11 (slide 16), 7.47 (slide 41).

Gordon AG, Lewis BV: Gynecological Endoscopy. JB Lippincott/ Gower Medical Publishing, Philadelphia/London, 1988: Figs 7.27A (p 6.21), 7.27B (p 6.23), 7.28A (p 6.24), 7.40 (p 9.8), 7.46 (p 6.10).

Price AB, Morson BC, Scheuer PJ, eds: Alimentary system. In Turk JL, Fletcher CDM, eds: RCSE Slide Atlas of Pathology. Gower Medical Publishing, London, 1986: Fig. 7.21A (slide 104).

Weiss MA, Mills SE: Atlas of Genitourinary Tract Disorders. Lippincott/ Gower Medical Publishing, Philadelphia/New York, 1988: Fig. 7.74 (p 19.11).

Woodruff JD, Parmley TH: Atlas of Gynecologic Pathology. Lippincott/ Gower Medical Publishing, Philadelphia/New York, 1988: Figs 7.3B (p 7.29), 7.5A (p 7.25), 7.5B (p 7.26), 7.7 (p 7.29), 7.10A (p 7.28), 7.10B (p 7.29), 7.12 (p 7.38), 7.13 (p 7.33), 7.15 (p 7.42), 7.17B (p 7.39), 7.18 (p 7.37), 7.20B (p 7.46), 7.21B (p 7.46), 7.37A (p 4.24), 7.37B (p 4.24), 7.37C (p 4.25), 7.38 (p 4.28), 7.48 (p 5.5), 7.52 (p 5.13), 7.55 (p 5.16), 7.61 (p 3.11), 7.64 (p 3.12), 7.65 (3.18), 7.72 (p 1.16), 7.73 (p 1.15), 7.75 (p 1.21), 7.76 (p1.17), 7.77 (p 2.13), 7.79 (p 2.12), 7.80 (p 2.13), 7.82 (p 2.6), 7.83 (p 6.22), 7.84 (6.21), 7.91 (p 8.24), 7.92 (p 8.20).

Breast cancer

Susana M. Campos, Daniel F. Hayes

8

Breast cancer is a major cause of morbidity and mortality in women over 45 years of age, especially in the United States. Each year over 185 000 new cases are diagnosed and more than 40 000 women die of the disease. It is a highly heterogeneous disease, both pathologically and clinically. Although age is the single most common risk factor for the development of breast cancer in women (*see* Fig. 8.12), several other epidemiological associations have been identified. These include a germline mutation (BRCA 1 and BRCA 2), positive family history, a prior history of breast cancer and a history of prolonged, uninterrupted menses (early menarche and late first full-term pregnancy) (*see* Table 8.2).

Much progress has been made in the diagnosis and treatment of primary and metastatic breast cancer in the last 20 years. The widespread use of routine mammography and ultrasonography has led to an increased incidence in the detection of early primary lesions, a factor that has contributed to a significant decrease in mortality (*see* Figs 8.38–8.41, 8.44) MRI of the breast has been useful in detecting smaller lesions not identified by either modality (Fig. 8.7). Moreover, less aggressive, conservative local therapy has been shown to be as effective as mastectomy in prolonging survival, while avoiding the cosmetic disfigurement associated with more extensive surgery. Newer techniques such as sentinel node biopsy (*see* Fig. 8.80) have in select patients decreased the morbidity associated with the traditional axillary node dissection. Adjuvant systemic therapy, such as chemotherapy and/or hormonal therapy, has also contributed to the prolonged survival of patients with early breast cancer. The identification of molecular targets such as the overexpression of Her 2 neu receptor has allowed newer therapies such as biological therapy to contribute to the management of metastatic breast cancer. The advent of biological therapy in combination with chemotherapy has improved survival in the metastatic setting.

INCIDENCE

Breast cancer incidence rates have remained level during the last decade. Breast cancer deaths are decreasing, primarily for white women and younger women. Although white women develop breast cancer more frequently, black women are most likely to die of the disease.

SCREENING

Routine mammographic screening allows better detection of primary breast cancers than physical examination. Mammographic screening has been shown to decrease mortality rates in women 50–69 years of age. A 26% decrease in the relative risk of breast cancer was noted with screening mammography in this group. The role of screening mammography in women 40–49 years of age remains controversial. Current imaging modalities include mammography, ultrasound and, recently, magnetic resonance imaging. Only mammography has been demonstrated to be a valuable tool.

Over half of all women will develop benign breast lesions. These include macro- and microcysts, adenosis, apocrine changes, intraductal papillomas, fibrosis, fibroadenomas and epithelial hyperplasias (*see* Figs 8.2–8.6, 8.8–8.11). Only the latter, however, particularly those showing dysplastic changes, are believed to be precursors to the development of malignancy. Benign lesions may present with pain, tenderness and nipples discharge, as well as masses and dimpling of the skin. Mammographic changes such as densities and microcalcifications are also noted in benign lesions. They may mimic malignancies.

HISTOLOGY
In situ breast cancers/non-invasive breast cancer

The enthusiasm for screening has led to the detection of small primary lesions that pose difficult diagnostic dilemmas when breast biopsies reveal premalignant histopathologic findings. The diagnosis of *in situ* carcinomas appears to be increasing in frequency. Non-invasive breast cancer includes ductal carcinoma *in situ* (DCIS) and lobular carcinoma *in situ* (LCIS). DCIS is described as the proliferation of malignant epithelial cells confined to the mammary ducts without evidence of invasion through the basement membrane (*see* Figs 8.13, 8.16–8.19, 8.21). It is considered a precursor lesion. DCIS (also called intraductal carcinoma) is more likely to be localized to a region within one breast. Variants include papillary carcinoma *in situ* (*see* Fig. 8.20) which may mimic benign atypical papillomatosis, and comedo carcinoma, which consists of a solid growth of neoplastic cells within the ducts, associated with centrally located necrotic debris.

In contrast, LCIS (*see* Figs 8.22, 8.23) tends to be diffusely distributed throughout both breasts. LCIS is considered a risk factor for breast cancer and is not a precursor lesion.

Intraductal carcinoma is more common, representing about 21% of cases. The prognosis for patients with *in situ* lesions is very good. Nonetheless, invasive lesions will develop in a certain fraction of patients with *in situ* carcinomas. Although mastectomy has been the treatment of choice for DCIS lesions, recent studies have suggested that in selected cases breast-conserving therapy has become an alternative to mastectomy. Management options for LCIS include careful observation or bilateral prophylactic simple mastectomy or, most recently, the use of tamoxifen.

Invasive breast cancers

Over 75% of all infiltrating breast cancers originate in the ductal system (*see* Figs 8.1, 8.26–28; Table 8.3). A number of histologic variants of ductal carcinoma have been described. Pure examples of these variants constitute only a small percentage of the total number of cases, but certain features of each may be seen within the main portions of tumors that exhibit the more common presentation designated invasive (or infiltrating) ductal carcinoma. Medullary carcinoma (*see* Fig. 8.31) is distinguished by poorly differentiated nuclei and infiltration by lymphocytes and plasma cells, while tubular carcinomas (*see* Fig. 8.30) are highly differentiated tumors that are marked, as their name suggests, by tubule formation. In mucinous (or colloid) carcinomas (*see* Fig. 8.32), nests of neoplastic epithelial cells are surrounded by a mucinous matrix. A few invasive ductal carcinomas exhibit papillary features, hence their designation as papillary carcinomas. Although the above variants may carry a more favorable prognosis than routine infiltrating ductal carcinomas, they are treated similarly, based on stage of disease.

About 5–10% of infiltrating cancers arise from the lobules (*see* Fig. 8.29). Histologically, neoplastic cells of these tumors manifest a distinctive 'single file' pattern. The prognosis and treatment of invasive lobular carcinoma are nearly identical to those of the invasive ductal type. Other unusual malignancies can develop in the breast, including apocrine, metaplastic, adenoid cystic and squamous cell carcinomas. The cell of origin of the latter three has been difficult to determine. Fibroepithelial malignancies, such as cystosarcoma phylloides, are occasionally found in the breast, arising from the mesenchymal stroma (*see* Fig. 8.33).

STAGING OF BREAST CANCER

Staging evaluation consists of a detailed history and physical examination. Particular attention is given to the size, consistency and fixation of the breast mass, skin changes such as erythema, edema, dimpling and satellite nodules, as well as nipple changes such as retraction, discharge and thickening. The status of axillary and infra- and supraclavicular lymph nodes is also evaluated. Posteroanterior and lateral chest radiographs are obtained and a complete blood cell count and blood chemistries are essential. Determination of biologic tumor markers (e.g. CEA, CA27, 29) may be useful in many patients, especially those with more advanced disease. A bone scan can be justified in node-positive disease. Chest and abdominal CT scans are performed in patients with node-positive disease and those with localizing symptoms. Head CTs are not routinely done unless patients are experiencing symptoms such as unusual headaches, nausea, cranial nerve deficits and/or gait disturbances.

Classically, staging systems are based on the findings of the clinical examination, in particular on the size of the primary lesion and the extent of metastases to regional lymph nodes (*see* Figs 8.35, 8.37). However, pathologic findings, such as microscopic lymph node metastases, are also important (*see* Fig. 8.50). Stage I breast cancers consist of small lesions (<2 cm) with no palpable adenopathy; these account for approximately 60% or more of all newly diagnosed breast cancers. Lesions are designated stage II by virtue of the presence of large primary tumors (> 2 cm) and/or palpable, freely movable axillary lymphadenopathy. Locally advanced tumors (stage III) are marked by T3 or T4 lesions and/or fixed axillary lymph nodes (N2) or any internal mammary nodal involvement (N3). T4 tumors, distinguished clinically by fixation to the chest wall, edema, peau d'orange (orange-peel appearance of the skin), skin ulcerations or nodules, or inflammatory breast cancer, which is marked by erythema and thickening of the skin, are particularly aggressive in terms of local recurrence and morbidity, as well as distant metastases and mortality. The diagnosis of inflammatory breast cancer is made on both clinical and pathologic grounds (*see* Figs 8.42–8.47). Patients are considered to have stage IV disease if they have supraclavicular lymphadenopathy or any evidence of distant metastases (*see* Fig. 8.51).

The heterogeneity of breast cancer is perhaps best illustrated by the wide confidence intervals surrounding the survival curves for each of the staging categories, with considerable overlap between categories. Nonetheless, the presence of metastases to axillary lymph nodes (designated pathologic stage II) is the single most important prognostic factor in patients with breast cancer. Over 70% of patients with stage I disease are alive 10 years after diagnosis. The survival rates at 5 years for patients with stage II and stage III breast cancer are 50–60% and 30–40%, respectively. Patients with metastatic disease are rarely, if ever, cured and fewer than 10–15% of stage IV patients are alive 5 years after metastases are detected (*see* Fig. 8.36).

PRIMARY TREATMENT

In the late 19th century, the technique of mastectomy was pioneered by Halsted and found to improve local control of breast cancer. For the next 50–75 years, the concept that breast cancer spread in an orderly fashion from the primary lesion to regional lymph nodes and then to distant organs dominated the treatment of early disease (*see* Figs 8.14, 8.15). During this time, radical mastectomy (the complete removal of the breast, pectoral muscles and axillary contents) was the treatment of choice. Subsequent studies have demonstrated that patients treated with less aggressive (modified radical) mastectomies have the same survival as those treated with radical mastectomies. In the last 15 years, breast-conserving therapy, in which the initial mass is removed by 'lumpectomy' or 'quadrantectomy', followed by primary radiation to the remainder of the breast, has been shown to produce survival rates similar to those seen with treatment by mastectomy. In most cases less aggressive, breast-conserving local therapy provides excellent cosmetic results (*see* Figs 8.71, 8.72).

There are also new advances in exploring the axilla for the determination of lymph node involvement. A sentinel axillary lymph node is the first area to receive lymph flow and is usually the first to harbor a metastasis from the breast cancer. In selected patients a sentinel node biopsy serves as a means of avoiding a complete axillary dissection. In experienced hands a sentinel node biopsy is the preferred manner to assess disease in the axilla. To localize the sentinel node, surgeons inject one or two markers, blue dye or as technetium sulfur colloid-TC 99m, around the tumor or biopsy cavity. The markers are taken up into the lymphatic channels surrounding the tumor site and travel to the nodal basin. In some situations lymphoscintigraphy is performed after the injection to map out the lymphatic drainage pattern. A positive sentinel node requires a full axillary dissection (*see* Fig. 8.80). If the sentinel node biopsy is negative a full axillary dissection can be spared, eliminating the known potential complications of a dissection such as lymph edema (*see* Fig. 8.79).

The completion of breast conservation therapy involves radiation therapy. The whole breast is treated using a pair of tangentially directed fields. The fields are designed to skim along the chest wall and thus irradiate the smallest amount of underlying lung. At the conclusion of the whole breast treatment a boost dose is often given to the tumor bed. Such conservative therapy, however, is not appropriate for all patients. Contraindications include multicentric disease, diffuse malignant microcalcifications and previous breast radiation therapy. For those who require or prefer mastectomies, remarkable advances have been made in recent years in reconstructive surgery (*see* Figs 8.73–8.77).

Advances in primary therapy have been complemented by the recent demonstration that adjuvant systemic therapy significantly prolongs survival compared with observation alone for certain subgroups of patients. Prognostic factors in stage I and II breast cancer include lymph node status, tumor size, estrogen/progesterone receptor, tumor kinetics and overexpression/overamplification of Her 2 neu (*see* Table 8.5).

METASTATIC BREAST CANCER/LOCALLY RECURRENT DISEASE

Locally recurrent disease is often manifested by subcutaneous nodules or a nodular cutaneous rash along the mastectomy site. Occasionally the subcutaneous nodules become confluent and extend across the chest wall. The confluence is called an 'en cuirasse' carcinoma (*see* Figs 8.48, 8.49).

Patients with metastatic breast cancer demonstrate considerable heterogeneity in the clinical course of their disease. Some patients have a rapidly progressing tumor that metastasizes to multiple vital organs and some have indolent disease. Fewer than 5% of newly diagnosed cases present with disseminated metastatic disease.

For patients with metastases recurring after primary breast treatment, median survival is approximately 3 years. The survival of all patients with metastatic disease varies according to certain prognostic factors: a long, disease-free interval after primary therapy is a more favorable prognostic factor than a short interval; non-visceral sites of metastases carry a better prognosis than visceral sites; and a single site of metastasis is more favorable than multiple sites. Estrogen receptor protein (ER) status of the primary tumor may be a good indicator of prognosis, with positive ER status more favorable than negative. ER also predicts response to hormone therapy (*see* Fig. 8.34).

Breast cancer can recur in almost every tissue and organ in the body. However, common sites of metastases include the ipsilateral chest wall and regional lymph nodes (local-regional recurrence), as well as bone, lung, pleura, liver, gastrointestinal tract and the central nervous system (*see* Figs 8.52–8.68). Approximately half of all patients who relapse will have local recurrences and 30–40% of all first relapses will be local-regional. It is of interest that local-regional recurrence is considered to represent metastatic (stage IV) disease and the prognosis for these patients is similar to that for patients with distant metastases. Manifestations of recurrence depend on the site and extent of recurrence, varying from asymptomatic findings on physical, serologic or radiologic examination to symptoms referable to the organ involved (for example, bone pain, shortness of breath, anorexia or motor and/or neurologic deficits). Hypercalcemia is almost always related to bone metastases and only rarely is it encountered as part of a paraneoplastic syndrome.

Hormonal therapy and chemotherapy have till recently formed the basis of treatment. Over the past several years new hormonal agents, SERMS (serum estrogen receptor modulators), SERDS (serum estrogen receptor down regulators), aromatase inhibitors and LHRH agonists, have contributed to the management of women with hormone-responsive disease. Newer chemotherapy agents, including oral agents, and old agents given new roles (liposomal anthracyclines, weekly taxanes) have changed the management of these patients. Complications of therapy can lead to myelosuppression, nausea, vomiting, alopecia, neurotoxicity and integumentary toxicity (*see* Fig. 8.82). Complications of radiation therapy include radiation pneumonitis (*see* Fig. 8.83). The most recent development is the approval of trastuzumab (Herceptin), a humanized monoclonal antibody to the 2-neu protein. The 2-neu protein is overexpressed in approximately 25–30% of breast cancers. Several methods of detection of her 2 neu are employed. Immunoperoxidase studies employ the use of antibodies directed at her 2-neu protein. A more accurate but labor-intensive method looking at the amplification of the gene is FISH (fluorescent *in situ* hybridization) (*see* Fig. 8.81). A randomized trial showed that the combination of Herceptin with chemotherapy was statistically superior to treatment with chemotherapy alone. Overall response rate, time to progression and 1-year survival were statistically superior.

Additionally selective use of surgery, radiation therapy and use of biphosphonates can provide significant palliation to patients with metastases. Monitoring of tumor markers – CEA or CA15-3 – is often helpful in monitoring disease course (*see* Fig. 8.69).

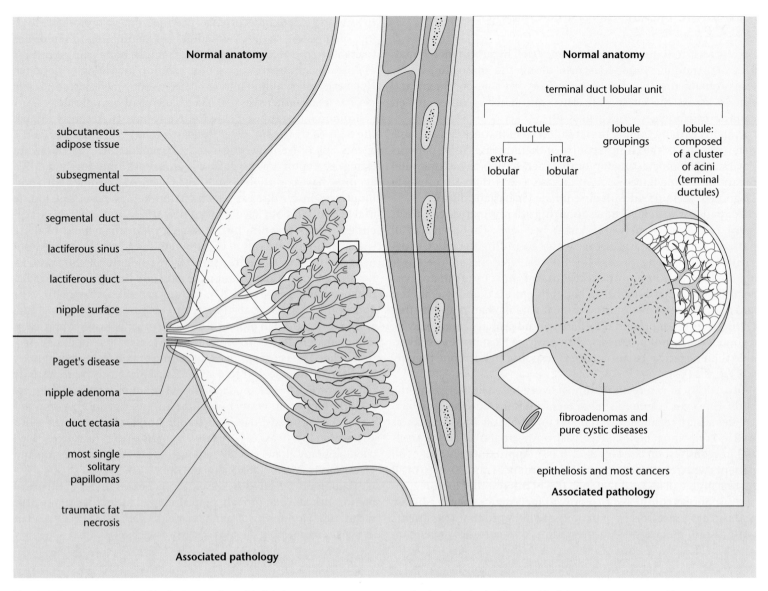

Normal anatomy

subcutaneous adipose tissue

subsegmental duct

segmental duct

lactiferous sinus

lactiferous duct

nipple surface

Paget's disease

nipple adenoma

duct ectasia

most single solitary papillomas

traumatic fat necrosis

Associated pathology

Normal anatomy

terminal duct lobular unit

ductule

extra-lobular

intra-lobular

lobule groupings

lobule: composed of a cluster of acini (terminal ductules)

fibroadenomas and pure cystic diseases

epitheliosis and most cancers

Associated pathology

Fig. 8.1 Breast anatomy. Within the breast, the epithelial elements are organized into lobular units consisting of acini that feed into ductules. The latter in turn coalesce into larger ducts that form a reservoir, or laciferous sinus, proximal to the nipple. These epithelial structures, supported by adipose and fibrous tissue, give rise to more than 95% of breast malignancies

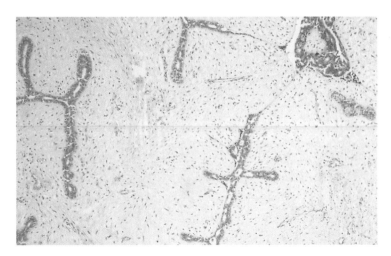

Fig. 8.2 Fibroadenoma. The tumor from which this histologic section was taken was a well-circumscribed, discoid mass, clearly demarcated from the surrounding breast tissue. High magnification reveals stroma compressing ducts so that they form slit-like curvilinear spaces. Note the low cellularity of the stroma, an important benign feature.

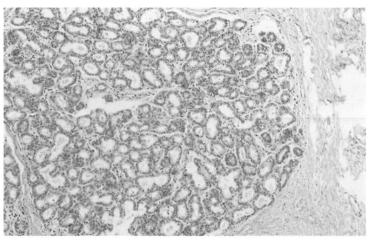

Fig. 8.3 Lactating adenoma. This well-circumscribed lesion has closely packed acini with prominent epithelial cells marked by large nuclei and abundant, pink, vacuolated cytoplasm. (Courtesy of Dr N. Weidner, Brigham and Women's Hospital, Boston, MA.)

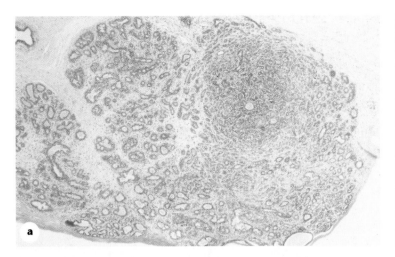
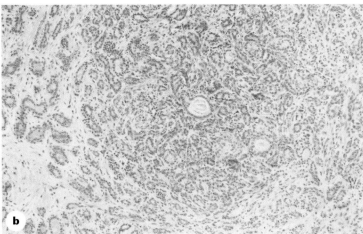

Fig. 8.4 Sclerosing adenosis. (**a**) Low-power microscopic section shows distortion of the lobular architecture; there is an increase in acini (terminal ductules), appearing in a whorled, expansile and vaguely defined pattern. The low-power view is very helpful in distinguishing this benign proliferation from malignancy. (**b**) Higher magnification shows that the acini are composed of a normal two-cell population.

Table 8.1 Differential diagnosis of papilloma vs non-invasive papillary carcinoma

Feature	Papilloma	Papillary carcinoma
Epithelial layer	Two-cell (composed of two cell types)	Single-cell
Nuclear chromatism	Normochromatic	Hyperchromatic
Nucleus/cytoplasm ratio	Low	High
Connective tissue stroma	Prominent	Delicate to absent

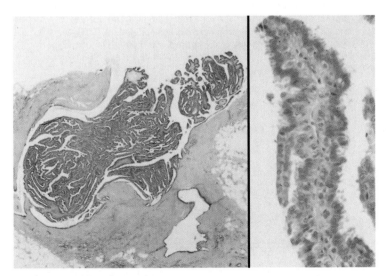
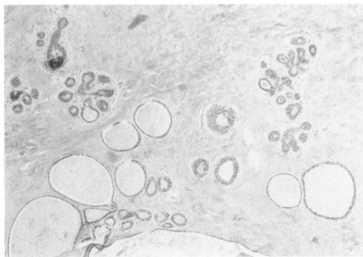

Fig. 8.5 Papilloma. Low-magnification view shows a large duct filled with a papillary proliferation. At higher power (inset), a papillary branch can be seen with a normal two-cell population covering a fibrovascular stalk. In this benign tumor, the lining epithelial cells can exhibit apocrine changes.

Fig. 8.6 Fibrocystic changes. These benign changes are the most common findings in breast biopsies. They are characterized by dense fibrosis intermixed with cystic areas.

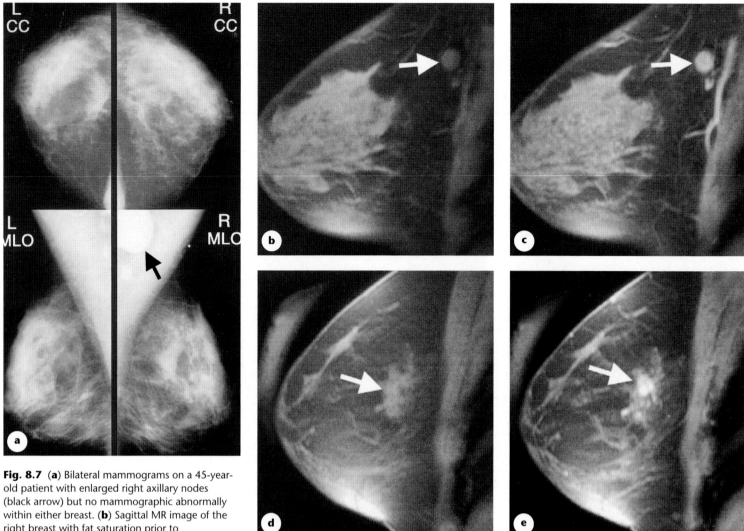

Fig. 8.7 (a) Bilateral mammograms on a 45-year-old patient with enlarged right axillary nodes (black arrow) but no mammographic abnormally within either breast. (b) Sagittal MR image of the right breast with fat saturation prior to administration of gadolinium. A rounded density represents an axillary node (white arrow). (c) Sagittal MR image at the same location as (b) after administration of gadolinium. Enhancement of the node is evident (white arrow). (d) Sagittal MR image of the right breast at a level slightly medial to (b) and (c). A patch of stromal density is evident deep in the breast prior to contrast administration (white arrow). Other retroareolar stromal densities with similar appearance are also present. (e) Sagittal MR image of the right breast in the same location as (d), after administration of gadolinium. The deep stroma is enhancing (white arrow) consistent with tumor, while the other stromal densities have not changed, consistent with normal breast tissue.

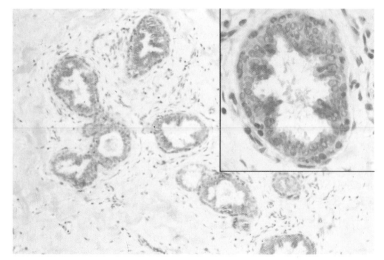

Fig. 8.8 Epithelial hyperplasia (mild). This lobular unit exhibits irregular areas of heaped-up cells lining the acini (terminal ductules). At high magnification (inset), the epithelial layer of one ductule is 3–4 cell layers thick and there is no bridging of cells across the acinar structure.

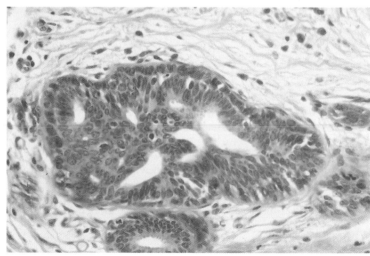

Fig. 8.9 Epithelial hyperplasia (moderate). At this stage, the acinar structure is distended by hyperplastic cells that frequently bridge the lumen, often filling as much as half of it.

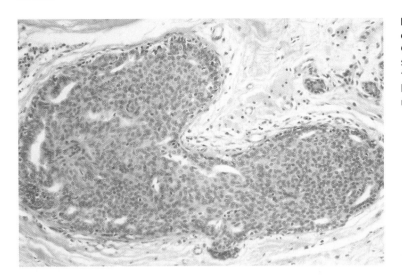

Fig. 8.10 Epithelial hyperplasia (florid). Involved spaces show marked distension by hyperplastic cells that occupy the majority of the lumen. Collapsed slit-like spaces are present, frequently at the periphery of the structure. These slits are surrounded by serpentine passages composed of 'flowing' cells, which often lack clear cell borders. Moderate and florid hyperplasias imply a slightly higher risk of subsequent invasive carcinoma than mild or no hyperplasia.

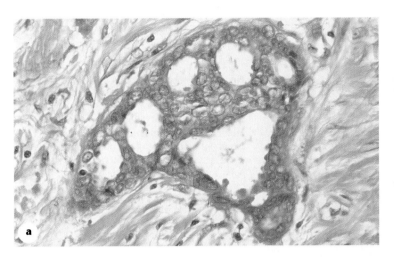

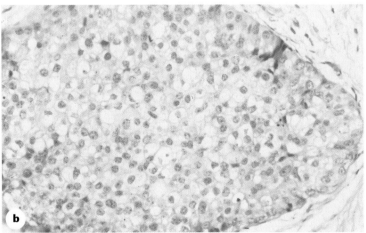

Fig. 8.11 Epithelial hyperplasia (atypical). (**a**) Atypical cases exhibit a non-uniform population of cells from normochromatic nuclei surrounding spaces that are not quite smooth-lined. It is these features that distinguish atypical epithelial (ductal) hyperplasia from ductal carcinoma *in situ*, in which smooth, geometric spaces are surrounded by a uniform cell population with hyperchromatic nuclei. (**b**) High magnification shows that these proliferating, relatively non-uniform cells lack the necessary degree of cell-to-cell rigidity. Atypical hyperplasia carries a relatively higher risk of subsequent development of invasive carcinoma than other types. This risk is further elevated in women with a family history of breast cancer in a first-degree relative.

Fig. 8.12 Age-specific incidence of breast cancer in the United States.

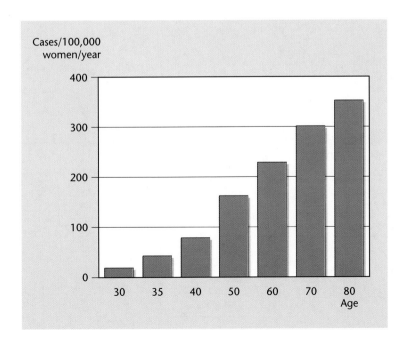

Table 8.2 Breast cancer risk factors.

Highly elevated risk (relative risk at least 4 times that of population without factor)	Moderately elevated risk (relative risk 2 to 4 times that of population without factor)	Slightly elevated risk (relative risk 1 to 2 times that of population without factor)
Female	Any first degree relative with history of breast cancer	Moderate alcohol intake
Age > 50	Upper social/economic class	Menarche <12 years old
Country of birth in North America, Northern Europe	Prolonged uninterrupted menses (late pregnancy, nulliparous)	Hormonal replacement therapy
Personal history of prior breast cancer	Postmenopausal obesity	Oral contraceptives
Family history of bilateral, pre-menopausal, or familial cancer syndrome	Personal history of prior carcinoma of ovary or endometrium	Diet
Atypical proliferative benign breast disease, especially with family history	Proliferative benign breast disease, if no atypia	

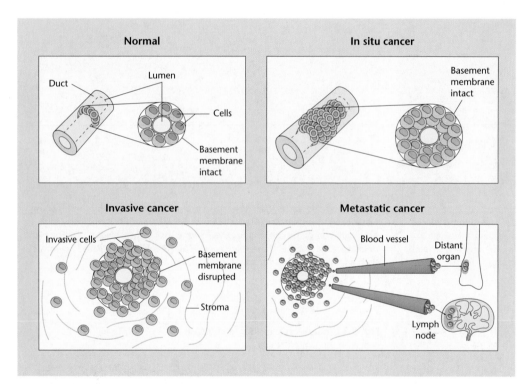

Fig. 8.13 Timeline of breast cancer suggesting probable heterogeneity. Primary breast cancers begin as single (or more) cells which have lost normal regulation of differentiation and proliferation but remain confined within the basement membrane of the duct or lobule. As these cells go through several doublings, at some point they invade through the basement membrane of the ductule or lobule and ultimately metastasize to distant organs.

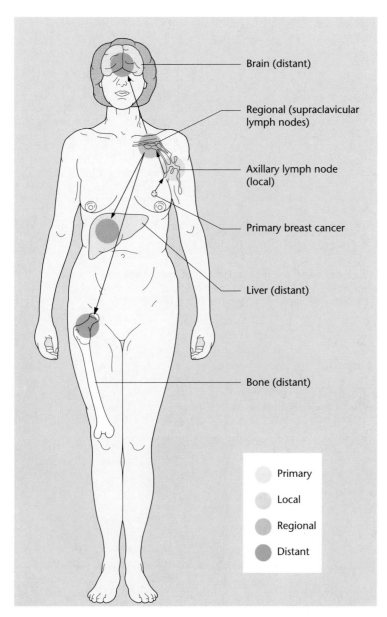

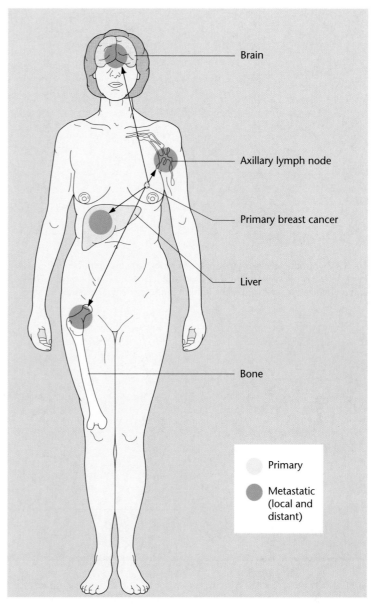

Fig. 8.14 Halsted theory of breast cancer spread. This theory suggests that breast cancer originates in the breast, eventually spreads to local skin and/or lymph nodes and then ultimately affects distant organs. This theory maintains that local/regional lymph nodes serve as 'barriers' to the spread of metastatic breast cancer. The implication of this theory is that more intensive local therapy should lead to an increased rate of cures.

Fig. 8.15 Systemic theory of breast cancer spread. This theory suggests that breast cancer becomes metastatic very early in its course, once invasion through the basement membrane of the duct or lobule has occurred. It maintains that local therapy will have few if any long-term effects on survival, since the disease is already systemic at the time of diagnosis.

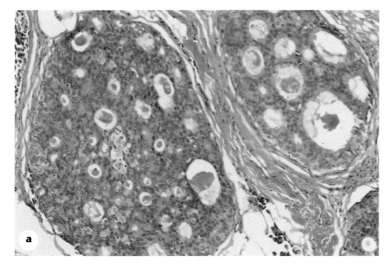

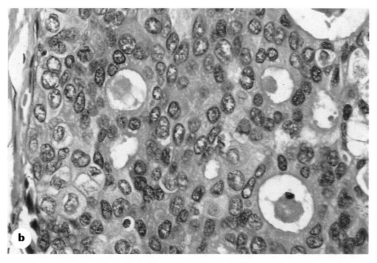

Fig. 8.16 Intraductal carcinoma (cribriform type). (**a**) Low- and (**b**) high-power photomicrographs demonstrate a cribriform pattern composed of a rather uniform tumor cell population with distinct cytoplasmic borders; the cells are rigidly arranged around crisp, circular holes. With this pattern, the risk for the subsequent development of invasive cancer increases 10–11-fold. (Courtesy of Dr N. Weidner, Brigham and Women's Hospital, Boston, MA.)

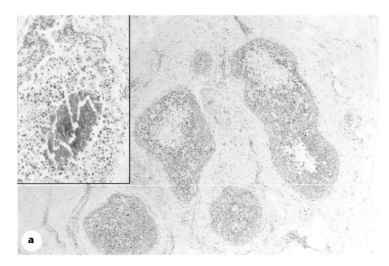

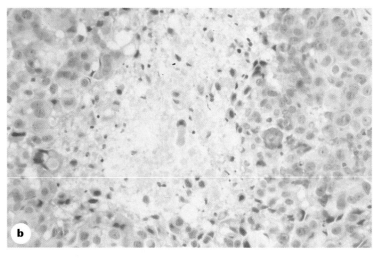

Fig. 8.17 Intraductal carcinoma (comedo type). (**a**) Low- and medium-power (inset) microscopic sections show expanded ducts with central necrosis. (**b**) At high magnification, cellular pleomorphism is also evident. This feature is seen to a greater extent and more commonly in the comedo type of ductal carcinoma *in situ*. Occult invasive elements may also be more common in the comedo than non-comedo types (*see* Figs 8.18–8.20).

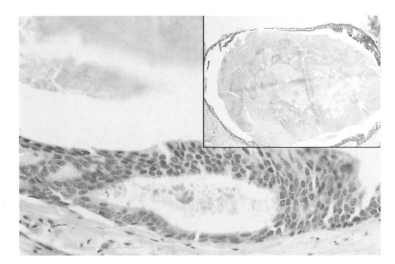

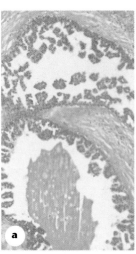

Fig. 8.18 Intraductal carcinoma ('clinging' type). Low- (inset) and high-power microscopic sections show tumor cells 'clinging' to the periphery of a duct. The clusters of basophilic malignant cells exhibit a high nucleus-to-cytoplasm ratio. Note the bridge-like structure formed by these cells on the high-power view.

Fig. 8.19 Intraductal carcinoma (micropapillary type). (**a**) Low magnification reveals expanded ducts with fronds of tumor characteristically extending toward the center of the lumina. (**b**) At high magnification, the bulbous fronds typically appear narrow at the base and expanded at the tip. (**a**: Courtesy of Dr N. Weidner, Brigham and Women's Hospital, Boston, MA.)

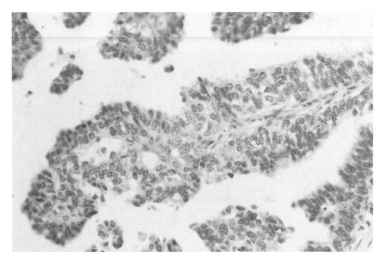

Fig. 8.20 Papillary carcinoma *in situ*. The architectural features of this *in situ* breast cancer are similar to those of a papilloma. The normal two-cell-layer epithelium covering the fibrovascular fronds is replaced by a uniform proliferation of cells with hyperchromatic nuclei.

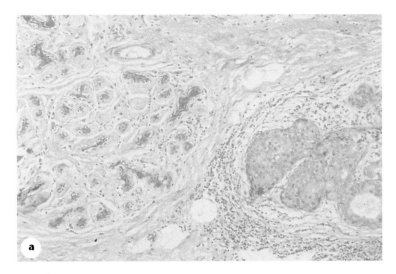

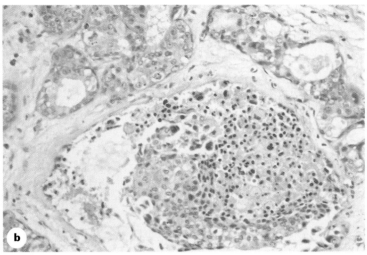

Fig. 8.21 Intraductal carcinoma. (**a**) Microscopic section shows a normal lobular unit on the left and 'cancerization of the lobules' on the right, where a ductal carcinoma has extended into the lobules. (**b**) High magnification demonstrates 'cancerization of the lobules' in the upper portion of the field, while the lower portion reveals a duct that has been expanded by an intraductal carcinoma with foci of necrosis. 'Cancerization of the lobules' carries no clinical significance except that it may mimic lobular carcinoma *in situ*. However, pleomorphism, tubule formation and necrosis, as seen here, are not encountered in lobular carcinoma.

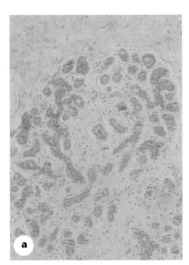

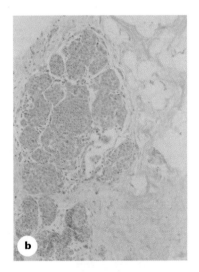

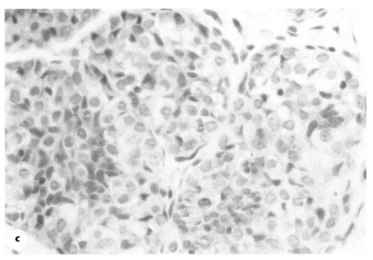

Fig. 8.22 Lobular carcinoma *in situ* (LCIS). Low-power photomicrographs show (**a**) the normal architecture of a lobular unit and (**b**) a distended lobular unit exhibiting the typical appearance of lobular carcinoma *in situ*. (**c**) At high magnification, the lobular unit is seen to be distended and distorted by characteristically uniform, round tumor cells with bland nuclei. LCIS is usually diffusely dispersed throughout the breast and is often bilateral. Rarely producing a mass or abnormality on mammography, it is commonly discovered coincidentally during a biopsy performed for other suspicious lesions. Women with LCIS have a slightly higher risk of developing invasive cancer, whether ductal or lobular in origin, in their lifetime.

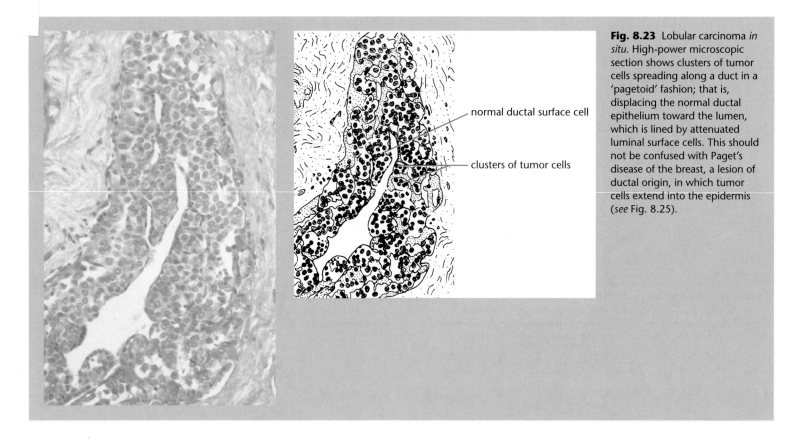

Fig. 8.23 Lobular carcinoma *in situ*. High-power microscopic section shows clusters of tumor cells spreading along a duct in a 'pagetoid' fashion; that is, displacing the normal ductal epithelium toward the lumen, which is lined by attenuated luminal surface cells. This should not be confused with Paget's disease of the breast, a lesion of ductal origin, in which tumor cells extend into the epidermis (*see* Fig. 8.25).

normal ductal surface cell

clusters of tumor cells

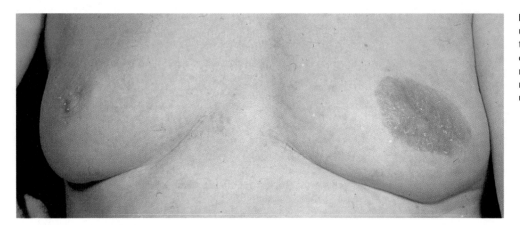

Fig. 8.24 Paget's disease of the breast. In this unique clinical entity, one of the main ducts leading to the nipple becomes engorged with neoplastic cells. Clinically, patients present with an eczematous rash that extends to and involves the areola. This rare condition may or may not be associated with an underlying invasive carcinoma.

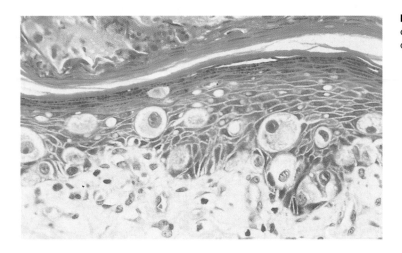

Fig. 8.25 Paget's disease of the breast. The irregular epidermis is infiltrated by characteristic cells with abundant pale-staining granular cytoplasm and large, oval, vesicular nuclei with prominent nucleoli.

Table 8.3 Incidence of histologic types of invasive breast cancer

Type	Frequency (%)
Pure tumor groups	68.1
Infilerating (Invasive) ductal	52.6
Medullary	6.2
Lobular invasive	4.9
Mucinous	2.4
Tubular	1.2
Adenocystic	0.4
Papillary	0.3
Carcinosarcoma	0.1
Paget's disease	2.3
Combinations of infiltrating ductal and other types	28.0
Miscellaneous combinations (e.g., tubular + papillary)	1.6

NSABP data; modified from Fisher *et al.*, 1975

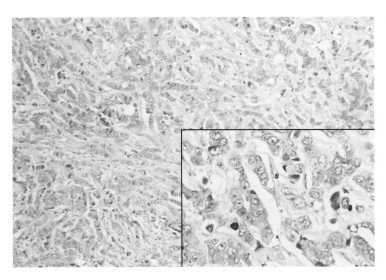

Fig. 8.26 Invasive ductal carcinoma. Low- and high-power (inset) photomicrographs of a poorly differentiated adenocarcinoma show that the stroma is infiltrated by pleomorphic tumor cells exhibiting a high mitotic rate. Note the necrosis and lack of tubule formation.

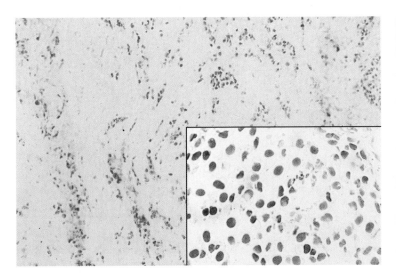

Fig. 8.27 Invasive ductal carcinoma. Low magnification of a breast biopsy specimen stained for estrogen receptor protein (ERP) using an immunocytochemical assay (ERICA) shows that most cells are positive (brown). ERICA allows for semiquantitation of ERP. High magnification (inset) reveals that the antibody is localized to the nuclei (brown). (Courtesy of Dr S.L. Khoury, Brigham and Women's Hospital, Boston, MA.)

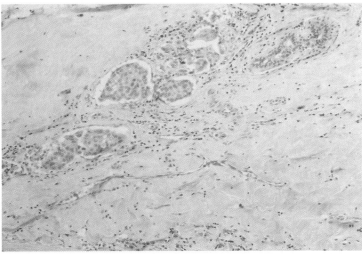

Fig. 8.28 Invasive ductal carcinoma. Photomicroscopic section of a breast biopsy specimen demonstrates an invasive ductal carcinoma in the lymphatic vessels of the breast parenchyma.

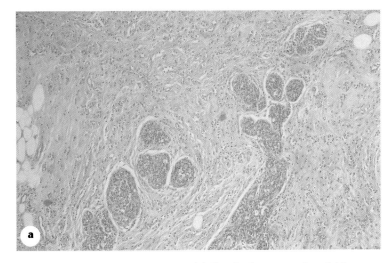

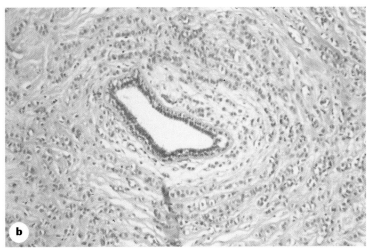

Fig. 8.29 Invasive lobular carcinoma. (**a**) The classic presentation of this tumor is marked by a 'single file' pattern of uniform malignant cells infiltrating the stroma. The invasive lesion surrounds foci of *in situ* tumor. (**b**) Single file tumor cells surround an involved duct, producing a target-like pattern.

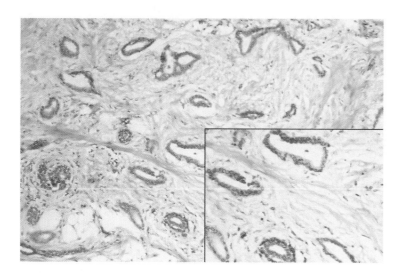

Fig. 8.30 Tubular carcinoma. Low- and high-power (inset) microscopic sections of this histologic variant of invasive ductal carcinoma show tubular structures infiltrating the stroma. The lumina of the tubules are lined by a single cell layer of well-differentiated cells. This type of breast cancer has a better prognosis than common infiltrating ductal carcinoma.

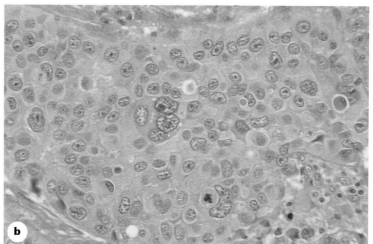

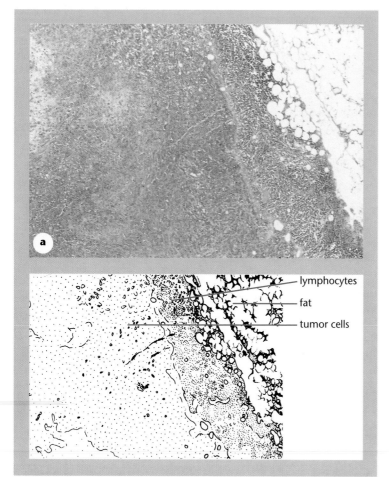

lymphocytes

fat

tumor cells

Fig. 8.31 Medullary carcinoma. (**a**) Low-power photomicrograph of this histologic variant of invasive ductal carcinoma demonstrates its characteristic syncytial growth pattern. The tumor has a smooth, well-circumscribed border and exhibits a prominent lymphocytic infiltrate. (**b**) At higher magnification, the classic pleomorphic cells with bizarre nuclei are evident. This malignancy has better 5- and 10-year survival rates than common ductal carcinoma. (Courtesy of Dr N. Weidner, Brigham and Women's Hospital, Boston, MA.)

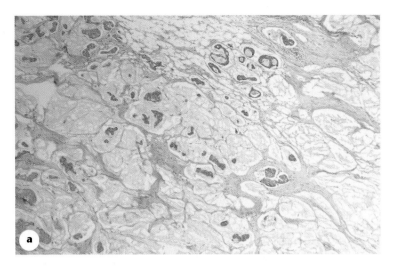

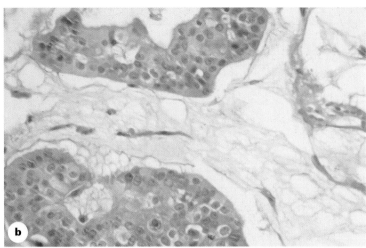

Fig. 8.32 Mucinous or colloid carcinoma. (**a**) Low-power microscopic section shows islands of tumor cells within a sea of mucin. (**b**) Higher magnification demonstrates sharply circumscribed tumor aggregates with characteristic smooth borders and a homogeneous cell population. Pure histologic forms of this variant have better prognoses than common ductal carcinoma.

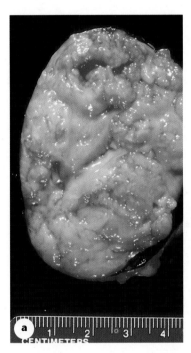

Fig. 8.33 Cystosarcoma phylloides. (**a**) The irregular cut surface of this tumor is marked by clefts that surround glistening gray to yellow islands of tumor intermixed with foci of necrosis (yellow). (**b**) Low-magnification study shows the classic leaf-like projection of hypercellular stroma into a benign ductal structure. At high magnification (**c**), hypercellular areas demonstrate osteosarcomatous differentiation with osteoid (pink) deposition. Scattered 'osteoclast-like' giant cells are also present. Typically, malignant stroma in these tumors appears fibro- or myxoliposarcomatous and less commonly like osteosarcoma, rhabdomysarcoma or chondrosarcoma. (Courtesy of Dr N. Weidner, Brigham and Women's Hospital, Boston, MA.)

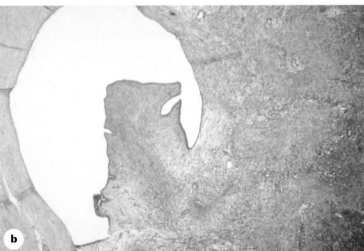

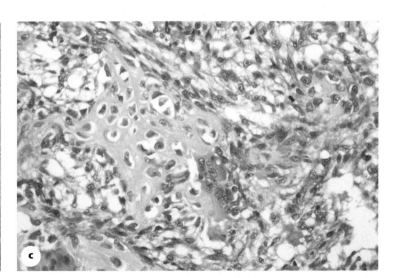

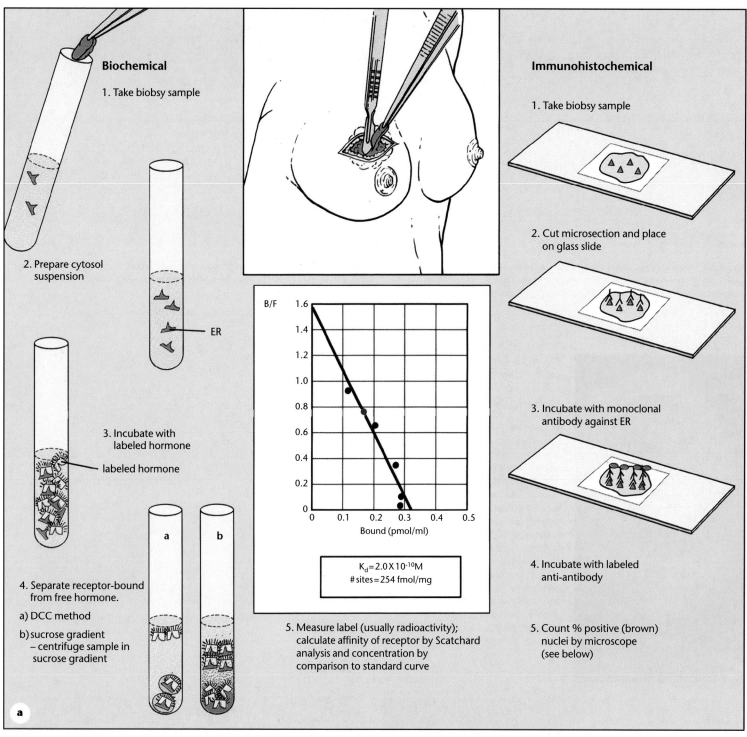

Biochemical

1. Take biobsy sample

2. Prepare cytosol suspension

ER

3. Incubate with labeled hormone

labeled hormone

4. Separate receptor-bound from free hormone.

a) DCC method

b) sucrose gradient – centrifuge sample in sucrose gradient

a

b

B/F

$K_d = 2.0 \times 10^{-10} M$
#sites = 254 fmol/mg

5. Measure label (usually radioactivity); calculate affinity of receptor by Scatchard analysis and concentration by comparison to standard curve

Immunohistochemical

1. Take biobsy sample

2. Cut microsection and place on glass slide

3. Incubate with monoclonal antibody against ER

4. Incubate with labeled anti-antibody

5. Count % positive (brown) nuclei by microscope (see below)

a

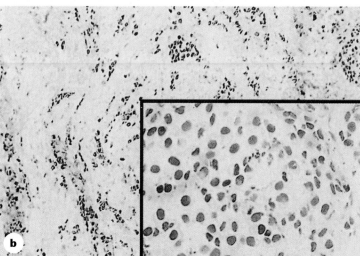

b

Fig. 8.34 (**a**) Assays for steroid hormone receptors. Scatchard analysis of [³H] estradiol binding to estrogen receptor (ER) in human breast cancer cytosol, determined by the multipoint DDC assay. The calculated binding affinity (K_d) and the quantitative receptor content are shown. (**b**) Localization of estrogen receptor protein using the estrogen receptor immunocytochemical assay (ERICA). In this frozen section of an infiltrating ductal carcinoma, a brown stain in the nucleus defines the presence of estrogen receptor. Although most cells in this tumor show immunoreactivity, there is heterogeneity in the degree of reactivity among the tumor cells.

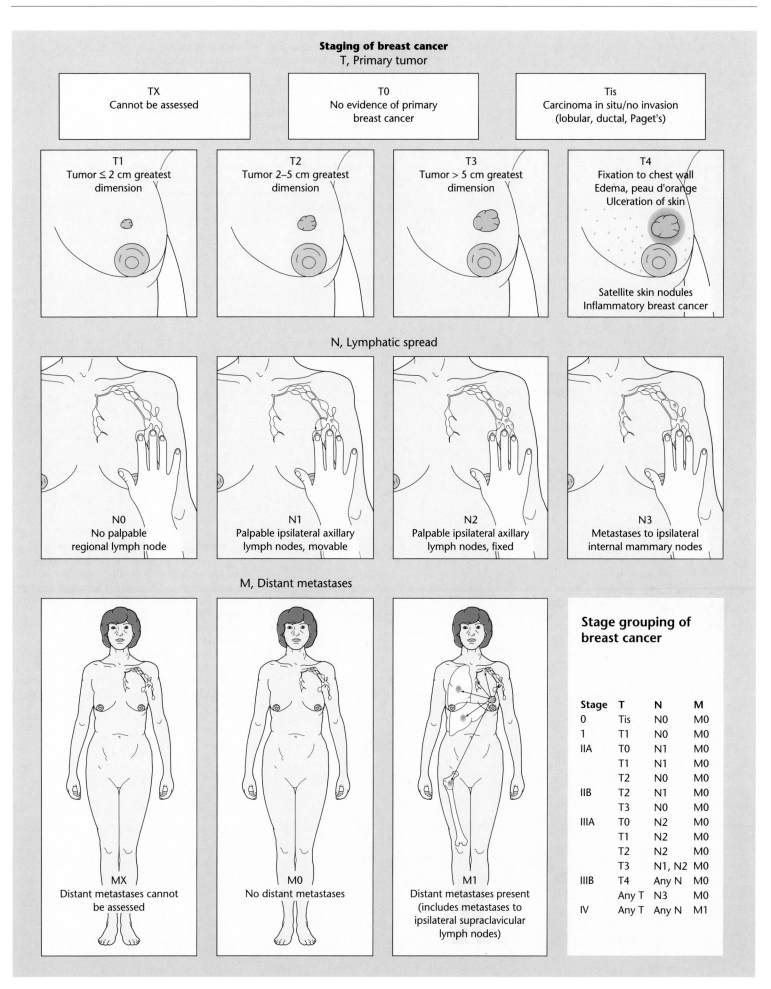

Staging of breast cancer
T, Primary tumor

TX
Cannot be assessed

T0
No evidence of primary
breast cancer

Tis
Carcinoma in situ/no invasion
(lobular, ductal, Paget's)

T1
Tumor ≤ 2 cm greatest
dimension

T2
Tumor 2–5 cm greatest
dimension

T3
Tumor > 5 cm greatest
dimension

T4
Fixation to chest wall
Edema, peau d'orange
Ulceration of skin

Satellite skin nodules
Inflammatory breast cancer

N, Lymphatic spread

N0
No palpable
regional lymph node

N1
Palpable ipsilateral axillary
lymph nodes, movable

N2
Palpable ipsilateral axillary
lymph nodes, fixed

N3
Metastases to ipsilateral
internal mammary nodes

M, Distant metastases

MX
Distant metastases cannot
be assessed

M0
No distant metastases

M1
Distant metastases present
(includes metastases to
ipsilateral supraclavicular
lymph nodes)

Stage grouping of breast cancer

Stage	T	N	M
0	Tis	N0	M0
1	T1	N0	M0
IIA	T0	N1	M0
	T1	N1	M0
	T2	N0	M0
IIB	T2	N1	M0
	T3	N0	M0
IIIA	T0	N2	M0
	T1	N2	M0
	T2	N2	M0
	T3	N1, N2	M0
IIIB	T4	Any N	M0
	Any T	N3	M0
IV	Any T	Any N	M1

Fig. 8.35 Breast cancer staging based on clinical characteristics (from AJCC:
Manual for Staging of Cancer, 4th edn. Lippincott, Philadelphia, 1993.)

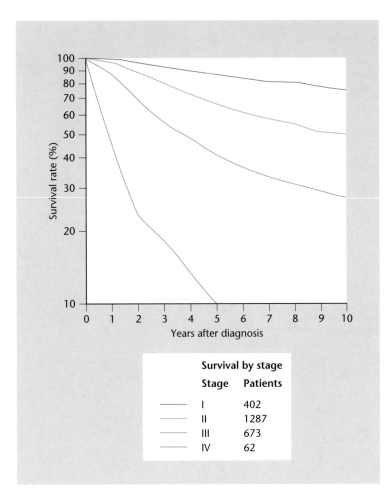

Survival by stage	
Stage	Patients
I	402
II	1287
III	673
IV	62

Fig. 8.36 Survival of breast cancer patients by stage at the time of diagnosis. The number of patients diagnosed with each stage is also given (adapted from Cutler, 1974).

Of note, the 2002 TNM Staging Classification system was modified as follows (Greene *et al*, 2002).
- Stratification of node staging by the number of involved lymph nodes (0, 1–3, 4–9, and, >9)
- Classification of supraclavicular nodes as N3 instead of M1
- Subclassification of nodes based on the extent of involvement and the method of pathologic evaluation (H & E vs. immunohistochemistry or molecular techniques)

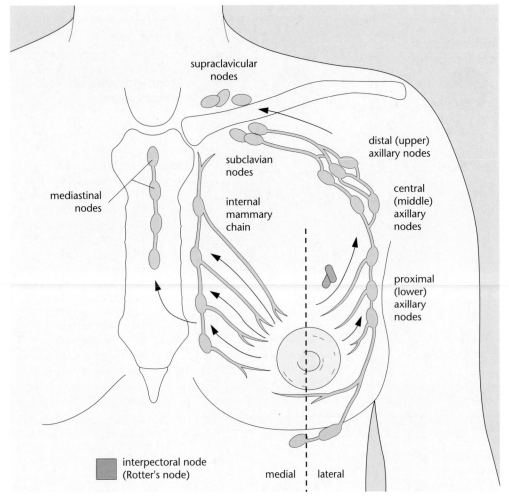

Fig. 8.37 Lymphatic spread of breast cancer. Lymph node metastases are present at the time of diagnosis in up to 60% of cases. In general, lateral lesions in the breast metastasize to axillary and supraclavicular nodes, whereas medial tumors tend to metastasize to the internal mammary and mediastinal lymph nodes, as well as the supraclavicular nodes. However, lymph node involvement is merely a marker for the probability that the cancer has spread from the breast. A positive finding implies that microdeposits of breast cancer will likely be present in other areas as well.

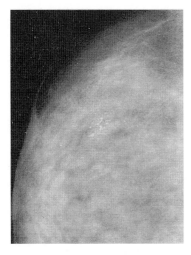

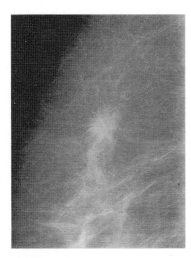

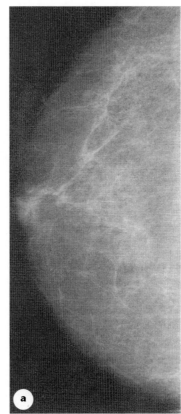

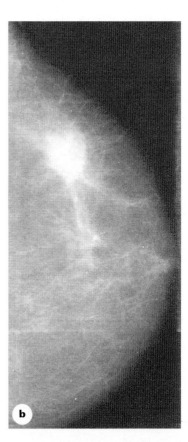

Fig. 8.38 Stage I (T1N0) breast cancer. Magnified view of a screening mammogram from a 52-year-old woman who had no palpable mass demonstrates the classic clustered microcalcifications of several shapes and sizes highly suggestive of carcinoma. Some exhibit linear branching, which is even more suggestive of a ductal lesion. Biopsy confirmed an early invasive ductal carcinoma. (Courtesy of Dr P. Stomper, Roswell Park Memorial Institute, Buffalo, NY.)

Fig. 8.39 Stage (T1N0) breast cancer. Magnified view of a mammogram from a 50-year-old woman with a history of 'lumpy' breasts shows a 1.0 cm stellate mass in the superior portion of the breast. The lesion was excised and found to be an invasive ductal carcinoma. (Courtesy of Dr P. Stomper, Roswell Park Memorial Institute, Buffalo, NY.)

Fig. 8.40 Stage IIA (T2N0) breast cancer. This mammogram from a 65-year-old woman shows that the breasts are not too dense; therefore, the 2.5 cm stellate mass in the upper outer quadrant of the right breast was easily palpated. Histologic examination following resection showed an invasive ductal carcinoma.

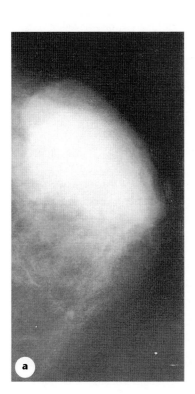

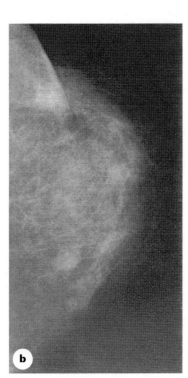

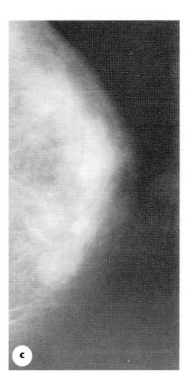

Fig. 8.41 Stage IIIB (T4N0) breast cancer. A 45-year-old woman presented with a very large (10 cm) primary tumor. There was an inflammatory component, but a distinct underlying mass was palpable and quite easily detected on the mammogram (**a**). (**b**) Following chemotherapy and radiotherapy, the mass completely disappeared, replaced only by the distortion artefact left by the biopsy. Three months later, the tumor recurred within the same breast. (**c**) The mammogram demonstrates multiple nodular tumor masses.

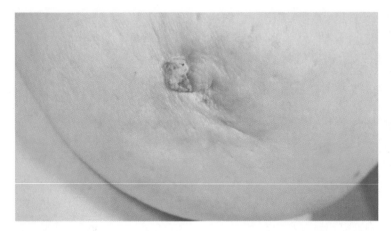

Fig. 8.42 Stage IIIB (T4) breast cancer. A common presentation at this stage is retraction, dimpling and thickening of the skin surrounding the nipple. This clinical finding is designated 'peau d'orange' a name deriving from the pitting and coloration of the skin like orange peel.

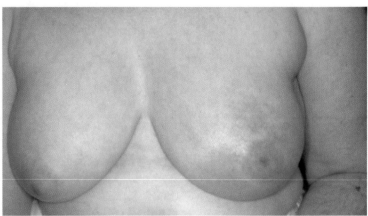

Fig. 8.43 Stage IIB (T4) breast cancer. Classically, inflammatory breast cancer does not present as a discrete mass, but rather as cutaneous erythema with overlying skin warmth, as illustrated in the left breast of this 63-year-old patient.

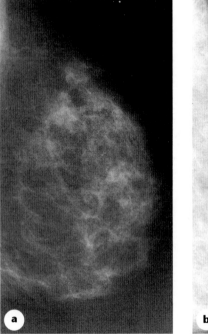
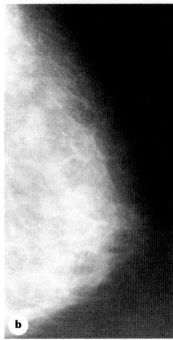

Fig. 8.44 Stage IIB (T4) breast cancer. Seven months after a normal baseline mammogram (**a**), a 35-year-old woman developed skin thickening and erythema of the breast. (**b**) At that time, her mammogram demonstrated a diffuse increase in density – a characteristic finding in inflammatory breast cancer corresponding to the lack of a distinct mass. Biopsy confirmed the diagnosis of inflammatory breast cancer.

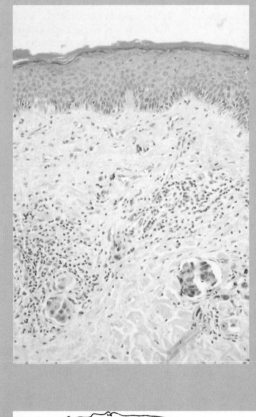

Fig. 8.45 Stage IIIB (T4) breast cancer. The clinical presentation of inflammatory breast cancer is sufficient to make a diagnosis. Yet pathologic confirmation of invasion of dermal lymphatics by malignant cells, as shown in this photomicrograph, can help distinguish this condition from benign mastitis. Note the absence of skin infiltration by inflammatory cells in cancer. The erythema and warmth observed clinically are due to obstruction of dermal lymphatics and subsequent cutaneous lymphedema.

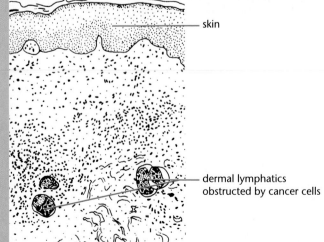

skin

dermal lymphatics obstructed by cancer cells

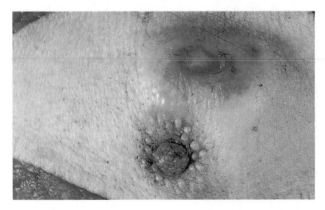

Fig. 8.46 Stage IIIB (T4) breast cancer. Advanced primary carcinomas can present with skin ulceration, as shown in this mastectomy specimen, in the area above the nipple, which is raised and ulcerated by an underlying tumor. Biopsy revealed an adenocarcinoma.

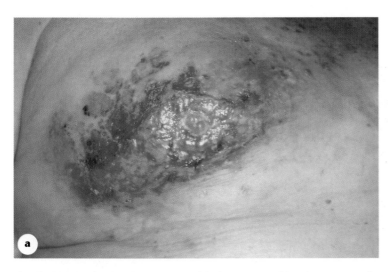

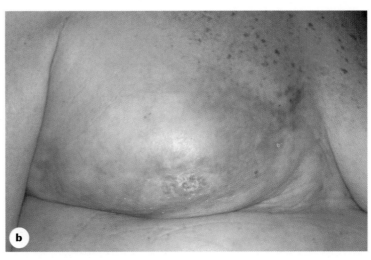

Fig. 8.47 Stage IIIB (T4) breast cancer. (**a**) This 66-year-old patient presented with a locally advanced carcinoma that had ulcerated through the skin, causing substantial morbidity. She was treated effectively with chemotherapy and over 5 months the ulceration decreased as the tumor regressed. (**b**) Ultimately, the skin healed completely.

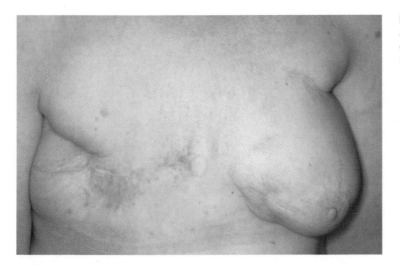

Fig. 8.48 Recurrent breast cancer. Locally recurrent disease can often present as very subtle subcutaneous nodules along the mastectomy scar or as a nodular cutaneous rash. This patient exhibits elements of both presentations. Biopsy revealed adenocarcinoma that resembled the primary carcinoma.

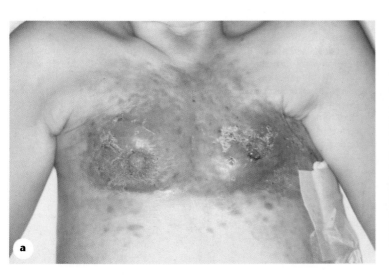

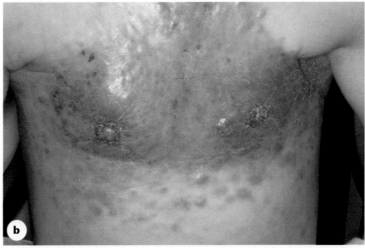

Fig. 8.49 Progressive breast cancer. In a few patients with regional metastases, local problems become the main source of morbidity. Occasionally, as in the case of this 60-year-old patient (**a**), the subcutaneous nodules become confluent and extend across the chest wall, as well as laterally and posteriorly. This pattern of confluence has been designated an 'en cuirasse' carcinoma. Advanced cancer has involved both breasts, resulting in 'auto-mastectomies'. For most of the course of her illness, this patient was plagued by a restriction in pulmonary function due to the band-like distribution of metastases involving the chest wall. (**b**) Six months later, the metastases have progressed despite therapy.

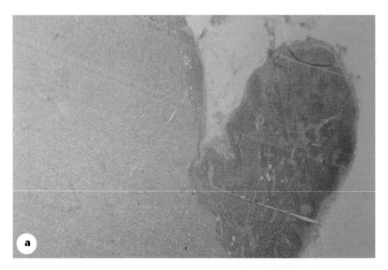

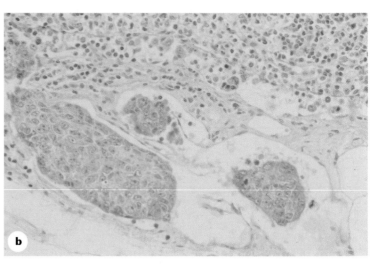

Fig. 8.50 Axillary lymph node metastases. The presence of metastases to the axillary lymph nodes is the single most important prognostic factor in patients with primary breast cancer. (**a**) This lymph node with metastatic breast cancer shows only a small residual area of lymphoid tissue. (**b**) At higher magnification, metastatic deposits can be seen in the subcapsular sinus, a common location for metastases.

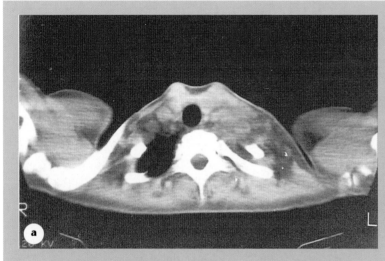

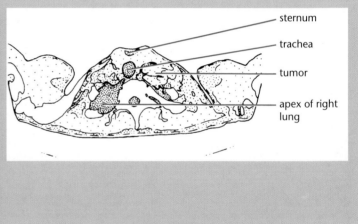

sternum

trachea

tumor

apex of right lung

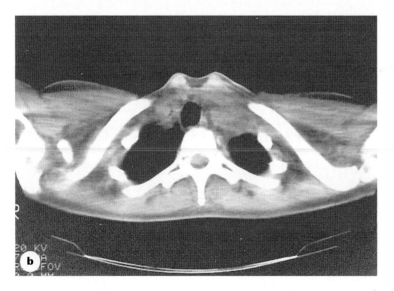

Fig. 8.51 Supraclavicular/mediastinal metastases. A 35-year-old woman who had undergone lumpectomy and radiotherapy for stage I breast cancer 2 years previously presented with left-sided Horner's syndrome and was found to have a 1 cm hard, fixed nodule in the left supraclavicular fossa. Her chest film demonstrated a soft tissue mass in the left aortopulmonary window. CT scans of the upper thorax show a soft tissue mass (**a**) filling the left supraclavicular fossa and (**b**) extending interiorly into the left anterior mediastinum. There was no evidence of distant disease. It was of interest that the primary lesion was located in the medial aspect of the left breast and axillary lymph nodes did not contain cancer. The pattern of recurrence shown here probably represents metastasis to the internal mammary lymph node chain.

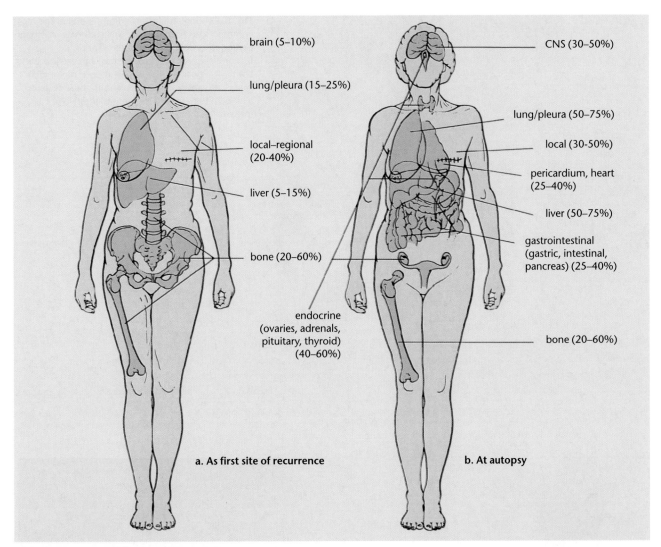

brain (5–10%)

lung/pleura (15–25%)

local–regional
(20-40%)

liver (5–15%)

bone (20–60%)

endocrine
(ovaries, adrenals,
pituitary, thyroid)
(40–60%)

CNS (30–50%)

lung/pleura (50–75%)

local (30-50%)

pericardium, heart
(25–40%)

liver (50–75%)

gastrointestinal
(gastric, intestinal,
pancreas) (25–40%)

bone (20–60%)

a. As first site of recurrence

b. At autopsy

Fig. 8.52 Frequency of breast cancer metastases. The most common first sites of recurrent breast cancer are the chest wall, the regional lymph nodes and/or bone. Liver, lung and central nervous system (CNS) are less common sites of recurrence. In patients with well-advanced disease, breast cancer can be found in almost any organ. Autopsy studies show that metastases are most commonly found in the chest wall and in the surrounding lymph nodes, as well as in the bones, liver, lung, pleura and CNS (brain, spinal cord, meninges). Metastases may also occur in gastrointestinal organs (pancreas, stomach, large and small intestine), endocrine organs (ovaries, adrenals, pituitary, thyroid) and in the cardiovascular system (pericardium, endocardium, myocardium).

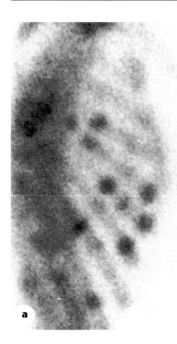

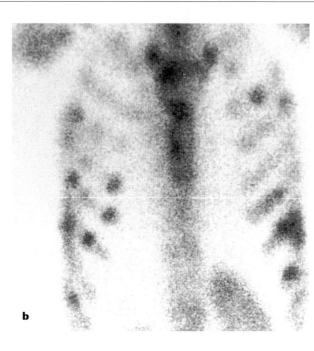

Fig. 8.53 Bone metastases. Bone is one of the most common sites of metastatic breast disease. Although benign disorders, such as osteoarthritis, osteomyelitis, or benign fractures, can cause a bone scan to be positive, the appearance of multiple 'hot spots', especially in the axial and thoracic skeleton, as shown here (**a, b**), is highly suggestive of metastases.

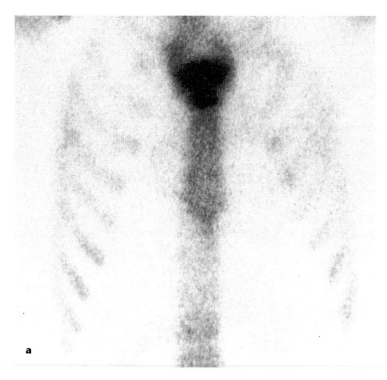

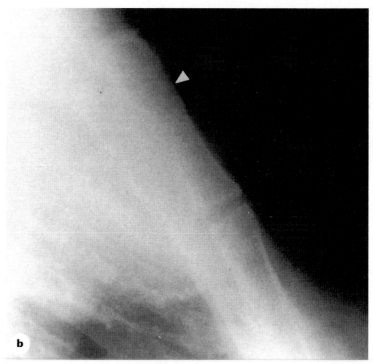

Fig. 8.54 Bone metastases. Bone metastases are not always multiple. (**a**) This bone scan demonstrates an isolated area of increased uptake in the manubrial-sternal area; there was no evidence of other abnormalities. Plain radiographs of suspected areas can help confirm the presence or absence of bone metastases.

Such films may show the presence of a benign lesion, which can explain an abnormal scan. On the other hand, lytic or blastic lesions are suggestive of an underlying carcinoma. (**b**) Plain film of the sternum reveals a lytic area (arrow) corresponding to the 'hot spot' on bone scan.

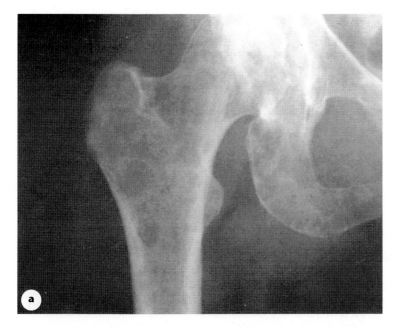

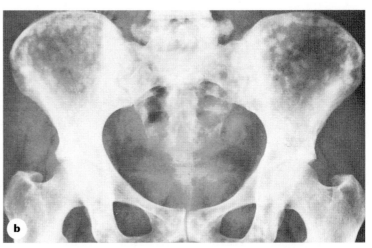

Fig. 8.55 Lytic vs blastic bone metastases. In general, lytic bone metastases are more common than osteoblastic lesions, although many patients exhibit mixed lytic lesions with areas of osteoblastic reaction. (**a**) Diffuse lytic lesions can be seen in this patient's right femoral head and ischial pubic ramus. Such lesions weaken the cortex, often resulting in pathologic fracture.

(**b**) Radiograph of the pelvis of a 45-year-old woman demonstrates widespread foci of increased bone density representing osteoblastic activity surrounding bone metastases of breast cancer. It is interesting to note that effective therapy may alter the nature of lytic bone metastases, converting them to sclerotic, blastic lesions.

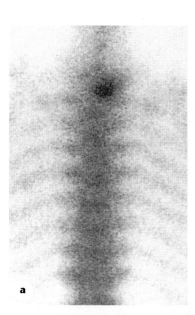

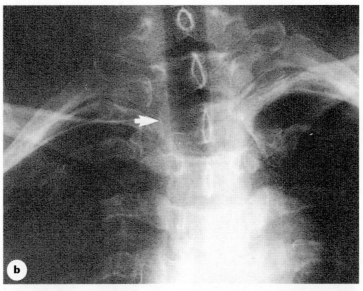

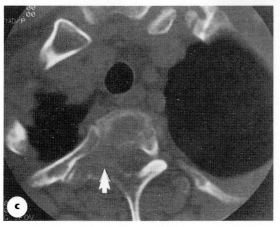

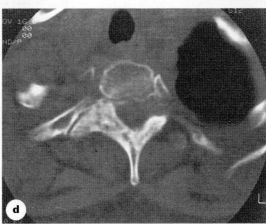

Fig. 8.56 Vertebral metastases. A common site of metastatic breast cancer is the vertebral column. Whereas a single area of increased uptake on bone scan in a long bone may represent a benign process, the same finding in the axial skeleton, as shown here (**a**) in the right side of the T2 vertebra in a 52-year-old patient, is highly suspicious for metastatic disease, especially if plain films do not show another etiology. (**b**) Plain radiograph reveals an absent right pedicle of T2 (arrow), the area corresponding to the 'hot spot' on bone scan. (**c**) CT scan demonstrates a large lytic region (arrow) with destruction of the right pedicle. (**d**) At the same horizontal section following successful radiation therapy, the previously lytic area shows sclerosis and recalcification.

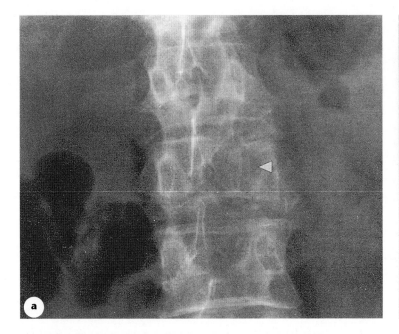

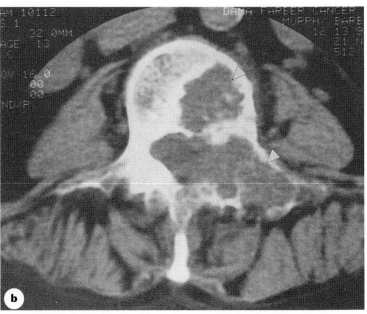

Fig. 8.57 Vertebral metastases. (**a**) Plain film of the lumbar spine demonstrates complete absence of the left pedicle of the L2 vertebra (arrow). (**b**) On CT scan, a large lytic lesion can be seen involving about half of the body of L2, including the left pedicle (arrow). In addition, a soft tissue mass extends into the spinal canal, compressing the spinal cord. Spinal cord compression is classified as an 'oncologic emergency', requiring either immediate decompression or radiation therapy. It can rapidly lead to neurologic deficits and even paraplegia.

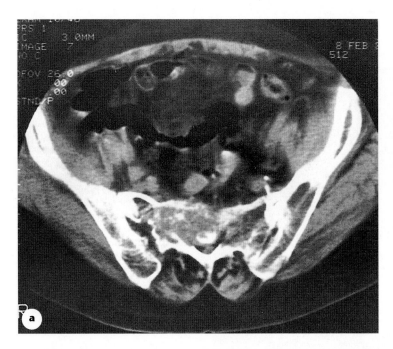

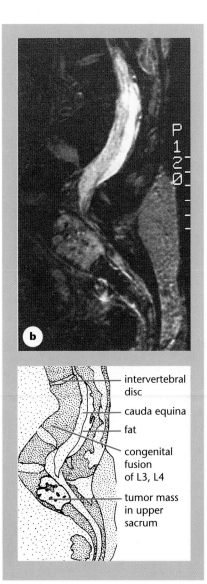

Fig. 8.58 Vertebral metastases. A postmenopausal woman receiving adjuvant chemotherapy for breast cancer developed pain in her left hip and buttock. Bone scan of the area indicated increased uptake across the left sacroiliac region, while a CT scan (**a**) reveals bilateral lytic lesions within the sacrum and iliac bones. The tumor appears to extend into the epidural canal and project superiorly toward the lumbar spine. (**b**) MR scan demonstrates that the superior extent of the tumor is well below the end of the spinal cord. As an incidental finding, congenital fusion of her lumbar vertebrae was also noted. Although metastases below L2 or L3 may cause significant symptoms, they do not cause spinal cord compression because these sites are at the level of the cauda equina or sacral nerve roots.

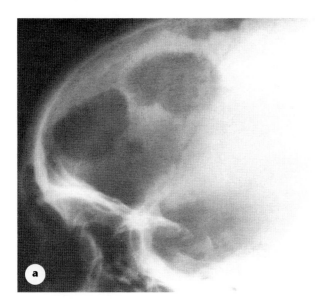

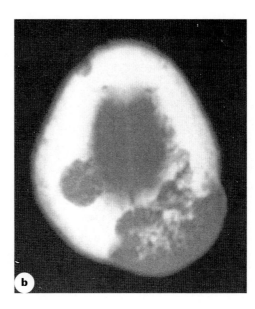

Fig. 8.59 Skull metastases. Breast cancer can metastasize to the skull without involving the brain parenchyma. (**a**) Plain radiograph demonstrates large lytic metastases in the bones of the cranium. (**b**) CT scan of another patient who had a palpable posterior skull metastasis shows a soft tissue mass with extension through the thickness of the bone. Although the brain parenchyma was compressed posteriorly, the patient had no neurologic symptoms.

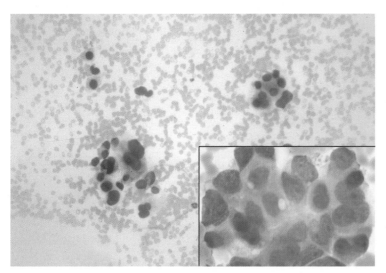

Fig. 8.60 Bone marrow metastases. Bone marrow metastases may develop with or without lytic or osteoblastic bone lesions. Anemia, leukopenia, thrombocytopenia or various combinations of these may be the presenting clues to underlying intramedullary metastases. This low-power microscopic section of a bone marrow aspirate shows several clumps of malignant cells. At high power (inset), one clump of tumor cells demonstrates the characteristic features of metastatic carcinoma: a syncytial pattern or clumping of cells, the variable size and shape of tumor cells and a high nucleus-to-cytoplasm ratio. The distinct, rather large, nucleoli seen here may not always be present. (Courtesy of P. Leavitt, Administrator of Clinical Laboratories, Dana-Farber Cancer Institute, Boston, MA.)

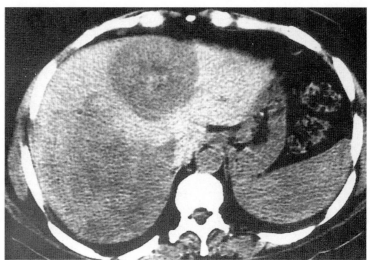

Fig. 8.61 Liver metastases. Liver metastases of breast cancer are usually suspected in the presence of abnormal liver function tests or elevated circulating tumor markers (e.g. CEA or CA15–3). This CT scan demonstrates two very large metastases.

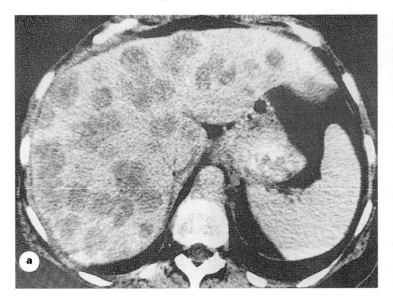

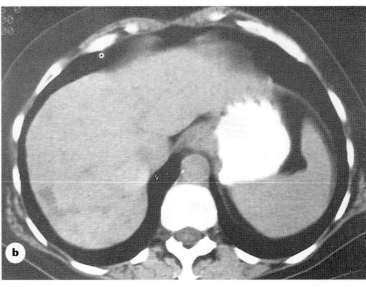

Fig. 8.62 Liver metastases. (**a**) CT scan of the abdomen in a 40-year-old patient shows multiple discrete lesions within the liver. (**b**) The response to chemotherapy can be impressive. After three courses of chemotherapy, the improvement in the patient's liver is remarkable.

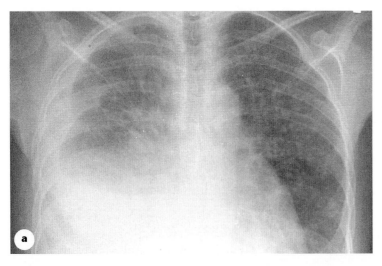

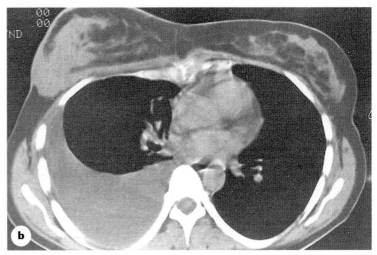

Fig. 8.63 Intrathoracic metastases. Intrathoracic metastases can be manifested in several ways. Among the more common is malignant pleural effusion, as demonstrated by the large right effusion on this chest film (**a**); multiple metastatic pulmonary nodules are also evident). (**b**) Chest CT scan confirms the pleural effusion; in addition, the advanced right breast cancer can also be seen.

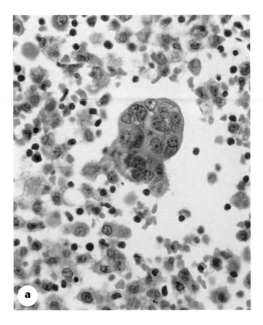

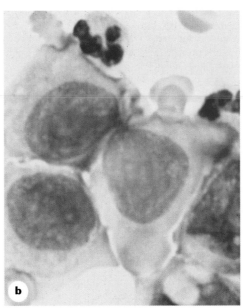

Fig. 8.64 Malignant pleural effusion. Pleural effusions are common in patients with breast cancer as a result of metastatic spread to the pleural surfaces or mediastinum. However, a correct diagnosis may require thoracocentesis with biochemical analysis and cytologic examination of pleural fluid. (**a**) Cytospin preparation from a malignant pleural effusion shows a cluster of highly pleomorphic breast cancer cells with distinct nucleoli. The surrounding cells are all normal mesothelial cells. (**b**) High-power view of a cytocentrifuge smear of pleural fluid shows a clump of large, bizarre, malignant cells with discrete nucleoli. (**a**: Courtesy of Dr A. Lukacher, Brigham and Women's Hospital, Boston, MA.)

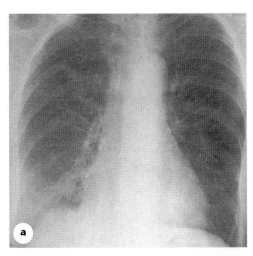

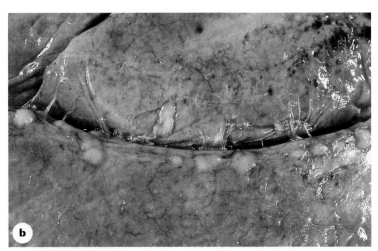

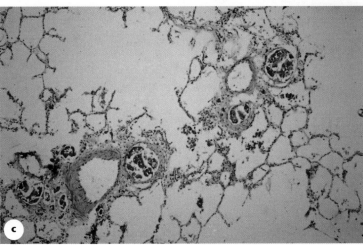

Fig. 8.65 Lymphangitic metastases. Two years after undergoing a left modified radical mastectomy, a 59-year-old patient developed shortness of breath. (**a**) Her chest film shows a diffuse, nodular-interstitial pattern consistent with lymphangitic metastases. (**b**) Macroscopically, lymphangitic metastases (from a different patient) appear as multiple yellow lesions involving lymphatic vessels. (**c**) Microscopically, metastatic tumor cells can be observed filling these vessels.

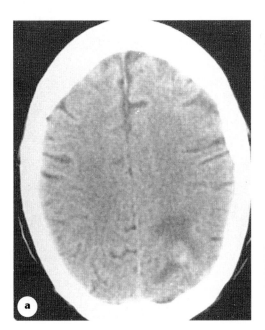

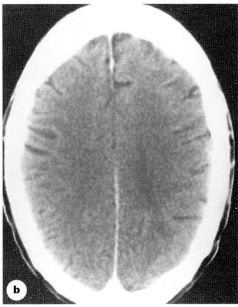

Fig. 8.66 Brain metastases. Breast cancer commonly spreads to the brain, causing neurologic morbidity related to the specific site of involvement. Metastases can be single, multiple or meningeal. (**a**) CT scan of the brain of a 62-year-old woman, who presented 6 years after having undergone a mastectomy and adjuvant chemotherapy for a stage II breast carcinoma, shows a well-circumscribed, enhancing lesion with surrounding edema in the left temporo-occipital region. She also had pulmonary and hepatic metastases. (**b**) Repeat CT scan taken 3 months after completion of successful radiotherapy reveals that the enhancing lesion is no longer evident and the edema has almost completely resolved. Her symptoms also totally resolved.

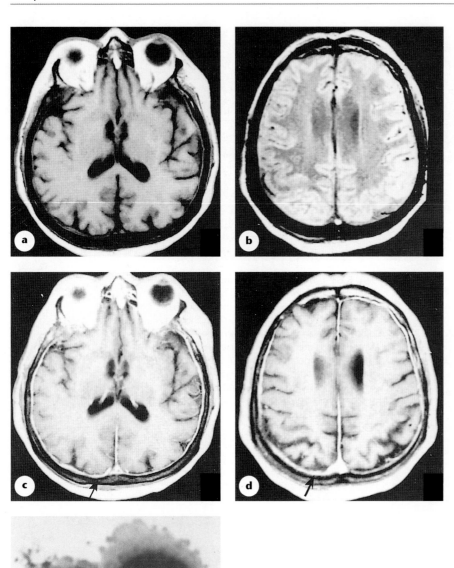

Fig. 8.67 Meningeal metastases. In addition to parenchymal CNS metastases, breast cancer can also spread to the leptomeninges. This 65-year-old woman with known metastatic breast cancer presented with a headache and multiple cranial nerve deficits. MRI without gadolinium was interpreted as normal (**a, b**). However, with gadolinium enhancement (**c, d**), the meningeal surface was found to be abnormally thickened (arrow). Lumbar puncture revealed the presence of metastatic breast cancer in the cerebrospinal fluid (**e**).

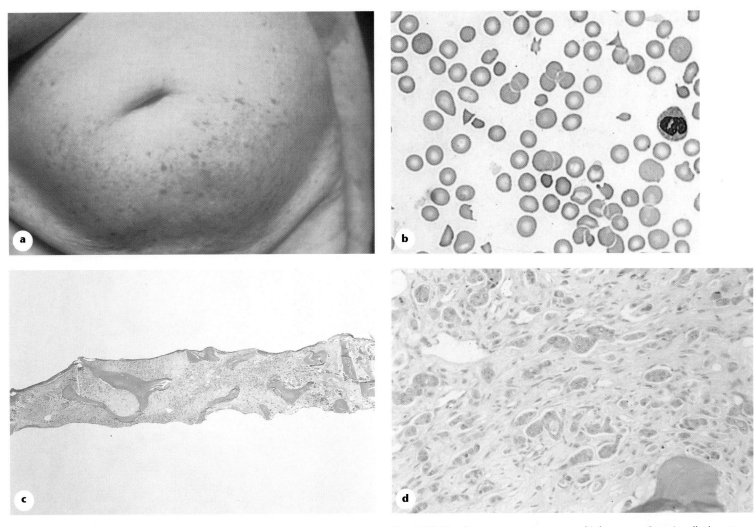

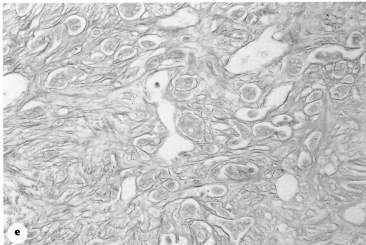

Fig. 8.68 Simultaneous metastases to multiple organs. Occasionally, breast cancer metastasizes to multiple organs simultaneously, resulting in complex syndromes that are diagnostically challenging. A 63-year-old patient presented 5 years after a left modified radical mastectomy with complaints of fatigue, malaise, nausea, vomiting, shortness of breath and multiple areas of bony pain. In addition, she noted bruising, hematuria and some blood in the stools. Physical examination revealed paleness and multiple petechiae and ecchymoses (**a**); she also had congestive heart failure and hepatomegaly. CT scan demonstrated diffuse hepatic metastases and bone scan showed multiple sites of increased uptake. Her chest film was highly suggestive of lymphangitic carcinomatosis. Laboratory evaluation revealed pancytopenia, as well as hepatic and renal insufficiency. (**b**) Evaluation of a peripheral blood smear demonstrates a 'red cell fragmentation syndrome' with numerous schistocytes and anisocytosis. Almost no platelets were seen and the leukocyte count was low. She had microangiopathic hemolytic anemia. (**c**) Bone marrow core biopsy examination reveals almost complete replacement of hematopoietic elements with metastatic breast cancer cells, together with marked fibrosis. (**d**) At higher magnification, nests of tumor cells are seen forming tubular structures within a dense fibrous stroma. (**e**) Silver-stained section shows that the nests of tumor cells are surrounded by reticulin fibers. All the patient's signs and symptoms could be related to widespread metastatic breast cancer.

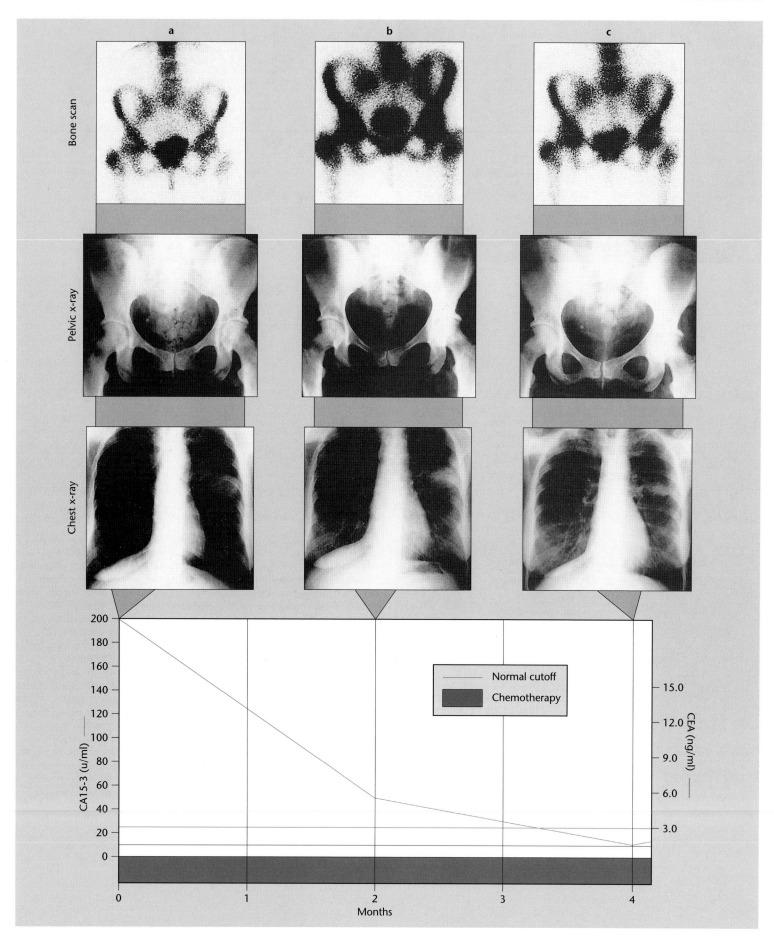

Fig. 8.69 Circulating tumor markers as monitors of disease course. The preceding figures have illustrated the importance of determining whether a patient is responding to therapy or whether her disease is progressing. History, physical examination and radiographic tests can be very helpful in determining which of these is occurring. However, circulating tumor markers can also correlate with clinical disease course and can be useful in monitoring patients during therapy. In this figure, a patient with metastatic breast cancer to bone and lung (**a**) was initially treated with chemotherapy. Her symptoms began to resolve during the first 2 months of therapy, but interpretations of her physical examination, chest X-ray and bone scans were equivocal (**b**). However, her CA15-3 levels decreased from an initial level of 200 U/ml to 50 U/ml. Her chemotherapy was continued and by the fourth month of therapy she was found to be responding, as determined by history, bone scan and chest X-ray findings (**c**). Of note is that the patient's CEA was never elevated and therefore in this patient was of no clinical utility.

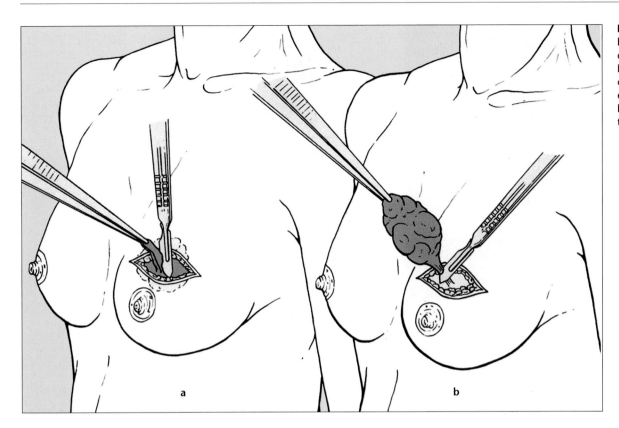

Fig. 8.70 (**a**) An incisional biopsy makes a definitive diagnosis. (**b**) Excisional biopsies, although diagnostic, can also be therapeutic by eliminating the need for further breast surgery when radiation therapy is performed.

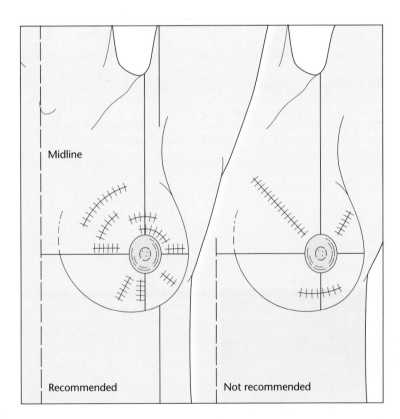

Fig. 8.71 Cosmesis is best maintained using circular incisions in the upper half of the breast and radial incisions in the lower half of the breast.

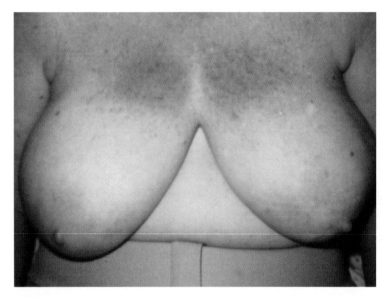

Fig. 8.72 The cosmetic results of conservative therapy are usually quite satisfactory. This 70-year-old patient had a stage I carcinoma of the left breast that was treated by excisional biopsy and primary irradiation. Although there is some asymmetry of the breast, as well as, on close inspection, some modest skin thickening and retraction due to the therapy, it is very difficult to determine which breast was treated.

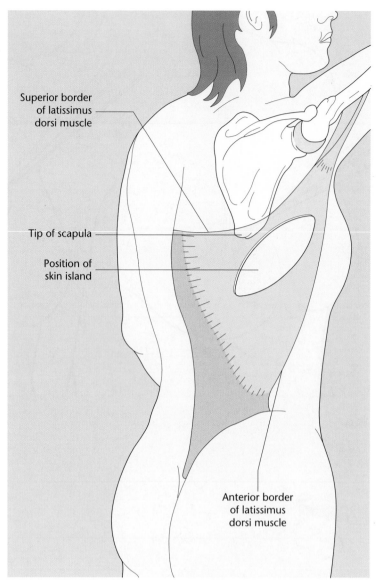

Fig. 8.73 Breast reconstructive surgery. The latissimus dorsi myocutaneous flap is based on the thoracodorsal artery and vein. This flap is rotated from the back and becomes the breast mound (from Vasconez *et al.*, 1991). Alternatively, a transverse rectus abdominis muscle (TRAM) flap can be used which is advantageous in large-breasted women when additional tissue coverage is needed.

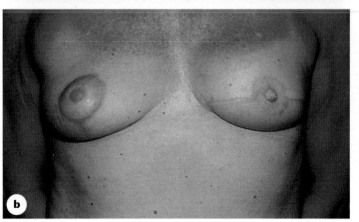

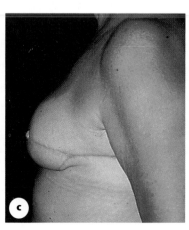

Fig. 8.74 (**a**) The resultant scar from harvesting a latissimus flap. (**b,c**) The resulting cosmetic effect after reconstruction with a latissimus flap.

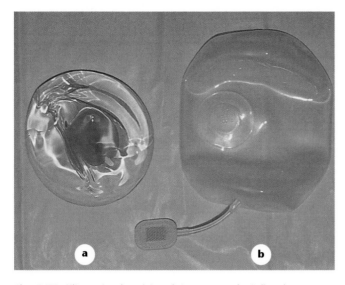

Table 8.4 Incidence of complications with TRAM flap versus tissue expander/implant reconstruction.

Type of complication	Incidence (%)	Tissue expander implant
Infection	1.1	0.7
Hematoma	1.1	3.1
Weak abdominal fascia	3.3	0
Chest flap necrosis	3.3	3.9
Flap necrosis < 20%	6.7	0
Cardiac	1.1	0

Fig. 8.75 Silicone implant (**a**) and tissue expander inflated with saline (**b**).

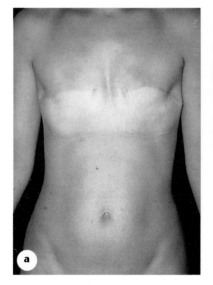

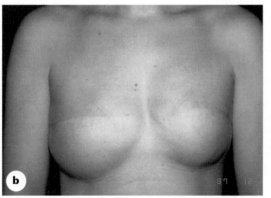

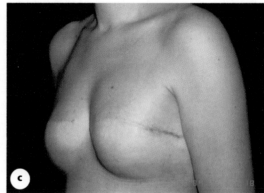

Fig. 8.76 (**a**) A patient with bilateral mastectomies. (**b,c**) Frontal and side views of the same patient after bilateral silicone implants.

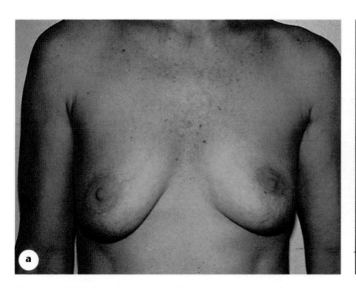

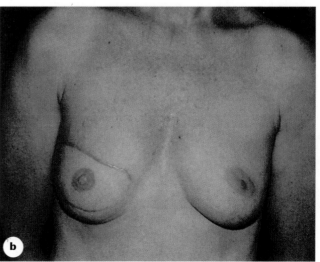

Fig. 8.77 (**a**) Before mastectomy. (**b**) The same patient after mastectomy and TRAM flap reconstruction.

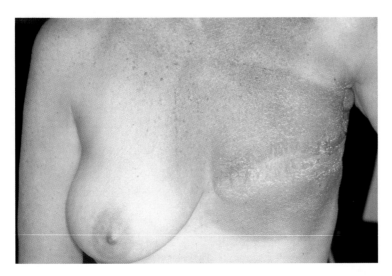

Fig. 8.78 Stage I and II breast cancer can be treated by conservative therapy or mastectomy. This 46-year-old patient had stage II disease and underwent a left modified radical mastectomy followed by radiation therapy to the chest wall. L-phenylalanine mustard was then administered, resulting in a geometrically shaped area of hyperpigmentation and thickening of the chest wall due to a radiation recall reaction in the skin. Adjuvant radiation to the chest after mastectomy is no longer indicated in most patients. Although it decreases local recurrence, it does not affect survival and may be associated with significant morbidity.

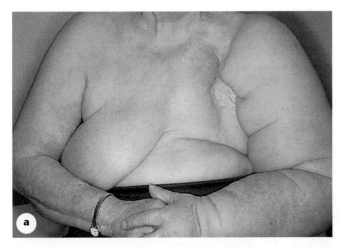

Fig. 8.79 (**a**) A 64-year-old patient with significant arm edema after a radical mastectomy, full axillary dissection and postoperative chest wall and axillary radiotherapy. The patient's left arm is immensely swollen in contrast to her unaffected, normal right arm. After subcutaneous injection of radionuclide into the dorsa of each hand, scintigrams were obtained (**b**). In the anterior views at 15 minutes and 2 hours, flow can easily be seen in normal channels in the right arm. However, only a 'blush' can be seen in the left arm because the normal lymph channels are occluded and the radionuclide is present only in small collateral channels that do not communicate with distal vessels. In the view of the thorax at 2.5 hours, flow can be seen on the right side in normal channels leading to axillary lymph nodes. In contrast, radionuclide has accumulated in the lower arm and is absent in the left axilla.

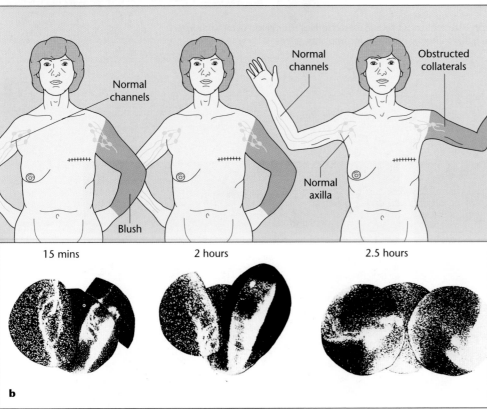

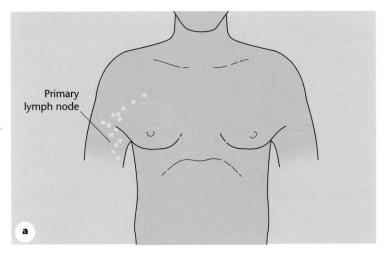

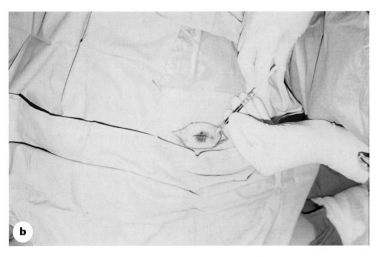

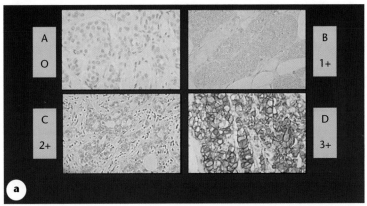

Fig. 8.80 Sentinel node biopsy. (**a**) Axillary lymph mapping. (**b**) Injection of blue dye in the tumor cavity. (**c**) Identification of the sentinel node (follow blue line).

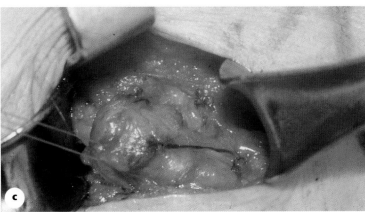

Fig. 8.81 (**a–b**) There are two methods to determine HER2 neu status of tumors: immunohistochemistry (IHC) and fluorescent *in situ* hybridization (FISH). HER2 neu overexpression is assessed by immunohistochemistry and is scored as 0, 1+, 2+ or 3+. Generally her 2 neu 2+ and above are considered positive. HER2 neu overamplification is assessed by FISH.

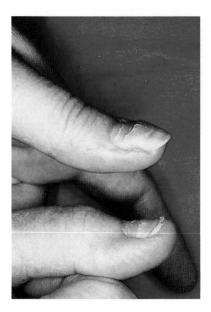

Fig. 8.82 Complications of chemotherapy. Chemotherapy can also produce integumentary toxicity. This patient had metastatic breast cancer and was treated with high-dose doxorubicin. After her first course she noticed change in her fingernails. She went on to develop onycholysis and onychomadesis. Although uncommon, this is a potential complication of doxorubicin.

Table 8.5 Adverse prognostic factors in breast cancer (adapted from Hayes, 1993, and McGuire and Clark, 1992)
Lymph node status   Negative < few positive < many positive

Larger tumor size
    Clinical features: fixation; ulceration; inflammation
    High histologic grade
    High nuclear grade

Estrogen- and progesterone-receptor content negative
Tumor kinetics   Thymidine labeling index; high S-phase fraction
DNA aneuploidy
Her 2-neu overexpression/overamplification

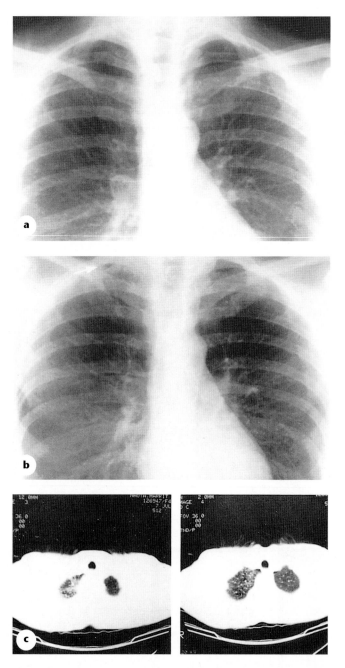

Fig. 8.83 Radiation pneumonitis. Radiation therapy can be associated with local tissue damage and toxicity. This patient presented with a T2N3 breast cancer with supraclavicular lymphadenopathy. She was treated by lumpectomy and radiotherapy to the breast, as well as radiation therapy to the supraclavicular fossa. At this time her chest X-ray was normal (**a**). Two years later the patient presented with a nagging, non-productive cough and some dyspnea on exertion. A chest X-ray (**b**) demonstrated a nodular, right upper lobe density and a CT scan (**c**) confirmed the presence of these apical nodules. Bronchoscopic evaluation failed to reveal any endobronchial lesions and a fine-needle aspiration of this area was also non-diagnostic. Over the next 5 years the patient did not develop any progressive symptoms or signs of malignancy. Therefore, the changes were considered to be secondary to her prior radiation, which included the right pulmonary apex.

REFERENCES

AJCC: Manual for Staging of Cancer, 4th edn. Lippincott, Philadelphia, 1993. Berg JW, Hutter RVP: Breast cancer, histology of cancer. Incidence and prognosis: SEER population-based data, 1973–1987. Cancer 1995; 75: 257–269.

Cutler SJ: Classification of extent of disease in breast cancer. Semin Oncol 1974; 1: 91.

Early Breast Cancer Trialists' Collaborative Group T: Systemic treatment of early breast cancer by hormonal, cytotoxic, or immune therapy: 133 randomized trials involving 31,000 recurrences and 24,000 deaths among 75,000 women. Lancet 1992; 339: 1–15, 71–85.

Fisher B, Costantino J, Redmond C, et al.: Lumpectomy compared with lumpectomy and radiation therapy for the treatment of intraductal breast cancer. N Engl J Med 1993; 328: 1581–1586.

Fisher B, Costantino J, Redmond C, et al.: Endometrial cancer in tamoxifen-treated breast cancer patients: findings from the National Surgical Adjuvant Breast and Bowel Project (NSAPBP). J Natl Cancer Inst 1994; 86: 527–537.

Fisher ER, Gregorio RM, Fisher B, et al.: The pathology of invasive breast cancer. A syllabus derived from findings of the National Surgical Adjuvant Breast Project (Protocol No. 4). Cancer 1975; 36: 1.

Gabriel S, O'Fallon W, Kurland L, et al.: Risk of connective-tissue disease and other disorders after breast implantation. N Engl J Med 1994; 330: 1697–1702.

Greenlee, R et al. Cancer Statistics, 2000. CA Vol 50(1) Jan/Feb 2000

Greene FL, Page DL, Fleming ID, et al.: AJCC Cancer Staging Manual, 6th edn. Springer-Verlag, New York, 2002.

Harris J, Hellman S, Henderson IC, et al.: Breast Diseases, 2nd edn. Lippincott, Philadelphia, 1990.

Harris JR, Lippman ME, Veronesi U, Willett W: Breast cancer, pt 1. N Engl J Med 1992; 327: 319–328.

Hayes DF, ed: Atlas of Breast Cancer. Mosby Europe, London, 1993.

Hayes DF; Tumor markers for breast cancer. Ann Oncol 1993; 4: 807–819.

Hayes DF, Henderson, IC, Shapiro, CL: Treatment of metastatic breast cancer: present and future prospect. Semin Oncol 1995; 22: 5–21.

Kelsey JL, Berkowitz GS: Breast cancer epidemiology. Cancer Res 1988; 48: 5615–5623.

Lumb G, Mackenzie DH: The incidence of metastases in adrenal glands and ovaries removed for cancer of the breast. Cancer 1959; 12: 521.

McGuire WL, Clark GM: Prognostic factors and treatment decisions in axillary node-negative breast cancer. N Engl J Med 1992; 326: 1756–1761.

Merkel DE, Osborne CK: Prognostic factors in breast cancer. Hematol Oncol Clin North Am 1989; 3: 641–652.

Miki Y, Shattuck-Eldens D, Futreal PA, et al.: Isolation of BRCA1, the 17q-linked breast and ovarian cancer susceptibility gene. Science 1994; 266: 61–71.

Schnitt SJ, Sadowsky NL, Connolly JL, et al.: Ductal carcinoma in situ (intraductal carcinoma) of the breast. N Engl J Med 1988; 318: 898–903.

Shapiro CL, Henderson IC: New Directions in Breast Cancer. Saunders, Philadelphia, 1994.

Smart C, Hendrick RE, Rutledge J, et al.: Benefit of mammography screening in women aged 40–49 years. Cancer 1995; 75: 1619–1626.

Stomper PC, Gelman RS: Mammography in symptomatic and asymptomatic patients. Hematol Oncol Clin North Am 1989; 3: 611–640.

Vasconez LO, LeJour H, Gamboa-Bobadilla M: Atlas of Breast Reconstruction. Gower, New York, 1991.

Verones U et al. Sentinel-node biopsy to avoid axillary dissection in breast cancer with clinically negative lymph nodes. Lancet 1997; 349: 1864–1867.

FIGURE CREDITS

The following books published by Gower Medical Publishing are sources of figures in the present chapter. The figure numbers given in the listing are those of the figures in the present chapter. The page numbers given in parentheses are those of the original publication.

Besser GM, Cudworth AG: Clinical Endocrinology. Lippincott/Gower Medical Publishing, Philadelphia/London, 1987: Fig. 8.64A (p. 21.25).

du Vivier A: Atlas of Clinical Dermatology. Churchill Livingstone/Gower Medical Publishing, Edinburgh/London, 1986: Figs 8.24 (p. 7.12), 8.25 (p. 7.13).

Fletcher CDM, McKee PH: An Atlas of Gross Pathology. Edward Arnold/Gower Medical Publishing, London, 1987: Figs 8.38 (p. 48), 8.47 (p. 47).

Hayes DF, ed: Atlas of Breast Cancer. Mosby Europe, London, 1993: Figs 8.12 (p. 2.2); 8.13 (p. 1.4); 8.14 (p. 1.3); 8.15 (p. 1.3); 8.34 (p. 6.5); 8.39 (p. 12.3); 8.52 (p. 12.6); 8.67 (p. 12.15); 8.69 (p. 12.24); 8.70 (p. 5.4); 8.71 (p. 5.5); 8.73 (p. 5.14); 8.74 (p. 5.14); 8.75 (p. 5.12); 8.76 (p. 5.12); 8.77 (p. 5.17); 8.73b (p. 5.11); 8.82 (p. 12.22); 8.83 (p. 12.22), Table 8.2 (p. 2.3), Table 8.4 (p. 5.12),

Hewitt PE: Blood Diseases (Pocket Picture Guides). Gower Medical Publishing, London, 1985: Fig. 8.69A (p. 58).

Hoffbrand AV, Pettit JE: Clinical Haematology Illustrated. Churchill Livingstone/Gower Medical Publishing, Edinburgh/London, 1987: Figs 8.56B (p. 15.3), 8.69B (p. 4.10).

9

Endocrine Tumors and Malignancies

Francis D. Moore Jr, Mark A. Socinski, Nancy E. Joste

CANCER OF THE THYROID GLAND

Cancer of the thyroid gland is a relatively uncommon malignancy, marked by slow growth, delayed symptoms and a low incidence of morbidity and mortality. In the United States, approximately 17 000 new cases are diagnosed each year and about 1 700 deaths occur. The incidence of thyroid cancer in women is twice that in men, with a peak occurring in the third and fourth decades. The prevalence of cancer in a solitary nodule is approximately 1%. The prevalence of microscopic foci of unsuspected thyroid malignancy in multinodular glands is approximately 10–15%.

The most well-documented risk factor for thyroid cancer is radiation administered during childhood for benign conditions of the head and neck or thymus. The risk appears to be dose related, with the greatest risk between 200 and 1000 rads. Thyroid cancer is thought to be less common after doses higher than 2000 rads, probably because few cells remain to undergo malignant degeneration after radiation-induced atrophy and fibrosis. However, thyroid cancer cases have been reported within the atypical nodular hyperplasia of the thyroid occurring after radiation for childhood Hodgkin's disease or rhabomyosarcoma of the neck. Papillary and follicular cancers are most commonly associated with prior radiation exposure. Other less well-defined risk factors for thyroid cancer include endemic goiter, high iodine intake, Graves' disease and Hashimoto's disease (papillary). I[131] therapy for hyperthyroidism does not appear to increase the risk of thyroid cancer. Medullary carcinoma of the thyroid can be sporadic or inherited as an autosomal dominant trait, either alone or in the context of multiple endocrine neoplasia (MEN) type II. Patients with Hashimoto's thyroiditis also are at increased risk for lymphoma of the thyroid.

HISTOLOGY
Papillary adenocarcinoma

Most malignancies of the thyroid gland originate in the glandular epithelium (*see* Table 9.1). Papillary adenocarcinoma is the most common type, representing more than 70% of adult thyroid cancers. It most often arises in young adults and shows a predilection for females (75%). Although often multicentric in origin on microscopic analysis, it usually manifests as a solitary thyroid nodule, with or without cervical lymph node metastases. The latter may occur in the absence of a clinically detectable thyroid nodule. Macroscopic lymph node involvement is seen in 40% of cases at presentation but does not signify a less favorable prognosis. Microscopic involvement may be universal in papillary carcinoma. Less than 10% of papillary carcinomas have metastasized outside the neck region at the time of presentation, the most common sites of metastases being lung and bone. The overall 10-year survival rate is about 93%.

Follicular adenocarcinoma

Follicular adenocarcinoma represents approximately 25% of thyroid malignancies. Somewhat more common in women, it tends to occur in middle age, with a clinical presentation similar to that of papillary adenocarcinoma. A propensity for local blood vessel invasion is a characteristic feature of this malignancy. Most commonplace is the minimally invasive form which, confined to the thyroid, demonstrates little capsular and no vascular invasion. It is otherwise difficult to distinguish from a benign follicular adenoma. Less frequently seen are widely invasive carcinomas which have a more aggressive behavior with extensive gross and microscopic spread at presentation. Follicular cancers may also be capable of absorbing ingested radioactive iodine as a treatment. A recognized variant of follicular adenocarcinoma, Hürthle cell adenocarcinoma, does not share this property. As a result, while 10-year survival for follicular carcinoma is 85%, it is less for Hürthle cell cancer at 75%.

Wider dissemination usually occurs via the hematogenous route, in contrast to the lymphatic spread of papillary carcinoma. Bone, lung and other visceral metastases may not become evident for years.

Undifferentiated (anaplastic) carcinomas

Constituting less than 5% of thyroid malignancies, undifferentiated (anaplastic) carcinomas are clinically quite distinct from papillary and follicular carcinomas. They occur in an older age group and are marked by rapid tumor growth and extensive local invasion (often with tracheal stenosis). They present as large, stony hard masses with little mobility and often, the hoarse voice of a recurrent laryngeal nerve palsy. Widespread metastatic disease is a typical finding. They are usually fatal within a year of diagnosis and may originate within long-standing, and neglected, papillary or follicular adenocarcinomas.

Medullary carcinoma

Medullary carcinoma is a neoplasm of the parafollicular C cells, accounting for 5–10% of thyroid malignancies. C cells are derived from the neural crest and secrete calcitonin, as well as other polypeptides, such as vasoactive intestinal polypeptide (VIP), carcinoembryonic antigen (CEA), somatostatin and corticotropin (ACTH). Tumor cells also show reactivity for panendocrine markers, including neuron-specific enolase and chromogranin. Immunohistochemical stains are consequently useful in the diagnosis of medullary carcinoma.

Medullary carcinoma usually presents as a solitary solid mass, often with encapsulation. Vascular invasion is common, as is involvement of regional lymph nodes. Severe watery diarrhea, an effect of VIP secretion, is present in some patients. The majority of cases are sporadic and occur in patients over the age of 40; the disease is usually unilateral. This malignancy also occurs as part of the MEN-II syndrome, in which case the incidence involves a younger age group and is uniformly bilateral. As a result of routine screening of family members for mutations within the RET oncogene and for elevated thyrocalcitonin levels, a progressively younger age group with smaller tumors or even preclinical C-cell hyperplasia is now being identified. A non-MEN familial type also exists; it is characteristically bilateral.

STAGING OF THYROID CANCER

The primary determinants of prognosis in thyroid cancer are tumor factors (size, local invasion, lymph node involvement, histology) and host factors (age and gender). In the staging system for thyroid cancers (see Fig. 9.1), stage I is marked by confinement of the tumor to the thyroid gland; involvement may be unilateral, bilateral or multifocal. With stage II disease, the tumor is localized to the gland, with movable regional lymph nodes. Direct local invasion or fixed regional nodes mark stage III tumors and the presence of distant metastases characterizes stage IV lesions.

Additional factors are taken into consideration in determining prognosis. With papillary carcinoma, presentation at an older age (generally greater than 50), tumor size and extent (extrathyroidal extension), cytologic atypia and lack of differentiation are all unfavorable prognostic factors. Follicular carcinomas which are minimally invasive carry a favorable prognosis. Extension beyond the thyroid, tumor size and an older age at presentation are likewise unfavorable prognostic features in follicular carcinoma, together with nodal involvement and spread to distant sites. In medullary carcinoma, patients with the sporadic form of the disease usually have a poorer prognosis than those with the familial form, perhaps owing to the earlier diagnosis of the latter. Other unfavorable prognostic factors include metastatic disease, tumor size, an older age at diagnosis, male sex, the presence of diarrhea and rapidly increasing calcitonin levels.

CLINICAL MANIFESTATIONS

Most patients (75%) present with a neck mass. Uncommon manifestations include rapid thyroid enlargement, neck pain, dysphagia, hoarseness and hyper- or hypothyroidism. The diagnostic approach to the incidentally discovered thyroid nodule is undergoing constant change. Because benign nodules greatly outnumber thyroid cancers, accurate diagnosis is imperative to avoid unnecessary surgery. With the exception of an elevated thyrocalcitonin level in medullary carcinoma, the only definitive diagnostic test is biopsy by needle aspiration. Lesions suspicious or diagnostic for malignancy can then be surgically evaluated.

Thyroid scanning is uncertain, because hypofunction is common in benign nodules and only 6–20% of 'cold' nodules are malignant. Conversely, if a nodule is hyperfunctional (i.e. 'hot') on thyroid scan, the likelihood of malignancy is very low but not absent. Because a cystic lesion is less likely to be malignant, ultrasonography has been used to distinguish benign from malignant nodules. Cystic lesions, however, represent only 10–25% of thyroid nodules. The cystic nature of the lesion must be confirmed by aspiration and cytologic examination. As most cysts arise from spontaneous bleeding into small solid lesions, even a negative cytologic exam does not erase the possibility that a cyst might have been caused by a subcentimeter carcinoma. The prevalence of cancer within a cyst ranges from 0.6% to 2%, the same incidence as in solid nodules overall.

MOLECULAR BIOLOGY

Determination of DNA ploidy status by flow cytometry or growth activity by Ki-67 are not of value in discriminating between follicular adenomas and well-differentiated follicular carcinomas. In frankly malignant tumors, however, the presence of aneuploidy portends a more aggressive behavior compared with diploid or polyploid carcinomas. This is also the case for the Hürthle cells, papillary, anaplastic and medullary carcinomas. About 10–20% of papillary carcinomas are associated with activation of an oncogene named papillary thyroid carcinoma (PTC). PTC is derived from a rearrangement of the *ret* proto-oncogene mapped to chromosome 10q11.2. Sequential dedifferentiation of follicular carcinomas is associated with overexpression of p53 gene mutations. In addition, *ras* genes are frequently mutated in these tumors. Mutations of mitochondrial DNA are reported in papillary carcinoma. Follicular adenocarcinoma of the thyroid has been noted recently to contain the PAX-PPAR chromosomal translocation oncogene, not seen with papillary carcinoma nor with follicular adenoma. Patients with familial medullary carcinoma would be expected to possess a mutation in the RET proto-oncogene as is seen in MEN II. Defects of this sort do not appear to be involved in the non-MEN sporadic medullary carcinoma.

TUMORS OF THE PARATHYROID GLANDS

Parathyroid tumors are most commonly benign and can be identified on the basis of the biochemical abnormality which they induce: hypercalcemia. Parathyroid tissue expresses extracellular calcium receptors. Parathyroid tumors are characterized by deficient expression of these receptors, resulting in impaired calcium regulation. In effect, the tumor senses that the serum ionized calcium concentration is lower than in reality, causing the tumor to secrete parathormone at a physiologically inappropriately elevated level. This high level of parathormone for a given calcium concentration causes the manifestations of the disease: hypercalcemia, bone resorption and osteoporosis, hypercalcuria and kidney stones.

Benign parathyroid disease is usually caused by solitary adenomas. These can be ectopically located anywhere from the angle of the jaw to the lower mediastinum. However, more than 99% are within the neck and can be identified based on mitochondrial uptake of radiolabeled sestamibi or on gross morphology alone. These cause an indolent disease extending over 5 or more years before detection. In contrast, parathyroid adenocarcinomas cause rapidly progressive hypercalcemia with higher calcium and parathormone concentrations than are seen customarily with the diagnosis of hyperparathyroidism. Furthermore, these malignancies are rock hard with local invasion, in contrast to the soft and nonadherent adenomas. Parathyroid carcinoma represents less than 1% of all cases of hyperparathyroidism. An entity of non-functioning parathyroid carcinoma is only anecdotal. Also, whereas a parathyroid adenoma may weigh only 100 mg, carcinomas are typically much larger. The adenoma is often dark brown, soft and uniform, with the carcinomas whitish, hard and with bands of fibrosis.

Table 9.1 Malignant tumors of the thyroid gland.

Epithelial tumors	Nonepithelial and miscellaneous tumors
Papillary or papillary-follicular adenocarcinoma	Lymphoma
Follicular adenocarcinoma	Sarcoma

Undifferentiated (anaplastic) carcinoma
    Small cell carcinoma
    Giant cell carcinoma
    Spindle cell carcinoma
	Metastatic tumor
	Malignant teratoma
	Unclassified tumors

Medullary carcinoma	
Squamous cell carcinoma	

Fig. 9.1 Staging of thyroid cancer (from Flemming *et al.*, 1997).

Staging of thyroid cancers

Definition of TNM

Primary tumor (T)
(Note: All categories may be subdivided into (a) solitary tumor and (b) multifocal tumor with the largest tumor determining the classification)

TX	Primary tumor cannot be assessed
T0	No evidence of primary tumor
T1	Tumor 1 cm or less in greatest dimension limited to the thyroid
T2	Tumor more than 1 cm, but not more than, 4 cm in greatest dimension limited to the thyroid
T3	Tumor more than 4 cm in greatest dimension limited to the thyroid
T4	Tumor of any size extending beyond the thyroid capsule

Regional lymph nodes (N)
(Regional lymph nodes are the cervical and upper mediastinal lymph nodes)

NX	Regional lymph nodes cannot be assessed
N0	No regional lymph node metastasis
N1	Regional lymph node metastasis
	N1a Metastasis in ipsilateral cervical lymph node(s)
	N1b Metastasis in bilateral, midline, or contralateral cervical or mediastinal lymph node(s)

Distant metastasis (M)

MX	Presence of distant metastasis cannot be assessed
M0	No distant metastasis
M1	Distant metastasis

Stage grouping

Separate stage groupings are recommended for papillary and follicular, medullary, and undifferentiated (anaplastic)

	Papillary or follicular	
	Under 45 years	*45 years and older*
Stage I	Any T, Any N, M0	T1, N0, M0
Stage II	Any T, Any N, M1	T2, N0, M0
		T3, N0, M0
Stage III		T4, N0, M0
		Any T, Any N1, M0
Stage IV		Any T N1, M0

	Medullary		
Stage I	T1	N0	M0
Stage II	T2	N0	M0
	T3	N0	M0
	T4	N0	M0
Stage III	Any T	N1	M0
Stage IV	Any T	Any N	M1

	Undifferentiated (anaplastic)		
All cases are stage IV			
Stage IV	Any T	Any N	Any M

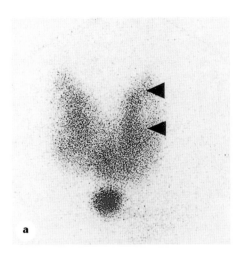

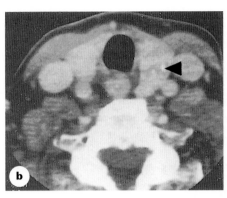

Fig. 9.2 Papillary adenocarcinoma. A 74-year-old woman presented with a thyroid nodule. (**a**) An I^{123} thyroid scan (anterior view) demonstrates a 'cold' nodule (arrows) in the upper portion of the left thyroid lobe. The 'hot' spot below the thyroid is a suprasternal marker. (**b**) An axial CT scan demonstrates an irregular density within the left thyroid lobe at the level of the lesion seen on the radionuclide scan. The lesion contains a single area of calcification (arrow) and is not sharply demarcated from normal thyroid tissue. At operation, there proved to be extracapsular extension.

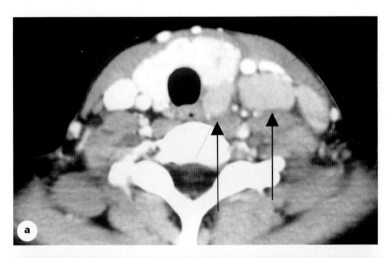

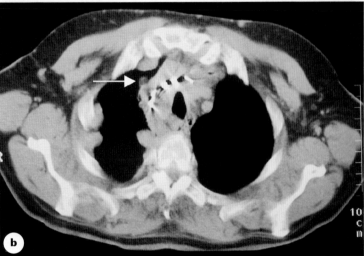

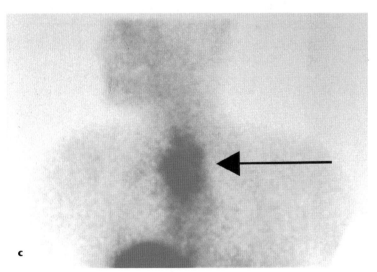

Fig. 9.3 Metastatic papillary adenocarinoma. A. CT scan showing presentation of tumor with involvement of local and regional lymph nodes of neck. Left arrow points to paratracheal lymph node involvement. Right arrow points to massively enlarged jugular nodes. (**b**) CT scanning showing recurrence of papillary carcinoma after treatment in mediastinal lymph nodes. Arrow points to area of involvement, recurrent after mediastinal lymph node dissection on the right. (**c**) Papillary adenocarcinoma may express somatostatin receptors. This is a radiolabeled somatostatin analogue scan of the patient in (**b**). Arrow points to massive mediastinal involvement.

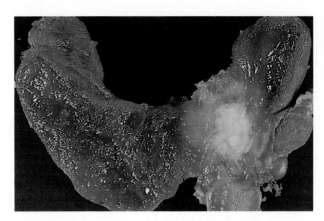

Fig. 9.4 Papillary adenocarcinoma. A pale, irregular neoplasm has arisen in the right lobe of an otherwise normal thyroid gland. A lymph node infiltrated by metastatic tumor is adherent to the lower pole.

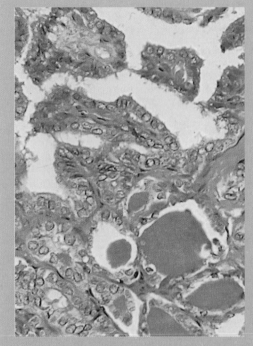

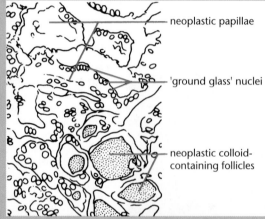

neoplastic papillae

'ground glass' nuclei

neoplastic colloid-containing follicles

Fig. 9.5 Papillary adenocarcinoma. There is a typical mixture of neoplastic papillae and neoplastic colloid-containing follicles. The diagnosis rests on cytologic, not architectural features. The nuclei are crowded, irregular in shape and appear empty, typically with nuclear membrane folding and nuclear pseudoinclusions.

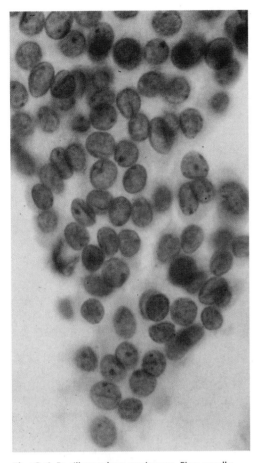

Fig. 9.6 Papillary adenocarcinoma. Fine-needle aspirate shows a neoplastic tissue fragment with characteristic nuclear features of powdery chromatin, nuclear membrane folds and macronucleoli.

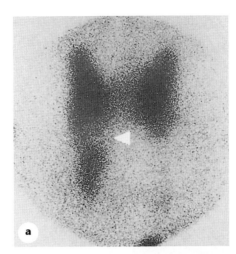

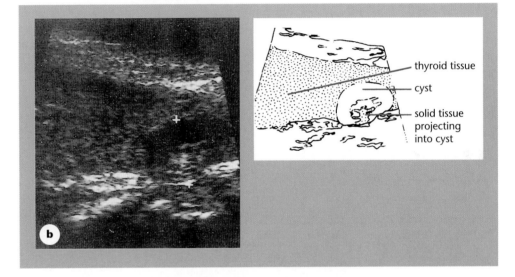

Fig. 9.7 Follicular adenoma. A 51-year-old woman with a history of previous irradiation of the neck had a thyroid scintiscan as a routine follow-up procedure. A mass could not be palpated. (**a**) Pertechnetate scan (anterior view) shows a 'cold' defect (arrow) in the medial aspect of the lower portion of the right thyroid lobe. The left lobe is much smaller than the right. (**b**) High-resolution sagittal sonogram of the right thyroid lobe shows a hypoechoic focus in the posteroinferior region, which corresponds to the 'cold' defect seen on the scintiscan. A mound of echogenic tissue projects into the lumen from the posterior wall of the predominantly cystic lesion (measuring 1.01 cm in diameter). Needle aspiration performed under ultrasonic guidance yielded the diagnosis.

thyroid tissue
cyst
solid tissue projecting into cyst

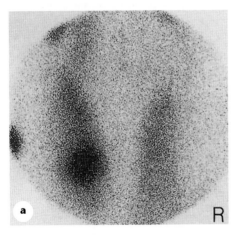

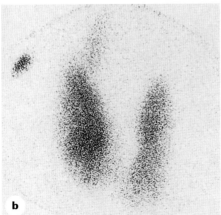

Fig. 9.8 Follicular adenoma. (**a**) Pertechnetate thyroid scan in a 56-year-old man who was found to have a thyroid nodule on routine physical examination shows a 'hot' area in the lower portion of the right thyroid lobe. (**b**) I123 scintiscan, obtained to ascertain whether the area represented functioning thyroid tissue, shows no difference in uptake between the nodule and the remainder of the right thyroid lobe, indicating no increase in synthesis of thyroid hormone. The benign nature of the lesion was confirmed at operation.

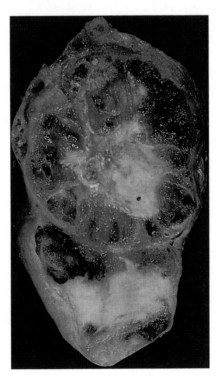

Fig. 9.9 Follicular adenocarcinoma. Within this lobe of the thyroid, which is distorted by a multinodular goiter, a pale infiltrative neoplasm is visible in the lower pole. Local infiltration and vascular spread are common with this neoplasm.

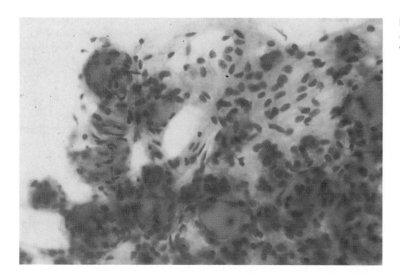

Fig. 9.10 Follicular adenocarcinoma. Fine-needle aspirate demonstrating neoplastic tissue fragments with a follicular architecture.

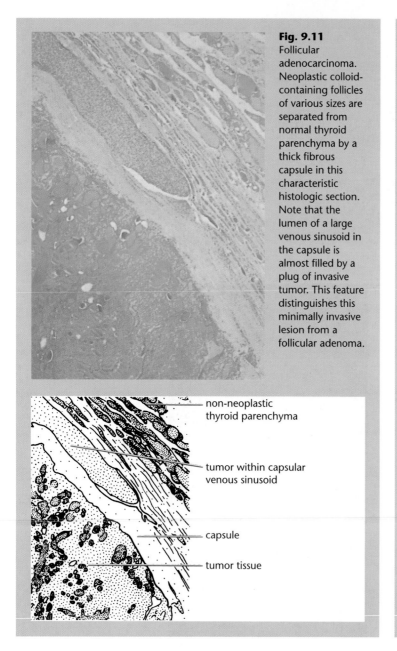

Fig. 9.11 Follicular adenocarcinoma. Neoplastic colloid-containing follicles of various sizes are separated from normal thyroid parenchyma by a thick fibrous capsule in this characteristic histologic section. Note that the lumen of a large venous sinusoid in the capsule is almost filled by a plug of invasive tumor. This feature distinguishes this minimally invasive lesion from a follicular adenoma.

non-neoplastic thyroid parenchyma

tumor within capsular venous sinusoid

capsule

tumor tissue

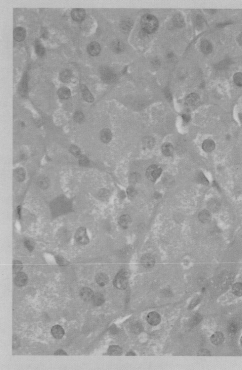

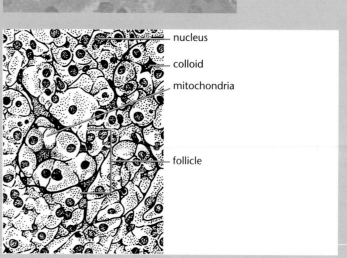

Fig. 9.12 Oxyphil follicular (Hürthle cell) adenocarcinoma. In this variant of follicular carcinoma, most neoplastic cells are large, like the polygonal cells seen here, with eosinophilic, granular cytoplasm due to proliferation of mitochondria.

nucleus

colloid

mitochondria

follicle

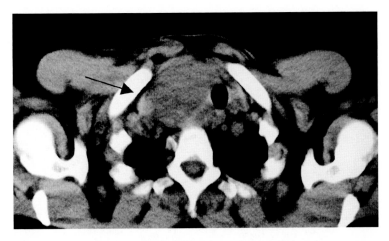

Fig. 9.13 CT scan of lymphoma of thyroid. Arrow points to lymphomatous mass which is deviating the trachea to the left. Uninvolved thyroid on the left is dense and scarred, consistent with known Hashimoto's disease.

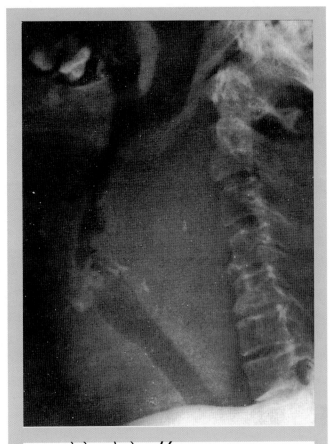

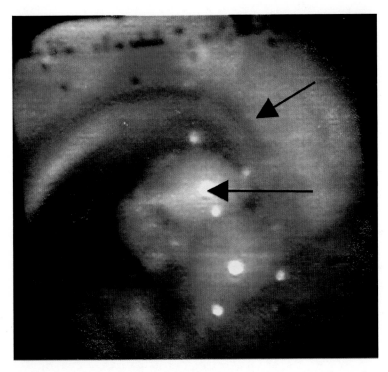

Fig. 9.14 Recurrent follicular carcinoma invading the trachea, bronchoscopic view. Outer arrow points to normal tracheal wall. Inner arrow points to exophytic tumor within the tracheal lumen.

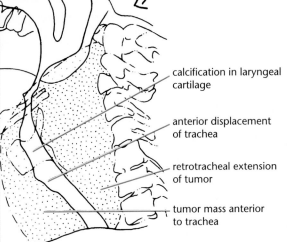

calcification in laryngeal cartilage

anterior displacement of trachea

retrotracheal extension of tumor

tumor mass anterior to trachea

Fig. 9.15 Anaplastic carcinoma. Lateral view of the neck shows massive soft tissue swelling with marked anterior displacement of the trachea, which is compressed in its anteroposterior diameter. The displacement is due to gross retrotracheal extension of the thyroid. The malignancy of the lesion was confirmed at operation.

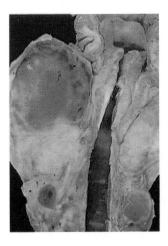

Fig. 9.16 Anaplastic carcinoma. This large, pale and focally hemorrhagic tumor has replaced most of the normal thyroid tissue and has extended directly into adjacent lymph nodes and the tracheal wall. There is an associated florid tracheitis. Extensive local invasion, often with tracheal stenosis, is a common feature of this tumor.

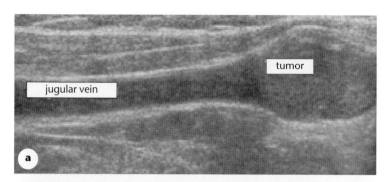

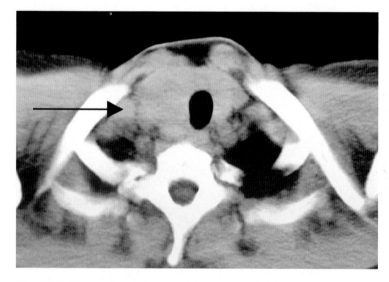

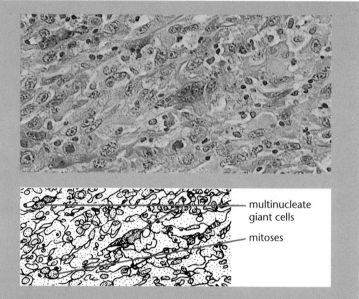

Fig. 9.18 Anaplastic carcinoma. Large spindle and giant cells with bizarre nuclei are characteristic of this type of undifferentiated carcinoma. Mitoses are numerous.

Fig. 9.17 Ultrasound of neck in patient with anaplastic thyroid carcinoma invading the right jugular vein. (**a**) Static image demonstrates the jugular vein with a large tumor thrombus. (**b**) Color Doppler showing blood flow slowed (blue) by tumor thrombus.

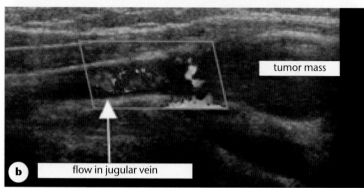

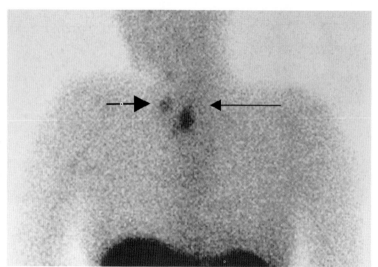

Fig. 9.19 CT scan of neck. Arrow points to metastatic leiomyosarcoma to the thyroid, with tracheal deviation to the left.

Fig. 9.20 Medullary carcinomas express somatostatin receptors. This is a scan with radiolabeled somatostatin analogue in a patient with metastatic medullary carcinoma at presentation. Short arrow points to an involved jugular lymph node. Long arrow points to the primary in the right lower lobe of the thyroid.

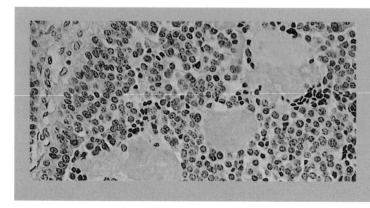

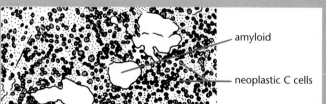

Fig. 9.21 Medullary carcinoma. The neoplastic C cells have round nuclei of regular appearance and finely granular cytoplasm. The chromatin appearance is speckled, typical of a neuroendocrine origin. Also present are amorphous intercellular masses of pink (Congo red-positive) amyloid deposits.

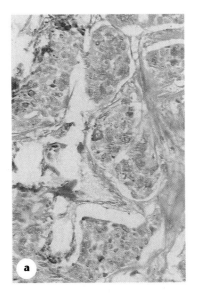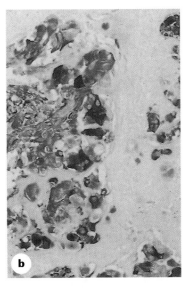

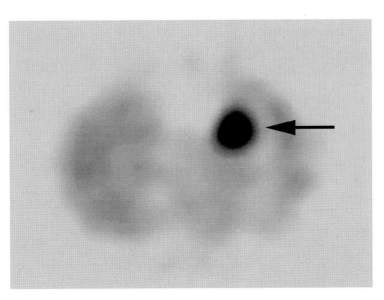

Fig. 9.22 Medullary carcinoma. Immunohistochemical stains are useful in the diagnosis of medullary carcinoma. Tumor cells are reactive for neuroendocrine markers such as (**a**) chromagranin and (**b**) calcitonin. Plasma calcitonin and CEA levels may be quite elevated.

Fig. 9.23 Medullary carcinomas may produce CEA. This is an axial view of a radiolabeled monocolonal anti-CEA scan in a woman with medullary carcinoma presenting with an enlarged mediastinal lymph node on the left and an occult primary. Arrow points to the involved mediastinal lymph node. Scan was obtained after serum CEA was noted to be elevated.

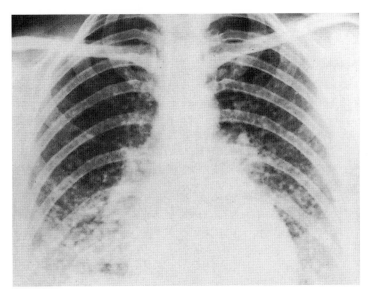

Fig. 9.24 Pulmonary metastases of thyroid cancer. This PA chest film shows many small nodular opacities throughout both lungs but most markedly at the bases. A 'snowstorm' appearance is characteristic of metastatic thyroid cancer, in this case a papillary carcinoma. Metastatic deposits may remain unchanged over a long period of time due to a very low grade of malignancy.

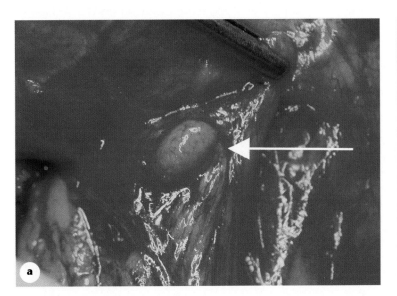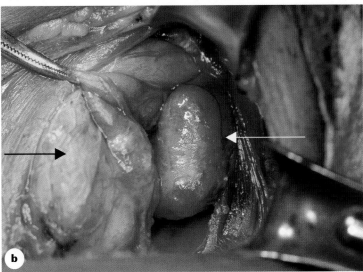

Fig. 9.25 Gross appearance of parathyroid tumors *in situ* (**a**) Arrow points to normal parathyroid gland, measuring 3 mm in longitudinal dimension. (**b**) White arrow points to a large left upper parathyroid adenoma measuring

over 1.5 cm in longitudinal dimension. Black arrow points to the normal thyroid gland.

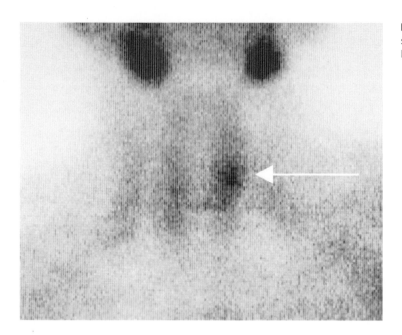

Fig. 9.26 AP view of (MIBI 99 m technetium 2-methoxy isobutylisonitrile) scan on the case in Fig. 9.25b. Arrow points to radio-intense focus in left neck. Residual MIBI can be seen in the thyroid in this delayed scan.

TUMORS OF THE ADRENAL GLAND

Tumors of the adrenal cortex can produce a wide variety of clinical syndromes, depending on the abnormal secretory ability of the particular neoplasm. The adrenal cortex may be hyperplastic or may harbor benign cortical adenomas or adrenocortical carcinomas. Hyperplasia may be diffuse or nodular and is usually bilateral. Benign adenomas are usually unilateral, as are carcinomas.

The incidence of benign adrenocortical tumors is poorly defined. However, autopsy series suggest that asymptomatic adrenal adenomas are present in 2% of adult patients, in approximately 30% of elderly, obese diabetic patients and in up to 20% of hypertensive patients. CT scans for other conditions identify unsuspected 'incidental' adenomas at the same rate. In familial MEN syndromes, the autopsy incidence of adrenal adenoma appears to be 33%. About 20% of patients with Cushing's syndrome have adrenal tumors, benign tumors being slightly more common than malignant tumors in the adult. An estimated 130 new cases of adrenocortical carcinoma are diagnosed each year in the United States, with the peak incidence occurring in the fourth and fifth decades.

MORPHOLOGY

Grossly, benign cortical adenomas are usually yellow-orange, rounded masses that may show areas of hemorrhage, cystic degeneration and calcification. Adrenocortical carcinomas are usually larger than 100 g and are often metastatic when diagnosed; they typically exhibit a considerable degree of hemorrhage, necrosis and calcification. The distinction between benign and malignant tumors is difficult to make on the basis of morphologic characteristics. However, vascular or capsular invasion and distant metastases are certain signs of malignancy, as is gross local invasion at the time of surgical resection. Although extensive necrosis, hemorrhage, numerous mitoses and cellular and nuclear pleomorphism are more likely to be seen in malignant tumors, these features are not reliable indicators of malignancy.

CLINICAL MANIFESTATIONS

Tumors of the adrenal cortex may be functional or non-functional in their ability to synthesize and secrete biologically active steroid molecules. Patients with non-functional tumors typically present with manifestations attributable to a large abdominal mass, which is palpable in less than 50% of cases. The most common presentation is on a CT scan for persistent back pain. This is typical of adrenocortical carcinomas, which are inefficient producers of steroids. Patients with functioning tumors present with features attributable to the predominant excess steroid produced (*see* Table 9.2). The hypothalamic-pituitary-adrenal (HPA) axis and the effects of its interaction with exogenous or endogenous steroids or ACTH are shown in Fig. 9.27. Also depicted are the effects on this axis of primary pituitary and adrenal tumors, as well as ectopic tumors.

Although in most cases Cushing's syndrome has either a primary pituitary or an adrenal etiology, ectopic elaboration of ACTH is also an important cause (*see* Fig. 9.27). Ectopic secretion of ACTH is usually associated with small cell lung cancer, although other tumors reported to secrete ectopic ACTH include carcinoid tumor, pheochromocytoma, medullary carcinoma of the thyroid and thymoma. Excess mineralocorticoid secretion is usually caused by benign cortical adenomas and is only rarely observed in association with adrenocortical carcinoma. Syndromes of virilization or feminization and precocious puberty are also seen in primary adrenal enzymatic disorders, as well as in primary hypothalamic, gonadal disorders and adrenal tumors.

Once the diagnosis of excess adrenocortical hormone secretion has been made, attempts at localization are undertaken. CT scanning is useful for localizing adrenal tumors and can exclude local extension from tumors of other abdominal organs. Adrenal hyperplasia is marked by bilateral enlargement, which is usually symmetric, whereas adrenal tumors are usually unilateral and can be quite massive. Examination of the inferior vena cava by CT scan can document venous invasion in some malignant tumors. Intravenous pyelography and ultrasonography have largely been supplanted by

CT. Angiography can be used to map the arterial supply of a tumor and may reveal hepatic metastases. Adrenal venous sampling, often employed when radiographic evaluation cannot localize the primary tumor, can accurately localize almost all aldosteronomas.

Recently, I^{131}-6-β-idomethylnorcholesterol (NP-59) has been used for radionuclide scanning of the adrenal gland, taking advantage of the accumulation of this cholesterol analogue in functioning adrenocortical tissue. Its major use may be in the evaluation of the solitary adrenal mass. Lateralization of the analogue to the side of the mass suggests a benign etiology; contralateral uptake is highly suggestive of a space-occupying adrenal mass, usually a metastasis. This technique can also be helpful in adrenal localization of ACTH-independent Cushing's syndrome; bilateral uptake in such cases suggests adrenocortical hyperplasia. Although a primary adrenal tumor must always be considered in the differential diagnosis of an adrenal mass, the adrenal glands are more commonly involved by metastatic disease from other primary neoplasms. The most common primary tumors metastatic to the adrenals are lung, breast, gastric, colorectal and melanoma. Although the involvement is usually unilateral, bilateral metastases sometimes occur. Adrenal insufficiency is uncommon and should be ruled out by an ACTH stimulation test. CT-guided fine-needle aspiration is of value in distinguishing between primary and metastatic tumors.

MOLECULAR BIOLOGY

Both adrenal cortical adenomas and carcinomas may contain abnormal DNA stem lines. Ploidy analyses, therefore, are not of benefit in discriminating between these two lesions. Ploidy abnormalities have been useful in predicting subsequent clinical behavior in known carcinomas. Aneuploid carcinomas are significantly associated with death from metastases while polyploid or diploid tumors are not.

Table 9.2 Clinical manifestations of functioning tumors of the adrenal cortex.

Major, steroid secreted	Clinical manifestations
Glucocorticoid	Cushing's syndrome (truncal obesity, moon facies, plethora buffalo hump, purple striae, hypertension, psychosis, impaired glucose tolerance, osteoporosis, thinning of the skin) Virilization may also occur
Mineralocorticoid	Conn's syndrome (hypertension and hypokalemic alkalosis) resulting from primary hyperaldosteronism
Androgen	Females: Virilization (clitoral hypertrophy, hirsutism, breast atrophy, deepening voice, decreased libido, and oligomenorrhea) Males: Precocious puberty
Estrogen	Males: Feminization (gynecomastia, testicular atrophy, decreased libido and impotence) Females: Precocious puberty

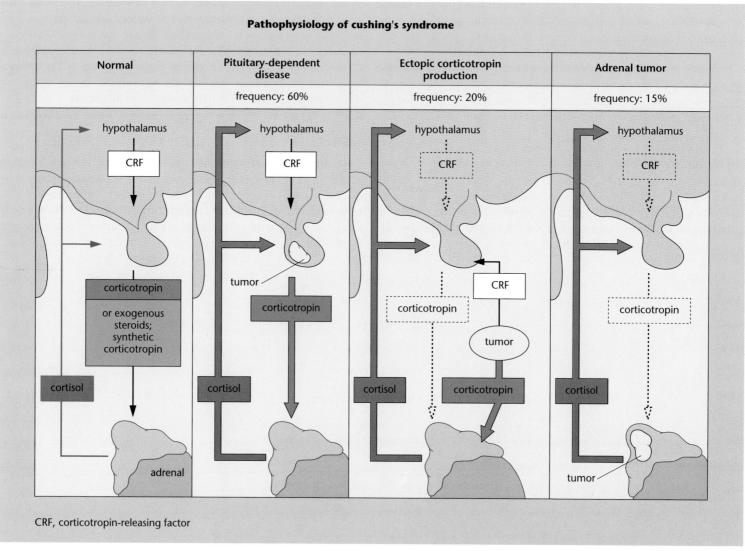

Fig. 9.27 Pathophysiology of Cushing's syndrome. (**a**) Cortisol, produced in the adrenals (or by an adrenal tumor), has a negative feedback effect on corticotropin (ACTH) production. Oral steroids have the same effect. Conversely, ACTH stimulates cortisol production and secretion, as do intramuscular injections of ACTH (as well as pituitary or ectopic tumors). (**b**) In pituitary-dependent Cushing's disease, caused by a basophil adenoma, a hypothalamic abnormality, or both, there is excessive production of ACTH. (**c**) Ectopic ACTH production by a tumor leads to enhanced cortisol production. (**d**) Raised cortisol levels are produced by an adrenal tumor.

Table 9.3 Comparison of the clinical features of pituitary and ectopic ACTH overproduction.

Features	Pituitary	Ectopic
Age	Usually under 50 years	Usually over 50 years
Sex	Predominantly women	Predominantly men
Anorexia	Rare	Always
Weight loss	Rare: often there is weight gain	Usual
Cushingoid features	Usual	Unusual
Hypertension	Occasional	Usual
Hyperpigmentation	Unusual except postadrenalectomy	Common
Serum potassium	Normal or low (usually 3–4 mmol/L)	Usually low (< 3.0 mmol/L)

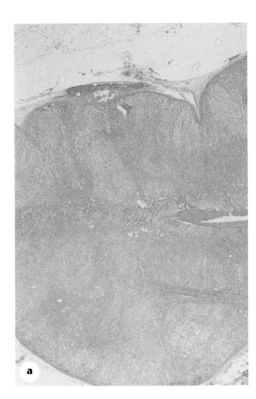
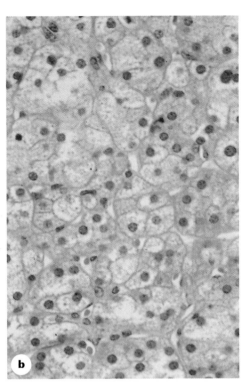

Fig. 9.28 Adrenocortical hyperplasia in Cushing's syndrome. (**a**) Low-power microscopic section shows expansion of the fasciculata and reticularis, producing a nodular and diffuse hyperplasia. (**b**) High-power view reveals a bland cytology; cells exhibit small, uniform nuclei and abundant clear cytoplasm.

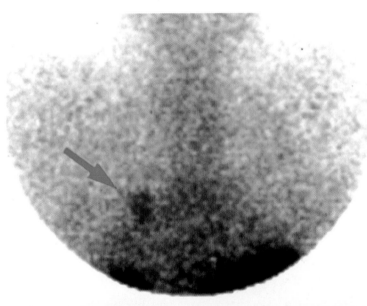

Fig. 9.29 Carcinoid tumors can express somatostatin receptors. This is an AP view of a scan with radiolabeled somatostatin analogue in a patient with ectopic ACTH syndrome. The arrow points to an occult bronchial carcinoid.

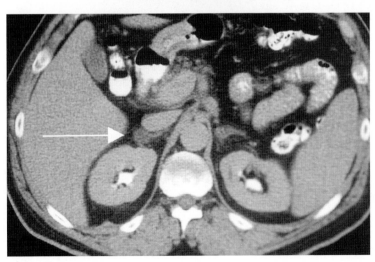

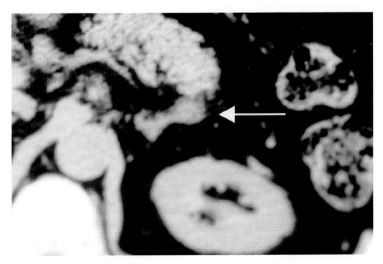

Fig. 9.30 Adrenocortical adenoma in Conn's syndrome. CT of aldosteronoma in right adrenal gland. Arrow points to lesion lying between the right kidney and the vena cava.

Fig. 9.31 Adrenal carcinoma in Conn's syndrome. Magnified CT of aldosteronoma of lateral limb of left adrenal gland. Arrow points to lesion immediately behind the pancreatic tail. In each case, the aldosteronoma was 1 cm in diameter.

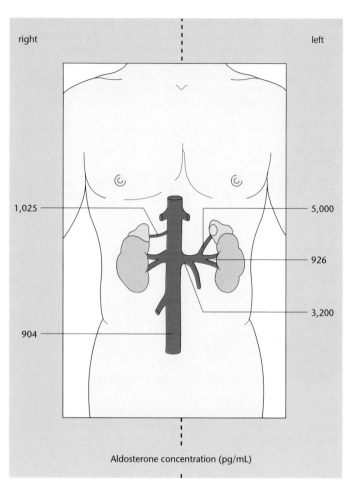

right

left

1,025

5,000

926

904

3,200

Aldosterone concentration (pg/mL)

Fig. 9.32 Adrenocortical adenoma. This diagram represents the results of an adrenal vein catheter study. The concentration of aldosterone (pg/ml) in the right adrenal vein is not significantly different from that found in the inferior vena cava. On the other hand, levels of aldosterone are high in the left adrenal vein. This patient had hypertension and hypokalemia and was subsequently cured after removal of a left adrenal tumor.

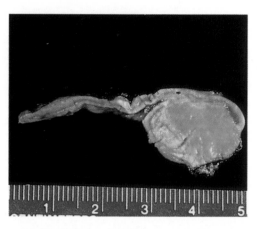

Fig. 9.33 Adrenocortical adenoma. A solitary yellow nodule arises from the thin overlying adrenal gland. The lesion is frequently encapsulated.

Fig. 9.34 Adrenocortical adenoma. Low power microscopic section shows the adrenal gland at the right overlaying adenomatous proliferations.

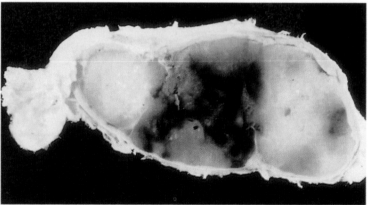

Fig. 9.35 Adrenal myelolipoma. This enlarged adrenal gland (measuring 4 × 2 × 2 cm) was an incidental finding at autopsy in a 46-year-old woman. It has been sectioned to show an attenuated rim of adrenal tissue around a well circumscribed mass of fatty tissue in which there are dark-red hemorrhagic areas, corresponding histologically to myeloid nodules. Adrenal myelolipomas are rare, usually asymptomatic, lesions, which may be detected when CT scanning is performed for staging of malignancies. CT scan often shows a low-attenuation area consistent with fat within the enlarged adrenal. Not true neoplasms, myelolipomas are believed to be hamartomatous malformations composed of adipose and hematopoietic tissue. There may be a familial tendency.

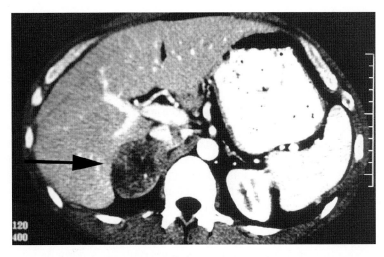

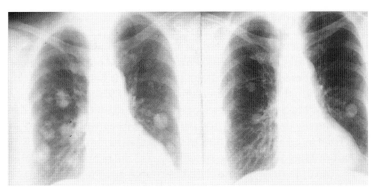

Fig. 9.37 Metastatic adrenocortical carcinoma. Chest radiograph along bilateral metastases (left). Marked decrease in metastases occurred 6 months after treatment with o,p'DDD (mitotane) (right). One year later, all metastases had regressed.

Fig. 9.36 Adrenocortical carcinoma. CT scan of 35 year-old male presenting with gynecomastia and decreased libido. Serum estrogen levels were increased. Resection of the large adrenal mass demonstrated on this CT produced instantaneous remission of his clinical syndrome.

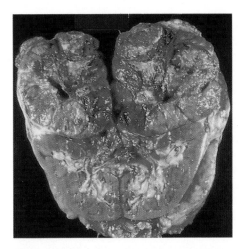

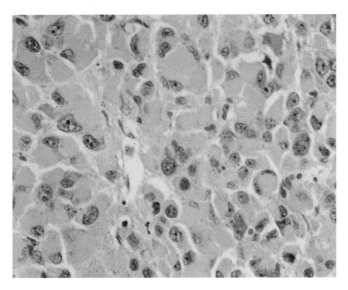

Fig. 9.39 Adrenocortical carcinoma. High-power photomicrograph shows large pleomorphic cells with abundant pink cytoplasm; the eccentric nuclei have prominent nucleoli.

Fig. 9.38 Adrenocortical carcinoma. This tumor consists of a necrotic, hemorrhagic lobular brown mass that compresses the upper pole of the kidney.

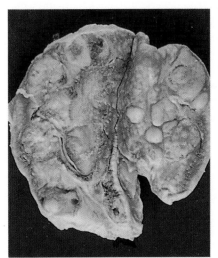

Fig. 9.40 Metastatic carcinoma. This partially bisected adrenal gland is distorted by many nodules of pale secondary tumor, some of which show necrosis or hemorrhage. The patient was a 60-year-old woman with poorly differentiated carcinoma of the lung.

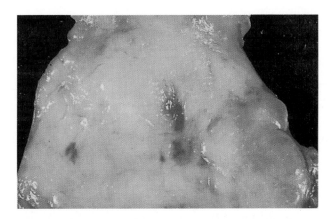

Fig. 9.41 Adrenal lymphoma. An irregular mass of pale yellowish-pink tissue has totally replaced this adrenal gland. Primary lymphoma of the adrenal gland, usually of the non-Hodgkin's type, is extremely rare. Even secondary involvement by any histologic type undergoing systemic dissemination is uncommon.

PHEOCHROMOCYTOMA

Pheochromocytoma is a neoplasm of the chromaffin cells of the sympathoadrenal system. It is, by definition, a paraganglioma of the adrenal medulla (see below). It occurs in 0.1–1% of hypertensive individuals, with an incidence rate of 0.95 per 100 000 person-years. The peak incidence occurs in the third to fifth decades, without a sex predilection. Ten percent of cases are familial and are inherited as an autosomal dominant trait, either independently or as part of MEN-II syndrome (in which case the neoplasm is bilateral in 70% of patients). Associated heritable disorders include von Recklinghausen's neurofibromatosis, von Hippel–Lindau syndrome and cerebellar hemangioblastoma.

Pheochromocytomas arise within the adrenal medulla in 90% of cases. Extra-adrenal pheochromocytomas usually occur intra-abdominally within the lower para-aortic sympathetic chains, also called the organs of Zuckerkandl. The tumors range in size from a few grams to 3 kg and are usually encapsulated, highly vascular and yellowish to reddish brown in color. Hemorrhage and/or necrosis are often present. Microscopically, the tumor is composed of clusters of finely granular and basophilic or eosinophilic cells separated by endothelium-lined spaces.

Electron microscopy identifies neuroendocrine granules containing norepinephrine or epinephrine. Only 5–10% of cases are malignant and malignancy can be confirmed only by the presence of direct extension into surrounding structures or distant metastases.

The diagnosis of pheochromocytoma is confirmed by the demonstration of excessive levels of catecholamines or their metabolites in urine or plasma. Measurements of 24-hour urinary catecholamines and their metabolites, vanyl mandelic acid (VMA) and metanephrines, remain the standard diagnostic tests. Metanephrine measurements are the most sensitive and are considered the best method of screening. One or more of these measurements are positive in 95% of cases. Pharmacologic tests, either provocative or suppressive, are rarely needed to make the diagnosis.

Localization of pheochromocytomas is most often accomplished non-invasively by use of CT or ultrasonography. Abdominal CT is positive in more than 90% of cases and allows localization of extra-adrenal pheochromocytomas. Chest radiographs may detect primary intrathoracic tumors or metastases from a malignant pheochromocytoma. I^{131}-labeled metaiodobenzyl guanidine (MIBG) scintigraphy has been very useful in localizing tumors. IMBG, an analogue of guanethidine, is taken up by adrenergic storage vesicles. Most pheochromocytomas express receptors for the hormone somatostatin. Thus, imaging with radiolabeled somatostatin analogue (octreotide) has also been useful.

The clinical manifestations of pheochromocytoma are attributable to increased release of catecholamines, mainly epinephrine. Hypertension, either sustained or episodic, is present in the majority of patients, often associated with headache, palpitations, excessive sweating, tremors, nausea/vomiting and flushing. Hypotension can be seen in some epinephrine-secreting tumors. A normal blood pressure may be associated with dopamine-secreting pheochromocytomas, which are mostly extra-adrenal. Other symptoms include orthostatic hypotension, atrial and ventricular arrhythmias, impaired glucose tolerance, constipation and symptoms of hypermetabolism such as heat intolerance and weight loss. In several studies, however, a significant proportion (15–20%) of pheochromocytomas were clinically unsuspected and diagnosed at autopsy.

PARAGANGLIOMA

The paraganglia consist of widely dispersed collections of the neural crest cells that arise in association with segmental or collateral autonomic ganglia throughout the body. The extra-adrenal paraganglionic system is divided into four anatomic groups. Tumors that arise in the branchiomeric or intravagal paraganglia are typically chromaffin negative and are therefore non-functional, whereas tumors in the aorticosympathetic paraganglia have variable chromaffinity and functional activity. Viscero-autonomic paraganglia are associated with viscera such as urinary bladder, gallbladder and intrathoracic structures.

Carotid body tumors (chemodectoma, non-chromaffin paraganglioma) are the most common of the extra-adrenal paragangliomas. They are highly vascular lesions, usually arising from and adherent to the bifurcation of the common carotid artery. They are inherited as an autosomal dominant trait. Patients typically present between the ages of 40 and 60 years with a painless, slowly enlarging mass in the upper neck below the angle of the jaw; the mass is bilateral in 2–5% of cases. The tumors are rarely functional and must be distinguished from an extra-adrenal paraganglioma arising in the cervical sympathetic chain. Although carotid body tumors are usually benign, in up to 10% of cases they may behave in a malignant fashion, invading locally.

Paragangliomas involving the temporal bone and middle ear (glomus jugulare tumors) constitute the second most common extra-adrenal paragangliomas. They usually occur in middle-aged women, who present with dizziness, tinnitus and conductive hearing loss. Cranial nerve palsies, seen in 40% of patients, result from tumor extension to the base of the brain. Less than 1% of the tumors are functional.

Vagal paragangliomas (vagal body or glomus vagale tumors) usually arise between the mastoid process and the angle of the jaw in the parapharyngeal space. Patients typically present with necrologic symptoms secondary to cranial nerve palsies (tongue weakness, vocal cord paralysis, hoarseness and Horner's syndrome). Vagal body tumors are more common in women and are multiple in 10–15% of cases. They are rarely functional and are often locally invasive, with lymph node metastases.

Mediastinal paragangliomas usually present as asymptomatic anterior or superior mediastinal masses. Posterior mediastinal paragangliomas are less common, typically occur in younger patients and are more often associated with functional activity. Metastases are seen in up to 10% of patients and locally aggressive disease in 20–30%.

Retroperitoneal paragangliomas, which typically arise adjacent to the adrenal glands, manifest in a younger age group (30–40 years) than head and neck paragangliomas. These can also occur at the aortic bifurcation in the organs of Zuckerkandl. Back pain and a palpable mass are the two most common symptoms, although 10% of patients present with metastatic disease. Functional symptoms caused by production of norepinephrine occur in 25–60% of patients. The tumors are typically large and chromaffin positive and they behave more aggressively than their adrenal counterparts. Metastases occur in 20–40% of patients, as compared with only 2–10% of patients with adrenal pheochromocytomas.

MOLECULAR BIOLOGY

Some studies have shown a greater propensity for aggressive pheochromocytomas or paragangliomas to have non-diploid DNA content. Others stress that aneuploid DNA content is also frequent in clinically benign tumors. The value of flow cytometry in the analysis of these lesions remains unclear. (See section on Tumors of the Pituitary Gland).

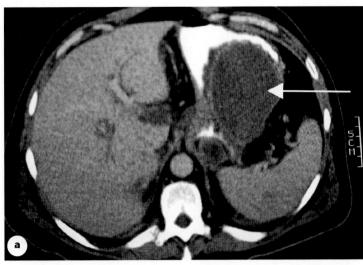

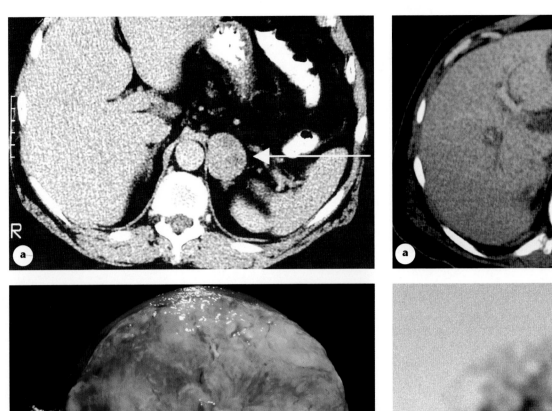

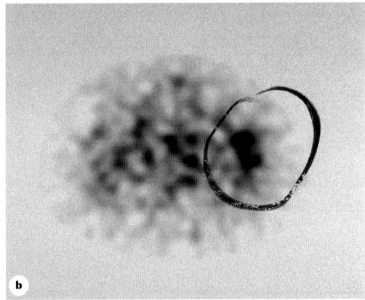

Fig. 9.42 Pheochromocytoma. (**a**) CT scan of left adrenal pheochromocytoma (arrow). Note variegated CT densities within the lesion. (**b**) Operative specimen showing well-encapsulated tumor.

Fig. 9.43 Cystic pheochromocytoma. (**a**) CT scan showing large retrogastric cystic mass (arrow). (**b**) Axial view of MIBG (123-iodine metaiodobenzylguanidine) scan showing that functional component (encircled) is lateral.

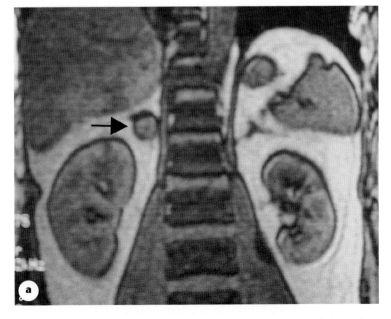

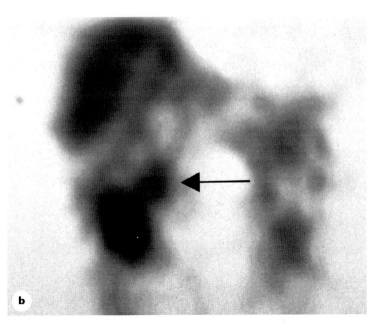

Fig. 9.44 Pheochromocytomas express somatostatin receptors. (**a**) Coronal view of MRI of right adrenal pheochromocytoma. (**b**) AP view of radiolabeled

somatostatin analogue scan demonstrating right adrenal lesion (arrow).

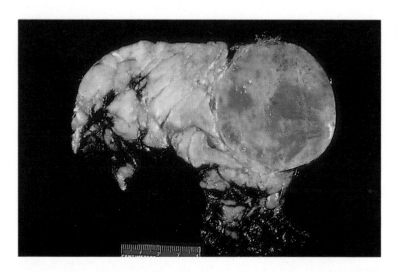

Fig. 9.45 Adrenal pheochromocytoma. A typically well-encapsulated tumor and adjacent fat (left) can be seen in this cut section of a right adrenal gland. The brown parenchyma shows areas of hemorrhage.

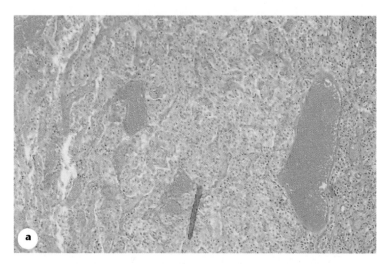

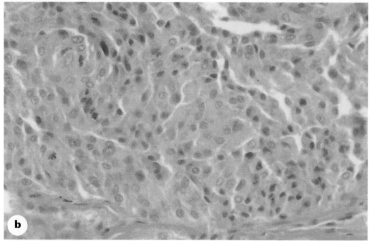

Fig. 9.46 Adrenal pheochromocytoma. (**a**) Low-power magnification shows nests of tumor cells (Zellballen) surrounded by a rich fibrovascular stroma. Dilated capillaries are packed with red blood cells. (**b**) Cells of the nests have abundant pink cytoplasm and uniform, bland nuclei. A wide range of cytologic pleomorphism may be seen.

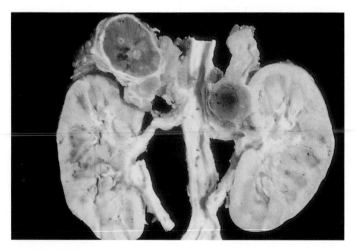

Fig. 9.47 Adrenal pheochromocytoma. This post-mortem specimen from an 11-year-old boy consists of both adrenals, with the kidneys, their vessels, and the aorta. In the medulla of each adrenal there is a typically rounded, dark-brown tumor over which is stretched a rim of normal yellow cortical tissue. Note also the atheromatous plaques in the aorta and at the origins of the arteries. The patient presented with a five-year history of intermittent attacks of acute abdominal pain associated with sweating and tachycardia. He was also found to have florid hypertensive retinopathy, marked but variable hypertension, and left ventricular hypertrophy. He died at laparotomy.

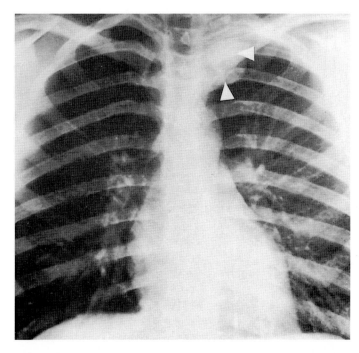

Fig. 9.48 Mediastinal paraganglioma. PA chest radiograph shows a mass with a well-defined margin in the left upper paravertebral region (arrows). The patient complained of occasional headaches and sweating but was normotensive. At operation, however, the blood pressure rose steeply while the tumor was being handled. Although histologic examination revealed what was thought to be a benign lesion, seven years later the tumor recurred in the chest and metastatic paraganglioma was found on biopsy of a skull lesion.

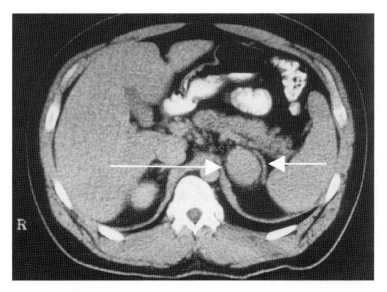

Fig. 9.49 Para-aortic paraganglioma. This CT scan demonstrates a 4 cm tumor lying to the left of the aorta just above the kidneys. Long arrow points to the tumor. Short arrow points to a laterally displaced, normal adrenal. This patient had signs and symptoms of pheochromocytoma. A benign paraganglioma was removed at surgery. If an adrenal tumor is not visible on CT scan in a patient with strong clinical evidence of a pheochromocytoma, it is probable that the tumor lies at an ectopic site along the sympathetic chain. Most such paragangliomas occur in the para-aortic region or around the renal hilum and may be visible on CT. To detect tumors at other ectopic sites or those too small to be seen on CT, venous sampling for catecholamine levels is required.

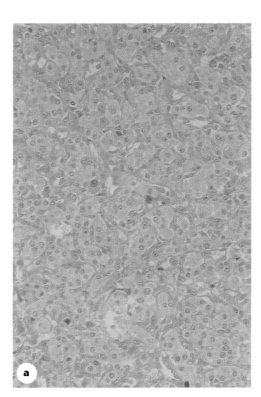

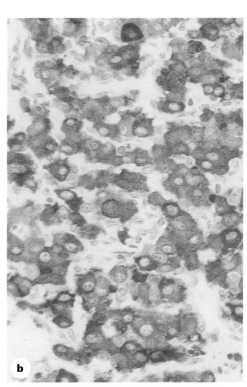

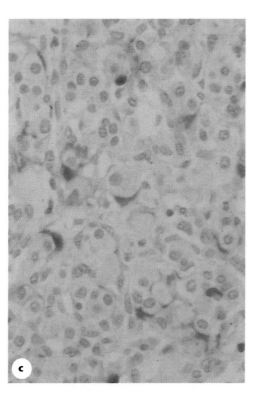

Fig. 9.50 Carotid body paraganglioma. (**a**) Nests of tumor cells (zellballen) with a well-vascularized fibrous stroma. (**b**) Immunohistochemical studies demonstrate strong positive staining for chromogranin by tumor cells.

(**c**) Supporting sustentacular cells envelope tumor nests and stain positive for S-100 protein.

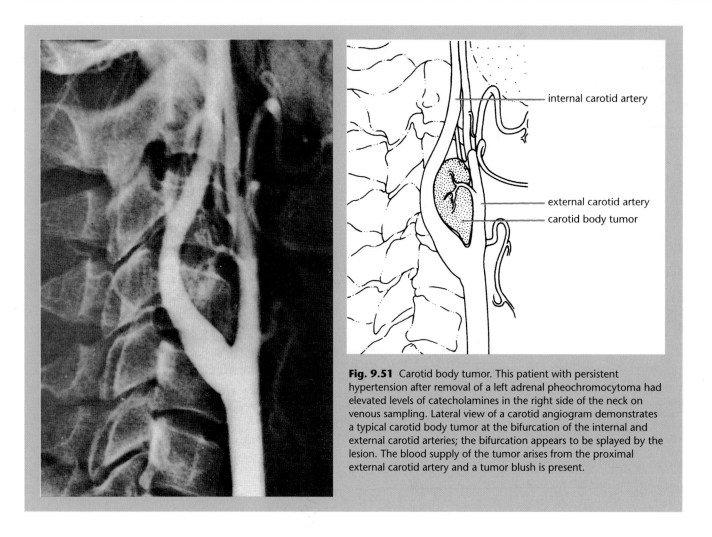

internal carotid artery

external carotid artery

carotid body tumor

Fig. 9.51 Carotid body tumor. This patient with persistent hypertension after removal of a left adrenal pheochromocytoma had elevated levels of catecholamines in the right side of the neck on venous sampling. Lateral view of a carotid angiogram demonstrates a typical carotid body tumor at the bifurcation of the internal and external carotid arteries; the bifurcation appears to be splayed by the lesion. The blood supply of the tumor arises from the proximal external carotid artery and a tumor blush is present.

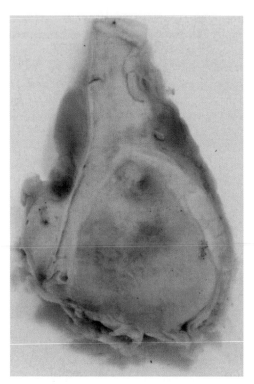

Fig. 9.52 Carotid body tumor. A 47-year-old woman had noticed a slow-growing tumor in the right side of the neck for 3 years. At surgery, this brownish, encapsulated tumor, measuring 3 cm in maximum diameter, was found to be firmly adherent to a portion of the carotid artery.

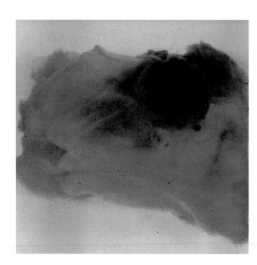

Fig. 9.53 Glomus jugulare tumor. This autopsy specimen is from a 76-year-old woman who died of bronchopneumonia. She had had a middle ear neoplasm, probably a glomus jugulare tumor, for 18 years, and had been treated with radiotherapy alone. A portion of the right petrous temporal bone is shown from which protrudes a small, rounded, pinkish tumor measuring 1 cm in diameter.

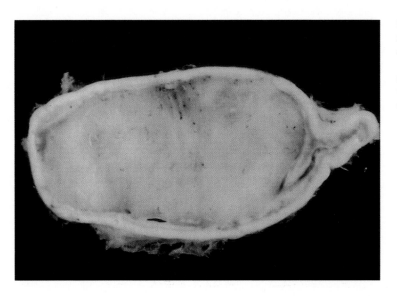

Fig. 9.54 Adrenal ganglioneuroma. This adrenal gland has been sectioned to show a well-circumscribed, grayish tumor, which was an incidental finding at autopsy of a 55-year-old man who died of bronchopneumonia. Measuring 3 × 15 × 1.5 cm, the tumor has expanded and replaced the medulla and is surrounded by a thin layer of normal cortical tissue. Ganglioneuroma is a benign adrenal medullary tumor derived from the non-chromaffin neural element. It more commonly arises elsewhere in the sympathetic chain.

TUMORS OF THE PITUITARY GLAND

The pituitary gland is of central importance because of its endocrinologic functions and its anatomic relationships. The hypothalamic-pituitary-adrenal axis (HPA) regulates the thyroid and adrenal glands as well as gonadal function, growth and development (*see* Fig. 9.27). Table 9.4 outlines the properties and biological actions of the various anterior pituitary hormones. The types of functioning and non-functioning pituitary tumors, as well as the parapituitary tumors, that must be considered in the differential diagnosis of sellar and parasellar masses are listed in Table 9.5.

Approximately 10% of symptomatic intracranial neoplasms are pituitary tumors. Asymptomatic adenomas are found at autopsy in 10–20% of presumably normal pituitary glands. The male-to-female ratio depends on the clinical syndrome produced with Cushing's syndrome and hyperprolactinemia being more common in females. Pituitary adenomas are seen in MEN I and are present in approximately 65% of cases.

HISTOLOGY

The traditional classification of pituitary tumors is based on light-microscopic evaluation of the staining properties of the cell cytoplasm and on electron microscopic and specific immunohistochemical techniques. The three recognized categories include chromophobe adenomas, which are assumed to be endocrinologically inactive, acidophilic or eosinophilic adenomas, which secrete growth hormone (GH) or prolactin and basophilic adenomas, which secret ACTH, thyroid-stimulating hormone (TSH), follicle-stimulating hormone (FSH) and β-melanocyte-stimulating hormone (β-MSH). The demonstration of hormone-specific granules in tumor cells does not necessarily correlate with secretion or with a clinical endocrinologic syndrome. Normal pituitary parenchyma is arranged in discrete nests, highlighted by reticulin stain. This architecture is disrupted in pituitary neoplasms.

CLINICAL MANIFESTATIONS

The clinical manifestations of pituitary tumors are due to one of three causes: (1) hypersecretion of a specific anterior pituitary hormone, (2) effects of an expanding mass in the sellar region or (3) symptoms related to a lack of anterior pituitary hormone secretion secondary to a compressive mass. Acromegaly, Cushing's disease and hyperprolactinemic syndrome are the most common clinical signs of hormone-producing pituitary adenomas. Mass-related symptoms are multiple because of the critical location of the pituitary adjacent to many important neural structures (*see* Fig. 9.55). Optic nerve compression with bilateral visual field loss (bitemporal hemianopsia) is the most common mass effect. Extraocular muscle dysfunction may occur as the result of compression of cranial nerves III, IV and VI. Headaches, increased intracranial pressure, seizures and cerebrospinal fluid rhinorrhea may be present. Hypothalamic dysfunction secondary to suprasellar extension of tumor may give rise to diabetes insipidus. Hypopituitarism may be due to either anterior pituitary compression or hypothalamic involvement. Sequential failure of hormone secretion leads initially to loss of gonadotropins and GH. Hypothyroidism or hypoadrenalism appear later as a result of secretory failure of TSH and ACTH, respectively. Non-functioning adenomas more commonly produce symptoms secondary to an enlarging mass. Functioning tumors are usually detected earlier because of the clinical syndromes they produce and are more likely to be microadenomas.

Pituitary adenomas are classically divided into either micro- or macroadenomas. Microadenomas are less than 10 mm in size and are usually encapsulated. Because they rarely cause local symptoms, they frequently become clinically suspected secondary to endocrine excess syndromes. Macroadenomas are greater than 10 mm in size and may be either encapsulated or invasive. These tumors are often characterized by suprasellar extension and are more likely to cause symptoms related to mass effect. Although macroadenomas may exhibit locally aggressive behavior, this does not imply malignancy. Features which may suggest a more aggressive behavior, such as necrosis or vascular invasion, are difficult to assess in the typically fragmented specimens from transsphenoidal resections. The presence of metastatic dissemination allows a clear-cut diagnosis of cancer.

The diagnosis of a pituitary adenoma is accomplished both endocrinologically and radiographically. Magnetic resonance imaging (MRI) is the modality of choice. Initially, all patients with a suspected or documented diagnosis of pituitary tumor should undergo adrenal, gonadal and thyroid function testing to evaluate the need for hormone replacement therapy. Specific stimulation and suppres-

sion tests are performed under certain circumstances for tumor detection, localization or determination of response to treatment.

MOLECULAR BIOLOGY

Ancillary studies offer little additional prognostic information beyond that gathered from histologic examination. In DNA studies, pituitary hyperplasia has been difficult to distinguish from adenomas. There has been no relationship demonstrated between ploidy and clinical behavior, including invasive growth or hormone secretion.

Table 9.4 Properties and biologic actions of anterior pituitary hormones.

Hormone	Cell type	Mean granule diameter (nm)*	Biologic action
Growth hormone (GH)	Acidophil	450	Growth of bone, muscle cartilage and connective tissue elevation of blood glucose
Prolactin (PRL)	Acidophil	550	Promotion of lactation
Follicle stimulating hormone (FSH)	Basophil	200	Female: Maturation of ovarian follicle and promotion of ovarian steroid formation Male: Promotion of spermatogenesis
Luteinizing hormone (LH)	Basophil	200	Female: Corpus luteum formation Male: Testosterone formation by interstitial cells of testis
Thyroid-stimulating hormone (TSH)	Basophil	135	Thyroid growth and hormone synthesis
Corticotropin (adrenocorticotrophic hormone) (ACTH)	Basophil	360	Adrenocortical growth and steroidogenesis
Melanocyte-stimulating hormone (MSH)	Basophil	360	Skin pigmentation; postulated role in onset of puberty

*Determined by electron-microscopic measurement.

Table 9.5 Pituitary and parapituitary tumors.

Anterior pituitary			Posterior pituitary	Parapituitary
Functioning	**Frequency (%)**	**Nonfunctioning***		
Prolactin-secreting	24	Adenoma	Ganglioneuroma	Pinealoma (ectopic)
GH-secreting	33	Carcinoma	Astrocytoma (very rare)	Craniopharyngioma
ACTH-secreting	14	Sarcoma		Chordoma
TSH- or gonadotropin-secreting	< 1			Optic nerve glioma Reticulosis Sphenoidal ridge meningioma Metastatic deposits (e.g. from breast and lung)

*Nonsecreting tumors represent the remaining 29% of anterior pituitary tumors.

Various symptoms of a pituitary tumor

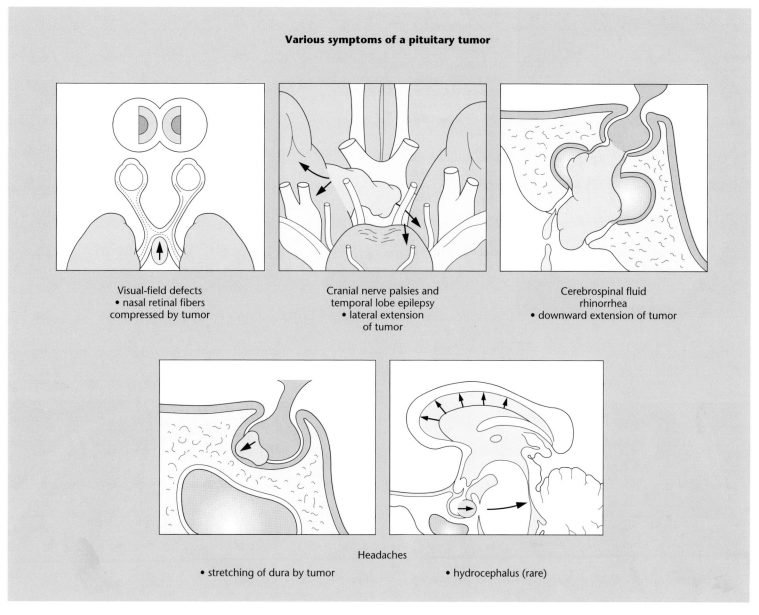

Visual-field defects
• nasal retinal fibers
compressed by tumor

Cranial nerve palsies and
temporal lobe epilepsy
• lateral extension
of tumor

Cerebrospinal fluid
rhinorrhea
• downward extension of tumor

Headaches
• stretching of dura by tumor
• hydrocephalus (rare)

Fig. 9.55 Symptoms of pituitary tumors. One source of symptoms involves the effects of an expanding mass in the sellar region. Symptoms are usually multiple because of the critical location of the pituitary to many important neural structures.

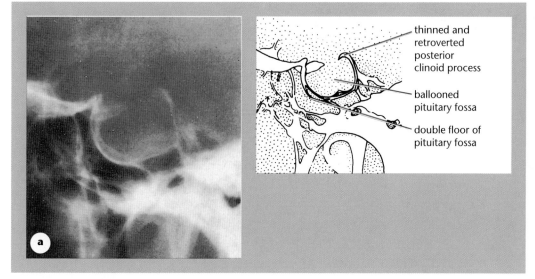

thinned and
retroverted
posterior
clinoid process

ballooned
pituitary fossa

double floor of
pituitary fossa

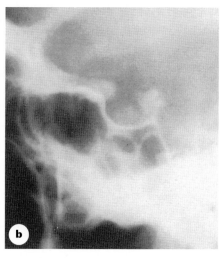

Fig. 9.56 Pituitary tumor. (**a**) Lateral skull radiograph shows ballooning of the floor of the pituitary fossa as a result of compression by an enlarging tumor mass. (**b**) The normal appearance of the pituitary fossa is shown for comparison.

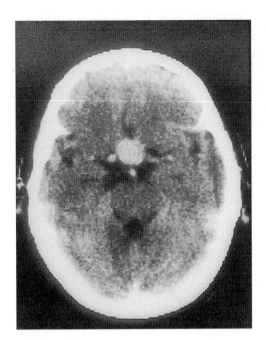

Fig. 9.57
Chromophobe adenoma. Contrast-enhanced CT scan shows a suprasellar mass in a 69-year-old man who complained of difficulty with vision in his left eye for several years. Examination suggested hypopituitarism, which was later confirmed, together with a central defect in the left eye extending temporally and reduced visual acuity. The tumor was resected.

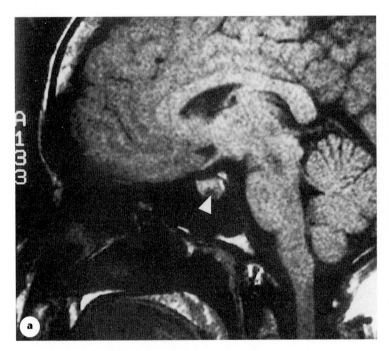

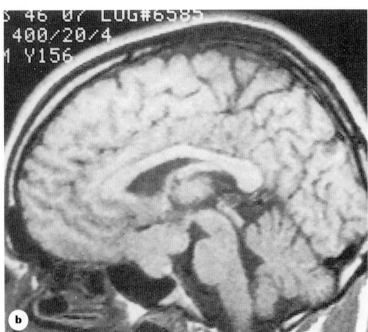

Fig. 9.58 Pituitary adenoma. (**a**) T$_1$-weighted midline sagittal MR image demonstrates a local hypointensity within the pituitary gland, representing a microadenoma (arrow). (**b**) A similar scan in another patient shows a large intrasellar mass (macroadenoma) with suprasellar extension.

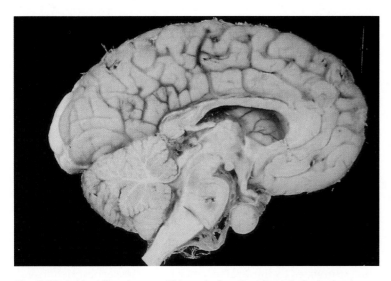

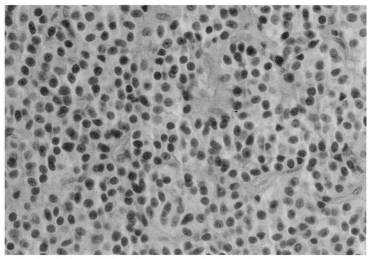

Fig. 9.59 Acidophilic adenoma. This sagittal section through the brain of a 64-year-old woman shows a well-demarcated, rounded pituitary tumor (1.5 cm in diameter) anterior to the mid-brain. The woman presented with a two-year history of visual disturbance and occipital headaches. She was found to be grossly acromegalic and hyperglycemic. Over the following 2 years she developed severe congestive heart failure and her persistent hyperglycemia became unresponsive to insulin. Eventually, she became comatose and died.

Fig. 9.60 Acidophilic adenoma. Nests of uniform cells are intermixed with a delicate vascular stroma.

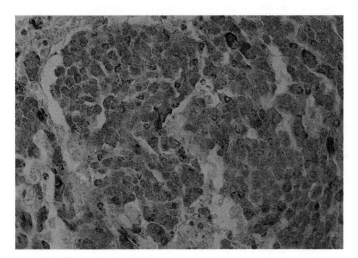

Fig. 9.61 Prolactinoma. Most of the tumor cells contain fine, brown cytoplasmic granules, thus indicating a positive immunoperoxidase reaction with anti-prolactin antibody (immunoperoxidase and hematoxylin). (Courtesy of Prof. I. Doniach).

CARCINOID TUMORS

Neuroendocrine neoplasms occur in every organ of the body, often sharing the common property of the amine precursor uptake and decarboxylation (APUD) reaction. They are a heterogeneous group of tumors, showing either neural differentiation (e.g. neuroblastomas, pheochromocytomas, paragangliomas) and/or epithelial differentiation (e.g. carcinoid tumors and neuroendocrine carcinomas). The epithelial types demonstrate a morphologic and biologic continuum, ranging from the least malignant, cytologically bland carcinoid tumors to the more aggressive, cytologically malignant, undifferentiated small cell (oat cell) carcinoma. The term 'neuroendocrine carcinoma' can be applied to the latter very aggressive small cell carcinomas; however, occasional tumors show features intermediate between carcinoid tumors and undifferentiated small cell carcinomas. These intermediate, yet aggressive tumors have been called well-differentiated neuroendocrine carcinoma, atypical carcinoid or malignant carcinoid: they are characterized by an increased mitotic rate and focal necrosis compared to typical carcinoids (*see also* Chapter 4).

Carcinoid tumors are neoplasms of argentaffin (Kulchitzky) cells, which are characterized by the APUD reaction. In 95% of cases, they arise in the GI tract but have also been reported in the larynx, lung, bronchus, thymus, esophagus, pancreas, stomach, ovary, testis and biliary tract. Autopsy series have suggested an incidence of GI carcinoids of approximately 1%, most of which are clinically occult. Within the GI tract, the most common site is the appendix, followed by the small bowel and rectum; in fact, carcinoid tumors are the most common neoplasms of the appendix and the second most common tumor of the small bowel. The incidence of malignant carcinoids is approximately 1 in 100 000, with women outnumbering men at a ratio of 1.5 : 1. Tumors may occur in any age group, but the majority of patients present in the seventh decade.

ETIOLOGY AND CLASSIFICATION

The sites of carcinoid tumors are divided according to their tissue of origin during embryologic development. Foregut carcinoids arise from the oral pharynx to the mid-duodenum; midgut carcinoids originate in the small bowel and proximal colon; and hindgut carcinoids originate in the descending colon and rectum. Foregut and midgut carcinoid tumors are frequently associated with the carcinoid syndrome, whereas hindgut tumors are only infrequently symptomatic. The small bowel is the most common site of origin of clinically significant carcinoids. Tumors smaller than 1 cm are unlikely to metastasize, whereas 80% of tumors larger than 2 cm are associated with metastatic disease, most commonly of liver, lung and bone.

CLINICAL MANIFESTATIONS

The classic symptoms of the carcinoid syndrome are flushing and diarrhea. For the syndrome to become clinically apparent, metastases to the liver from a bowel primary must be present. In the absence of hepatic metastases, the biologically active tumor products are metabolized by the liver and rendered inactive. Exceptions to this are bronchial and ovarian carcinoids, which may manifest the syndrome owing to the systemic venous drainage that bypasses the liver. It is estimated that even when liver metastases are present only about half of patients will exhibit the carcinoid syndrome. Of those patients with the carcinoid syndrome up to 50% develop cardiac complications. The average interval between the diagnosis of metastatic carcinoid tumor and the development of clinically apparent heart disease is 5 years. Although usually involvement is limited to the right heart, most often characterized by fibrosis of the right cardiac valves and endocardium, the left heart may be affected, manifesting with mitral valve disease.

Carcinoid tumors secrete a wide variety of endocrinologically active substances, including serotonin, histamine, bradykinin, prostaglandins, and vasoactive intestinal polypeptide (VIP). The predominant substance produced is serotonin, which is derived from tryptophan by hydroxylation followed by a decarboxylation step. The major metabolite of serotonin is 5-hydroxyindoleacetic acid (5-HIAA), which is excreted in the urine. Although not responsible for all the symptoms of the carcinoid syndrome, serotonin is considered to be the probable cause of the diarrhea. The carcinoid flush is caused predominantly by bradykinins. In addition to these substances, carcinoid tumors have been documented to secrete GH, ACTH and calcitonin.

The symptoms produced by carcinoid tumors may be caused by the primary tumor or by metastases. Because many of these symptoms are non-specific and are associated with no clearly abnormal physical and radiographic findings, the duration of symptoms prior to diagnosis averages 2–4 years and may be as long as 20 years. Symptoms characteristic of small bowel carcinoids include abdominal pain, nausea and vomiting. Intermittent intestinal obstruction may occur as a result of intussusception. The tumors are typically submucosal in location and the extensive desmoplastic reaction often stimulated by these tumors may lead to bowel obstruction and, rarely, to vascular compromise of the bowel. GI bleeding is unusual.

The diagnosis of functioning carcinoids, with or without the carcinoid syndrome, can be achieved by documenting elevated levels of biologically active substances produced by the tumor. The most useful test is the measurement of 5-HIAA in a 24-hour urine collection. A urine level of 5-HIAA greater than 30 mg/24 h confirms the diagnosis. In the rare patient with a foregut carcinoid that lacks the ability to decarboxylate 5-hydroxytryptophan, chromatographic measurement of 5- hydroxytryptophan can be diagnostic. Diagnosis of non-functioning carcinoids is more difficult. Abdominal masses are present in only 20% of cases. GI radiographic studies and CT scanning are useful once local symptoms have appeared. Most carcinoid tumors express somatostatin receptors, making imaging with radiolabeled somatostatin analogue a useful localization and staging modality.

MOLECULAR BIOLOGY

Studies investigating DNA content and behavior of carcinoids are infrequent. Aneuploidy does appear to be significantly associated with tumor size, nuclear atypia and lymph node and vascular involvement.

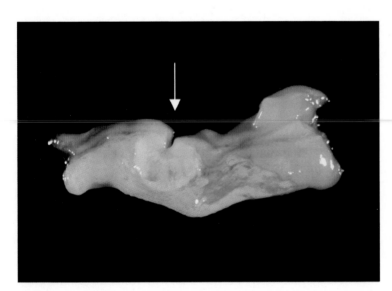

Fig. 9.62 Carcinoid tumor of distal ileum. Gross specimen shows thickening, together with angulation and tethering of mucosal folds. A nodular mass has invaded the bowel wall (arrow), causing an extensive fibroblastic response.

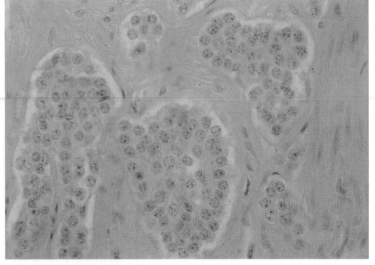

Fig. 9.63 Carcinoid tumor of small intestine. High magnification reveals characteristic solid nests of monomorphic tumor cells with ample cytoplasm. Nuclei are strikingly uniform, and chromatin is deeply stippled.

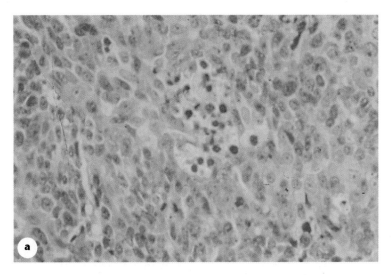

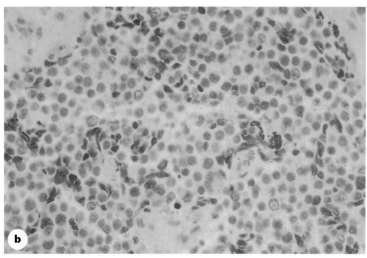

Fig. 9.64 Neuroendocrine carcinoma. (**a**) Tumor cells arranged in nests exhibit scanty cytoplasm and cell pleomorphism. Many mitotic figures and areas of focal necrosis can be seen. (**b**) Tumor cells in this extrapulmonary small cell undifferentiated (oat cell) carcinoma are marked by scanty cytoplasm and lack of a nucleolus. Note the crush artefact.

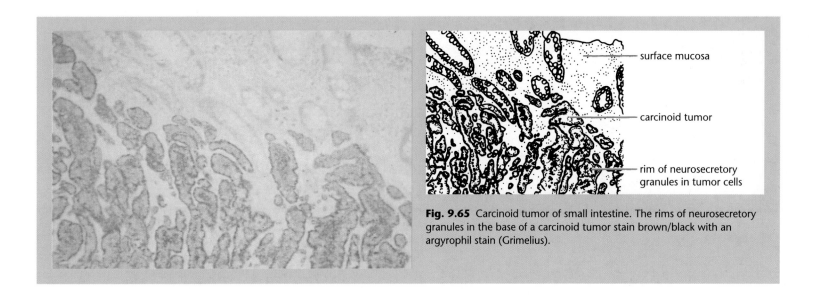

surface mucosa

carcinoid tumor

rim of neurosecretory granules in tumor cells

Fig. 9.65 Carcinoid tumor of small intestine. The rims of neurosecretory granules in the base of a carcinoid tumor stain brown/black with an argyrophil stain (Grimelius).

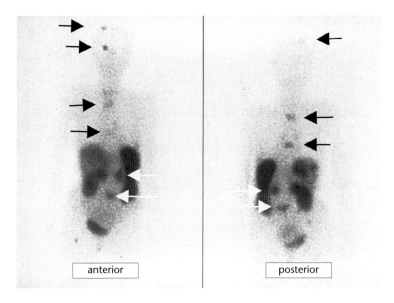

anterior

posterior

Fig. 9.66 Carcinoid tumors express somatostatin receptors. AP view of radiolabeled somatostatin receptor analogue scan in patient with widely metastatic carcinoid. White arrows indicate intra-abdominal disease, of which the lower was the ileal primary. Black arrows point to distant metastatic disease.

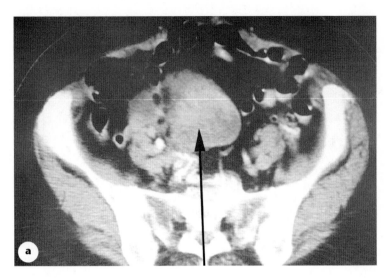

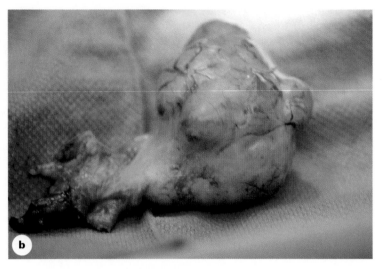

Fig. 9.67 Ovarian carcinoid. (**a**) CT scan of pelvis in older woman with flagrant carcinoid syndrome and tricuspid insufficiency. Arrow points to midline mass in low pelvis. (**b**) Operative specimen. There were no liver metastases.

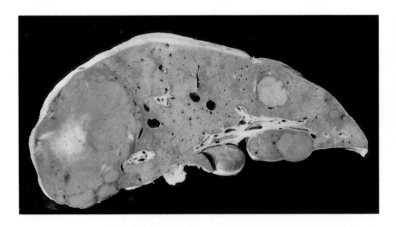

Fig. 9.68 Liver metastases. This liver specimen is from a 66-year-old woman who presented with a 30-month history of facial flushing and recent onset of swelling of the hands and feet and desquamation of the skin. She was found to have hepatomegaly and large amounts of 5-HIAA in the urine. She rapidly developed signs of tricuspid incompetence, jaundice and ascites and died shortly afterwards. At autopsy, there were carcinoid tumors in the ileum and within a Meckel's diverticulum and metastases were present in the liver and lungs. Within the liver are several discrete, rounded secondary deposits of typically yellow-brown metastatic tumor. The largest metastasis shows evidence of necrosis at its center.

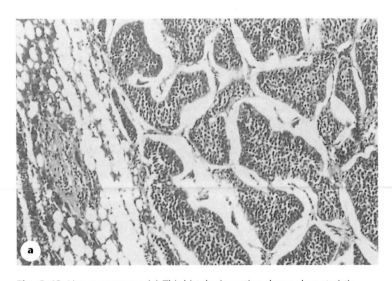

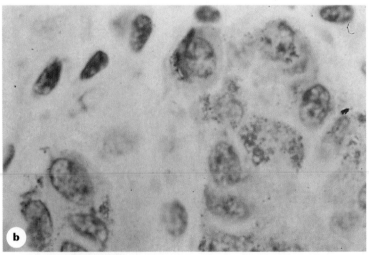

Fig. 9.69 Liver metastases. (**a**) This histologic section shows characteristic regular islands of metastatic carcinoid tumor. (**b**) With higher magnification and an alkaline diazo reaction, red-brown neurosecretory granules of a carcinoid tumor can be seen.

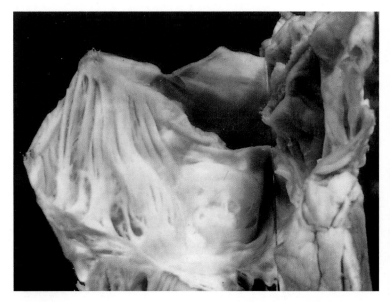

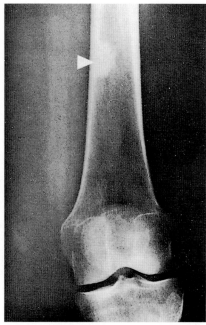

Fig. 9.71 Bone metastasis. AP radiograph of the distal femur and knee shows the typical appearance of an intramedullary blastic metastasis (arrow) from a malignant carcinoid tumor. Lytic metastatic lesions have also been described.

Fig. 9.70 Cardiac metastases. The right atrium of this postmortem specimen from a 62-year-old man has been opened to show patchy, pale endocardial thickening. The tricuspid valve (bottom right) shows similar changes. The patient presented with a one-year history of intermittent diarrhea and reddish-blue discoloration of the face. Examination revealed irregular hepatomegaly and a variable cardiac murmur. Urinary 5-HIAA was grossly elevated, presumably due to a small intestinal primary tumor with liver metastases. The patient died 15 months later. (Courtesy of the Gordon Museum, Guy's Hospital Medical School, London, UK.)

ISLET CELL TUMORS

The endocrine pancreas contains at least five types of cells, each of which produces its own polypeptide. The clinical manifestations of tumors arising from islet cells, therefore, vary according to the cell of origin (*see* Table 9.6). Islet cells are believed to be neuroectodermal in origin and are included in the APUD system.

The prevalence and incidence of islet cell tumors are poorly documented. Estimates indicate that 250 new cases are diagnosed each year in the United States and there appears to be no sex predilection. Islet cell tumors have been identified in up to 1.5% of autopsies and in the majority of cases were not clinically apparent. The peak incidence is seen in the 40–60 year age group.

Islet cell tumors of the pancreas may present with excessive hormone production or a mass effect as a result of increasing size. Of the functioning lesions, up to 70% are β-cell tumors that secrete insulin (insulinoma). A further 15% are of α-cell origin (glucagonoma) and γ-and δ-cell tumors (gastrinoma and somatostatinoma, respectively) account for up to 10%. A much smaller group of tumors secretes pancreatic polypeptide (PP) or VIP, the latter giving rise to the watery diarrhea, hypokalemia; achlorhydria (WDHA or Verner–Morrison) syndrome.

Pancreatic islet cell tumors may be multiple and may form part of the MEN-1 (Wermer's) syndrome. They are only rarely malignant. The most common malignant islet cell tumors are of probable γ-cell origin; up to 90% of gastrinomas, for example, are malignant.

The histopathologic diagnosis of malignancy is difficult and unequivocal determination requires evidence of either local invasion or distant metastases. It has become increasingly apparent that islet cell tumors often secrete multiple hormones. Immunoperoxidase histochemical techniques are useful in the diagnosis, as well as for assessment of the hormone(s) synthesized by tumors. As the tumors grow, the clinical symptoms may change because of alterations in the pattern of hormones they secrete. The clinical syndromes observed may be caused by a benign adenoma, malignant carcinoma or sometimes by adenomatous hyperplasia.

Both benign and malignant pancreatic neuroendocrine tumors may exhibit aneuploid DNA patterns. DNA ploidy analyses are unlikely to provide useful prognostic information in these tumors.

Table 9.6 Characteristics of endocrine tumors of the pancreas

Tumor type	Major, clinical symptoms	Predominant hormone	Islet cell type	Malignant (%)	Localization	Other clinical features
Insulinoma	Hypoglycemia (fasting or nocturnal)	Insulin	β	10	Usually pancreatic; rarely extrapancreatic	Catecholamine excess
Glucagonoma	Diabetes mellitus Migratory necrolytic erythema	Glucagon	α	90	Usually pancreatic; rarely extrapancreatic	Panhypoamino-aciduria Thromboembolism Weight loss
Gastrinoma	Recurrent peptic ulcer disease	Gastrin	γ	90	Usually pancreatic, but frequently extrapancreatic	Diarrhea/steatorrhea
Somatostatinoma	Diabetes mellitus Diarrhea, steatorrhea	Somatostatin	δ	80	Pancreatic and duodenal	Hypochlorhydria Weight loss Gallbladder disease
VIPoma	Watery diarrhea hypokalemia, achlorhydria (WDHA syndrome)	Vasoactive intestinal polypeptide (VIP)	δ	50	Usually pancreatic, but frequently extrapancreatic	Metabolic acidosis Hyperglycemia Hypercalcemia Flushing
PPoma	Hepatomegaly Abdominal pain	Pancreatic polypeptide (PP)	PP cells	80	Usually pancreatic; rarely extrapancreatic	Occasional watery diarrhea

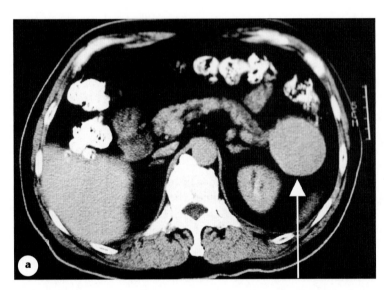

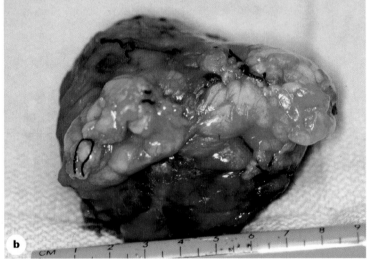

Fig. 9.72 Insulinoma. (**a**) This CT scan shows a large mass in the tail of the pancreas in a patient with symptomatic hypoglycemia and elevated insulin levels. (**b**) Operative specimen from same patient. Most insulinomas are smaller than this.

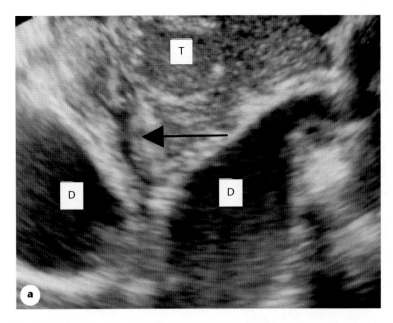

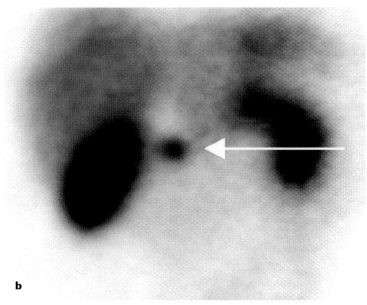

Fig. 9.73 Insulinomas are well identified by intraoperative ultrasound. Some of these lesions also express somatostatin receptors. (**a**) Intraoperative ultrasound of insulinoma of head of pancreas. T designates the tumor. D designates the duodenum. The arrow points to the distal common duct. (**b**) AP view of radiolabeled somatostatin analogue scan from same patient. Arrow points to the insulinoma.

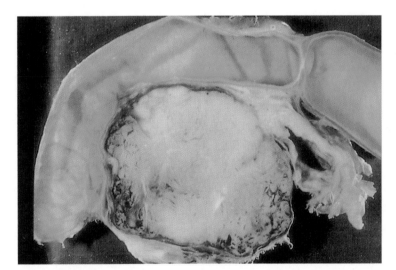

Fig. 9.74 Islet cell tumor. This specimen, comprising the pyloric canal, proximal duodenum and head of the pancreas, is from a 35-year-old woman who presented with an 8-month history of backache and intermittent abdominal pain. Following surgery, she developed hepatorenal failure and died. The head of the pancreas has been completely replaced by a circumscribed tumor measuring 7 cm in diameter and showing foci of necrosis and hemorrhage. There is no infiltration of the duodenal wall. Note the cystic dilatation of the pancreatic duct in the body of the pancreas (right) due to obstruction by tumor.

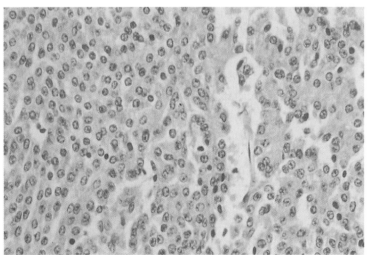

Fig. 9.75 Islet cell tumor. High-power photomicrograph shows a solid pattern of tumor cells. Malignant potential cannot be determined solely on the basis of the histopathologic features.

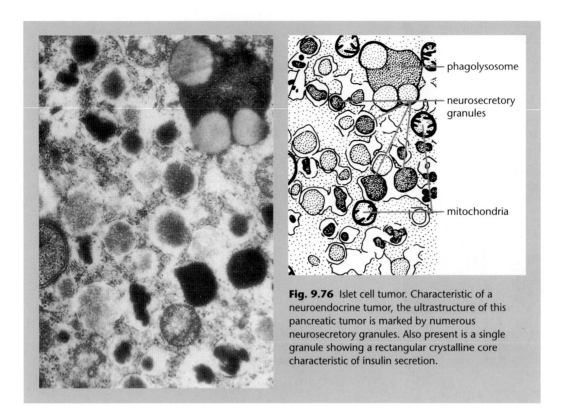

Fig. 9.76 Islet cell tumor. Characteristic of a neuroendocrine tumor, the ultrastructure of this pancreatic tumor is marked by numerous neurosecretory granules. Also present is a single granule showing a rectangular crystalline core characteristic of insulin secretion.

MULTIPLE ENDOCRINE NEOPLASIA SYNDROME

Multiple endocrine neoplasia (MEN), a syndrome inherited as an autosoma dominant trait, is characterized by tumors affecting multiple endocrine glands. Three forms of the syndrome have been identified (MEN I, MEN IIA and MEN IIB) (*see* Table 9.7). The individual endocrine neoplasms involved in the syndrome have been discussed in earlier sections.

MEN I involves principally the parathyroid and pituitary glands and pancreatic islet cells, and less commonly the adrenal and thyroid glands. Approximately 70% of patients have adenomas of two or more systems and 20% of patients develop adenomas of three or more systems. Parathyroid involvement is manifested as hypercalcemia resulting from parathyroid hyperplasia. The symptoms caused by pituitary adenomas are usually secondary to a mass effect and only a minority of patients present with acromegaly, Cushing's syndrome or hyperprolactinemia. Pancreatic islet cell tumors in MEN I are often malignant. Cushing's syndrome may be due either to a pituitary or to an adrenal tumor or to ectopic elaboration of ACTH by an islet cell tumor. Affected individuals may present with simultaneous involvement of multiple endocrine glands or several glands may become sequentially affected over a period of months to years. Continuing surveillance is necessary to evaluate each patient for new manifestations of the disease. Once a patient has been diagnosed with MEN, all family members should undergo screening.

MEN IIA, also known as Stipple's syndrome, consists of medullary carcinoma of the thyroid, which is usually bilateral, together with often bilateral pheochromocytomas of the adrenal gland in about 50% of patients. The pheochromocytoma is occasionally extra-adrenal. Associated with these in a minority of cases is parathyroid hyperplasia. Symptoms at the initial presentation are usually caused either by medullary carcinoma of the thyroid or by pheochromocytoma; only rarely are symptoms the result of hyperparathyroidism.

MEN IIB shares with MEN IIA the frequency of medullary carcinoma of the thyroid and pheochromocytomas. However, MEN IIB patients also exhibit dysmorphic features consisting of mucosal neuromas and a marfanoid body habitus. The neuromas may be found in the conjunctival, buccal mucosa and tongue, labia, larynx and GI tract. In some cases, café-au-lait spots and cutaneous neuromas are also present. Family members should be screened for serum calcitonin levels or the RET proto-oncogene, with the hope of identifying C-cell hyperplasia of the thyroid before the development of overt medullary carcinoma.

MOLECULAR BIOLOGY

A tumor suppression gene thought to be responsible for MEN I has been localized to the pericentromeric region of the long arm of chromosome 11. The gene for the MEN IIA syndrome has been mapped to a locus (or loci) spanning the centromere of chromosome 10. Restriction fragment length polymorphism analyses using polymorphic DNA probes to this region can identify carriers for this syndrome.

Table 9.7 Syndromes of multiple endocrine neoplasia (MEN).

Type	Organ	Neoplasm	Patients Affected (%)
I	Parathyroid	Hyperplasia	90
	Pituitary	Adenoma	65
	Pancreas	Islet cell	75
	Adrenal	Cortical adenoma	Rare
	Thyroid	Adenoma	Rare
	Adipocyte	Lipoma	Rare
	Multiple	Carcinoid	Rare
IIA	Thyroid	Medullary carcinoma	100
	Adrenal	Pheochromocytoma	50
	Parathyroid	Hyperplasia	20
IIB	Thyroid	Medullary carcinoma	75
	Adrenal	Pheochromocytoma	50
	Parathyroid	Hyperplasia	5
	Neuron	Mucosal neuromas; intestinal ganglioneuromas	100

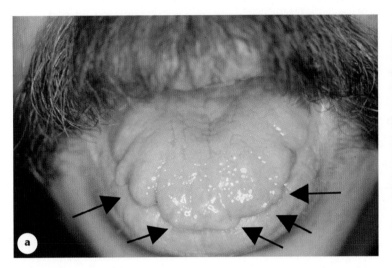

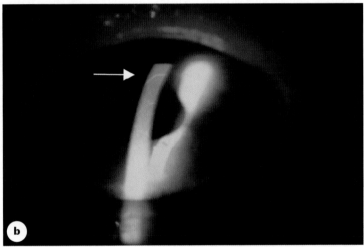

Fig. 9.77 MEN IIB. (**a**) In this patient, neuromas of lips and tongue were associated with medullary carcinoma of the thyroid and adrenal pheochromocytomas. (**b**) Prominent corneal nerves were visible with slit lamp exam (arrow).

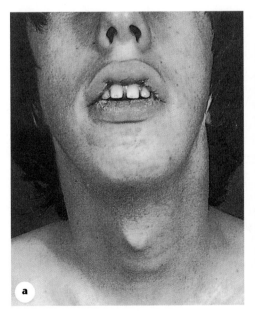

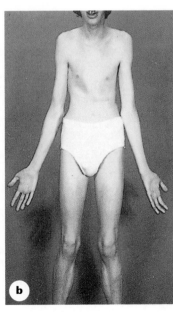

Fig. 9.78 MEN-IIB. In this patient with thyroid swelling caused by medullary carcinoma, (**a**) the lips are typically swollen and (**b**) there is a marfanoid body habitus. (Courtesy of Mr K.F. Moos.)

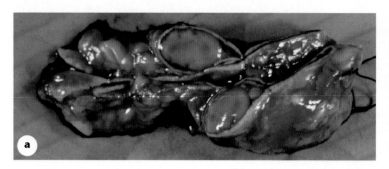
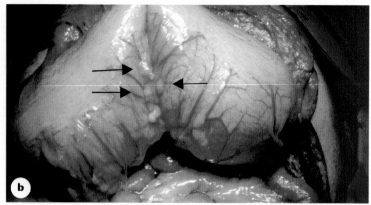

Fig. 9.79 MEN II-B. (**a**) Operative specimen showing multiple adrenal pheochromocytomas. (**b**) Operative photograph showing neuromas of a megacolon (arrows).

REFERENCES

Benker G, Olbricht T, Reinwein D, *et al.*: Survival rates in patients with differentiated thyroid carcinoma. Cancer 1990; 65 : 1517–1520.

Boggild MD, Jenkinson S, Pistorella M, *et al.*: Molecular genetic studies of sporadic pituitary tumors. J Clin Endocrinol Metab 1994; 78 : 387–392.

Bystrom C, Larsson C, Blomberg C, *et al.*: Localization of the MEN I gene to a small region within chromosome 11q13 by deletion mapping in tumors. Proc Natl Acad Sci USA 1990; 87 : 1968–1972.

Copeland RM: The incidentally discovered adrenal mass. Ann Intern Med 1983; 98 : 940–945.

Dobashi Y, Sugimura H, Sakamoto A, *et al.*: Stepwise participation of p53 gene mutation during dedifferentiation of human thyroid carcinomas. Diagn Mol Pathol 1994; 3 : 9–14.

Eng C, Smith DP, Mulligan LM, *et al.*: A novel point mutation in the tyrosine kinase domain of the RET proto-oncogene in sporadic medullary thyroid carcinoma and in a family with FMTC. Oncogene 1995; 10(3):509–513.

Flemming I, Cooper J, Henson D, *et al.*: AJCC Cancer, Staging Manual, 5th edn. Lippincott, Philadelphia, 1997.

Friesen SR: Tumors of the endocrine pancreas. N Engl J Med 1982; 306 : 508–590.

Jhiang SM, Mazzaferri EL: The ret/PTC oncogene in papillary thyroid carcinoma. J Lab Clin Med 1994; 123 : 331–337.

Katoh R, Bray CE, Suzuki K, *et al.*: Growth activity in hyperplastic and neoplastic human thyroid determined by an immunohistochemical staining procedure using monoclonal antibody MIB-I. Human Pathol 1995; 26 : 139–146.

Keren DF, Hanson CA, Hurtubise PE: Flow Cytometry and Clinical Diagnosis. American Society of Clinical Pathology, Chicago, 1994.

Kifor O, Moore FD Jr, Wang P, *et al.*: Reduced expression of the extracellular Ca^{2+}-sensing receptor in primary and uremic secondary hyperparathyroidism. J Clin Endo Metab 1996; 81 : 1598–1606.

Lack EE: Pathology of Adrenal and Extra-Adrenal Paraganglia. Major Problems in Pathology, vol 29. Saunders, Philadelphia, 1994.

Luton JP, Cerdas S, Billaud L: Clinical features of adrenocortical carcinoma, prognostic factors, and the effects of mitotane therapy. N Engl J Med 1990;322 : 1195–1201.

Mikhail RA, Moore JB, Reed DN, *et al.*: Malignant retroperitoneal paragangliomas. J Surg Oncol 1986; 5 : 1503–1522.

Moertel CA: An odyssey in the land of small tumors. J Clin Oncol 1987; 1503–1522.

Mulligan LM, Gardner E, Smith BA, *et al.*: Genetic events in tumour initiation and progression in multiple endocrine neoplasia type 2. Genes Chrom Cancer 1993; 6 : 166–177.

Nilsson O, Wangberg B, Kolby L, *et al.*: Expression of transforming growth factor alpha and its receptor in human neuroendocrine tumors. Int J Cancer 1995; 60 : 645–651.

Pilato FP, D'Adda T, Banchini E, *et al.*: Nonrandom expression of polypeptide hormones in pancreatic endocrine tumors. Cancer 1988; 61 : 1815–1820.

Pipeleers-Marichal M, Somers G, Willems G, *et al.*: Gastrinomas in the duodenums of patients with multiple endocrine neoplasia type I and Zollinger-Ellison syndrome. N Engl J Med 1990; 322 : 723–727.

Redman BG, Pazdur R, Zingas AP, *et al.*: Prospective evaluation of adrenal insufficiency in patients with adrenal metastasis. Cancer 1987; 60 : 103–107.

Remick SC, Hafez GR, Carbone PP: Extrapulmonary small cell carcinoma: a review of the literature with emphasis on therapy and outcome. Med 1987; 66 : 457–471.

Saad MF, Ordonez NG, Rashid RK, *et al.*: Medullary carcinoma of the thyroid. A study of the clinical features and prognostic factors in 161 patients. Medicine 1984; 63 : 319–342.

Samaan NA, Hickey RC: Adrenal cortical carcinoma. Semin Oncol 1987; 14 : 292–296.

Samaan NA, Hickey RC: Pheochromocytoma. Semin Oncol 1987; 14 : 297–305.

Sobol H, Narod SA, Nakamura Y, *et al.*: Screening for multiple endocrine neoplasia type 2a with DNA-polymorphism analysis. N Engl J Med 1989; 31 : 996–1000.

Simpson WJ, McKinney SE, Carruthers JS, *et al.*: Papillary and follicular thyroid cancer: prognostic factors in 1,578 patients. Am J Med 1989;83: 479–488.

Wolfe MM, Jensen RT: Zollinger-Ellison syndrome. N Engl J Med 1987; 317 : 1200–1209.

Yeh JJ, Lunetta KL, van Orsouw NJ, *et al.*: Somatic mitochondrial DNA (mtDNA) in papillary thyroid carcinomas and differential mtDNA sequence variants in malignant and benign thyroid tumors. Oncogene 2000; 19 : 2060.

FIGURE CREDITS

The following books published by Gower Medical Publishing are sources of figures in the present chapter. The figure numbers given in the listing are those of the figures in the present chapter. The page numbers (or slide numbers) given in parentheses are those of the original publication.

Besser GM, Cudworth AG: Clinical Endocrinology. Lippincott/Gower Medical Publishing, Philadelphia/London, 1987: Figs 9.5 (p 14.4), 9.9 (p 14.4), 9.10 (p 14.4), 9.11 (p 14.5), 9.12 (p 20.19), 9.15 (p 14.6), 9.14 (p 14.6), 9.22 (p 20.20), 9.28 (p 9.4), 9.34 (p 20.10), 9.40 (p 9.8), 9.46 (p 20.13), 9.42 (p 20.12), 9.53 (p 2.2), 9.54 (p 2.8), 9.58 (p 2.3), 9.59 (p 20.16), 9.63 (p 20.11), 9.64 (p 20.16), 9.62 (p 20.16), 9.71 (p 20.15), 9.75 (p 9.7), Table 9.2 (p 19.5), Table 9.3 (p. 9.4), Table 9.4 (p 2.9), Table 9.6 (p 20.15).

Cawson RA, Eveson JW: Oral Pathology and Diagnosis. Heinemann Medical Books/Gower Medical Publishing, London, 1987: Fig. 9.76 (p 10.13).

Fletcher CDM, McKee PH: An Atlas of Gross Pathology. Edward Arnold/Gower Medical Publishing, London, 1987: Figs 9.4 (p 57), 9.8 (p 57), 9.16 (p 58), 9.38 (p 60), 9.39 (p 61).

Kassner EG (ed): Atlas of Radiologic Imaging. Lippincott/Gower Medical Publishing, Philadelphia/New York, 1989: Figs 9.2 (p 12.34), 9.3 (p 12.45), 9.6 (p 12.33), 9.7 (p 12.33) Fig 9.35 (p 8.28).

Perkin GD, Rose FC, Blackwood W, *et al.*: Atlas of Clinical Neurology. Lippincott/Gower Medical Publishing, Philadelphia/London, 1986: Table 9.5 (p 9.16)

Price AB, Morson BC, Scheuer PJ (eds): Alimentary system. In: Turk JL, Fletcher CDM, eds: RCSE Slide Atlas of Pathology. Gower Medical Publishing, London, 1986: Fig. 9.63 (slide 323).

Sommers SC (ed): Endocrine system. In: Turk JL, Fletcher CDM, eds: RCSE Slide Atlas of Pathology. Gower Medical Publishing, London, 1986: Figs 9.33 (slide 50), 9.45 (slide 44), 9.48 (slide 48) 9.50 (slide 53), 9.51 (slide 55), 9.56 (slide 3), 9.65 (slide 323), 9.70 (slide 56).

Sarcomas of soft tissue and bone

George D. Demetri, Karen H. Antman

10

SARCOMAS

Sarcomas are a complex and heterogeneous family of malignancies which have histologic origins in mesenchymal tissues. As opposed to carcinomas, which represent malignancies of epithelial tissues, sarcomas are neoplastic disorders which differentiate into lineages related to so-called 'connective tissues', broadly including bone, fat, stromal supportive cells (such as fibroblasts), cartilage and blood vessels. The term 'sarcoma' is derived from the Greek root *sarc* (flesh) and the suffix *-oma* (tumor). Sarcasm, a flesh-tearing criticism, and sarcophagus, a carrier for a body, are based on the same root.

Although uncommon, sarcomas are highly informative about the mechanisms of human neoplasia. Virtually no class of human solid tumors has yielded as many tumor-specific clues as to specific molecular aberrancies linked to the tumor as in the field of sarcoma research. Tumor-selective and even tumor-specific chromosomal translocations have been defined for several different types of sarcomas. Identification of these molecular pathways of cancer has had both diagnostic and therapeutic impact. For example, the relationship between Ewing's sarcoma and primitive neuroectodermal tumor was identified because these entities shared a common cytogenetic aberrancy. The best example of the therapeutic impact of this knowledge has been the development of STI571 (Imatinib mesylate, Gleevec) as a novel molecularly targeted treatment for the previously untreatable gastrointestinal stromal tumors (GISTs) (Tuveson *et al.*, 2001; Joensuu *et al.*, 2001; Blanke *et al.*, 2001; van Oosterom *et al.*, 2001). It is hoped that with additional knowledge of these mechanisms derived from sarcomas, lessons will be learned which will have an impact on developing therapies for other types of malignancies beyond sarcomas themselves.

Sarcomas of soft tissue and bone currently represent 1% of adult malignancies but disproportionately affect children, comprising 15% of pediatric malignancies. The sex predominantly affected differs considerably among the histologic variants. For example, 70% of patients with Kaposi's sarcoma are male, as are 60% of those with liposarcoma and embryonal rhabdomyosarcoma, 35% with leiomyosarcoma and 10% with lymphangiosarcoma. Sarcomas develop in individuals of all ages. Embryonal rhabdomyosarcoma generally occurs in children and adolescents under 20 years of age; synovial sarcoma, osteosarcoma, alveolar rhabdomyosarcoma and Ewing's sarcoma arise in adolescents and young adults, while leiomyosarcoma, chondrosarcoma and gastrointestinal stromal tumors typically occur in patients over 50 years of age.

Sarcomas are traditionally classified in two major groupings: those arising in bone or cartilage and those originating in soft tissue. Soft tissue sarcomas can be further subdivided based upon the anatomic site of origin: for example, those that develop in the extremities and retroperitoneum versus those arising in visceral and parenchymal organs (such as gastrointestinal and gynecologic sarcomas). Clinicopathologic entities such as the sporadic variant of Kaposi's sarcoma, the HIV-associated Kaposi's sarcoma and mesotheliomas are often grouped with soft tissue sarcomas. However, these entities have distinct presentations and characteristic natural histories.

Table 10.1 Most common histologies of bone and soft tissue sarcomas[a].

Bone sarcomas	Frequency (%)	Soft tissue sarcomas	Frequency (%)
Osteosarcoma	45	Leiomyosarcoma	29
Chondrosarcoma	22	Malignant fibrous histiocytoma	20
Ewing's sarcoma	13	Liposarcoma	8
Chordoma	9	Fibrosarcoma	6
Fibrosarcoma	7	Synovial sarcoma	5
Malignant fibrous histiocytoma	2	Rhabdomyosarcoma	5
Angiosarcoma	1	Carcinosarcoma	5
Other	1	Malignant giant cell tumor	4
		Malignant schwannoma	4
		Endometrial stromal sarcoma	4
		Mixed mesodermal sarcoma	3
		Angiosarcoma	2
		Other[b]	5

[a]The relative percentages of bone sarcomas are from patients with bone sarcoma described by Dahlin (1978).
The percentages of soft tissue sarcomas are taken from unpublished data from the Dana–Farber, Cancer Institute.
[b]≤ 1% each: hemangiopericytoma, extraskeletal chondrosarcoma, extraskeletal osteosarcoma, mesenchymoma.

Table 10.2 Classification of malignant tumors and tumor-like lesions of bone and soft tissue by tissue of origin.

Tissue of origin	Benign lesion	Malignant lesion
Bone-forming	Osteoma Osteoid osteoma Osteoblastoma	Osteosarcoma (and variants) Juxtacortical osteosarcoma (and variants)

Cartilage-forming	Enchondroma (chondroma)
	Periosteal (juxtacortical chondroma)
	Enchondromatosis (Ollier's disease)
	Osteochondroma
	Osteocartaginous exostosis
	Chondromyxoid fibroma
	Chondroblastoma
		Chondrosarcoma (central)
		  Conventional
		  Mesenchymal
		  Clear cell
		  Dedifferentiated
		Chondrosarcoma (peripheral)
		  Periosteal (juxtacortical)

Fibrous and fibrohistiocytic	Fibrous cortical defect (metaphyseal fibrous defect) Nonossifying fibroma Benign fibrous histiocytoma Fibrous dysplasia Periosteal desmold Desmoplastic fibroma Osteofibrous dysplasia Ossifying fibrona (Sissons' lesion)	Fibrosarcoma Malignant fibrous histiocytoma
Vascular	Hemangioma Glomus tumor Hemangiopericytoma Cystic angiomatosis	Angiosarcoma Hemangioendothelioma Hemangiopericytoma Kaposi's sarcoma
Bone marrow (hematopoietic and lymphatic)	Giant cell tumor (osteoclastoma) Eosinophilic granuloma Lymphangioma Histiocytosis X	Malignant giant cell tumor Non-Hodgkin's lymphoma Hodgkin's disease Leukemia (myeloid or lymphoid) Myeloma (plasmacytoma) Lymphangiosarcoma Malignant histiocytosis
Neural	Neurofibroma Neurilemmoma Neurofibromatosis	Malignant schwannoma (and other malignant peripheral nerve sheath tumors) Peripheral neuroectodermal tumor Ewing's sarcoma Desmoplastic small round cell tumor Others*
Notochord		Chordoma
Smooth muscle	Leiomyoma (fibroid)	Leiomyosarcoma
Striated muscle	Rhabdomyoma	Rhabdomyosarcoma
Fat	Lipoma	Liposarcoma
Synovium	Synovial chondromatosis	Synovial sarcoma
Mesothelium	Benign mesothelioma	Malignant mesothelioma
Unknown	Simple bone cyst Aneurysmal bone cyst Intraosseous ganglion	Adamantinoma

*Askin's tumor of chest wall; ganglioneuroma; neuroblastoma; pheochromocytoma; malignant neuroepithelioma

Table 10.3 Molecular biologic and cytogenetic abnormalities of sarcomas.

Tumor type	Cytogenic aberrancy	Molecular genetic abnormality
Ewing's sarcoma (EWS) pNET Askin tumor	t (11;22) in 80% of cases	Novel fusion protein chimera of EWS and FL-1
Desmoplastic small round cell tumor (DSRCT)	(21,22) rearrangement	Hybrid chimeric EWS and WTI in DSRCT
Clear cell sarcoma (former misnomer was malignant melanoma of soft parts)	t (12;22)	Unknown
Lipoma	t (12; variety)	Unknown
Myxoid liposarcoma	t (12;16)	Fusion transcript of GADD153 (also known as CHOP) with FUS (homologous to EWS)
Synovial sarcoma	t (X;18)	Unknown
Poor-prognosis soft tissue sarcomas	Loss of heterozygosity at p53 locus (chromosome 17p13.1)	p53 mutations (overexpression)
Alveolar rhabdomyosarcomas	t (2;13) in 50% of cases	Rearrangement and chimeric fusion of PAX3 DNA-binding domain to a chromosome 13 gene of unknown function
Embryonal rhabdomyosarcoma	Loss of 11p15.5 locus	Loss of chromosome tumor-suppressor gene function
Malignant peripheral nerve sheath tumors		
• with neurofibromatosis 1	t (17; variety)	Loss of function of NFI tumor-suppressor gene and neurofibromin
• with neurofibromatosis 2	t (22; variety)	Loss of function of unknown tumor suppressor gene

Definition of TNM

Primary tumor (T)

TX   Primary tumor cannot be assessed

T0   No evidence of primary tumor

T1   Tumor confined within the cortex

T2   Tumor invades beyond the cortex

Regional lymph nodes (N)

NX   Regional lymph nodes cannot be assessed

N0   No regional lymph node metastasis

N1   Regional lymph node metastasis

Distant metastasis

MX   Presence of distant metastasis cannot be assessed

M0   No distant metastasis

M1   Distant metastasis

Histopathologic grade (G)

GX   Grade cannot be assessed
G1   Well differentiated
G2   Moderately differentiated
G3   Poorly differentiated
G4   Undifferentiated

Histopathologic type

Tumors included in the analysis are listed below

A   Bone forming
    Osteosarcoma (osteogenic sarcoma)
B   Cartilage-forming
    Chondrosarcoma
    Mesenchymal chondrosarcoma
C   Giant cell tumor
D   Ewing's sarcoma
E   Vascular tumors
    Hemangioendothelioma
    Hemangiopericytoma
    Angiosarcoma
F   Connective Tissue tumors
    Fibrosarcoma
    Liposarcoma
    Malignant mesenchymoma
    Undifferentiated sarcoma
G   Other tumors
    Chordoma
    Adamatinoma of long bones

Stage grouping

Stage 1A	G1,2	T1	N0	M0
Stage 1B	G1,2	T2	N0	M0
Stage IIA	G3,4	T1	N0	M0
Stage IIB	G3,4	T2	N0	M0
Stage III		Not defined		
Stage IVA	Any G	Any T	N1	M0
Stage IVB	Any G	Any T	Any N	M1

The TNM staging system is based upon determination of the tumor type and histologic grade of the primary tumor, and if submitted, regional lymph nodes or distant metastases (From AJCC: Manual for Staging of Cancer, 4th edn. Lippincott, Philadelphia, 1993.)

Fig. 10.1 Staging of sarcomas of bone. The TNM staging system is based upon determination of the tumor type and histologic grade of the primary tumor and, if examined, regional lymph nodes as well as the presence or absence of distant metastases.

Definition of TNM

Primary tumor (T)

TX   Primary tumor cannot be assessed
T0   No evidence of primary tumor
T1   Tumor 5cm or less in greatest dimension
T2   Tumor more than 5cm in greatest dimension

Regional lymph nodes (N)

NX   Regional lymph nodes cannot be assessed
N0   No regional lymph node metastasis
N1   Regional lymph node metastsis

Distant metastasis (M)

MX   Presence of distant metastasis cannot be assessed
M0   No distant metastasis
M1   Distant metastasis

Histopathologic grade (G)

After the histologic type has been determined, the tumor should be graded according to morphologic criteria of malignancy, including cellularity, cellular pleiomorphism, mitotic activity, and necrosis. The amount of intercellular substance, such as collagen or mucoid material, should be considered in assessing grade.

GX   Grade cannot be assessed
G1   Well differentiated
G2   Moderately differentiated
G3   Poorly differentiated
G4   Undifferentiated

Histopathologic type

Commonly used categories for histopathologic type are listed below:
Alveolar soft-part sarcoma
Angiosarcoma
Epithelioid sarcoma
Extraskeletal chondrosarcoma
Extraskeletal osteosarcoma
Fibrosarcoma
Leiomyosarcoma
Liposarcoma
Malignant fibrous histiocytoma
Malignant hemangiopericytoma
Malignant mesenchymoma
Malignant schwannoma
Rhabdomyosarcoma
Synovial sarcoma
Sarcoma, NOS

Stage grouping

Stage IA	G1	T1	N0	M0
Stage IB	G1	T2	N0	M0
Stage IIA	G2	T1	N0	M0
Stage IIB	G2	T2	N0	M0
Stage IIIA	G3,4	T1	N0	M0
Stage IIIB	G3,4	T2	N0	M0
Stage IVA	Any G	Any T	N1	M0
Stage IVB	Any G	Any T	Any N	M1

The TNM staging system is based upon determination of the tumor type and histologic grade of the primary tumor, and if submitted, regional lymph nodes or distant metastases (From AJCC: Manual for Staging of Cancer, 4th edn. Lippincott, Philadelphia, 1993.)

Fig. 10.2 Staging of sarcomas of soft tissue. The TNM staging system is based upon determination of the tumor type and histologic grade of the primary tumor and, if examined, regional lymph nodes as well as the presence or absence of distant metastases.

SARCOMAS OF BONE AND CARTILAGE

As with any soft tissue mass, tumors of bone may also be benign or malignant. Primary malignant lesions and secondary malignancies (i.e. those arising in association with a prior benign tumor) must be distinguished from metastatic lesions. Each of the structural components of bone may give rise to benign or malignant neoplasms and it is important to recognize that certain benign lesions have the potential for malignant transformation. Radiographs of a lesion can help in the assessment of whether a lesion is benign or malignant and in some cases such imaging studies can even suggest the histopathologic subtype of the bone tumor.

OSTEOSARCOMA

Defined as an osteoid-producing primary malignancy of bone, osteosarcoma is the most common sarcoma of bone and the second most common primary bone tumor after myeloma. It develops in men slightly more frequently than in women, with an incidence ratio of 1.5 : 1. The distribution by age is bimodal. During adolescence, osteosarcoma arises in areas of rapid growth, e.g. around the epiphyses of long bones. In some studies, adolescents with this tumor have been found to be taller than age-matched controls. In the second peak in incidence, among older patients, osteosarcoma

develops most frequently in areas of prior benign bone lesions or in previously irradiated sites. For example, solitary lesions of osteochondroma rarely give rise to osteosarcoma, but in patients with multiple lesions (enchondromatosis or Ollier's disease) osteosarcoma develops with more frequency. In 0.2% of patients with Paget's disease, osteosarcoma arises in pagetoid bone. Multicentric tumors have developed in patients with prior chronic radium ingestion, such as watch-dial painters, and occasionally in the absence of any known risk factors, usually in children under age 10. Patients with familial retinoblastoma (i.e. those who have inherited deficiencies of the Rb tumor suppressor gene) have a greatly increased risk of developing osteosarcoma (nearly a 10% lifetime risk, hundreds of times higher than the risk in the general population).

Patients present with symptoms of severe bone pain, usually of relatively short duration, and often with a firm, rock-hard mass. The overlying skin is often stretched and shiny, with prominent vasculature. Alkaline phosphatase levels are generally elevated, except in very undifferentiated osteosarcoma, and they have prognostic value; elevated values after amputation herald residual or relapsing disease. (It should be remembered that normal values in children are higher than in adults.)

Characteristic radiographs and CT scans of primary lesions reveal osteolysis and periosteal new bone formation; later stage tumors may exhibit cortical destruction and breakthrough into soft tissues.

The telangiectatic variant of osteosarcoma is almost entirely lytic. Periosteal elevation results in the classic 'Codman's triangle' on radiography (*see* Fig. 10.9). Ossification may be slight, moderate or densely sclerotic. Another pattern of periosteal reaction can be identified by a 'sunburst' appearance of ossification. This phenomenon results from newly formed bone spicules oriented at right angles to the cortical soft tissue extension. (In the gross specimens shown among the figures that follow, it is instructive to note the morphology that results in the characteristic radiographic appearance of osteosarcoma.) In addition to plain radiography, CT examination, including scans of the chest, is essential to evaluate the stage of a lesion; CT scans of the chest help detect pulmonary metastases, the most likely site of disseminated disease. Radionuclide bone scan imaging is useful in the staging evaluation of osteosarcoma. Radionuclide bone scan, which generally reveals intense uptake within the lesion, may detect skip lesions of bone, metastases or a multicentric primary tumor. Uptake in the lungs on bone scan may identify early pulmonary lesions. Initial careful radiologic imaging of the chest is required to rule out the presence of occult metastases at diagnosis.

The demonstration of 'malignant osteoid' (i.e. non-calcified bony substance produced by the tumor cells themselves) is required for a histologic diagnosis of osteosarcoma. Based on the predominant cell type, osteosarcomas are divided into osteoblastic (45% of cases), chondroblastic (27%), anaplastic (17%), fibroblastic (9%) and telangiectatic (1%) variants. Although most reports have shown that the various subclassifications have little prognostic value, histologic grade appears to correlate with tumor behavior.

Juxtacortical (parosteal) osteosarcomas (*see* Fig. 10.7) are relatively uncommon (3–4%), often low-grade variants that arise equally in either sex. Patients with these tumors are about a decade older than patients with higher-grade types. Gross examination shows that the tumors are bulky and tend to encircle the cortex of bone, generally the distal femur and less commonly the proximal humerus. The radiologic differential diagnosis includes osteochondroma and myositis ossificans.

Preoperative ('neoadjuvant') and/or postoperative ('adjuvant') chemotherapy for osteosarcoma is now accepted as standard treatment. Histologic evidence of tumor necrosis following preoperative chemotherapy is among the most powerful prognostic factors for survival of patients with osteosarcoma. Doxorubicin and cisplatin are the core of adjuvant regimens in osteosarcoma, but ifosfamide and methotrexate may also have useful roles. Although these aggressive combination chemotherapy regimens can be associated with considerable toxicity, disease-free survival at 2 years in randomized studies of the combined modality approach is approximately 56–59%, as compared to 18–40% after amputation alone.

Besides the routine use of adjuvant chemotherapy, in osteosarcoma management function-sparing surgery has been shown to be completely equivalent in overall survival outcomes to more debilitating amputations, which were the standard of care prior to the 1970s. Current treatment approaches combine chemotherapy with local resection rather than amputation, with encouraging results in terms of survival rates and the functional status of affected limbs. Intensive chemotherapy with surgical intervention should be considered if metastases develop in the lung. Some patients who present initially with radiographically evident metastatic disease in the lung are now being cured by resection of both the primary lesion and pulmonary metastases, combined with systemic chemotherapy.

In sites of prior Paget's disease or irradiation, osteosarcoma appears to be responsive to the usual therapeutic methods. However, because of its more central location and the vascularity of pagetoid bone, it tends to be difficult to resect for cure.

EWING'S SARCOMA

Ewing's sarcoma is currently thought to be possibly of neurogenic origin, although the histopathology of the primitive, small, round blue cells which comprise this tumor does not allow a more lineage-specific attribution. Importantly, Ewing's sarcoma was once considered primarily a bone tumor, but it is increasingly recognized as a primary malignancy of soft tissues as well. Cytogenetically, it is frequently characterized by chromosomal translocations involving chromosome 22 (most often an 11;22 translocation, identical to that found in peripheral neuroectodermal tumors) (*see* Chapter 16). The molecular identity of Ewing's sarcoma with peripheral neuroectodermal tumors has led to a change in the classification of these diseases into a new grouping known as the Ewing's family of tumors based on the molecular pathology. Ewing's sarcoma accounts for about 10–14% of primary malignant bone tumors in whites, but it is rare in blacks. Its incidence peaks between the ages of 10 and 25 years (range 2 to 65), with a 2 : 1 male to female ratio. Both Ewing's sarcoma and osteosarcoma occur primarily in the same sex and age group, but they can be clinically distinguished by other characteristics (*see* Table 10.5). The common sites of occurrence include the femur (27%), pelvis (18%) and tibia or fibula (17%).

Patients with primary Ewing's sarcoma of bone often present with pain, a rapidly enlarging mass and often fever, leukocytosis and an elevated erythrocyte sedimentation rate (sometimes mimicking osteomyelitis). Early diagnosis of Ewing's sarcoma involving the pelvic bones is frequently delayed because of poorly localized pain and a clinically inapparent mass. Patients may also have pulmonary symptoms, indicating lung metastases, or spinal cord compression, resulting from metastatic deposits in vertebrae. Radiographically, Ewing's sarcoma characteristically presents as a fusiform enlargement of the long bones with central mottling ('cracked ice'), indicating a permeative type of bone destruction, and 'onion-skin' layering of the periosteal reaction. Initial diagnostic evaluation should definitely include CT and/or MRI scans of the primary site, as well as imaging of the chest and liver, since those are common sites of disease spread. Additionally, baseline bone scan should be obtained to rule out occult metastases at diagnosis. Ewing's sarcoma can be imaged by 18FDG-positron emision tomography (PET scans) as well as by labeled octreotide scans, although the supplemental value of these more sophisticated imaging studies needs further clarification.

Microscopic examination of biopsy specimens typically reveals small, blue-stained cells arranged in clusters bordered by fibrous septa. In contrast to lymphoma, the reticulin stain outlines clusters of cells. The periodic acid–Schiff (PAS) stain is positive for glycogen, which can be digested by the diastase reaction. Electron microscopy can confirm the presence of large quantities of glycogen. Since the 11;22 translocation appears pathognomonic for this clinical entity, cytogenetic evaluation of the resected tumor or biopsy specimen is now a critical diagnostic step. Other translocations of the *EWS* gene on chromosome 22 are also consistent with Ewing's sarcoma (so, for example, a 9;22 translocation can be found with this diagnosis in the proper histopathologic setting).

Current aggressive multimodality treatment results in long-term disease-free survival in about 70% of children under 16 years of age who present with localized Ewing's sarcoma. Perhaps a quarter of patients with metastases can also be cured. Combination chemotherapy is given before or concurrent with radiotherapy to involved bone. Expendable bones such as the ribs or tibia should be resected rather than irradiated. Metastases most frequently involve the lung, bone, bone marrow and spinal cord. Survival rates correlate inversely with age; 70% of patients under 10 years of age survive as compared with 46% of those 16 years and older. This may be due to differences in the resectability of the disease and a disproportionate finding of unresectable pelvic and proximal sites of disease in adults, rather than because the underlying biology of the tumor cells is different in adults.

CHONDROSARCOMA

Malignant stromal tumors of bone that produce cartilage but no osteoid are defined as chondrosarcomas. They account for 17–22% of primary malignant bone tumors and are the second most common bone sarcoma. Their incidence increases steadily with age. Extraskeletal chondrosarcomas, arising totally within soft tissue, by definition have no attachment to bone or cartilage. Primary lesions occur in previously normal bone, whereas secondary chondrosarcomas arise in prior benign lesions, most frequently enchondromas. Malignant degeneration in multiple enchondromatosis (Ollier's disease) is reported in patients with this condition alone or in association with soft tissue hemangiomas (Maffucci's disease). Although chondrosarcomas in patients with multiple enchondromatosis are generally low grade, those associated with soft tissue hemangiomas are more frequently high-grade lesions. About a tenth of radiation-associated sarcomas are chondrosarcomas and secondary tumors may arise in bone affected by Paget's disease. The most common sites of involvement for primary chondrosarcoma are the pelvis (31%), femur (21%), shoulder (13%), ribs (9%) and face (9%). Lesions may be painful, especially if they increase rapidly in size, or they may present as a painless mass.

Radiographically, central chondrosarcomas exhibit fluffy, 'popcorn'-like calcifications. Peripheral tumors, on the other hand, tend to have long, lightly calcified spicules radiating from the cortex to a flattened outer surface, with little evidence of cortical or medullary involvement. A faint Codman's triangle may be evident as a result of lipping of the periosteum. Chondrosarcomas tend to take up radionuclides avidly during bone scanning. In their gross aspect, chondrosarcomas have translucent, bluish-white, mucoid surfaces; reactive new bone formation is seen in slow-growing lesions or cortical destruction may be evident, marking high-grade, rapidly enlarging lesions. Its microscopic appearance is characterized by the appearance of cartilage with malignant chondrocytes. Especially in low-grade lesions, the histologic character of a tumor is an unreliable predictor of biologic behavior, since similar lesions may behave differently depending on age, site of origin, lesion size and particularly radiographic appearance. Variants based on predominant cell type include clear cell chondrosarcoma and mesenchymal chondrosarcoma. The clear cell type, which occurs predominantly in the femoral head or humeral head of adult men, is marked by local recurrences and eventual metastases. Mesenchymal chondrosarcoma is characterized histologically by a small round cell component. This tumor tends to arise in the ribs, mandible, maxilla, skull and extraskeletal sites.

Because local recurrences appear to increase with histologic aggressiveness and because chondrosarcomas are relatively resistant to both radiotherapy and chemotherapy, every effort should be made to resect the primary lesion adequately when it first appears. Thus, radical resection is indicated, particularly of eminently curable, low-grade chondrosarcomas.

GIANT CELL TUMOR OF BONE (OSTEOCLASTOMA)

Constituting 5% of primary tumors of bone, giant cell tumor of bone is an unusual lesion that may behave locally in a very aggressive manner but is considered to have low metastatic potential. Incidence of the lesion peaks in the third decade, with a range of 5 to 73 years. Fifty-five percent of affected individuals are women. Half of giant cell tumors of bone are located around the knee, arising in the distal femur, patella or proximal tibia or fibula. Lesions may be associated with areas of active Paget's disease.

Radiographically, giant cell tumors are generally eccentrically situated, epiphyseal lesions having a central lucency and increasing density toward the periphery. No new bone formation is present in actively growing lesions. Grossly, the tumor may appear solid despite a cystic appearance on radiography. Microscopically, it is marked by prominent, multinucleated giant cells dispersed throughout well-vascularized stromal tumor tissue. Inconspicuous stromal cells separating the multinucleated giant cells have nuclei identical to those of the giant cells. Large fields of dense collagenous scarring within the lesion, or a prominent stroma with relatively diminished numbers of giant cells, suggests malignant behavior. Mitotic figures may be present. A fully malignant stroma resembles fibrosarcoma. Although fewer than 10% of these tumors are malignant on first presentation, up to 30% assume a malignant behavior after multiple recurrences.

The prognosis of these tumors is often difficult to predict. A recurrence rate of 50% or more has been reported after curettage; most patients require multiple therapeutic interventions before disease is successfully eradicated. Wound implantation results in recurrences in soft tissue. Sarcomatous transformation develops an average of 9 years after initial treatment and may be related to prior radiotherapy. Case reports of putatively 'antiangiogenic' therapy being useful in the management of metastatic, unresectable giant cell tumor of bone suggest that this tumor type may be sensitive to agents such as recombinant human interferon-α.

CHORDOMA

Chordoma, representing 1% of malignant bone tumors, arises from remnants of the embryologic notochord, generally in the cervical or sacral area. Patients at presentation range from 2 to 74 years of age, with peak incidence in the fifth to seventh decades. Sacral lesions generally occur in older patients, with a median age of 56 years as compared with 47 years for cervical lesions. Sacral lesions result in pain, usually of over a year's duration before diagnosis; the pain is sometimes referred to the hip or knee. Neurologic bowel or bladder symptoms may be the presenting manifestations. Eighty percent of patients with cranial chordomas report headache. Cranial nerve signs, chiasmal involvement or endocrine abnormalities may be present. Nasopharyngeal chordomas present as a mass with nasal obstruction before neurologic involvement. Osteolysis of one or more vertebral bodies and a soft tissue mass herald the presence of a sacral chordoma. Cranial chordomas present with destruction of the sella, the clinoid, the clivus and the apices of the petrous bones. On gross examination, chordomas are lobulated, pseudoencapsulated masses varying in consistency from jelly-like to cartilaginous. Microscopically, intracellular and extracellular mucin production is prominent, as are physaliferous ('bubble') cells and 'signet ring' forms. Multinucleated giant cells may be present, but mitotic figures are uncommon.

Treatment consists of resection and radiotherapy, including promising data using newer radiotherapeutic techniques such as highly focused radiotherapy via proton beam accelerators. Complete resection is seldom possible. Local failure is common and 5–43% of these tumors eventually metastasize. The median survival is about 6 years.

Table 10.4 Benign bone lesions with potential for malignant transformation.

Benign lesion	Resultant malignancy
Enchondroma: in long or flat bones; in short tubular bones only in Maffucci's syndrome or Ollier's disease	Chondrosarcoma
Osteochrondroma: one of the many lesion of multiple cartilaginous exostoses	Peripheral chondrosarcoma
Fibrous dysplasia: usually polyostotic and secondary to radiation treatment	Fibrosarcoma Malignant fibrous histiocytoma Osteosarcoma
Bone infarct	Fibrosarcoma Malignant fibrous histiocytoma
Osteomyelitis with chronic draining sinus tract: usually of more than 15 to 20 years, duration	Squamous cell carcinoma Fibrosarcoma
Paget's disease	Osteosarcoma Chondrosarcoma Fibrosarcoma Malignant fibrous histiocytoma
Osteofibrous dysplasia (Kempson–Campanacci lesion)	Adamantinoma*
Neurofibroma: in plexiform neurofibromatosis	Malignant schwannoma Liposarcoma Malignant mesenchymoma*

*Some authorities believe that this does not result from a transformation but rather represents the development of a true malignancy, within a benign condition.

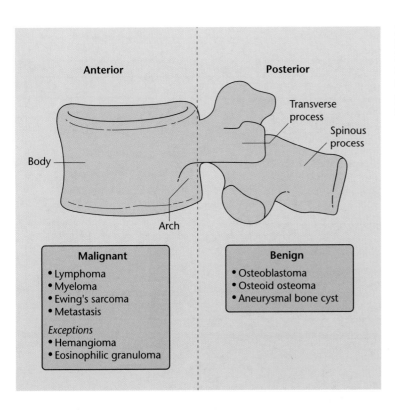

Fig. 10.3 Tumors and tumor-like lesions in a vertebra. Malignant lesions are seen predominantly in the anterior part of a vertebra (body), whereas benign lesions predominate in the posterior elements (neural arch).

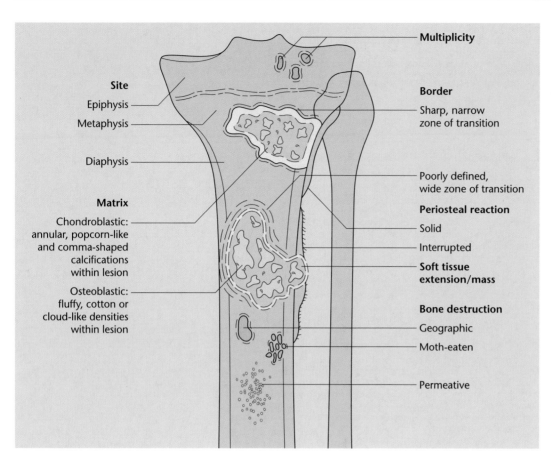

Fig. 10.4 Radiographic evaluation of tumors and tumor-like lesions of bone. Several features have been identified that help characterize bone tumors and tumor-like lesions. These features include the site of the lesion, its borders and matrix, the presence or absence of soft tissue extension or mass, the type of periosteal reaction (if present), the type of bone destruction and whether the lesion is singular or multiple.

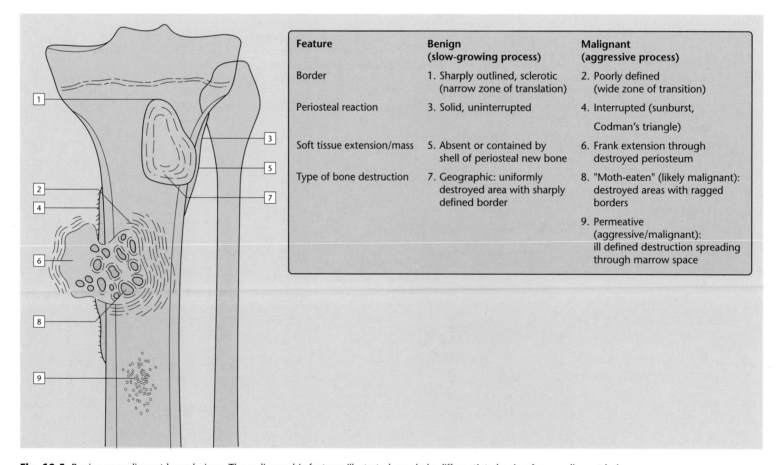

Fig. 10.5 Benign vs malignant bone lesions. The radiographic features illustrated may help differentiate benign from malignant lesions.

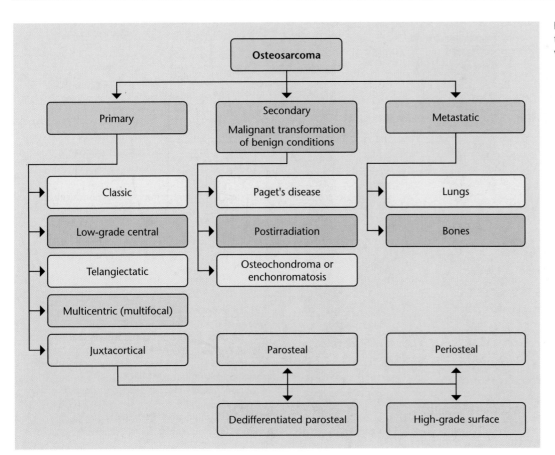

Fig. 10.6 Osteosarcoma. Classification of the type of osteosarcoma, with specific variants of juxtacortical osteosarcoma.

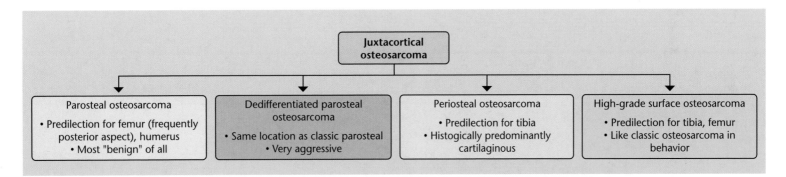

Fig. 10.7 Juxtacortical osteosarcoma. Features distinguishing the variants of juxtacortical osteosarcoma.

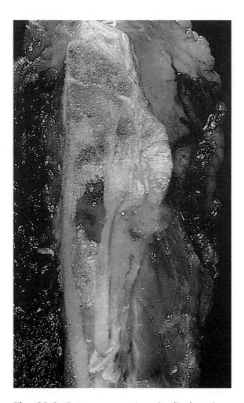

Fig. 10.8 Osteosarcoma. Longitudinal section through the proximal fibula was made after resection of the bone in a 13-year-old girl. Note the extension of the tumor through the cortex into adjacent soft tissues.

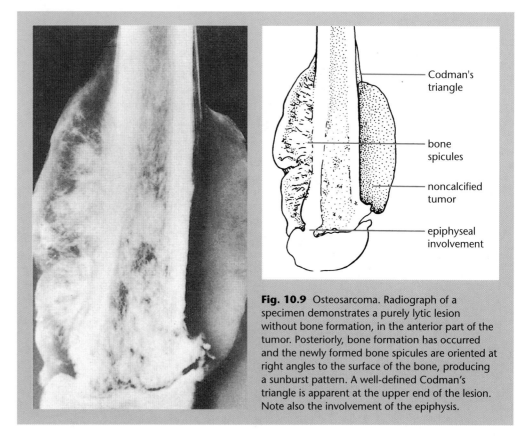

Fig. 10.9 Osteosarcoma. Radiograph of a specimen demonstrates a purely lytic lesion without bone formation, in the anterior part of the tumor. Posteriorly, bone formation has occurred and the newly formed bone spicules are oriented at right angles to the surface of the bone, producing a sunburst pattern. A well-defined Codman's triangle is apparent at the upper end of the lesion. Note also the involvement of the epiphysis.

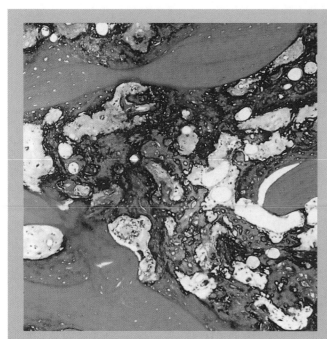

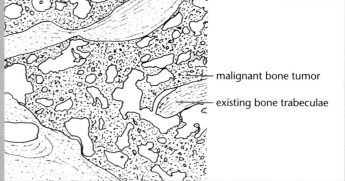

Fig. 10.10 Osteosarcoma. A characteristic feature of osteosarcoma is the formation of an abundant mineralized matrix and infiltration of the tumor through the marrow spaces between the existing bone trabeculae. As seen in this photomicrograph, the malignant tumor tissue becomes firmly applied to the surface of the existing bone.

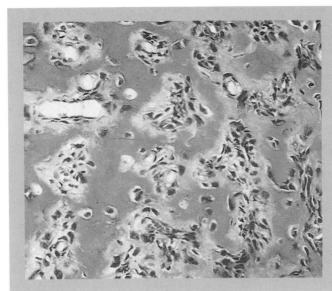

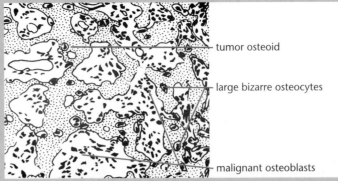

tumor osteoid

large bizarre osteocytes

malignant osteoblasts

Fig. 10.11 Osteosarcoma. Tumor bone has been deposited in a sarcomatous stroma. Note the pleomorphic pattern of malignant cells, many with dark-staining nuclei.

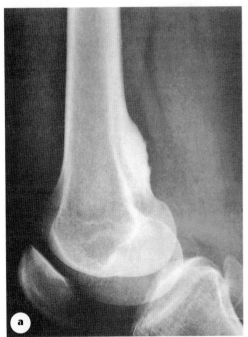

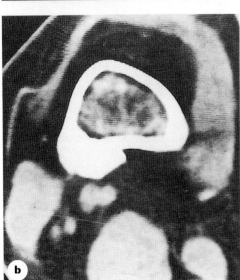

Fig. 10.12 Parosteal osteosarcoma. (**a**) Lateral radiograph of the knee of a 37-year-old woman shows an ossific mass attached to the posterior cortex of the distal femur. Its location and appearance are typical of parosteal osteosarcoma. (**b**) CT section demonstrates lack of invasion of the medullary portion of the bone.

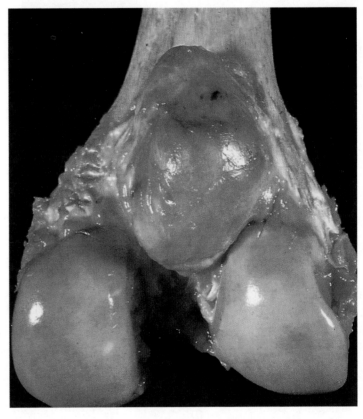

Fig. 10.13 Parosteal osteosarcoma. Specimen photograph of the lower end of the femur shows a large mass on the cortex of the bone just above and between the two femoral condyles. This location is typical for parosteal osteosarcoma.

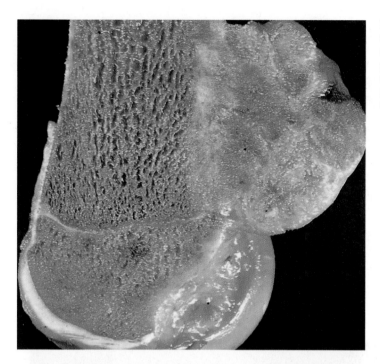

Fig. 10.14 Parosteal osteosarcoma. Photograph of a sagittal section through the specimen shown in Figure 10.13 demonstrates that the lesion is well encapsulated and formed of bone-producing tissue. As in the case shown here, parosteal osteosarcoma frequently extends for a short distance through the cortex into the medullary cavity. For this reason, when surgical treatment is planned, medullary extension should be carefully sought and taken into account if local recurrence is to be prevented.

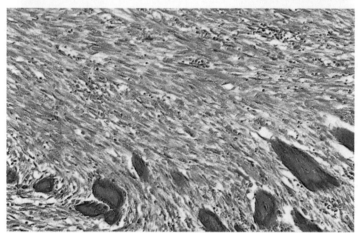

Fig. 10.15 Juxtacortical osteosarcoma. High-power photomicrograph shows islands of bone tissue within the cellular, though unremarkable, fibrous stroma of this tumor.

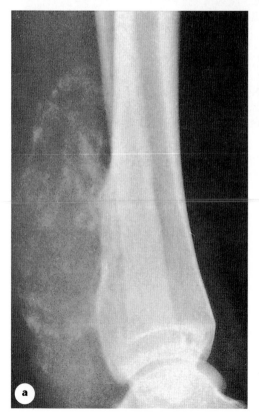

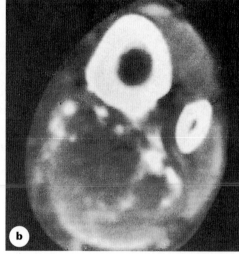

Fig. 10.16 High-grade surface osteosarcoma. (**a**) Lateral view of the lower leg demonstrates a high-grade surface osteosarcoma attached to the posterior cortex of the distal tibia in a 24-year-old man. Ill-defined ossific foci are seen within a large soft tissue mass. (**b**) CT section demonstrates the extent of the lesion. Characteristically, the marrow cavity is not affected.

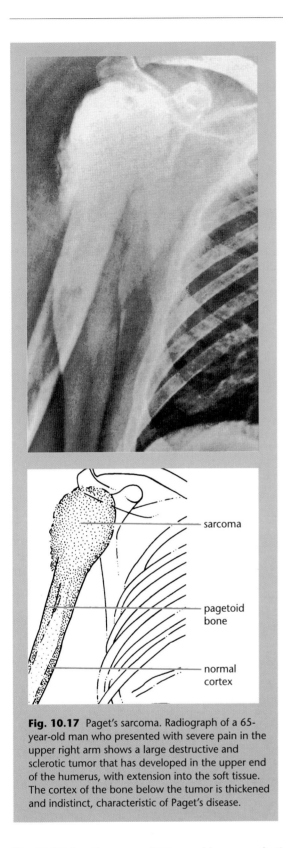

Fig. 10.17 Paget's sarcoma. Radiograph of a 65-year-old man who presented with severe pain in the upper right arm shows a large destructive and sclerotic tumor that has developed in the upper end of the humerus, with extension into the soft tissue. The cortex of the bone below the tumor is thickened and indistinct, characteristic of Paget's disease.

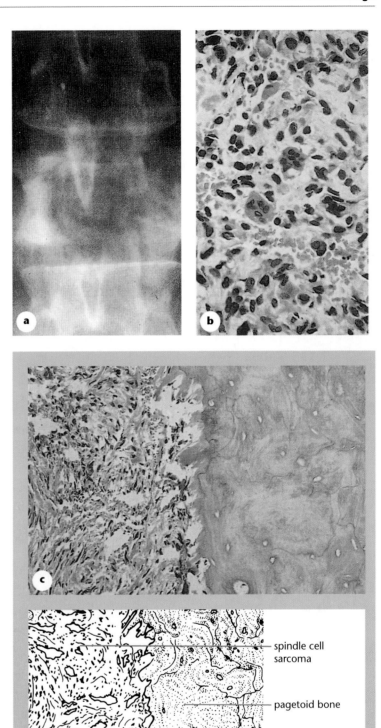

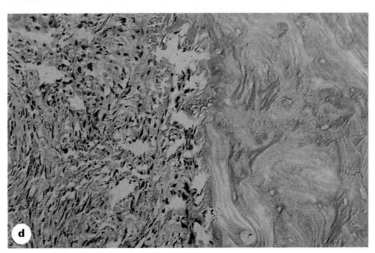

Fig. 10.18 Paget's sarcoma. A 58-year-old woman, who 14 years earlier had undergone a hysterectomy for cervical carcinoma, presented with a 2-month history of lower back pain. (**a**) Spiral radiograph of the lumbar spine shows a patchy sclerotic and lytic appearance interpreted to be consistent with metastatic disease. However, there is some widening of the body which is unusual in metastasis. (**b**) Photomicrograph of a needle biopsy specimen shows an anaplastic tumor with many giant cells, consistent with Paget's sarcoma. Foci of bone obtained with this biopsy shows the typical mosaic pattern of Paget's sarcoma. The patient died about 4 months later. Autopsy revealed local extension of the tumor, which involved T12 and L2. Extensive lung metastases had the pattern of a Paget's sarcoma. (**c**) H&E-stained section of bone adjacent to the tumor shows an increased number of cement lines within the bone. (**d**) In a polarized section of the same field, the disorganized bony architecture is obvious. This case is significant because it demonstrates that even in monostotic Paget's disease, a sarcoma may rarely occur as a complication.

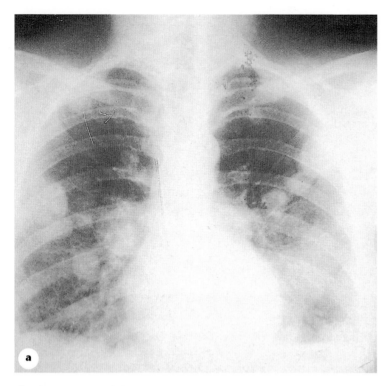
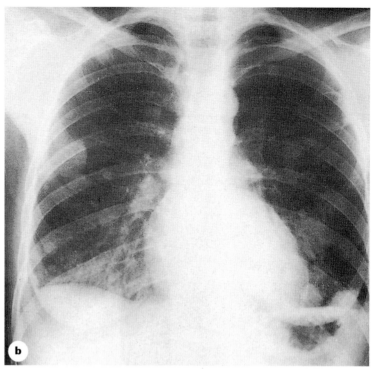

Fig. 10.19 'Cannonball' lung metastases of sarcoma. (**a**) The appearance of such metastatic deposits on chest films is characteristic. As many as half of patients who die of metastatic sarcoma have disease confined to the lungs at autopsy. Because metastatic sarcoma is commonly subpleural in location, resection of slow-growing lesions in selected patients results in a 5-year disease-free survival of 15–30%. (**b**) In this patient with a leiomyosarcoma, combination chemotherapy has resulted in a partial response.

Table 10.5 Osteosarcoma and Ewing's sarcoma: Distinguishing characteristics		
Feature	Osteosarcoma	Ewing's sarcoma
Site of involvement		
Long bone	Metaphysis	Diaphysis
Flat bone	Rare	Common
Medullary cavity	Rare	Common (moth-eaten appearance)
New bone formation	Common	Only secondary
Periosteal reaction	Codman's triangle spiculation (sunburst)	Lamellated ('onion-skinning')
Soft tissue mass	Less prominent	Large, common
Radiation associated	Yes	No
Precursor lesions	Yes	No

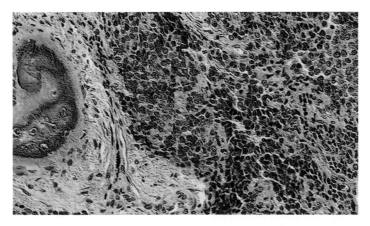

Fig. 10.21 Ewing's sarcoma. Photomicrograph shows the typical small vesicular nuclei with scant, poorly defined cytoplasm and scattered foci of pyknotic nuclei throughout.

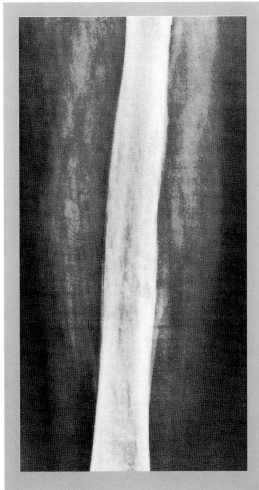

permeative tumor

"onion skinning" periosteal reaction

Fig. 10.20 Ewing's sarcoma. Radiograph of the femur in a 13-year-old child who complained of pain in the thigh shows an extensive permeative lesion in the midshaft. The overlying periosteum has been elevated and new bone has formed in several layers, giving the periosteum an onion-skin appearance.

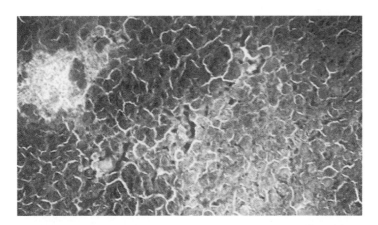

Fig. 10.22 Ewing's sarcoma. Low-power photomicrograph of a PAS-stained section shows strong positivity due to the presence of glycogen in tumor cells.

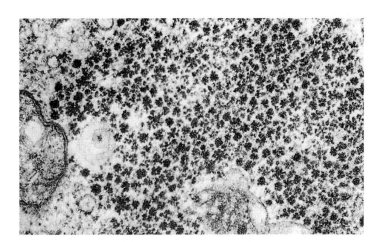

Fig. 10.23 Ewing's sarcoma. Electron photomicrograph of a tumor cell shows packing of the cytoplasm with glycogen granules.

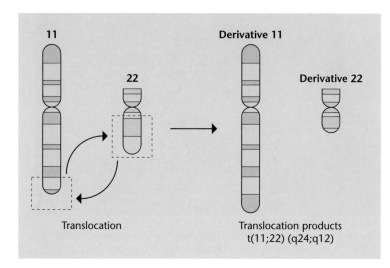

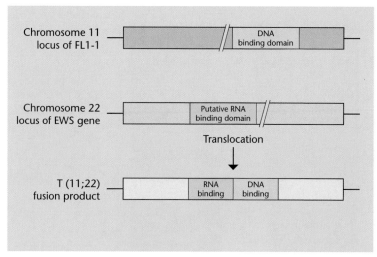

Fig. 10.24 Ewing's sarcoma. Characteristic chromosomal rearrangement in Ewing's sarcoma.

Fig. 10.25 Genetic recombination of DNA in Ewing's sarcoma: creation of novel fusion transcript.

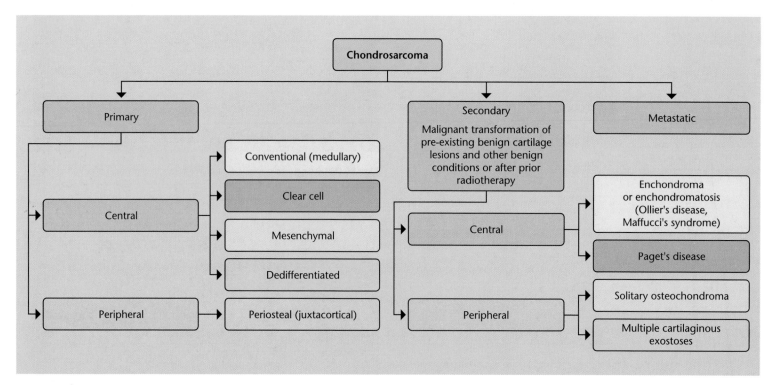

Fig. 10.26 Chondrosarcoma. Classification of the types of chondrosarcoma.

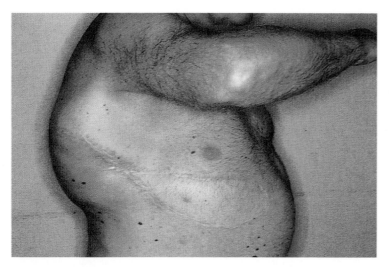

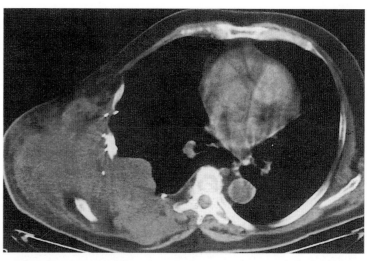

Fig. 10.27 Chondrosarcoma. In this 64-year-old man with a long-standing low-grade chondrosarcoma of the chest wall, there is local recurrence despite several radical surgical procedures.

Fig. 10.28 Chondrosarcoma. Chest CT scan of the patient shown in Figure 10.27 shows a large, right chest wall mass extending through the ribs and into the pleural space. Surgical clips from previous resections are also seen.

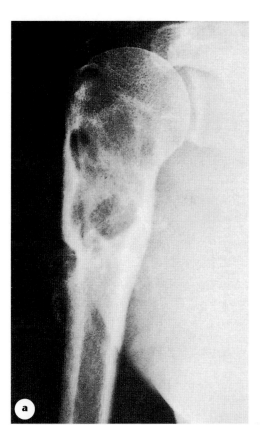

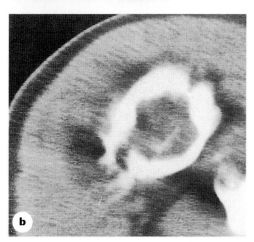

Fig. 10.29 Chondrosarcoma. (**a**) AP plain film of the right proximal humerus of a 62-year-old man is not adequate for demonstrating the soft tissue extension of a chondrosarcoma in the proximal humerus. (**b**) CT section through the lesion demonstrates cortical destruction and an extensive soft tissue mass. Marked irregular destruction, expansion and cystic areas of the bone are evident.

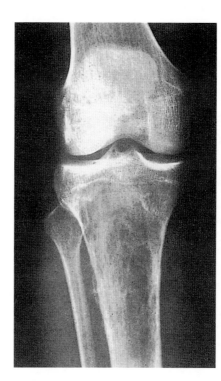

Fig. 10.30 Chondrosarcoma. Radiograph of the knee of a 27-year-old man shows a large, irregular lytic lesion of the proximal tibia.

Fig. 10.31 Chondrosarcoma. Photomicrograph shows a moderately cellular tumor composed of chondrocytes separated by abundant chondroid matrix. Cellular pleomorphism and mild nuclear hyperchromatism are evident.

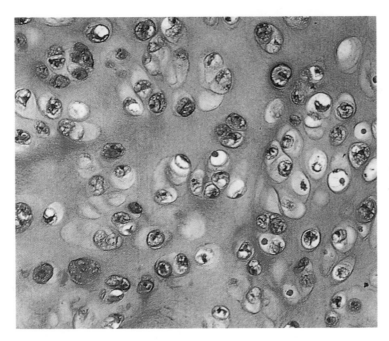

Fig. 10.32 Chondrosarcoma. Photomicrograph of a fully malignant, anaplastic tumor shows marked cellular atypia and crowding.

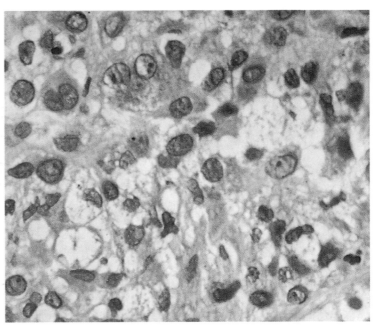

Fig. 10.33 Clear cell chondrosarcoma. Photomicrograph of an area within a tumor shows numerous cells with abundant, clear, vacuolated cytoplasm. Some nuclear variation and occasional giant cells are present.

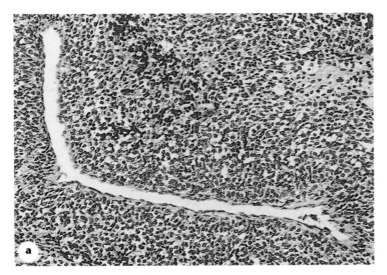

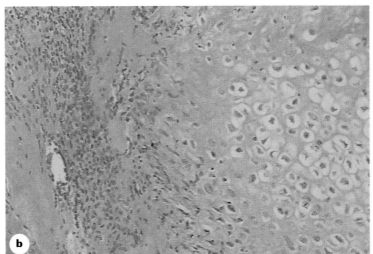

Fig. 10.34 Mesenchymal chondrosarcoma. Photomicrographs reveal the typical biphasic pattern of this type of chondrosarcoma. (**a**) Large areas of undifferentiated small cells, resembling those of Ewing's sarcoma, are interspersed between vascular spaces. (**b**) In this photomicrograph, low-grade malignant cartilage can also be seen.

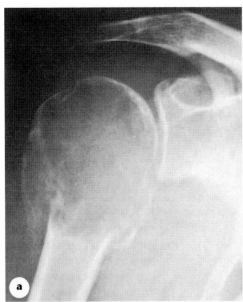

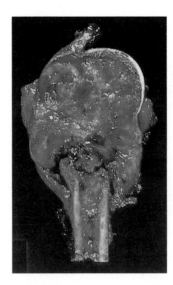

Fig. 10.35 Giant cell tumor of bone. (**a**) Plain film of the shoulder of a 27-year-old woman shows a tumor destroying almost the entire proximal end of the humerus. (**b**) Wide resection was performed and the humerus was reconstructed by means of allograft.

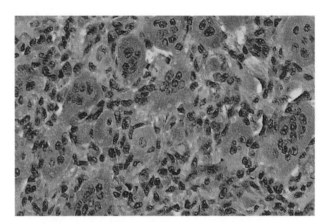

Fig. 10.36 Giant cell tumor of bone. Specimen photograph shows the right proximal humerus, which has been sectioned longitudinally, after resection in a 25-year-old man. Note the extension of well-vascularized loculations of tumor outside the bone.

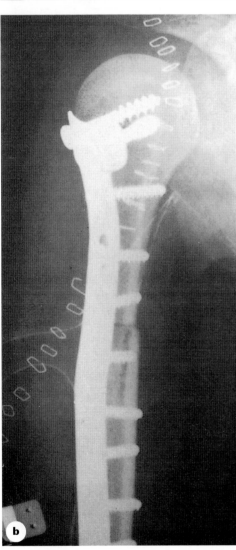

Fig. 10.37 Giant cell tumor of bone. Photomicrograph of a conventional giant cell tumor demonstrates evenly spaced and crowded giant cells, with intervening polygonal stromal cells.

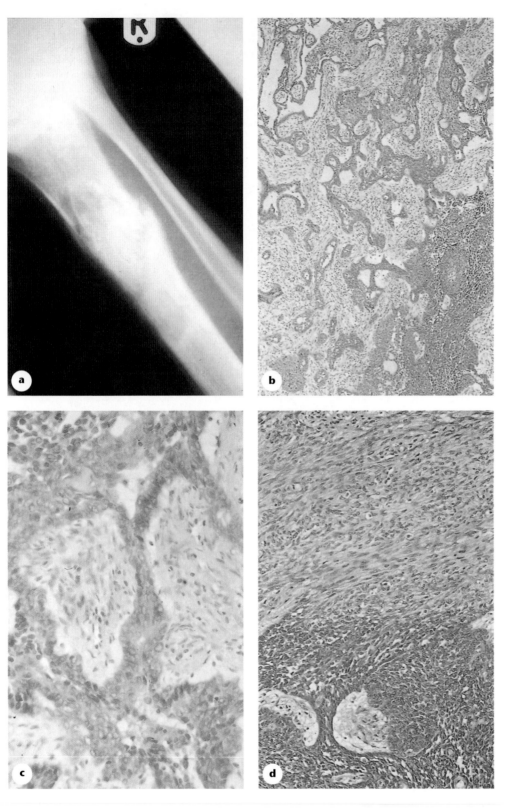

Fig. 10.38 Adamantinoma of distal tibia. Adamantinomas typically produce an eccentric, sharply defined osteolytic defect, frequently with infiltration of bone and hemorrhagic and cystic areas. (**a**) Postoperative features related to placement of bone chips after a bone graft. (**b, c**) Histologically, the tumor is composed of epithelial elements within a fibrous stroma. There is extensive diversity of these epithelial elements, with the four major histologic patterns being squamoid, basaloid, tubular and spindled. These express epithelial antigens, e.g. cytokeratins, which may be critical in recognition of the spindled variants. (**d**) The risk of local recurrence and metastatic disease is significant, with lymph node metastases in approximately 10% of patients. Lung metastases are also common and can occur up to 15 years after diagnosis, necessitating long-term surveillance.

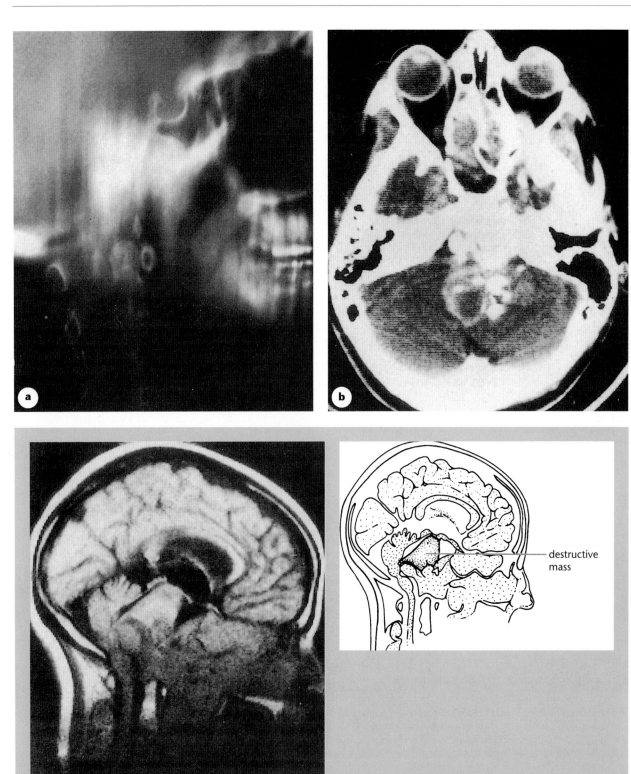

destructive
mass

Fig. 10.39 Chondroid chordoma. (**a**) Lateral tomogram of the skull of a woman with a chordoma of the clivus that was partially removed 2 years previously shows a large, dense, midline mass. The lesion, which extends anteriorly into the nasopharynx and posteriorly into the posterior fossa, is seen destroying the inferior clivus. (**b**) Contrast-enhanced CT section demonstrates several areas of calcification within the posterior fossa and a large mass occupying the region where the brainstem is normally seen. (**c**) MR scan shows an enormous mass that fills the nasal cavity and ethmoid sinus anteriorly. It has obliterated the nasopharynx, extending into the hypopharynx. It also extends into the cranial cavity, completely destroying the clivus. It has displaced the brainstem, extending to the fourth ventricle.

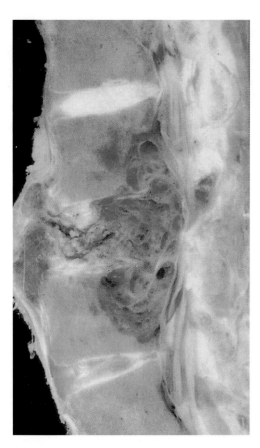

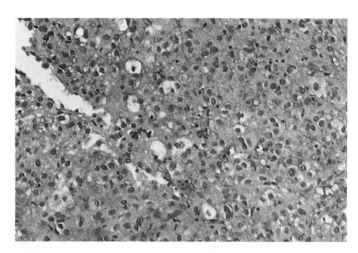

Fig. 10.40 Chordoma. Specimen photograph shows a sagittal section through the lumbar spine of a 70-year-old man who clinically was thought to have metastatic disease. He died with paraplegia and an intractable urinary infection. The specimen exhibits a destructive hemorrhagic lesion in L3 that involves the bodies of L2 and L4. The lesion has extended posteriorly, compressing the cauda equina. Histologic study revealed a typical chordoma. The lumbar spine is a rare site of involvement for this neoplasm. (Courtesy of the Royal College of Surgeons of England, London, UK.)

Fig. 10.41 Chondroid chordoma. Some chordomas arising in the area of the clivus show a distinctly chondroid appearance, as seen in this photomicrograph. This pattern is important to recognize, since the prognosis for chondroid chordomas in the base of the skull is much better than for tumors in that area that have a conventional pattern. Physaliferous or 'bubble' cells, as seen here, are characteristic of chordoma; these cells are remnants of the notochord and are of ectodermal origin (i.e. keratin positive).

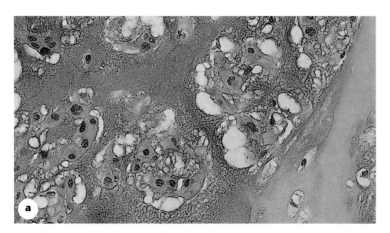

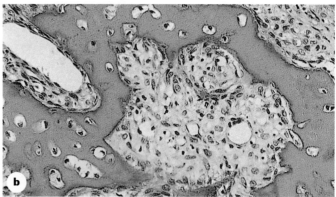

Fig. 10.42 Chondroid chordoma and osteosarcoma. (**a**) Photomicrograph of the nasopharyngeal mass, resected at the first intervention from the patient shown in Figure 10.39, exhibits cords of cells with basophilic, round nuclei and abundant, focally vacuolated cytoplasm. The cords are set in a basophilic matrix which is focally vacuolated but in many areas has a more uniform, chondroid appearance. The lesion was diagnosed as a chondroid chordoma. (**b**) At the second intervention, similar tissue was resected but it exhibits areas that show neoplastic osteoid surrounded by malignant spindle cells; it was diagnosed as osteosarcoma.

SARCOMAS OF SOFT TISSUES

Soft tissue sarcomas are found in all age groups; they range from orbital rhabdomyosarcoma, which peaks in incidence at 4 years, to liposarcoma, the most common sarcoma in adults over age 50. Forty percent of soft tissue sarcomas develop in the lower extremities, most commonly in the thigh; these tumors may also arise in virtually any site of the body, such as the trunk, head or neck, arm and retroperitoneum (*see* Table 10.6). Patients usually present with a solitary, painless, palpable mass on the extremities or trunk. Intra-abdominal and retroperitoneal primary tumors, when advanced and large, may cause symptoms related to invasion or displacement of organs, weight loss and pain. The duration of symptoms ranges from a few weeks to decades, with a median of 1–3 months. Hypoglycemia is rare, associated predominantly with large, retroperitoneal sarcomas (and probably due to tumor-derived production of insulin-like growth factor). Soft tissue sarcomas have developed within ports of prior radiotherapy delivered 2–20 years earlier (median about 10 years). Many histologic types have been observed, including fibrosarcoma, angiosarcoma, undifferentiated spindle cell sarcoma and mesothelioma. Fibrosarcoma, in particular, has developed in scars of prior burns or major trauma, often after an interval of 30 years or more.

Preoperative evaluation requires CT or MR scan of the primary lesion to assess the anatomic extent of disease involvement locally. If the lesion abuts bone, MRI scanning may be particularly helpful to determine whether there is periosteal invasion or reaction. Uptake of radionuclide on bone scan is usually not documentation of involvement by tumor but rather indication of a reaction; however, if this is documented at a site distal to the primary, the presence of occult bony metastases should be considered in sarcomas which have a predilection to spread to the bones, such as myxoid liposarcoma, endometrial stromal sarcoma and angiosarcoma. Staging is directed at determining whether distal spread of disease has occurred and this should be performed prior to definitive local therapy. Staging generally requires a CT scan of lungs and liver, the two most common sites of metastasis for soft tissue sarcomas.

The gross appearance of many soft tissue sarcomas is not particularly distinctive. The histopathology, however, varies greatly with the specific subtype of sarcoma and these distinctions can be subtle. There is no substitute for having pathology reviewed by a pathologist with a specialty expertise in the diagnosis of soft tissue sarcomas. Grossly, soft tissue sarcomas are often pseudoencapsulated, fleshy tumors that grow along physiologic tissue planes, thus requiring wide excision beyond the apparent border of the grossly evident disease for local control. Low-grade tumors have a lobulated appearance, pushing aside contiguous structures; high-grade tumors are characterized by invasion of adjacent organs and prominent areas of necrosis, particularly central, as the tumor outgrows its blood supply and as apoptotic areas of the tumors condense upon themselves. Because of microscopic projections of tumor beyond the apparent capsule, local recurrence follows a 'shelling out' procedure in about 80% of cases (*see* Fig. 10.43). Therefore, it is critical to have a proper surgical re-resection considered in situations where a margin-positive 'shelling out' surgical procedure had previously been performed.

A summary of the American Joint Cancer Committee staging system for soft tissue sarcomas is shown in Table 10.7. Tumor stage, which is determined by both grade and size, correlates with survival. The 5-year survival rate for soft tissue sarcomas arising in various anatomic locations is similar when it is adjusted for grade. The exceptions to this pattern are intra-abdominal and retroperitoneal primary tumors; these lesions, even if low grade, tend to be large and at the time of diagnosis they have often already invaded vital organs.

The behavior and treatment of the histologic variants of soft tissue sarcomas as a group are generally similar grade for grade. However, important new insights continue to be made considering relevant differences between various histopathologic subtypes (van Glabbeke *et al.*, 1999). The major exceptions to this are embryonal rhabdomyosarcoma, Kaposi's sarcoma and mesothelioma, which are discussed below. The goal of treatment of soft tissue sarcomas is to achieve local control and to manage metastases if they develop. In this regard, it is critical to distinguish between clinical scenarios where there is some reasonable potential for curative therapy versus those settings in which palliation is the goal. For primary surgical management of sarcomas, wide excision (2–5 cm of normal tissue) is generally considered optimal, particularly for abdominal or low-grade lesions, to minimize the risks of recurrence due to residual locoregional disease. Limb-sparing surgery, resulting in carefully documented, negative margins pathologically, is preferable if function can be spared. Additional consideration must be given to whether adequate radiotherapy (generally considered high dosing, in the range of 6.6 Gy) is indicated and whether it can be delivered. Radiotherapy may be delivered by traditional external beam approach, focused computer-generated fields such as IMRT (intensity-modulated radiotherapy) or by local implants via 'brachytherapy', although the latter approach is generally not recommended for low-grade lesions. Careful pathologic examination and documentation of the surgical margins is essential to document adequate resection and to locate any involved margins for further resection.

Adjuvant chemotherapy following complete resection of the primary disease site remains of unclear overall clinical benefit for patients with soft tissue sarcomas. Several well-conducted prospective randomized clinical trials have documented that adjuvant doxorubicin-based chemotherapy improves disease-free survival of patients with sarcomas of soft tissues, but that this benefit does not apparently translate into a benefit for overall survival (Bramwell, 2001). A single recent trial has demonstrated an overall as well as disease-free survival benefit, but this study is not sufficiently powered to recommend a global change in the standard of care in this regard (Frustacl *et al.*, 2001; Bramwell, 2001). Therefore, the risks and potential benefits of adjuvant chemotherapy need to be considered and discussed individually with patients based on unique characteristics of presentation, co-morbidities and risks. Whenever possible, patients should be offered the participation in well-designed clinical investigations to study the impact of adjuvant treatment strategies. Resection of up to six subpleural metastases, especially in patients with relatively slow-growing lesions (doubling time >40 days) and a long disease-free interval (>12 months), may result in long-term disease-free survival in about 20% of patients.

DISAPPEARANCE OF 'MALIGNANT FIBROUS HISTIOCYTOMA (MFH)' AS A USEFUL DIAGNOSTIC CLASSIFICATION

Characterized as a distinct clinicopathologic entity in 1963, MFH rose to become the most common histologic diagnosis of soft tissue sarcoma in adults in the 1970s. MFH was thought to be derived from cells of fibroblastic origin (based on light microscopy and immunohistochemical staining). It is now clear that a significant subset of what previously would have been called 'MFH' can now be classified under the rubric of other sarcoma terms, using more sophisticated techniques of cytogenetic testing, more appropriate tissue sampling and immunostaining (Fletcher *et al.*, 2001). For example, 'MFH' of the retroperitoneum can nearly always be found to be de-differentiated liposarcoma, with the high-grade non-adipocytic elements essentially hiding the abnormal lipoblasts and well-differentiated sarcomatous cells of that disease. There is an entity known as 'inflammatory MFH' which is still recognized as a distinct histopathologic entity, and this may also be considered a variant of myxofibrosarcoma with inflammatory infiltrates. Other forms of MFH can often be reclassified as leiomyosarcomas using newer techniques of immunohistochemical analysis.

In short, the term 'MFH' is not objectively definable and therefore it is probably preferable to call any such difficult-to-classify tumors undifferentiated sarcomas or high-grade spindle cell sarcomas, not otherwise specifiable.

FIBROSARCOMA

The continuum of neoplasms of fibrous origin ranges from totally benign, encapsulated fibromas of the breast and subcutaneous tissue to locally invasive but borderline lesions, such as fibromatosis and Dupytren's contracture, to highly malignant fibrosarcomas. In the older literature, fibrosarcomas were quite common; however, larger numbers of lesions classified within this category in the past are now reclassified as de-differentiated liposarcomas, spindle cell sarcomas, spindle cell carcinomas, malignant schwannomas or even amelanotic melanomas. Fibrosarcoma tends to originate from inter- and intramuscular fibrous tissue, fascia, tendons and aponeuroses. An infantile variant generally arises in the first year of life, although some cases have been congenital; males predominate. Wide excision results in a cure in 80% of very young children. Histologically, fairly uniform fusiform or spindle-shaped cells are characteristic; cell borders are indistinct and variable mitotic activity, cellularity and collagen production are present. Interlacing fascicles sometimes form a classic herringbone pattern.

It is important to separate out one entity known as dermatofibrosarcoma protuberans (DFSP). This clinicopathologic entity nearly always affects the skin and can be curable by appropriate wide margin surgical excision. DFSP is characterized by a pathognomonic chromosomal translocation involving a fusion of genes encoding the platelet-derived growth factor B-chain and collagen type I (α-1). New data suggest that this leads to altered cell signaling and that this may contribute to the malignant cell proliferation in this disease and also that interruption of this signaling by inhibitors of PDGF signaling (such as by Imatinib mesylate, STI571) may be therapeutically useful (Sjoblom et al., 2001). Although the incidence of unresectable DFSP is exceedingly low, for such patients this will need to be tested in well-designed clinical trials.

Myxofibrosarcoma, also known occasionally as 'myxoid MFH', has, as its name indicates, a prominent myxoid component with branching blood vessels, as well as spindle cell elements (see Fig. 10.51).

LIPOSARCOMA

Tumors of malignant lipoblasts are the most common soft tissue sarcoma in adults. There is considerable variation in tumor behavior, ranging from low-grade, well-differentiated and myxoid liposarcomas to high-grade round cell and pleomorphic liposarcomas (McCormick et al., 1994). Patients are generally in their sixth decade at diagnosis, with somewhat more than half of liposarcomas affecting men. Most develop in the thigh or retroperitoneum and are unicentric in origin, but some may be multicentric, particularly in the abdominal cavity. They rarely, if ever, arise from benign lipomas. The cytogenetic distinctions between lipomas and liposarcomas also support a different pathophysiology between these two neoplastic processes (see Table 10.3). However, certain recent data also point to potential similarities, in certain molecular pathways shared between benign lipomas and well-differentiated liposarcomas (Tallini et al., 1997).

Examination of their gross aspect reveals that liposarcomas are often quite large, with a lobulated surface which, in high-grade tumors, may be sufficiently convoluted as to resemble cerebral cortex. On section, the tumor is yellowish-white and usually has a slimy appearance. Histologically, almost half of tumors have mucinous and fatty features which are histologically composed of lipoblasts, branching, thin-walled capillaries and a myxoid matrix. A poorly differentiated myxoid liposarcoma composed of small, round cells has an aggressive clinical course, despite a paucity of mitotic activity; this entity has a characteristic translocation between chromosomes 12 and 16. The round cell component appears to become more prominent in such myxoid liposarcomas with subsequent recurrences. Well-differentiated liposarcomas are deceptively similar to lipomas in appearance, but with a greater variation in adipocyte size and shape. Cytogenetics typically reveal giant marker chromosomes and often have abnormal ring chromosomes with expansion of genetic material derived from chromosome 12. Inflammatory and sclerosing variants have been described. Well-differentiated liposarcomas may contain de-differentiated areas (which can appear as bizarre, pleomorphic cells or as spindle cell fascicles), often with abrupt changes between the areas containing different elements (see Fig. 10.55). Frequently, in de-differentiated liposarcomas, it is only these pleomorphic components which appear in metastatic lesions, without any hint of the adipocytic elements from which they arose. Pleomorphic liposarcomas are characterized by the presence of large giant cells, which may contain lipid-containing vacuoles. Mitoses are frequent in this form of tumor and an aggressive clinical course is the rule. Multimodality therapy, including chemotherapy, should be considered for high-grade forms of liposarcoma, since these seem to exhibit sensitivity to chemotherapy in a substantial subset of cases (van Glabbeke et al., 1999).

Certain liposarcomas can contain malignant elements of other differentiation pathways, such as bone (osteosarcomatous elements), smooth muscle (leiomyosarcomatous elements), cartilage (chondrosarcomatous elements) or skeletal muscle (rhabdoid bodies or rhabdomyosarcomatous elements). These multicomponent tumors were once typically described as 'malignant mesenchymomas' if they had three or more lineages of differentiated malignancy within them (see Fig. 10.56). The presence of such elements does not obviously impact upon survival, nor should it necessarily trigger a therapeutic change. For example, there is no reason to treat resected well-differentiated liposarcoma with osteosarcomatous elements with adjuvant chemotherapy, as would be the standard of care for primary high-grade osteosarcomas.

SYNOVIAL SARCOMA

Synovial sarcoma is predominantly a tumor of older adolescents and young adults, with a median age of 27 years at diagnosis. It is somewhat more common in men than women. The tumor was named due to a pathological resemblance of the tumor cells to tendosynovial tissue, although the tumor does not necessarily have anything to do with normal synovium. Unlike patients with other localized soft tissue sarcomas (who are often asymptomatic at presentation), about half of patients with synovial sarcoma report pain or tenderness. These tumors can arise anywhere in the body and not simply around joint capsules, as was once thought. In particular, it is now recognized that a primary pulmonary and pleural variant of synovial sarcoma is possible and this should be considered in the differential diagnosis of difficult-to-classify chest malignancies.

Radiographically, about one-third of these tumors contain calcification, from fine stippling to radiopaque masses. Periosteal proliferation or invasion is less common. Gross examination reveals that the tumor is usually firmly adherent to surrounding tissues. Cystic areas may be prominent. Histologically, synovial sarcomas can be monophasic or biphasic, with epithelial or spindle cell components or both (*see* Fig. 10.61). The malignant cells therefore have the potential to differentiate aberrantly into both lineages, since each component can harbor the translocation of the X chromosome and chromosome 18 which characterizes synovial sarcoma. Most pathologists consider all synovial sarcomas to be high grade by definition. Synovial sarcoma appears to be particularly sensitive to combination chemotherapy and therefore this sensitivity should be considered in developing a comprehensive management plan for any individual patient with this disease (van Glabbeke *et al.*, 1999).

MALIGNANT PERIPHERAL NERVE SHEATH TUMOR (NEUROSARCOMA)

Malignant peripheral nerve sheath tumors (MPNSTs), also known in the older literature as neurosarcomas or malignant schwannomas, which constitute 5% of soft tissue sarcomas, differ from other sarcomas in that they are of ectodermal embryologic origin. Fifty percent of patients with neurosarcomas have von Recklinghausen's neurofibromatosis. Of patients with von Recklinghausen's disease, 80% are male, as compared with 56% of those with sporadic malignant schwannoma. The development of pain or the sudden enlargement of a pre-existing mass in a patient with neurofibromatosis should prompt immediate biopsy.

Generally arising as a large fusiform mass within a major nerve, MPNSTs tend to extend within the nerve sheath. Thus, most develop in the proximal extremity or trunk and larger surgical and radiotherapeutic margins are required to ensure local control. Although somewhat similar in organization to the spindle cells of fibrosarcomas, malignant Schwann cells have more irregular cell borders; their nuclei are waxy or buckled if sectioned parallel to the cell or oval if sectioned across the cell.

VASCULAR SARCOMAS

Several types of vascular malignancies, as well as their differential diagnostic features, are noted in Table 10.8. Like their benign counterparts, malignancies of vascular endothelium may produce microangiopathic hemolytic anemia (Kassabach–Merritt syndrome), presumably secondary to traumatic injury of red blood cells traversing the extensive vascular tumor bed with abnormal shear forces.

Hemangioendothelioma

The term 'hemangioendothelioma' is generally applied to a vascular tumor of intermediate malignancy between a benign hemangioma and conventional angiosarcoma. This relatively rare lesion affects men and women about equally and rarely develops in childhood. The epithelioid variant differs from the benign epithelioid hemangioma in that the vascular cells are more primitive. Rather than distinct vascular channels, the tumor forms small intracellular lumina, which occasionally contain erythrocytes. There is little mitotic activity. If the tumor contains areas with more than one mitosis per 10 high-power fields or significant necrosis, the course may be more aggressive. A spindle cell variant occurs in younger patients, predominantly males, and principally involves the skin, generally of the hand; it tends to be locally and regionally recurrent. Metastatic hemangioendothelioma can remain remarkably indolent even in the presence of extensive unresectable metastases in liver and/or lung. The utility of chemotherapy or other systemic treatments (such as putatively 'antiangiogenic' approaches with agents such as interferon-α) remains unclear, given the fact that this disease can exhibit indolent progression or even prolonged periods of stability even without treatment.

Angiosarcoma

Angiosarcomas are malignant lesions of vascular endothelium and vary considerably in differentiation. Described in the older literature under a variety of names, angiosarcomas include tumors previously called hemangiosarcoma, lymphangiosarcoma and hemangioblastoma, since immunoperoxidase stains do not show differences in cell of origin among them. These tumors frequently express the vascular antigen CD34 (an antigen which is shared with hematopoietic stem cells), but the most definitive immunohistochemical assay is the CD31 antigen.

Of these rare lesions (1% of sarcomas), about one-third arise in the skin typically as multicentric scalp lesions in elderly men, or as multiple chest and arm lesions in women with chronic lymphedema after mastectomy and radical lymph node dissection for breast cancer. The impact of prior radiation therapy is also increasingly recognized, since many postradiation sarcomas of the chest wall in women with previous breast cancer treated with locoregional irradiation can be secondary angiosarcomas. One quarter of these tumors develop in soft tissue sites and another quarter arise in organs such as the breast, liver and lungs. Primary angiosarcomas of the breast occur in young and middle-aged women; those of the liver arise in infants or, more often, in adults. Adult cases are associated with exposure to thorium dioxide (an outdated reagent used in angiography), arsenic (insecticides) and polyvinyl chloride (plastics). Angiosarcomas represent the most common primary malignant tumors of the heart. As noted above, angiosarcomas are also at risk to arise in sites of prior radiotherapy (for breast cancer, Hodgkin's disease, cervical cancer and other conditions) and have been reported at the site of an extensive foreign body reaction or prior herpes zoster infection.

Postmastectomy lymphangiosarcoma (Stewart–Treves syndrome) is a comparatively rare complication of radical mastectomy that usually manifests more than 10 years after the development of lymphedema. Although its origin is unclear, it is assumed to arise from lymphatics in the arm after dissection of axillary lymph nodes. Prior radiotherapy may also be associated. The prognosis is generally poor; repeated local recurrence and eventual dissemination are the rule.

On gross examination, angiosarcomas may appear to be single, but multiple clustered bruises are noted in about half of cases. Tumors infiltrate substantially beyond their apparent gross extent. Microscopically, many moderately to well-differentiated lesions form anastomosing vascular channels. Undifferentiated angiosarcomas may be difficult to distinguish from carcinomas or other sarcomas. Immunoperoxidase studies for factor VIII are positive in 50–85% of cases, whereas binding of the *Ulex europaeus* lectin is more common (80–100% of cases) but less specific. Angiosarcomas that appear deceptively benign under the microscope can be difficult to control locally, in part because of the tendency to be multifocal and in part because of their extensive invasion and high metastatic rate. In summary, it is not clear that the pathologic features of angiosarcoma predict clinical behavior as well as in other subtypes of soft tissue sarcomas. The prognosis is poor overall, especially for advanced disease. Chemotherapy can be effective for palliation of advanced disease and besides the conventional agents of doxorubicin and ifosfamide, microtubule poisons such as paclitaxel and vinorelbine have also been reported to have important activity in this disease.

Kaposi's sarcoma

This subtype of vascular sarcoma has classically presented as multiple blue-red nodes that progress in an indolent manner up the lower legs; it generally occurs in elderly men of Mediterranean origin. Secondary tumors, especially lymphomas, are common. A second variant of Kaposi's sarcoma occurs in about 0.4% of renal transplant patients; interestingly, this form is also more common in men of Mediterranean extraction. Developing a mean of 16 months after transplantation, Kaposi's sarcoma may respond to a decrease in immunosuppressive therapy. A more aggressive endemic form of lymphadenopathic Kaposi's sarcoma has been described in Africa, particularly in young children.

A highly aggressive form of Kaposi's sarcoma has been associated with HIV-I associated acquired immune deficiency syndrome (AIDS). The lesions involve the mucous membranes of the mouth, stomach, lungs, skin and lymph nodes. Coexistent opportunistic infections portend a short survival. Lesions progress from flat to plaque-like and then coalesce to form nodular lesions that may ulcerate. The fatality of this disease often resulted from uncontrolled disease in the lungs and gastrointestinal tract. In the era of more modern highly effective combination retroviral therapy, this disease has become less prevalent. The etiology of Kaposi's sarcoma remains unclear although the role of human herpesvirus 8 (HHV8) is increasingly recognized as an important pathogenetic mechanism in both the HIV-associated type as well as the sporadic type of this disease (Landau *et al.*, 2001; Froehner and Wirth, 2001).

Hemangiopericytoma

A malignancy of vascular pericytes which normally are found adjacent to blood vessel endothelium, hemangiopericytoma should not be confused with angiosarcoma or hemangioendothelioma. The incidence of hemangiopericytomas peaks in the fifth decade of life. Thirty-five percent of tumors are found in the thigh and 25% in the retroperitoneum, often in a perirenal location. These richly vascular tumors may lead to substantial arteriovenous shunting and bleeding. Hypoglycemia has been associated with large retroperitoneal tumors. Intracranial hemangiopericytomas (formerly designated angioblastic meningiomas) grow along the sinuses, locally recur and may metastasize.

The histologic appearance of hemangiopericytomas is marked by a dilated 'antler' or 'staghorn' configuration of anastomosing vascular channels lined by a single layer of flattened endothelial cells. Surrounding tumor cells do not stain for factor VIII or *Ulex europaeus* lectin, as angiosarcomas do. It is important to recognize that the 'staghorn' vascular channels which have been described in pathology depictions of hemangiopericytoma are not necessarily unique to this disease; it is not uncommon for a sarcoma specialty pathologist to reclassify tumors which were initially diagnosed as hemangiopericytoma simply on the basis of vascular pattern, since other types of sarcomas can have these same sort of abnormal tumor-associated vascular patterns.

SARCOMAS OF MUSCLE AND RELATED STROMAL TISSUE
Leiomyosarcomas and gastrointestinal stromal tumors (GISTs)

Exhibiting differentiation along the smooth muscle lineage, leiomyosarcomas frequently develop in the GI tract, uterus or retroperitoneum. GI or gynecologic leiomyosarcomas are excluded from many series, in which case leiomyosarcomas account for about 7% of soft tissue sarcomas. In other series that include leiomyosarcomas arising in the GI tract or the uterus, these tumors are among the most common histologic type of soft tissue sarcoma.

The median age of affected patients is 60 years. Leiomyosarcomas of the retroperitoneum and of the vena cava most commonly arise in women and their growth may be exacerbated during pregnancy. Tumors originating in other large veins affect the sexes equally. Cutaneous and subcutaneous leiomyosarcomas are more common in men. Perhaps because of their superficial location and early diagnosis when they are relatively small, these tumors carry a good prognosis with surgical resection alone.

Although more than half of GI tract sarcomas occur in the stomach, only 1–3% of gastric malignancies are sarcomas. Of GI tract sarcomas, 29% arise in the small bowel (constituting 20% of all small intestine malignancies) and 10% in the large bowel (only 0.1% of colorectal neoplasms). Patients with GI or uterine leiomyosarcomas may be asymptomatic, mimicking fibroids in the uterus, or they may present with pain and life-threatening bleeding. Characteristic findings on upper GI series frequently suggest the diagnosis before histologic confirmation. In more than half of patients, intraperitoneal seeding, liver metastases and lung nodules eventually develop. Multiple cutaneous leiomyosarcomas should suggest metastases from an occult retroperitoneal or intra-abdominal primary tumor.

It has been observed that children with AIDS have a greatly increased risk of developing smooth muscle tumors, including leiomyomas and leiomyosarcomas. Similarly, an increased risk of such tumors has been observed in chronically immunosuppressed patients following liver transplantation. Recent studies have detected clonal portions of the Epstein–Barr virus (EBV) genome within the malignant smooth muscle cells, suggesting a potential causative role for EBV in the etiologic development of these immunosuppression-related tumors. Histologically, on hematoxylin and eosin stain for light microscopy, the pink-to-red cells are elongated, with a centrally located, cigar-shaped nucleus (sometimes indented by a cytoplasmic vacuole). Mitoses are common. An epithelioid variant of leiomyosarcoma, characterized by rounder, vacuolated (clear cell) features, has also been called leiomyoblastoma.

The phrase 'gastrointestinal stromal tumor' (GIST) once was commonly used to refer to a variety of spindle cell tumors of the gastrointestinal tract. Specifically, prior to the year 2000, there was commonly a frequent blurring of the clinical or biologic distinction between true leiomyosarcomas of the GI tract and GISTs. It is now clear that GISTs can be differentiated from other spindle cell malignancies of the GI tract by the fact that GISTs express the CD117 antigen (*see* Fig. 10.81). CD117 is an epitope of the extracellular domain of the KIT protein, a transmembrane receptor tyrosine kinase. Differentiation of KIT-positive GIST from other spindle cell malignancies in the GI tract (such as leiomyosarcomas or de-differentiated liposarcomas, all of which are KIT negative) is important since it now may have therapeutic relevance. A key element of GIST pathogenesis is the aberrant signaling through uncontrolled kinase activity of the

KIT molecule. The majority of GISTs possess activating mutations in the c-*kit* proto-oncogene which encodes the KIT protein; even without mutations, it has been shown that all GISTs have aberrantly activated KIT (Rubin, 2001). The importance of constitutive KIT activation to the malignant phenotype has been documented by *in vitro* studies on human GIST cells: blocking KIT enzymatic action by the selective inhibitor Imatinib mesylate (STI-571, Gleevec) stops tumor cell proliferation and ultimately leads to death of the GIST cells by apoptosis (Tuveson *et al.*, 2001). This finding has now been confirmed in patients with GIST and this has led to the recognition that blocking the key signaling aberrancy in GIST with STI-571 is an important new systemic therapy for this disease (Joensuu *et al.*, 2001; Blanke *et al.*, 2001; van Oosterom *et al.*, 2001).

Endometrial stromal sarcomas

Endometrial stromal sarcomas are gynecologic sarcomas for which quite different natural histories can be observed depending on the grade of the tumor. These range from benign endometrial stromal tumors which can mimic leiomyomas, to low-grade endometrial stromal sarcomas, to high-grade ('undifferentiated') endometrial stromal sarcomas. The important new finding is that there is a chromosomal translocation between chromosomes 7 and 17 which is common to each of these subtypes of uterine sarcomas (Koontz *et al.*, 2001). These tumors can be viewed as stromal proliferations of varying degrees of malignancy: low-grade endometrial stromal sarcomas can exhibit a very indolent natural history and can often be cured by appropriate surgery alone, whereas the high-grade endometrial stromal sarcomas typically have very aggressive behavior with a predilection to metastasize early and widely. Additionally, the low-grade variant commonly expresses high levels of estrogen and progesterone receptors which can be therapeutically important, since these tumors can be managed by antiestrogens (e.g. tamoxifen) or progestins (e.g. megasterol acetate) (*see* Fig. 10.83). High-grade endometrial stromal sarcomas can be transiently responsive to chemotherapy but often acquired resistance develops rapidly and the tumors progress inexorably. These tumors can spread to bony sites with some frequency, unlike other subtypes of soft tissue sarcomas.

Rhabdomyosarcomas

These sarcomas, derived from striated muscle cells, appear as embryonal, alveolar and pleomorphic variants. Systemic as well as locoregional lymph node metastases are common. The peak incidence for embryonal rhabdomyosarcomas of the orbit occurs at age 4 and for those of the GI tract the peak is in childhood and adolescence. Alveolar rhabdomyosarcomas, which arise most commonly in the extremities of adolescents and young adults, carry a more serious prognosis. An important cytogenetic feature of alveolar rhabdomyosarcomas is the common translocation of the transcription factors PAX3 and FKHR. This may contribute to the malignant phenotype by providing an antiapoptotic signal via increased production of BCL-XL, an antiapoptotic protein (Margue *et al.*, 2000). Pleomorphic mabdomyosarcomas are rarely diagnosed, generally in older patients.

Without a multimodality approach to treatment, 80% of rhabdomyosarcomas would recur systemically. Patients are generally given combination chemotherapy including vincristine, actinomycin D and cyclophosphamide or ifosfamide. Doxorubicin is also frequently included. Resection is followed by regional radiotherapy. Embryonal rhabdomyosarcomas of the orbit and GU tract are highly sensitive to chemotherapy and radiotherapy.

MESOTHELIOMA

Defined as a primary malignancy of serosal surfaces, malignant mesothelioma is an uncommon tumor that develops in the parietal or visceral pleura, peritoneum, the tunica vaginalis of the testis or pericardium. It characteristically affects men 50–70 years old. A history of workplace exposure to asbestos has been elicited in 10–70% of patients in various series. Children with the disease have been reported, but a convincing history of asbestos exposure in these cases is rare. Patients with peritoneal primary lesions first note increased abdominal girth or pain. Those with pleural primary tumors report shortness of breath or pain and chest radiography reveals a unilateral effusion in 75% of patients. Asbestos or pleural calcifications are evident on chest films in only 20% of patients with pleural mesothelioma and in about half of those with peritoneal primary tumors.

Sampling of recurrent pleural effusions or ascites may or may not initially reveal malignant cells. Thoracotomy or laparotomy is often required to establish the diagnosis. Three histologic variants have been identified. Mesotheliomas may be epithelial (50–60% of cases), sarcomatous (20–25%) or mixed. A biphasic pattern is virtually pathognomic of malignant mesothelioma. It is important to differentiate malignant mesothelioma from adenocarcinoma of the lung and other common epithelial neoplasms which often metastasize to the pleura, resulting in a malignant pleural effusion.

The peritoneal variant of mesothelioma appears somewhat more treatable than the pleural. Debulking surgery, intraperitoneal cisplatin and doxorubicin, and whole abdominal radiotherapy have resulted in significant palliation and 5-year disease-free survival in a substantial percentage of selected patients with peritoneal disease. Patients with peritoneal disease in whom treatment fails die of respiratory failure or of inanition from small bowel obstruction.

Table 10.6 Soft tissue sarcomas: Distribution of primary sites of occurrence.

Site	Frequency (%)
Lower extremity	
Thigh	31
Below knee	10
Trunk	18
Head and neck	15
Retroperitoneum	13
Upper extremity	13

Table 10.7 Summary of the American Joint Committee (AJC) staging system for soft tissue sarcomas.[a] **See also updated TNM staging classification system (Fig. 10.2)**

Stage[b]	Grade	Comments	Five-year survival (%) AJC (1954–1968)	DFCI[c] (1978–1985)
1	Low	<1 mitosis/10 HPF[d]	76	85
2	Intermediate	1–4 mitoses/10 HPF	56	66
3	High	≥ 5 mitoses/10 HPF	26	54
4A		Gross invasion of bone, major vessels; or nerve	50	NA[e]
4B		Metastases	4	<20

[a]From Russel *et al.* 1977.
[b]For stages 1 to 3, subcategories designated A, B, and C have been defined: A represents a lesion < 5 cm in size, and B represents a lesion > 5 cm. A stage designated C denotes positive lymph nodes in a tumor of any grade.
[c]DFCI: from the Soft Tissue Sarcoma Registry, Data–Farber Cancer Institute, Boston, MA.
[d]HPF high-power field.
[e]NA: not available.

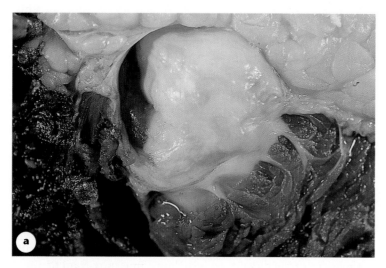

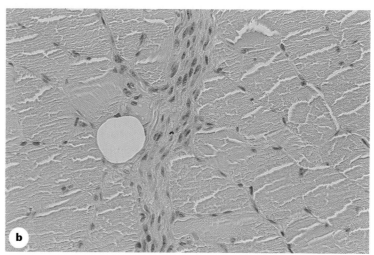

Fig. 10.43 Leiomyosarcoma. (**a**) Careful gross examination shows thin bands of tumor tissue focally infiltrating skeletal muscle at the edge of an otherwise circumscribed leiomyosarcoma. (**b**) Microscopic examination more clearly demonstrates the inconspicuous fascicles of tumor cells infiltrating skeletal muscle (note mitosis at center).

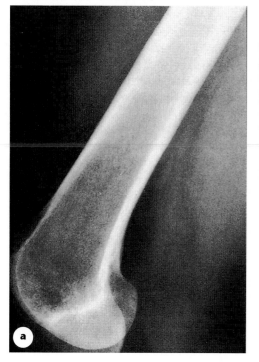

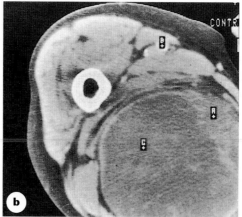

Fig. 10.44 Malignant fibrous histiocytoma. An 86-year-old woman presented with a soft tissue mass on the posteromedial aspect of the right thigh. (**a**) Lateral plain film of the femur demonstrates only a soft tissue prominence posteriorly. (**b**) CT scan shows an axial image of the mass, which is contained by a fibrotic capsule. The overlying skin is not infiltrated. Despite the benign appearance, the mass proved on biopsy to be a malignant fibrous histiocytoma.

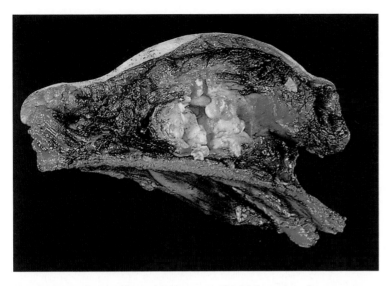

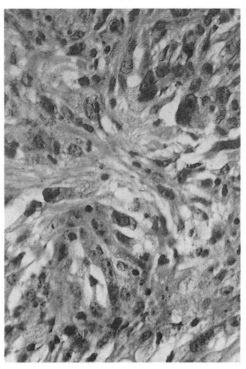

Fig. 10.46 Malignant fibrous histiocytoma. Photomicrograph demonstrates the characteristic storiform arrangement of spindle cells. The cells appear more histiocyte-like rather than fibroblast-like and exhibit considerable pleomorphism.

Fig. 10.45 Malignant fibrous histiocytoma. This high-grade malignancy was resected from the right upper chest wall of a 60-year-old woman. Note the localized, lobulated, soft tissue mass and adjacent ribs. The black material is India ink used to identify surgical margins. (Courtesy of Pathology Department, Brigham and Women's Hospital, Boston, MA.)

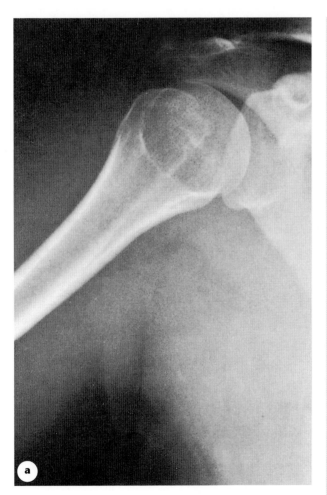

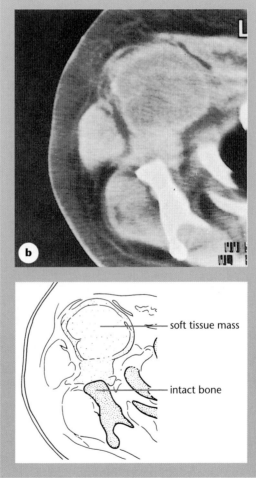

soft tissue mass

intact bone

Fig. 10.47 Fibrosarcoma. (**a**) AP plain film of the shoulder of a 40-year-old woman with a history of an enlarging mass in the right axilla shows an ill-defined mass adjacent to the lateral border of the scapula. (**b**) CT section with contrast enhancement shows the extent of the mass and the lack of bone involvement. The tumor proved to be a fibrosarcoma.

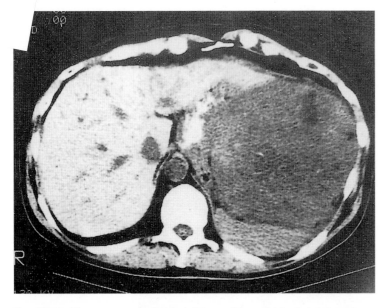

Fig. 10.48 Fibrosarcoma. Abdominal CT scan shows a large, heterogeneous, soft tissue mass in the left upper quadrant. The mass displaces the spleen posteriorly.

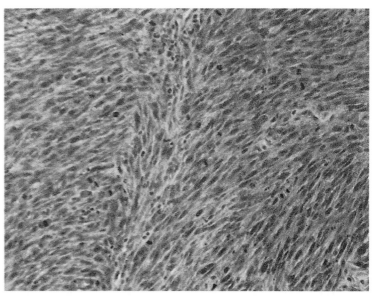

Fig. 10.49 Fibrosarcoma. Photomicrograph demonstrates well-differentiated malignant fibroblasts proliferating in parallel and forming interlacing bands. This appearance is known as a herringbone pattern.

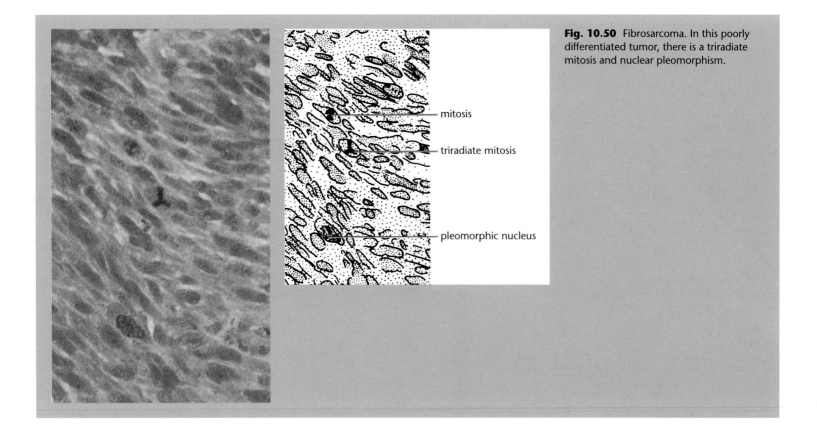

Fig. 10.50 Fibrosarcoma. In this poorly differentiated tumor, there is a triradiate mitosis and nuclear pleomorphism.

mitosis

triradiate mitosis

pleomorphic nucleus

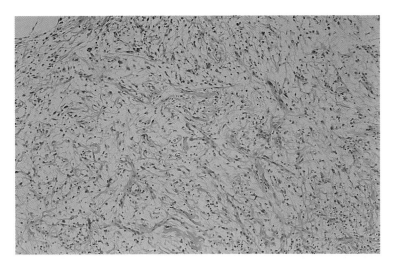

Fig. 10.51 Myxofibrosarcoma is characterized by atypical spindle cells set in a myxoid stroma with curvilinear vessels.

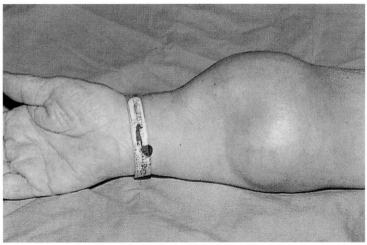

Fig. 10.52 Liposarcoma. This slow-growing tumor of the forearm of a 75-year-old woman was diagnosed as a liposarcoma. Radical resection was carried out with preservation of hand function. Postoperative radiotherapy was also administered. Such patients have a significant chance of remaining disease free for more than 5 years following local resection, as was the case with this patient.

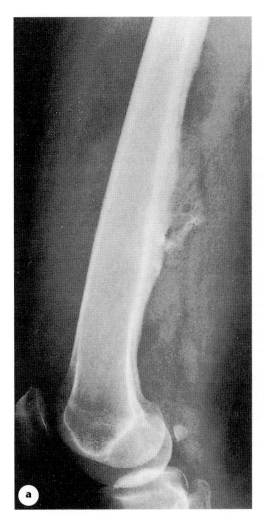

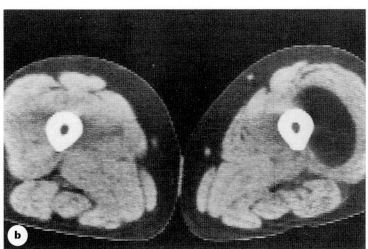

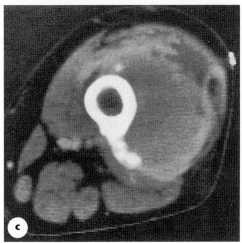

Fig. 10.53 Liposarcoma. (**a**) Lateral plain film of a 54-year-old man with a slowly enlarging mass on the posterior aspect of the thigh demonstrates a poorly defined soft tissue mass with radiolucent areas and bone formation at the posterior cortex of the femur. (**b**) CT section at the level of the radiolucency confirms the presence of fatty tissue. (**c**) A section through the bone formation discloses a denser mass infiltrating surrounding muscular structures. Liposarcoma, suggested as a possible diagnosis, was later confirmed on biopsy.

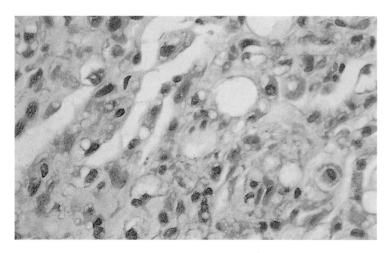

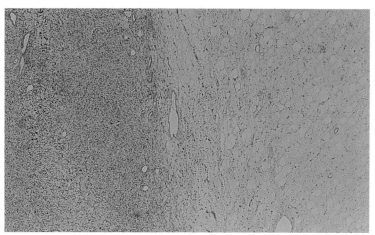

Fig. 10.54 Liposarcoma. In contrast to the microscopic appearance of lipoma, liposarcoma is highly cellular; it also contains much less fat in the signet ring cells (lipoblasts) and within the nuclei, giving it a foamy appearance.

Fig. 10.55 De-differentiated liposarcoma (left) is a cellular spindle cell neoplasm without obvious adipocytic differentiation; adjacent areas of well-differentiated liposarcoma (right) showing prominent intracellular lipid accumulation may coexist.

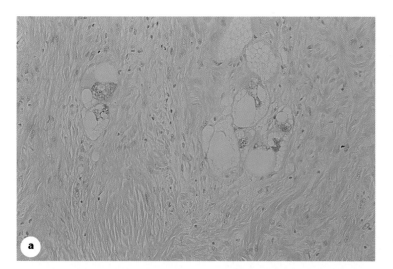

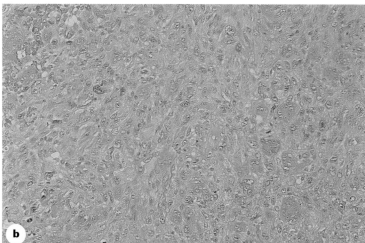

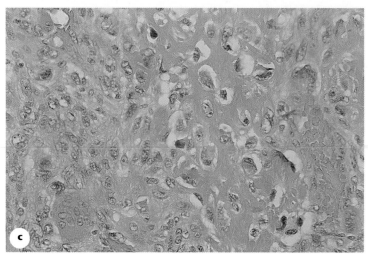

Fig. 10.56 A malignant spindle cell neoplasm showing combined lipogenic (**a**), myogenic (**b**) and osteogenic (**c**) differentiation would once have been regarded as 'malignant mesenchymoma'.

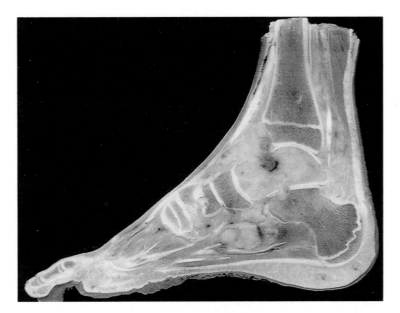

Fig. 10.57 Synovial sarcoma. This is an amputation specimen from a 13-year-old boy who reported a painful right ankle for 2½ years. The discomfort had become progressively worse and rapid swelling had developed during the previous 6 months. The specimen has been sectioned to show ill-defined, pale tumor masses, which were in continuity *in vivo* but are now apparent in the sole of the foot, beneath the calcaneal tendon, and on the upper surface of the talus. The tumor has widely invaded bone and soft tissues.

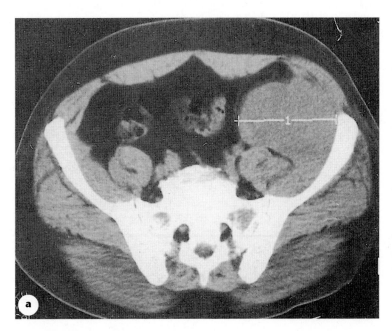

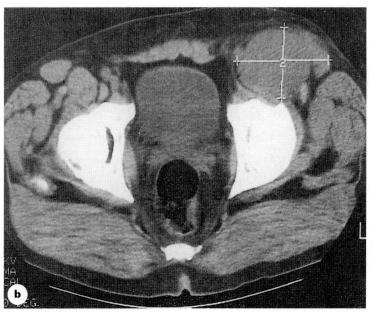

Fig. 10.58 Synovial sarcoma metastases. CT sections show soft tissue metastases to the pelvis (**a**) and groin (**b**) in a 22-year-old man with synovial sarcoma originating in the thigh.

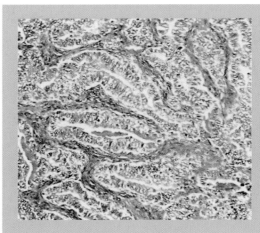

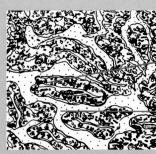

glandular epithelial component

fibrosarcomatous component

Fig. 10.59 Synovial sarcoma. Photomicrograph demonstrates the biphasic appearance of such lesions. Gland-like spaces lined by tall columnar epithelial cells are seen, as are fibrosarcomatous stromata. The ratio of these two components may vary considerably; in this example, the glandular component predominates.

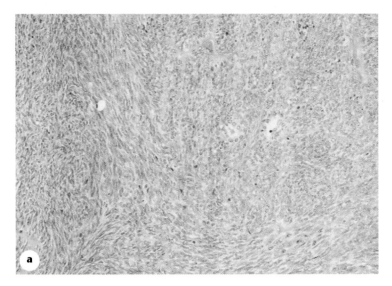

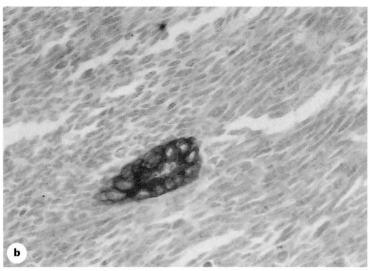

Fig. 10.60 Synovial sarcoma. Synovial sarcoma is a relatively common sarcoma whose tissue of origin is unknown. Its name derives from frequent occurrence in para-articular regions and occasional histologic resemblance to synovium. It most commonly occurs in the extremities of adolescents and young adults. (**a**) The classic biphasic histology is composed of epithelial and spindle cell components. Monophasic fibrous (spindle cell) and epithelial types may be difficult to discriminate from fibrosarcoma and carcinoma, respectively. Both spindle cell and epithelial components express cytokeratins. (**b**) Nested epithelioid cells, strongly positive (immunohistochemical stain for AE1/AE3, brown color). The tumor has a characteristic balanced chromosomal translocation, t(Xp;18q), in the majority of cases.

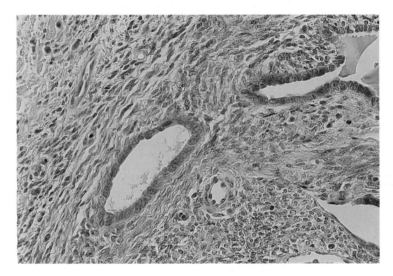

Fig. 10.61 Biphasic synovial sarcoma shows glandular elements in a background of relatively bland spindle cells and so-called 'wiry' collagen.

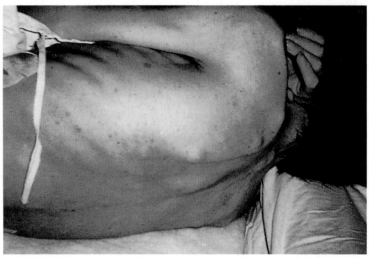

Fig. 10.62 Neurofibromatosis. Clinical photograph of a 70-year-old woman with von Recklinghausen's disease shows multiple cutaneous neurofibromas. An abdominal neurosarcoma had been resected.

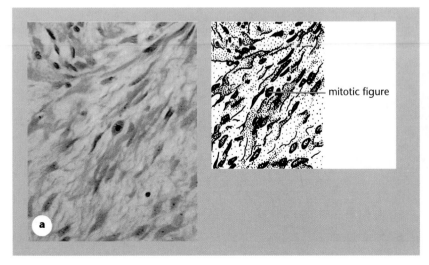

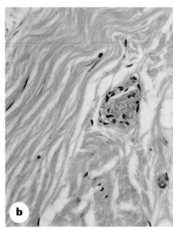

Fig. 10.63 Neurofibrosarcoma. (**a**) The connective tissue fibers are sinuous, as in neurofibroma, but the nuclei are more pleomorphic and may show mitoses. (**b**) Neural elements (neurites) may be present. Note that this area is strikingly acellular.

mitotic figure

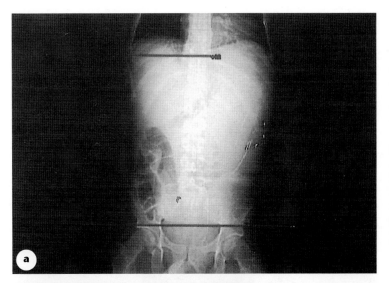

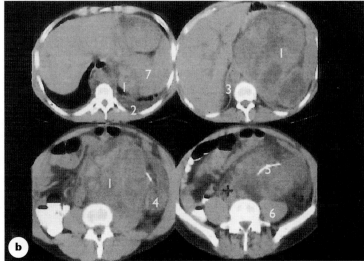

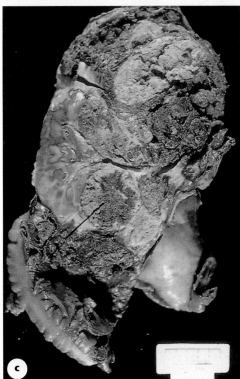

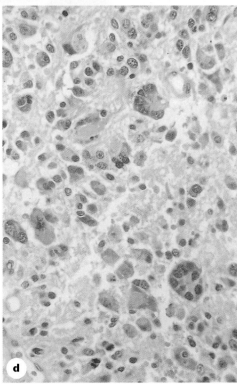

Fig. 10.64 Neuroblastoma. This neuroblastoma presented in a young man aged 28, with acute abdominal pain. Plain film and CT scan revealed a large retroperitoneal mass. (**a**) Localizing image for CT shows displacement of bowel into the right abdomen. Black lines indicate the superior and inferior margins of the large mass. (**b**) CT scan reveals a large heterogeneous tumor mass (1) extending into the lower abdomen. A small left pleural effusion is present (2). A right retrocrural lymph node mass is also evident (3). Lateral displacement of the left kidney is evident (4) with a ureteral stent in place (5). Note compression of the left psoas muscle (6) by the large tumor mass. Spleen (7) is evident in left upper quadrant. (**c**) Needle biopsy revealed a poorly differentiated malignancy, suggestive of sarcoma. Immunoperoxidase studies showed the tumor to be focally positive for chromogranin, synaptophysin and neurofilament proteins. These results and the neurofibrillary stroma raised the possibility of pleomorphic neuroblastoma, an unusual subtype of neuroblastoma. Following one cycle of combination chemotherapy, tumor necrosis resulted in a large retroperitoneal bleed. (**d**) The large tumor was resected and extensive histologic sampling showed some areas with small tumor cells, typical of classic neuroblastoma. The patient continued toward a stable, partial remission.

Table 10.8 Differential diagnosis of vascular malignancies.

Malignancy	Cell of origin	Diagnostic features
Anglosarcoma Hemangloendothelioma	Vascular endothelium	Hyperchromatic nuclei Papillations or piling up of cells
Lymphangiosarcoma	Vascular or lymphatic endothelium	Similar to angiosarcoma but with proliferation of small lymphatics
Kaposi's sarcoma	Vascular or lymphatic endothelium	Slit-like endothelium-lined channels Extravasation of red blood cells Stromal spindle-cell proliferation
Hemangiopericytoma	Pericyte	'Staghorn' vascular proliferation

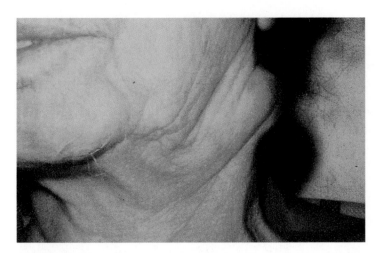

Fig. 10.65 Angiosarcoma. Fatal metastatic disease eventually developed from the angiosarcoma of the left upper neck in this 75-year-old woman.

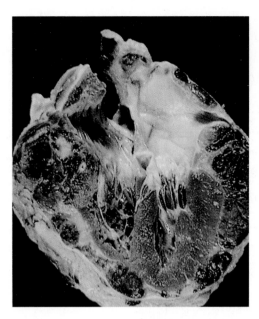

Fig. 10.66 Myocardial angiosarcoma. Specimen photograph shows numerous metastases throughout the heart. Angiosarcoma is the most common primary malignancy of the myocardium. (Courtesy of Pathology Department, Brigham and Women's Hospital, Boston, MA.)

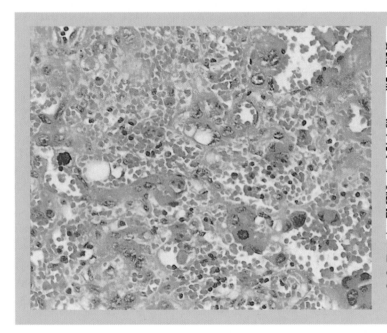

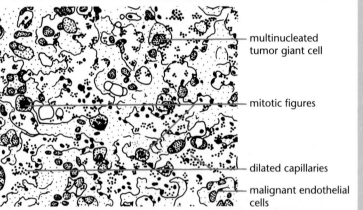

multinucleated tumor giant cell

mitotic figures

dilated capillaries

malignant endothelial cells

Fig. 10.67 Angiosarcoma. High-power photomicrograph shows well-differentiated areas consisting of irregular vascular channels lined by atypical endothelial cells; some cells show mitotic activity.

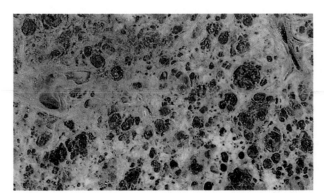

Fig. 10.68 Hepatic angiosarcoma. Specimen photograph shows the hepatic parenchyma largely replaced by a diffuse hemorrhagic neoplasm in which multiple small vascular channels are visible.

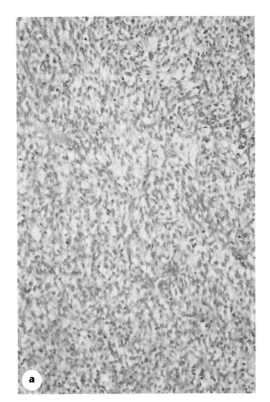
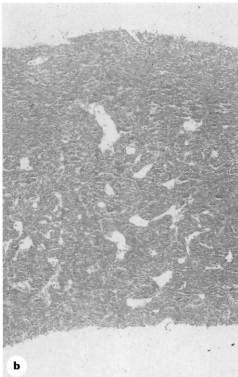

Fig. 10.69 Hemangiopericytoma. This 24-year-old patient presented with massive hepatic metastases. Needle biopsy of liver showed a cellular process composed of haphazardly arranged cells with oval nuclei and indistinct clear cytoplasm (**a**). Elsewhere, the characteristic 'staghorn' or antler-like gaping vascular channels were present (**b**). Immunoperoxidase studies showed the tumor to be positive for CD34 antigen (**c**), a marker of vascular tumors, some other mesenchymal tumors, and non-neoplastic hematopoietic stem and progenitor cells.

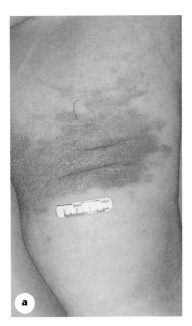
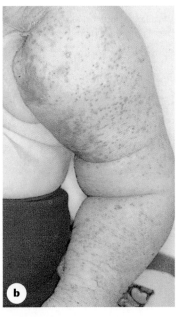
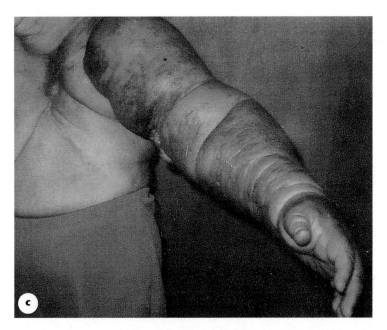

Fig. 10.70 Postmastectomy lymphangiosarcoma. This 65-year-old woman had undergone left radical mastectomy 9 years previously. Massive lymphedema of the left arm had been present since the operation and in recent months she had noticed the appearance of purplish, ulcerated nodules in the skin of the upper arm. (**a**) The cluster of lesions projects from an irregular area of dusky discoloration. (**b**) Six months later, numerous lesions have appeared on her arm. (**c**) Within 5 months, the entire arm is involved by metastatic disease.

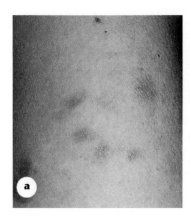

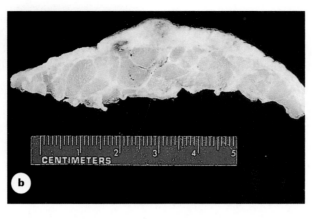

Fig. 10.71 Lymphangiosarcoma. (**a**) Multiple small lesions are diagnostic of early lymphangiosarcoma. This 48-year-old woman had a history of Hodgkin's disease treated 13 years previously by irradiation. At age 45, she underwent bilateral mastectomies for stage I breast cancer. Postoperative radiotherapy was not given. The patient did not have arm edema. (**b**) The resected tumor shows extension into the subcutaneous tissue.

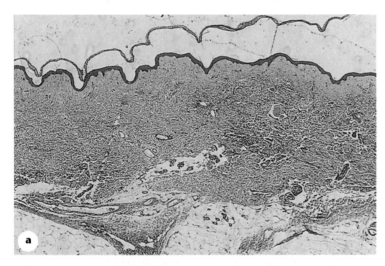

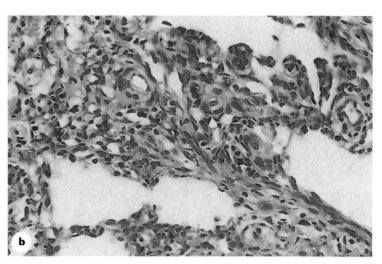

Fig. 10.72 Lymphangiosarcoma. (**a**) Low-power photomicrograph of a skin biopsy from a patient shown in Figure 10.70 exhibits extensive proliferation of vascular endothelial and lymphatic cells. (**b**) Higher-power view shows papillation of cells with hyperchromatic nuclei.

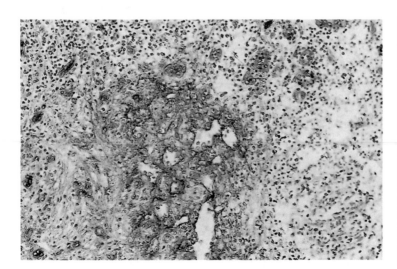

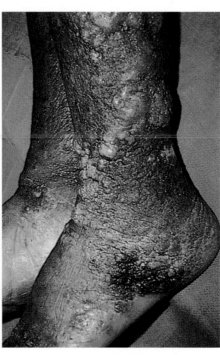

Fig. 10.74 Kaposi's sarcoma. Purplish, hyperpigmented plaques and nodules in association with edema of the lower extremities are characteristic cutaneous manifestations of Kaposi's sarcoma.

Fig. 10.73 Vascular malignancy. Proliferating endothelial cells of vascular malignancies show positive immunoperoxidase reactivity to factor VIII. (Courtesy of Pathology Department, Brigham and Women's Hospital, Boston, MA.)

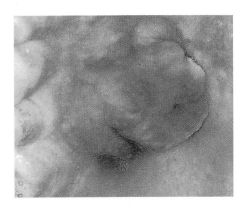

Fig. 10.75 Kaposi's sarcoma. The palate, lips and tongue are the most common sites of intraoral involvement. The patient whose palate is shown here was an African with a previous renal transplant.

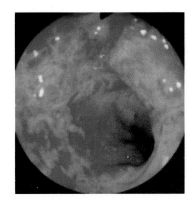

Fig. 10.76 Kaposi's sarcoma. Endoscopic view shows extensive Kaposi's sarcoma of the rectum in an AIDS patient. This is rarely seen.

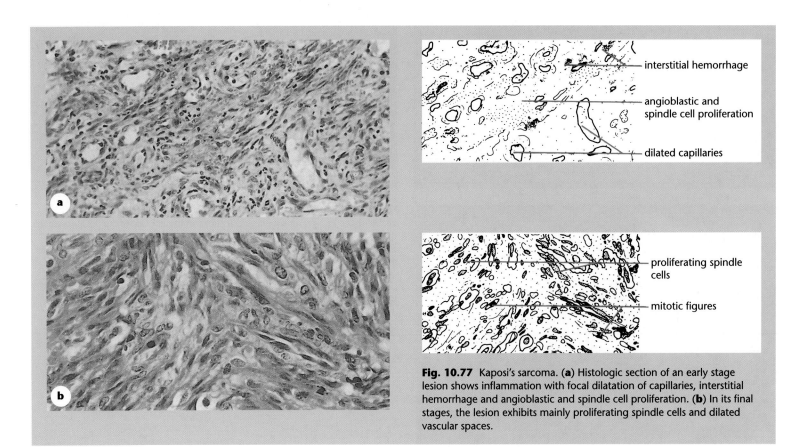

interstitial hemorrhage

angioblastic and spindle cell proliferation

dilated capillaries

proliferating spindle cells

mitotic figures

Fig. 10.77 Kaposi's sarcoma. (**a**) Histologic section of an early stage lesion shows inflammation with focal dilatation of capillaries, interstitial hemorrhage and angioblastic and spindle cell proliferation. (**b**) In its final stages, the lesion exhibits mainly proliferating spindle cells and dilated vascular spaces.

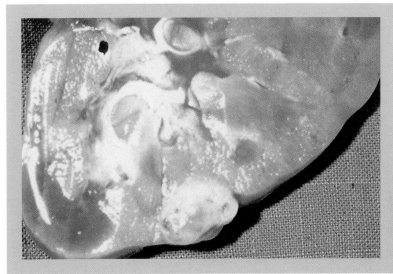

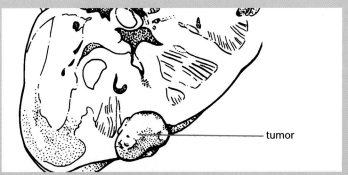

tumor

Fig. 10.78 Hemangiopericytoma. The small tumor at the lower pole of this kidney produced excessive quantities of renin, causing hypertension. (Courtesy of Dr JJ Brown.)

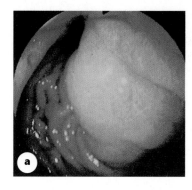

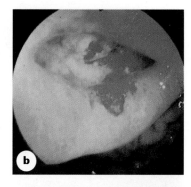

Fig. 10.79 Leiomyosarcoma. (**a**) Endoscopic view shows a large leiomyosarcoma protruding into the proximal gastric lumen. (**b**) With further insertion of the endoscope, necrosis can be seen in the center of the mass, presenting as a deep depression or ulcer. The ulcer is friable.

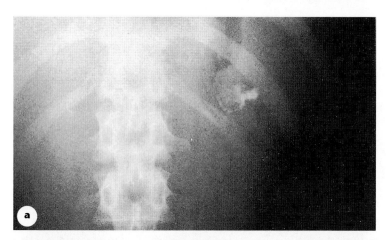

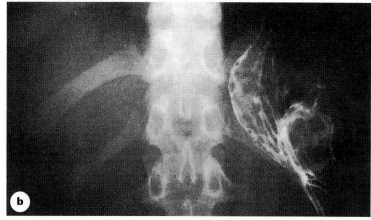

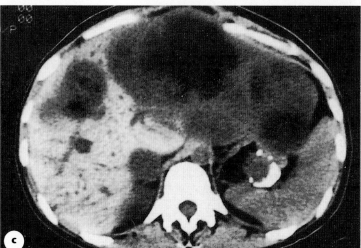

Fig. 10.80 Leiomyosarcoma. (**a**) KUB study from a 62-year-old man with a gastric leiomyosarcoma shows calcifications in the left upper quadrant lateral to the gastric air. (**b**) On upper GI series, barium outlines a large, predominantly submucosal lobular mass in the body of the stomach. The mass corresponds to the region of calcifications seen on the KUB. (**c**) Large, heterogeneous metastases are seen in both lobes of the liver on abdominal CT scan. The calcified mass posterior to the left lobe of the liver is the gastric leiomyosarcoma.

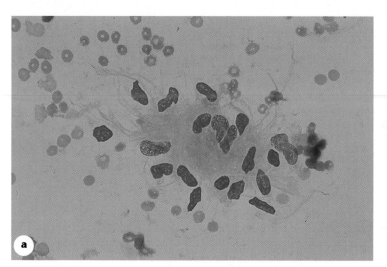

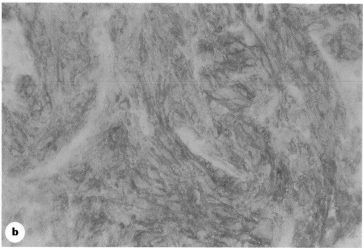

Fig. 10.81 Gastrointestinal stromal tumor (GIST). The characteristic morphologic features of GIST (typically bland spindle cells with abundant delicate cytoplasmic processes) make it possible to make a primary diagnosis by fine-needle aspiration (**a**), when supported by immunohistochemical positivity for c-*kit*, performed on cell block tissue (**b**).

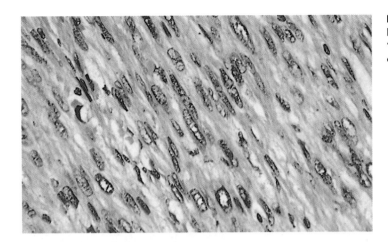

Fig. 10.82 Leiomyosarcoma. These malignant tumors are recognized mainly by their cellular pleomorphism, high mitotic rate and the appearance of 'boxcar' or cigar-shaped nuclei. Low-power magnification (not shown) revealed characteristic fascicles of cells at right angles.

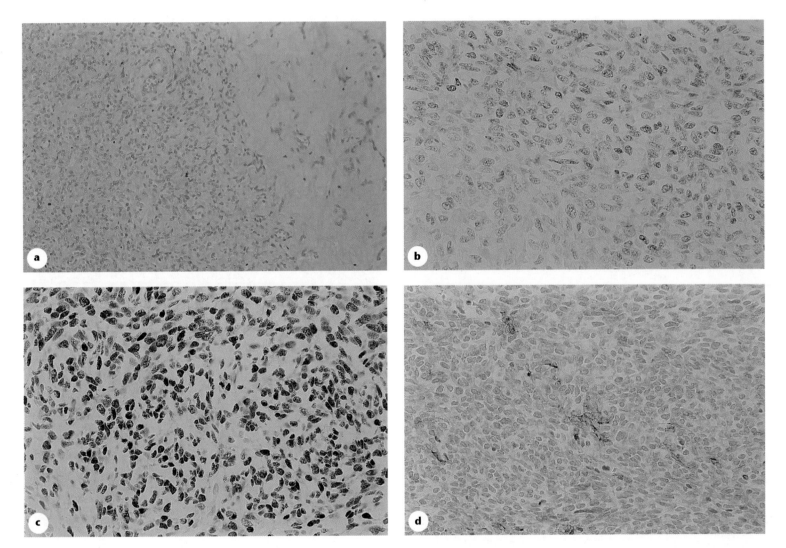

Fig. 10.83 (**a**) Characteristic features of endometrial stromal sarcoma include numerous capillary-like blood vessels (upper left center), hyaline nodules (upper right) and uniform ovoid cells with scant cytoplasm.

Immunohistochemical positivity for (**b**) estrogen receptor, (**c**) progesterone receptor and (**d**) CD10 (or CALLA – the common acute lymphocytic leukemia antigen) may be present.

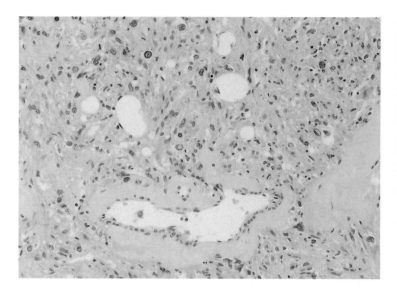

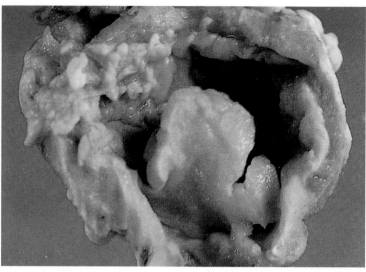

Fig. 10.84 Angiomyolipoma. Angiomyolipoma is a hamartomatous lesion that generally arises in one or both kidneys and is associated with tuberous sclerosis. Grossly the tumor is a yellow to gray fatty mass within the renal pelvis. Occasionally, the tumor may become pedunculated and very large examples may become attached to adjacent diaphragm or liver. Histologically, the tumor is composed of three tissue types in variable proportions: mature adipose tissue with variability in nuclear cytology and cellular size, convoluted thick-walled blood vessels, and irregular bundles of smooth muscle, often with a prominent perivascular arrangement. Angiomyolipoma can occasionally be misinterpreted as a malignant lesion due to striking pleomorphism (as occurred initially in this case) and, rarely, intravascular growth or infiltration of retroperitoneal lymph nodes. Despite these features, the tumor is benign. Review of the pathology resulted in a revision of the diagnosis to angiomyolipoma with extensive pleomorphism and, in the example shown, the 56-year-old woman is disease free following resection of this massive perinephric tumor. This unusual case underscores the critical importance of an experienced pathologist in reviewing the diagnosis.

Fig. 10.85 Botryoid embryonal rhabdomyosarcoma. As seen in this bladder specimen, in which the walls have been cut away, the botryoid type of embryonal rhabdomyosarcoma produces broad-based, translucent, polypoid masses.

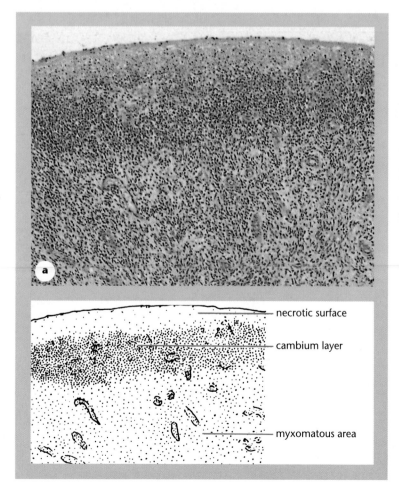

necrotic surface

cambium layer

myxomatous area

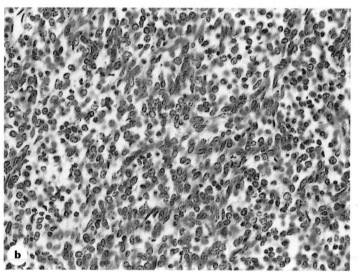

Fig. 10.86 Botryoid embryonal rhabdomyosarcoma. The grape-like masses occurring in botryoid sarcomas are hypocellular and appear myxomatous. (**a**) A cambium layer, consisting of a submucosal zone of markedly increased cellularity, is a characteristic feature. (**b**) On high-power view, the lesion is seen to contain primitive, round to oval mesenchymal cells.

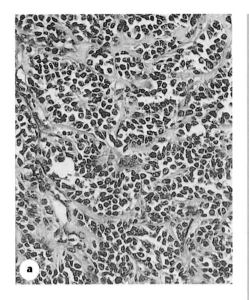

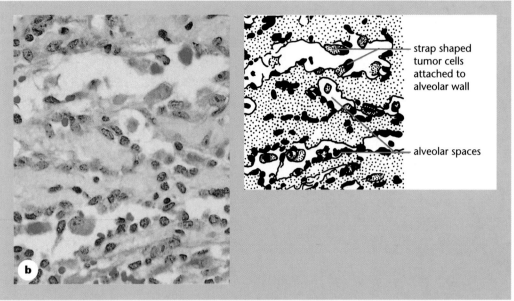

strap shaped
tumor cells
attached to
alveolar wall

alveolar spaces

Fig. 10.87 Alveolar rhabdomyosarcoma. (**a**) Low-power photomicrograph demonstrates fibrous septa separating slit-like spaces that have tumor cells hanging from their walls; these can be better appreciated on higher-power view (**b**). Elsewhere, the tumor had a less distinctive appearance, consisting of unbroken sheets of small, dark-staining cells.

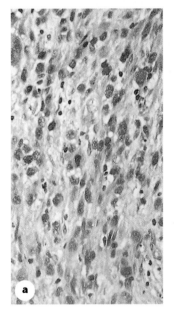

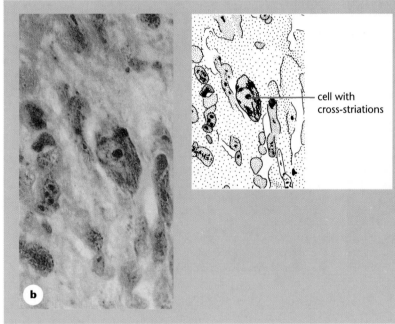

cell with
cross-striations

Fig. 10.88
Embryonal/pleomorphic rhabdomyosarcoma. (**a**) This section of tumor shows such a pleomorphic cellular picture that it hardly suggests the diagnosis of rhabdomyosarcoma. (**b**) But a single cell with cross-striations, a typical rhabdomyoblastic feature, was found on phosphotungstic acid–hematoxylin staining.

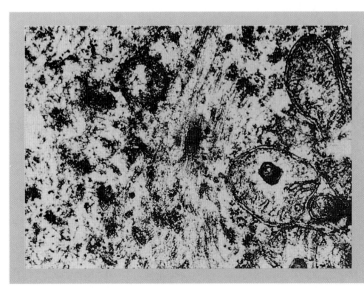

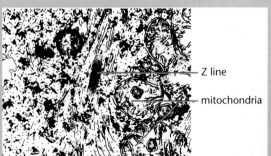

Z line

mitochondria

Fig. 10.89 Embryonal/pleomorphic rhabdomyosarcoma. Electron micrograph of the same specimen as shown in Figure 10.88 demonstrates the characteristic Z-line densities, confirming the nature of this tumor (× 6900). (Courtesy of Prof. PG Toner.)

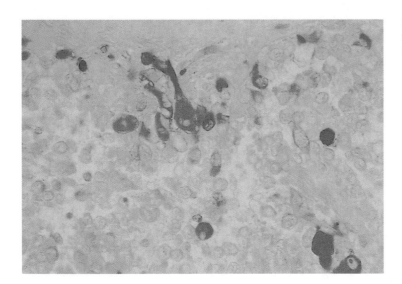

Fig. 10.90 Rhabdomyosarcoma. Immunoperoxidase reactivity of tumor cells to myoglobin is positive in this microscopic section. (Courtesy of Pathology Department, Brigham and Women's Hospital, Boston, MA.)

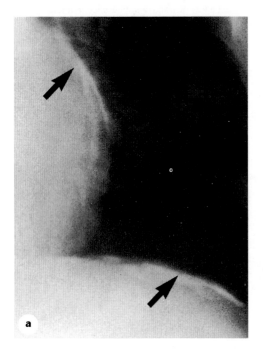

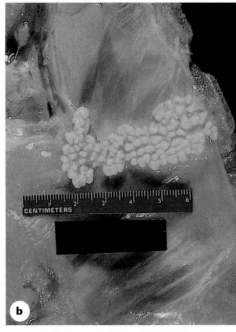

Fig. 10.91 Mesothelioma. (**a**) Chest radiograph showing the left lower lung of a 57-year-old man demonstrates pericardial and pleural plaques (arrows), representing fibrous thickening. These features are common findings indicating pulmonary asbestosis. (**b**) Autopsy features of calcified pleural plaques are quite striking. This specimen from a patient with mesothelioma shows focal calcifications on the lateral pleural surface. (Courtesy of Pathology Department, Brigham and Women's Hospital, Boston, MA.)

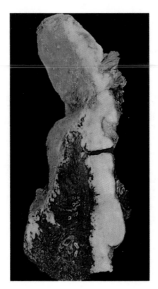

Fig. 10.92 Mesothelioma. Specimen photograph shows the apical portion of a lung that is encased in pale, infiltrative tumor arising from the pleura. Involvement of the soft tissues at the apex is also apparent.

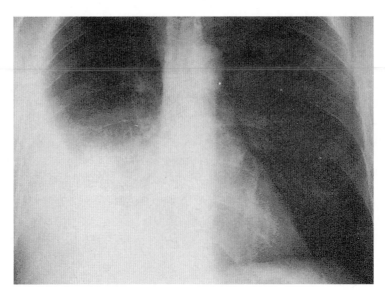

Fig. 10.93 Mesothelioma. A 60-year-old shipyard worker developed increasing dyspnea. On chest radiography, he was found to have a large right pleural effusion. Pleural biopsy confirmed a diagnosis of malignant mesothelioma.

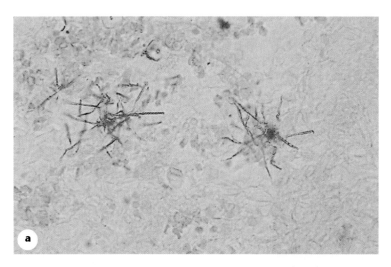

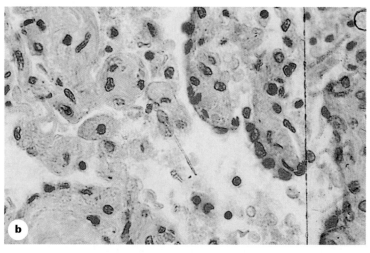

Fig. 10.94 Mesothelioma. Asbestos bodies can be counted in properly prepared specimens and are generally expressed as the number of fibers per gram of wet weight lung. Although urban dwellers commonly have 500 fibers/g, some workers with significant industrial exposure have counts in the millions. Microscopic sections shown here exhibit asbestos fibers within lung tissue (**a**) and within a mesothelioma (**b**), an extremely rare finding. A ferruginous body (not shown) is an iron-coated asbestos fiber. (Courtesy of Pathology Department, Brigham and Women's Hospital, Boston, MA.)

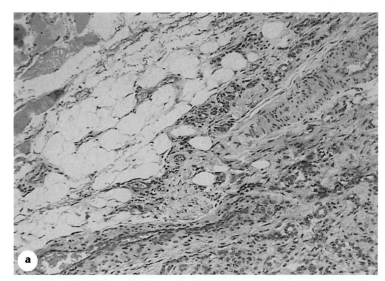

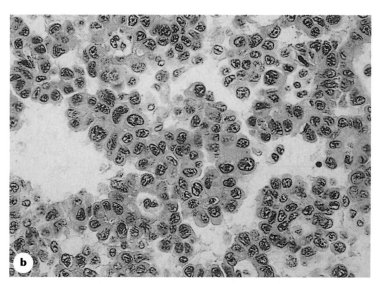

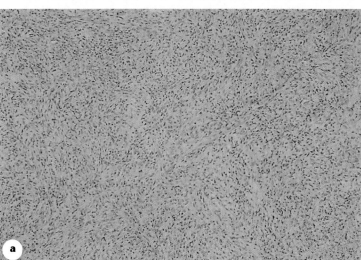

Fig. 10.95 Mesothelioma. Microscopically, the epithelial variant may be tubular (**a**), papillary (**b**), solid or vacuolated (**c**). Tumor cells of the sarcomatoid (fibrous) variant are ovoid to spindle shaped; their cellularity and hyperchromatism are similar to those of fibrosarcoma. In the biphastic or mixed type (not shown), both epithelial and sarcomatoid patterns are present, although extensive sampling may be required to demonstrate the minor component. (Courtesy of Pathology Department, Brigham and Women's Hospital, Boston, MA.)

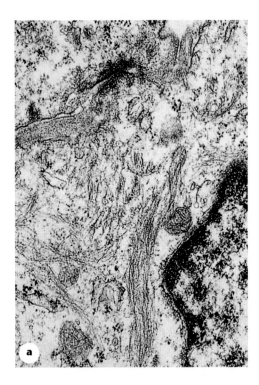
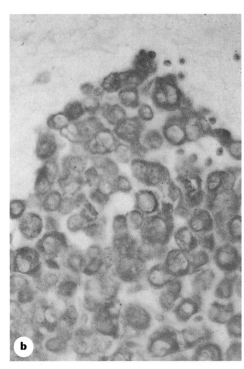

Fig. 10.96 Mesothelioma. (a) Electron microscopy reveals the cells of the epithelial variant to be polygonal with numerous long, slender, branching surface microvilli, abundant tonofilaments, desmosomes and intracellular lumen formation. In contrast, adenocarcinomas have short, stubby surface microvilli, fewer tonofilaments and microvillous rootlets or lamellar bodies. (b) Immunoperoxidase stain for keratin is markedly positive, especially in the perinuclear area of mesothelioma cells, and CEA reactivity is negative. In adenocarcinoma, keratin may be positive in the cell periphery, whereas CEA is strongly positive. Calretinin is positive in mesothelioma while negative in lung adenocarcinoma (see also Fig. 1.3). (Courtesy of Pathology Department, Brigham and Women's Hospital, Boston, MA.)

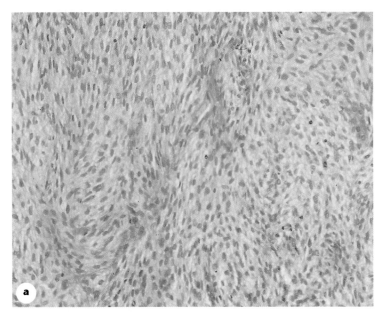
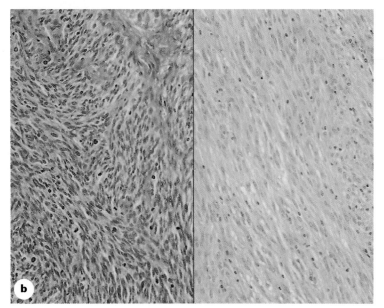

Fig. 10.97 Imitators of soft tissue sarcomas. The sarcomatoid variant of renal cell carcinoma, an epithelial malignancy, displays extensive spindle cell morphology. This can mislead the unwary toward a misdiagnosis of sarcoma. Note the comparison of sarcomatoid renal cell carcinoma (a) with a true sarcoma, a gastrointestinal stromal tumor (b). Careful pathologic evaluation in conjunction with clinical data and additional studies, e.g. immunocytochemistry, electron microscopy and cytogenetics, is essential for accurate diagnosis. Pathologists should be consulted prior to biopsy of such lesions, so that tissue can be handled appropriately. Improper tissue preparation can restrict the array of studies that can be performed and thus limit the ability of the pathologist to arrive at the correct diagnosis.

REFERENCES

Akwari OE, Dozois RR, Weiland LH, *et al.*: Leiomyosarcoma of the small and large bowel. Cancer 1978; 42 : 1375–1384.

Antman K, Corson J, Greenberger J, Wilson R: Multi-modality therapy in the management of angiosarcoma of the breast. Cancer 1982; 50 : 2000–2003.

Antman K, Klegar K, Pomfret E, *et al.*: Early peritoneal mesothelioma: a treatable malignancy. Lancet 1985; ii:977–982.

Antman K, Shemin R, Ryan L, *et al.*: Malignant mesothelioma: prognostic variables in a registry of 180 patients. The Dana-Farber Cancer Institute and Brigham and Women's Hospital, experience over two decades. 1965–1985. J Clin Oncol 1988; 6 : 147–153.

Blanke CD, von Mehren M, Joensuu H, *et al.*: Evaluation of the safety and efficacy of an oral molecularly targeted therapy, STI571, in patients (Pts) with unresectable or metastatic gastrointestinal stromal tumors (GISTS) expressing C-KIT (CD117). Proc ASCO 2001; 20: abstract 1, 1a.

Bramwell VH: Adjuvant chemotherapy for adult soft tissue sarcoma: is there a standard of care? J Clin Oncol 2001; 19(5):1235–1237.

Dahlin D, Beabout JW: Dedifferentiation of low-grade chondrosarcomas. Cancer 1971; 28 : 461–466.

Dahlin D: Bone Tumors: General Aspects and Data on 6,221 Cases, 3rd edn. Charles C. Thomas, Springfield, IL, 1978.

Delattre O, Zucman J, Melot T, *et al.*: The Ewing family of tumors – a sub-group of small-round cell tumors defined by specific chimeric transcript. N Engl J Med 1994; 331 : 294–299.

Enzinger FM, Weiss SW: Soft Tissue Tumors, 2nd edn. CV Mosby, St Louis, 1988.

Fletcher CD: Soft tissue tumors. In: Fletcher CD *et al.* (eds) Diagnostic Histopathology of Tumors, 2nd edn. Churchill Livingstone, Edinburgh, 1473–1540.

Fletcher CD, Gustafson P, Rydholm A, Willen H, Akerman M: Clinicopathologic re-evaluation of 100 malignant fibrous histiocytomas: prognostic relevance of subclassification. J Clin Oncol 2001; 19(12):3045–3050.

Frappaz D, Bouffet E, Dolbeau SD, *et al.*: Desmoplastic small round cell tumors of the abdomen. Cancer 1994; 73 : 1753–1756.

Froehner M, Wirth MP: Etiologic factors in soft tissue sarcomas. Onkologie 2001; 24(2):139–142.

Frustaci S, Gherlinzoni F, De Paoli A, *et al.*: Adjuvant chemotherapy for adult soft tissue sarcomas of the extremities and girdles: results of the Italian Randomized Cooperative Trial. J Clin Oncol 2001; 19(5):1238–1247.

Ho L, Sugarbaker D, Skarin AT: Malignant mesothelioma. In: Cancer Treatment and Research. In: Thoracic Oncology, D. Ettinger (Ed). Kluwer Academic Publishers, Boston, Part V, 327–373, 2000.

Huvos AG: Ewing's sarcoma. In: Bone Tumors: Diagnosis, Treatment, and Prognosis. Saunders, Philadelphia, 1979, 322–344.

Ioachim H, Adsay V, Giancotti F, *et al.*: Kaposi's sarcoma of internal organs. Cancer 1995; 75 : 1376–1385.

Janigan DT, Husain A, Robinson NA: Cardiac angiosarcomas: a review and a case report. Cancer 1986; 57 : 852–859.

Joensuu H, Roberts PJ, Sarlomo-Rikala M, *et al.*: Clinical response induced by the tyrosine kinase inhibitor STI571 in metastatic gastrointestinal stromal tumor expressing a mutant c-kit proto-oncogene. N Engl J Med 2001; 344 : 1052–1056.

Koontz JI, Soreng AL, Nucci M, *et al.*: Frequent fusion of the JAZF1 and JJAZ1 genes in endometrial stromal tumors. Proc Natl Acad Sci USA 2001; 98(11):6348–6353.

Kruzelock RP, Hansen MF: Molecular genetics and cytogenetics of sarcomas. Hematol Oncol Clin North Am 1995; 9 : 513–540.

Landau HJ, Poiesz BJ, Dube S, Bogart JA, Weiner LB, Souid AK: Classic Kaposi's sarcoma associated with human herpesvirus 8 infection in a 13-year-old male: a case report. Clin Cancer Res 2001; 7(8):2263–2268.

Lee ES, Locker J, Nalesnk M, *et al.*: The association of Epstein–Barr virus with smooth muscle tumors occurring after organ transplantation. N Engl J Med 1995; 332 : 19–25.

Margue CM, Bernasconi M, Barr FG, Schafer BW: Transcriptional modulation of the anti-apoptotic protein BCL-XL by the paired box transcription factors PAX3 and PAX3/FKHR. Oncogene 2000; 19(25):2921–2929.

McClain KL, Leach CT, Jensen HB, *et al.*: Association of Epstein–Barr virus with leiomyosarcomas in young people with AIDS. N Engl J Med 1995; 332 : 12–18.

McCormick D, Mentzel T, Beham A, Fletcher CD: Dedifferentiated liposarco-ma. Clinicopathologic analysis of 32 cases suggesting a better prognostic subgroup among pleomorphic sarcomas. Am J Surg Pathol 1994; 18(12):1213–1223.

Poon MC, Durant JR, Norgard MJ, *et al.*: Inflammatory fibrous histiocytoma: an important variant of malignant fibrous histiocytoma highly responsive to chemotherapy. Ann Intern Med 1982; 97 : 858–863.

Rubin B: KIT activation is a ubiquitous feature of gastrointestinal stromal tumors. Cancer Res 2001; 61:8118–8121.

Russel WO, Cohen J, Enzinger FM, *et al.*: A clinical and pathologic stagings system for soft tissue sarcomas. Cancer 1977; 40 : 1562–1570.

Shipley J, Crew J, Guterson B: The molecular biology of soft tissue sarcomas. Eur J Cancer 1993; 29a:2054–2058.

Sawyer JR, Tryka AF, Lewis JM: A novel reciprocal chromosome translocation t(11;22) (p13;q12) in an intraabdominal desmoplastic small round-cell tumor. Am J Surg Pathol 1992; 16 : 4411–4416.

Schajowicz F, Sissons, H, Sobin L: The World Health Organization's histologic classification of bone tumors. Cancer 1995; 75 : 1208–1214.

Silverberg E, Boring C, Squires T: Cancer statistics. Cancer 1990; 40 : 9–28.

Sjoblom T, Shimizu A, O'Brien KP, *et al.*: Growth inhibition of dermatofi-brosarcoma protuberans tumors by the platelet-derived growth factor receptor antagonist STI571 through induction of apoptosis. Cancer Res 2001; 61(15):5778–5783.

Tallini G, Dal Cin P, Rhoden KJ, *et al.*: Expression of HMGI-C and HMGI(Y) in ordinary lipoma and atypical lipomatous tumors: immunohistochemical reactivity correlates with karyotypic alterations. Am J Pathol 1997; 151(1):37–43.

Tucker MA, Fraumeni JF: Soft tissue. In: Schottenfeld D, Fraumeni JF, eds: Cancer Epidemiology. Saunders, Philadelphia, 1982, 827–836.

Tuveson DA, Willis NA, Jacks T, *et al.*: STI571 inactivation of the gastroin-testinal stromal tumor c-KIT oncoprotein: biological and clinical implica-tions. Oncogene 2001; 20(36):5054–5058.

Van Glabbeke M, van Oosterom AT, Oosterhuis JW, *et al.*: Prognostic factors for the outcome of chemotherapy in advanced soft tissue sarcoma: an analysis of 2,185 patients treated with anthracycline-containing first-line regimens – a European Organization for Research and Treatment of Cancer Soft Tissue and Bone Sarcoma Group Study. J Clin Oncol 1999; 17 : 150.

Van Oosterom AT, Judson I, Verweij J, *et al.*: STI 571, an active drug in metastatic gastrointestinal stromal tumors (GIST): an EORTC Phase I Study. Proc ASCO 2001; 20:abstract 2, 2a.

FIGURE CREDITS

The following books published by Gower Medical Publishing are sources of figures in the present chapter. The figure numbers given in the listing are those of the figures given in the present chapter. The page numbers (or slide numbers) given in parentheses are those of the original publication.

Asscher AW, Moffatt DB, Sanders E: Nephrology Illustrated. Pergamon Medical Publications/Gower Medical Publishing, Oxford /London, 1982: Fig. 10.69 (p. 9.12).

Bullough PG, Vigorita VJ: Atlas of Orthopedic Pathology. University Park Press/Gower Medical Publishing, Baltimore/New York, 1984: Figs 8.6 (p. 12.7), 10.7 (p. 12.8), 10.10 (p. 12.10), 10.11 (p. 12.11), 10.12 (p. 12.11), 10.14 (p. 12.12), 10.18 (p. 13.4), Table 10.5 (p. 13.6), 10.20 (p. 13.6), 10.27, (p. 12.20), 10.28 (p. 12.23), 10.35 (p. 13.11), 10.50 (p. 13.14).

Bullough PG, Boachie-Adjei O: Atlas of Spinal Diseases. Lippincott/Gower Medical Publishing, Philadelphia/New York, 1988: Figs 10.15 (p. 153), 10.19 (p. 203), 10.32 (p. 174), 10.33 (p. 196), 10.34 (p. 195), 10.36 (p. 197).

Cawson RA, Eveson JW: Oral Pathology and Diagnosis. Heinemann Medical Books/Gower Medical Publishing, London, 1987: Figs 10.8 (p. 7.5), 10.41 (p. 10.9), Table 10.7 (p. 10.8), 10.44 (p. 10.8), 10.47 (p. 10.15), 10.53 (p. 10.14), 10.59 (p. 17.13), 10.66 (p. 17.13), 10.68 (p. 17.14), 10.72 (p. 7.11), 10.75 (p. 10.20), 10.76 (p. 10.21), 10.77 (p. 17.21).

Fletcher CDM, McKee PHG: Atlas of Gross Pathology. Edward Arnold/Gower Medical Publishing, London, 1987: Figs 10.60 (p. 41), 10.80 (p. 22).

Greenspan A: Orthopedic Radiology. Lippincott/Gower Medical Publishing, Philadelphia/New York, 1988: Table 10.2 (p. 13.2), Table 10.3 (p. 13.3), 10.1 (p. 13.14), 10.2 (pp. 13.13, 13.16), Table 10.4 (pp. 13.14, 13.16, 13.19, 13.21), 10.3 (pp. 16.2, 16.6), 10.4 (p. 16.6), 10.9 (p. 16.7), 10.13 (p. 16.9), 10.21 (p. 16.10), 10.24 (p. 16.11), 10.30 (p. 15.18), 10.33 (p. 13.7), 10.42 (p. 13.27), 10.46 (p. 13.27).

Louis MM, Bone Tumor Surgery. Lippincott/Gower Medical Publishing, Philadelphia/New York, 1988: Figs 10.5 (p. 4.31), 10.25 (p. 4.2), 10.26 (p. 2.14), 10.31 (p. 2.11).

McKee PH, ed.: Skin, Soft Tissues subsection of slide volume (Endocrine System/Haemopoietic and Lymphoreticular Systems/Skin Soft Tissues). In: Turk JL, Fletcher CDM, eds.: RCSE Slide Atlas of Pathology. Gower Medical Publishing, London 1986: Fig. 10.48 (Soft Tissues slide no. 34).

Silverstein FE, Tytgat GNJ: Atlas of Gastrointestinal Endoscopy. Saunders/Gower Medical Publishing, Philadelphia/New York, 1987: Figs 10.67 (p. 10.20), 10.70 (p. 6.13).

Weiss MA, Mills SE: Atlas of Genitourinary Tract Disorders. Lippincott/Gower Medical Publishing, Philadelphia/New York, 1988: Figs 10.73 (p. 12.40), 10.74 (p. 12.41).

Zitelli BJ, Davis HW: Atlas of Pediatric Physical Diagnosis. CV Mosby/Gower Medical Publishing, St Louis/New York, 1987: Fig. 10.65 (p. 4.20).

11

Skin Cancer

F. Stephen Hodi, Michael M. Wick

Cancer of the skin is the most common human malignancy. There are about 600 000 cases of skin cancer annually in the United States, with melanoma representing about 47 700 cases and about 95% of the deaths due to skin cancer. The incidence of melanoma, currently the eighth most common tumor in the US, is rising worldwide with WHO statistics confirming that it is the most rapidly increasing cancer. Although the majority of deaths due to skin cancer are caused by malignant melanoma, non-melanoma skin cancer is responsible for significant morbidity. Even with cure rates of more than 90%, the high incidence of this disease means that 30 000–60 000 patients will have recurrent skin cancer – a much more serious condition. Since these cancers occur on the surface of the skin and are readily diagnosed, a knowledge of their clinical appearance, biology and treatment should logically lead to major reductions in morbidity and mortality.

The major environmental factors involved in the development of skin cancer today appear to be a combination of environmental ultraviolet light exposure and the ability to tan as controlled by genetic differences in skin color. These observations explain the high incidence of skin cancer in fair-skinned individuals and in those living in lower latitudes and higher altitudes. Dark skin, as in the black patient, is highly protective against the development of skin cancer. Exposure to ionizing radiation, either as part of therapy for a variety of benign disorders or as an occupational risk (e.g. for dentists, radiologists), has also been implicated in the development of squamous cell carcinoma. Arsenic, which is used in insecticides, has continued to be a significant cause of skin cancer in farmers and industrial workers. Finally, each of these causes may be enhanced by genetic defects in the body's ability to repair damage to DNA. Two disorders, xeroderma pigmentosum and the basal cell–nevus syndrome, are important, genetically transmitted conditions characterized by a much higher than average incidence of skin cancer.

Since skin cancer occurs on the body surface, careful inspection is the first step toward early diagnosis. Although each tumor described below demonstrates certain typical features that aid diagnosis, any lesion that shows biologic activity – as indicated by change in size, shape or color – should be considered suspicious. Bleeding and ulceration are generally found in more advanced lesions.

BENIGN SKIN TUMORS

The heterogeneity of skin with respect to resident cell types is apparent from the multiple kinds of benign tumors arising from skin. It is most important to identify these tumors in order to distinguish them from malignancies. Furthermore, it should be noted that many of these tumors are capable of causing functional disturbances, as well as cosmetic problems.

One of the most common benign skin tumors is keratoacanthoma. This lesion of the surface epithelium presents as a dome-shaped tumor with a central keratotic plug; it can appear suddenly and grow rapidly. It is somewhat difficult to distinguish from squamous cell carcinoma when a biopsy specimen is small, in which case conservative re-excision is indicated. Histologic sections characteristically show cup-shaped invagination of the epidermis, with lip-like lateral extension over the edge of a crater. Large cells with pale, eosinophilic cytoplasm are present, along with a well-demarcated base. The natural course of this tumor usually leads to spontaneous involution, but surgical excision is often chosen. If the lesion is not excised completely, it can recur. Large keratoacanthomas can be locally destructive to contiguous structures and should be treated early.

Among systemic disorders producing tumors of the skin, mastocytosis may present as isolated lesions or generalized eruptions. In this condition, also known as urticaria pigmentosa, systemic involvement may include pulmonary and gastrointestinal lesions, adenopathy and, rarely, a leukemic phase or the development of lymphoma. Its cutaneous manifestations include pigmented macules, papules or plaques that urticate with slight pressure (Darier's sign).

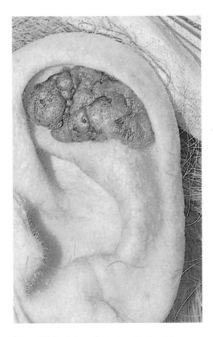

Fig. 11.1 Seborrheic keratosis. A large, dark brown tumor appears to have been 'stuck on' the upper portion of the antihelix. Fine cystic inclusions of keratin ('horn cysts') appear as black pits.

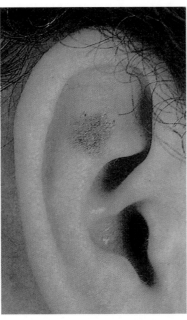

Fig. 11.2 Seborrheic keratosis. A brown, circumscribed lesion is located on the upper portion of the antihelix.

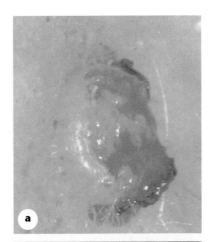

Fig. 11.3 Keratoacanthoma. (**a**) A small, early keratoacanthoma has arisen on a sun-exposed portion of the ear. Cup-like hyperplastic epithelium can be seen around the base and the central crater is granular and friable. (**b**) A larger, more mature keratoacanthoma, also in the conchal bowl, shows a central crater filled with keratinous material and a deep surrounding cuff of hyperplastic epithelium.

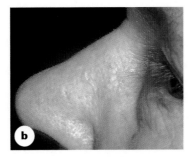

Fig. 11.4 Keratoacanthoma. (**a**) These fairly common and important lesions can arise very rapidly and thus have often been regarded as highly malignant carcinomas. They are in fact benign and, if left alone, will disappear spontaneously, as in this case (**b**).

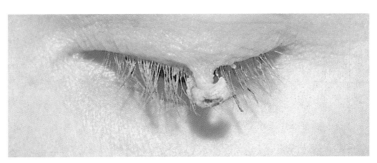

Fig. 11.5 Squamous papilloma. This lesion is a benign overgrowth of squamous epithelium. Keratin may build up on the surface of a lesion to form a cutaneous horn, as shown here. Usually, the lesion can be simply excised.

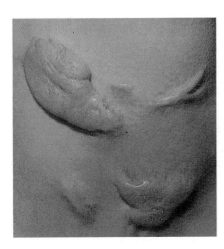

Fig. 11.6 Keloids. These tumors represent an abnormal reparative reaction to skin injury. Their frequent extension beyond the original injury distinguishes them from hypertrophic scars, which are confined to the wound margins. Histologically, they are characterized by proliferation of fibroblasts and collagen.

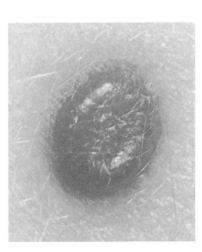

Fig. 11.7 Juvenile melanoma (Spitz nevus). This symmetrical lesion has a red-brown color and commonly occurs on the cheek of a young child.

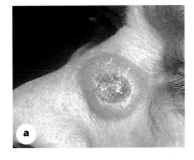

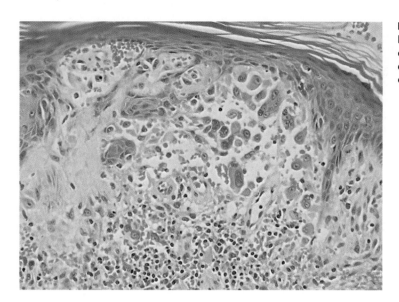

Fig. 11.8 Juvenile melanoma (Spitz nevus). The epitheliod type of this benign lesion is marked by epitheliod melanocytes, which are seen scattered in the center of the microscopic field. The melanocytes are characterized by abundant eosinophilic cytoplasm, large vesicular nuclei and prominent nucleoli. (Courtesy of Dr Philip H. McKee, London, UK.)

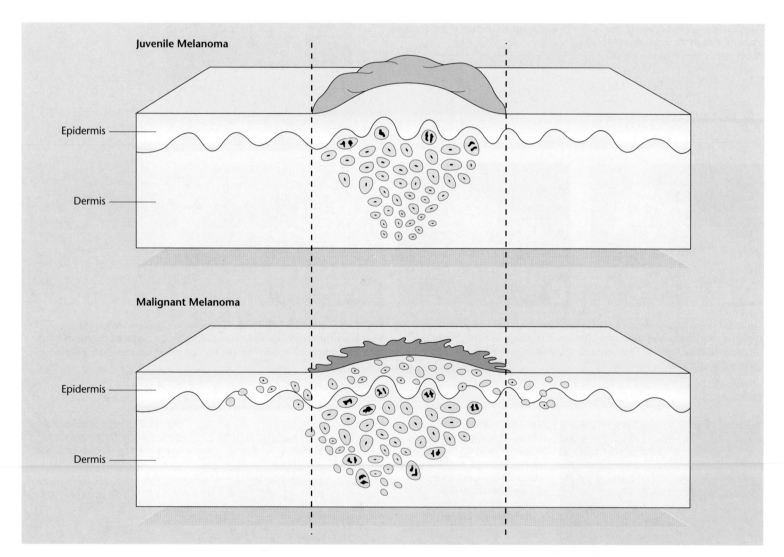

Fig. 11.9 Juvenile melanoma and malignant melanoma. A comparison between these two entities reveals that juvenile melanoma does not involve the epidermis and melanocytic proliferation is confined within the lateral borders of the lesion. Mitotic activity may be seen in juvenile melanoma, but only in the superficial component of the tumor. Moreover, cells show evidence of maturation (i.e become smaller) with increasing depth. The Spitz nevus is not malignant and surgery is curative.

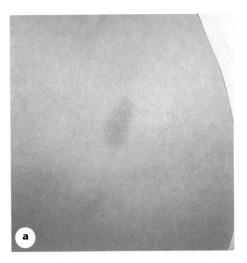

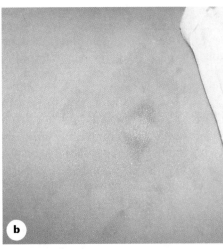

Fig. 11.10 Mastocytoma. (**a**) Isolated lesions, representing dermal accumulations of mast cells, may be seen in neonates and infants. They are usually skin colored, slightly indurated, infiltrated plaques 1–2 cm in size. (**b**) The clue to the diagnosis is a wheal-and-flare reaction following slight pressure on the lesions (Darier's sign). This response results from the effects on the local vasculature of histamine released from infiltrating mast cells.

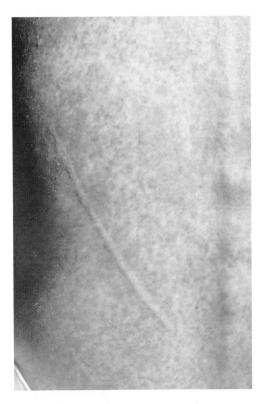

Fig. 11.11 Systemic mast cell disease (mastocytosis). This 48-year-old woman had a generalized hyperpigmented macular skin eruption. A pronounced urticarial reaction (Darier's sign) occurred after the skin was stroked with a pointed object.

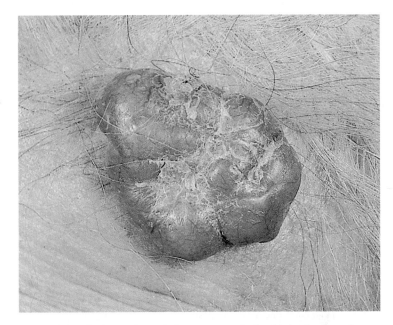

Fig. 11.12 Cylindroma the scalp is a common site for this benign apocrine gland tumor. The nodule has a smooth surface and telangiectasa may be present.

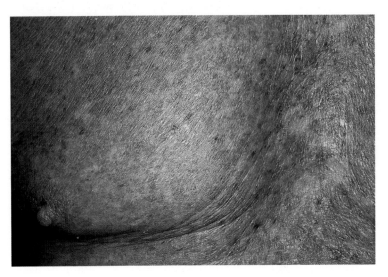

Fig. 11.13 Solar keratoses. Chronic skin changes on the chest of a 76-year-old man with long-standing sun exposure. Close-up shows numerous thin, scaly, red lesions and hyperpigmented areas. Use of modern sunscreens would prevent development of these skin changes.

PREMALIGNANT SKIN TUMORS

Solar keratoses, also called actinic keratoses, appear as thin, scaly, red lesions with epidermal hyperplasia and cellular atypia. Although they are allegedly premalignant lesions, most do not proceed to frank malignancy and conservative treatment is indicated. Non-scarring methods of destruction, such as cryosurgery, electrodesiccation or topical 5-fluorouracil cream, are usually adequate. Lesions that persist after treatment should be biopsied to determine whether invasive squamous cell carcinoma has developed. Recent studies have shown topical sunscreens to be effective in preventing the development of new lesions.

Arsenical keratoses are small, hard, punctate tumors that usually occur on the hands and feet. Lesions that increase in depth or diameter, or that ulcerate, have usually developed into squamous cell carcinomas.

Xeroderma pigmentosum is an autosomal-recessive disorder characterized by the inability to repair ultraviolet light-induced DNA damage and, consequently, a pronounced cutaneous hypersensitivity to the effects of the sun's rays. The disease, which starts in childhood, primarily affects the exposed parts of the body; lesions on the trunk may occur late in the course of disease. Dryness, desquamation and freckling are followed first by atrophic and telangiectatic spots, then by verrucous and keratotic lesions. Within 6 months to 2 years these lesions ulcerate and become malignant. The malignancy is most often basal cell carcinoma; less commonly it may be squamous cell carcinoma and only rarely a sarcoma or malignant melanoma.

Bowen's disease is a term used to describe a clinically characteristic lesion that presents as a well-demarcated, scaly, red plaque. Its histologic appearance demonstrates squamous cell carcinoma *in situ*. Bowen's disease can be associated with internal malignancies, particularly occult tumors of the GI tract, GU system or lung. The lesion appears to be capable of developing into an invasive malignancy. Removal by simple excision is adequate treatment.

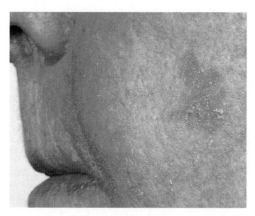

Fig. 11.14 Solar keratosis. This tumor appears as either a well-defined, raised red papule or, as shown here, a raised red plaque with an adherent scale.

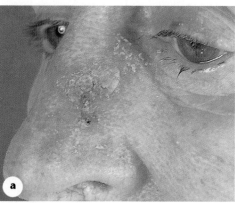

Fig. 11.15 Solar keratosis. This patient's scaly plaque (**a**) was treated successfully with 5-fluorouracil cream (**b**). (Courtesy of St Mary's Hospital, London, UK.)

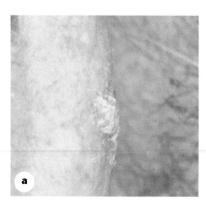

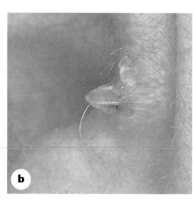

Fig. 11.16 Solar keratosis. (**a**) Ultraviolet light exposure has produced a dry, elevated, white, scaly lesion on the posterior helical rim. (**b**) A solar keratosis arising from the antihelix has produced a small keratin horn.

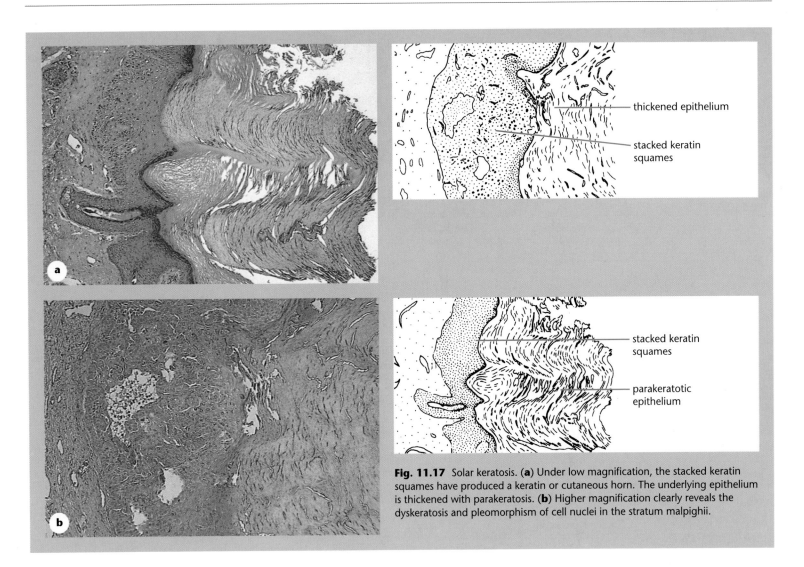

Fig. 11.17 Solar keratosis. (**a**) Under low magnification, the stacked keratin squames have produced a keratin or cutaneous horn. The underlying epithelium is thickened with parakeratosis. (**b**) Higher magnification clearly reveals the dyskeratosis and pleomorphism of cell nuclei in the stratum malpighii.

thickened epithelium

stacked keratin squames

stacked keratin squames

parakeratotic epithelium

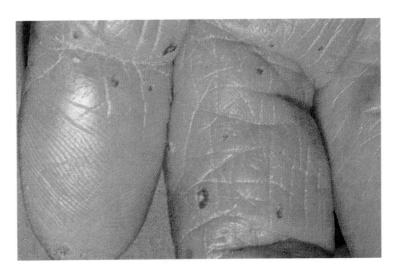

Fig. 11.18 Arsenical keratosis. Exposure to arsenic, often as a pesticide, produces keratoses on the palms and fingers.

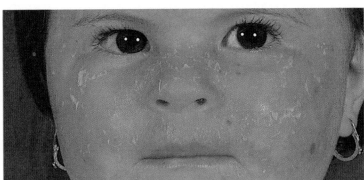

Fig. 11.19 Xeroderma pigmentosum. Extreme photosensitivity is the key feature of this condition. Persistent erythema occurs after seemingly innocent solar exposure. Multiple premalignant keratoses are evident.

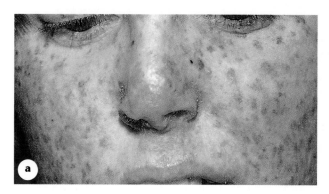

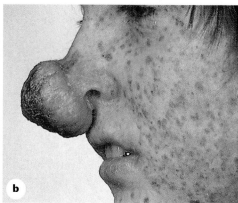

Fig. 11.20 Xeroderma pigmentation. (**a**) After solar exposure, permanent freckling of exposed skin quickly ensures. Malignant change occurs early in life. This patient had her first squamous cell carcinoma at the age of 2 years. (**b**) This keratoacanthoma developed when she was 12 years old. The lesion resolved spontaneously.

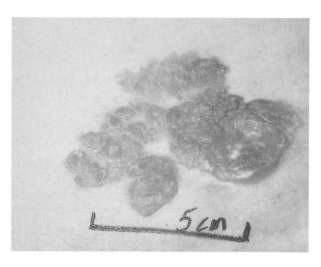

Fig. 11.21 Bowen's disease. This more specific type of premalignant lesion, or intradermal cancer, consists of defined, erythematous, scaly plaques that often resemble psoriasis. In this patient, the right side of the lesion has already undergone transformation into an invasive squamous cell carcinoma.

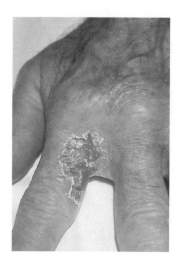

Fig. 11.22 Bowen's disease. Involvement of the hands is quite common and can present diagnostic and therapeutic problems.

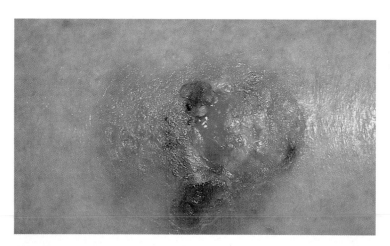

Fig. 11.23 Bowen's disease. The surface of the lesion, seen here in its characteristic presentation as a well-defined, slightly raised, red patch with an adherent scale, may become eroded.

COMMON SKIN CANCERS

BASAL CELL CARCINOMA

This malignancy can present in many forms, but usually appears as a pearly gray nodule with prominent telangiectasia. The majority of tumors are located on the face, neck and dorsum of the hands. Basal cell carcinomas usually invade locally, with only about 100 cases of metastatic disease reported in the world's literature. Histologically, the lesion consists of small, undifferentiated basal cells with minimal nuclear atypia. It can be treated by either surgery, radiotherapy or cryotherapy, all of which are effective, the choice depending on the site of the lesion and the physician's preference. Recurrence after treatment usually indicates that the tumor was not completely resected. Since basal cell carcinoma is such a fastidious tumor in growth requirements, 75% of cases are still considered to be cured even when there is microscopic tumor at a treatment margin. However, recurrent tumors incur serious complications. Treating cutaneous malignancy in a combined clinic, comprising a dermatologist, plastic surgeon and radiotherapist, is recommended.

The basal cell–nevus syndrome (Gorlin's syndrome) refers to an autosomal-dominant disorder characterized by multiple basal cell carcinomas, associated with jaw cysts and skeletal anomalies. Patients have unusual cutaneous pits in the palms and soles; the pits have the histologic features of miniature basal cell carcinomas.

SQUAMOUS CELL CARCINOMA

In contrast to basal cell carcinoma, squamous cell carcinoma usually presents as a scaly, keratotic, slightly elevated lesion that may or may not have a cutaneous horn. This tumor shows a tendency to appear in light-skinned individuals with sun-damaged skin; sun-induced squamous cell carcinomas behave similarly to basal cell carcinomas. In patients with xeroderma pigmentosum, squamous cell carcinomas may arise *de novo* or from a pre-existing senile keratosis or keratoacanthoma. Treatment is usually by surgical excision. Most squamous cell carcinomas have an excellent prognosis if the concept of growth by contiguity is kept in mind and all tumor is removed. All squamous cell carcinomas, however, have a propensity for metastasis, with 2–3% spreading to regional lymph nodes. Distant metastases are generally rare. Exceptions to this rule are squamous cell carcinomas that arise in a scar, a chronically ulcerated area or the site of radiation damage, as well as those appearing in immunosuppressed patients. In these cases, distant metastases may occur.

MALIGNANT MELANOMA

Malignant melanoma is a highly aggressive tumor whose cell of origin is the melanocyte. Arising embryologically from the neural crest, melanocytes possess a unique biochemical feature, the enzymatic conversion of L-dopa to melanin by tyrosinase. The normal melanocyte responds to ultraviolet light (tanning) and also to a variety of hormonal agents, such as melanocyte-stimulating hormone (MSH), corticotropin (ACTH) (Addison's disease), estrogens (increased pigmentation during pregnancy) and progestins (melasma developing in patients who take oral contraceptives). Melanoma cells may possess none, all or only part of the above responses found in their normal counterparts.

Approximately 47 000 new cases of malignant melanoma were expected in the US in 2000, accounting for 7700 deaths. The incidence in the US varies by region, but is approximately 15 per 100 000. In Australia, where the risk for developing malignant melanoma has been reported as high as 1 in 20, public health initiatives focused on sun protection and early detection have contributed to the leveling off in incidence. Given the relatively young age of peak incidence, malignant melanoma is a significant cause of loss of expected years of life. Unusual non-cutaneous melanomas may arise in the anal canal, vulva and eye, as well as the mucous membranes of the mouth, nose, pharynx and esophagus. A review of the pertinent features of cutaneous melanoma has been summarized in the NIH Consensus Statement Vol 10, #1, 1992. The importance of screening for early melanoma has been emphasized by the American Cancer Society and techniques have been published (Koh *et al.*, 1992).

The major risk factors for the development of malignant melanoma are genetic and sun exposure history. First-degree relatives with a history of melanoma, significant intermittent sun exposures and sun exposure in early adulthood have been determined to be particularly important. Recent evidence implicates exposure to UV-B radiation. Phenotypes of blue eyes, blonde or red hair, tendency to freckle or burn increase the risk for developing melanoma. Approximately 10% of patients have a family history of melanoma and specific inherited susceptibility genes have been identified. The dysplastic nevus syndrome refers to individuals with atypical moles or nevi, marked by irregularities in outline and pigmentation, who are at increased risk for developing malignant melanoma. The nevi may be acquired or occur in a familial melanoma syndrome. The benign lesions tend to be larger and more numerous than common moles and occur in sun-shielded skin such as the scalp and bathing suit area. Owing to the high risk of subsequent malignancy (up to 60%), these patients must be closely followed. The malignant potential of the isolated dysplastic nevus is less well established and complicated by the lack of concordance among pathologists in the identification of dysplasia. However, the patient with multiple dysplastic nevi and a family history of more than one first-degree family member having melanoma has a lifetime risk for developing melanoma nearing 100%.

Table 11.2 shows the major clinical–histologic types of malignant melanoma. Superficial spreading melanoma is the most common type, representing approximately 70% of cases. It is typified by a radial growth phase lasting from 1 to 7 years followed by a vertical growth phase in which the melanoma becomes increasingly invasive. This emphasizes the importance for early detection of these lesions in determining prognosis. Nodular melanoma, presenting as an elevated nodule, arises without a radial growth phase and therefore frequently presents as a deeper primary lesion. Although nodular and superficial spreading melanoma can be distinguished clinically, they have a similar prognosis, level for level. The sun-induced lentigo maligna melanoma (or 'Hutchinson's freckle'), level for level, has a markedly better prognosis. This relatively uncommon lesion, comprising 5–10% of melanomas, occurs typically on the sun-exposed areas such as the cheek of older individuals, arising in a lentigo maligna. Acral lentiginous melanoma is also uncommon, having less of a relationship to sun exposure, occurring on palms, soles and subungal regions. Desmoplastic (neurotropic) melanoma is rare, arising in elderly individuals typically as a deep primary, frequently amelanotic with histologic features of spindles and nerve infiltration and frequent local recurrences. Rarely melanomas can arise from areas other than the skin and include ocular melanomas as well as mucosal melanomas.

Favorable prognostic factors include female sex and location of the primary lesion on an extremity. The most important factors involved in determining the overall prognosis of a patient with malignant melanoma are the depth of the primary lesion and lymph node status. Levels of invasion may be determined anatomically by the Clark technique or micrometrically by the Breslow technique (*see* Fig. 11.47 and Table 11.3). The more useful measure is Breslow's, because it is not as dependent on histologic interpretation as the anatomic Clark technique. Examination of 5-year survival by either level or thickness indicates that melanomas fall into two basic categories: (1) early or thin lesions (corresponding to Clark level II or Breslow thickness <0.75 mm), which are essentially curable by simple excision, and (2) late or thick lesions (level III or higher with thickness >0.75 mm), which carry survival rates ranging from less than 25% to 70%.

Features that characterize early melanoma have been quantified in an effort to increase early diagnosis. The average size of a level II melanoma is 17×15 mm, as compared with 28×23 mm for level V lesions. In the majority of patients with early lesions, an increase in size and a darkening in color are present. Changes such as nodularity, ulceration or bleeding correspond to the development of histologically late or advanced lesions, with correspondingly poorer prognoses. Other adverse prognostic features include advanced age, male gender, head and neck primary sites, increased mitotic rate (>6/hpf), lack of inflammatory lymphoid infiltrate below the primary lesions, satellite lesions and abnormalities on chromosomes 7 and 11 (Dhawan and Kirkwi, 1994; Trent *et al.*, 1990).

Treatment of a primary melanoma includes wide local excision with appropriate margins for depth of primary. Recommended margins are 0.5–1 cm for *in situ* melanoma, 1 cm for lesions <1 mm deep, 2–3 cm for those >1 mm deep and 1 cm for lentigo maligna melanoma. The lack of efficacy for elective lymph node dissections led to the development of the technique to identify and biopsy the sentinel, or first draining lymph node from the region of skin. The procedure involves injection of a blue dye and intraoperative lymphoscintigraphy with radiolabeled Tc-99 dextran or sulfur colloid into the region of the primary site prior to wide excision. The use of a hand held probe localizes the radiolabel and the lymph node identification is assisted by the blue dye uptake. Recently, sentinel lymph node status has been found, along with depth of the primary lesion, to be the most important prognostic factors. Stage of disease is assessed by clinical evaluation, as well as by histologic documentation. Recently, an updated AJCC staging system has been proposed (Fig. 11.48a) which includes ulceration of the primary lesion, the number of involved lymph nodes in stage III disease and sites of disease and LDH level in stage IV disease as important prognostic factors. (*see* Fig. 11.48b)

Patients with deep primaries and/or lymph node disease have significant risk for developing disseminated disease. Adjuvant chemotherapy and non-specific immunotherapies with BCG of *Coryne bacterium parvum* have not revealed significant efficacy to warrant widespread administration. Positive results from randomized prospective trials of high-dose interferon α-2b in the adjuvant setting have led to FDA approval for patients with AJCC stage IIB and III disease.

The most common sites of metastases for patients with stage IV disease are the brain, lung and liver, but virtually any area can be involved. The histologic findings of metastatic melanoma vary considerably, from heavily pigmented cells to poorly differentiated amelanotic cells that may mimic lymphoma, carcinoma or sarcoma. Some patients may have no history of a primary skin lesion or may have had a melanoma removed many years earlier. The prognosis for a patient with metastatic melanoma is in general poor. Patients with metastatic disease limited to the lungs, soft tissues, lymph nodes and skin have a tendency for a slightly better prognosis than

patients with disease elsewhere such as the liver or brain. In-transit metastases frequently present a problem of local control of the disease. If in-transit metastases are limited to a limb, success for local control has occurred with various isolated limb perfusion strategies that include use of hyperthermia with infusions of chemotherapy or cytokines, with complete response rates reported ranging from 36% to 89%.

Once melanoma metastasizes beyond the local region it is difficult to treat and is almost uniformly fatal. While recent technological advances such as PET scanning improve the ability for detection, early detection of metastatic disease has not been demonstrated to improve patient outcome significantly. Melanoma is typically a relatively chemoresistant and radioresistant disease. The most active compound against melanoma is dacarbazine (DTIC), having response rates as a single agent of 19–25%. Other compounds with activity against melanoma include the nitrosureas, taxanes, platinum compounds and vinca alkaloids. Cytokines such as interferon and interleukin-2 have been widely used for the treatment of metastatic melanoma, offering response rates of 20% or less. In attempts to combine the effects of therapies, chemo immunotherapy or biochemotherapy regimens have reported response rates approaching 60%, but with increased side-effects. Given the poor prognosis for patients who develop metastatic disease, numerous experimental therapies are being investigated. Considerable progress has been made in the molecular biology of malignant melanoma, including the role of growth factors (*see* Figs 11.45 and 11.46 and Table 11.1) and over 60 different cell surface antigens have been identified. A primary focus of investigation has been the use of immunotherapies, particularly the study of vaccines. The basis for such investigation centers on an understanding of the role the immune system can play in responding to melanoma and the observation that melanoma can undergo spontaneous regression. Technical advances in both biochemistry and molecular biology have led to the discovery of numerous melanoma rejection antigens. Vaccination strategies include the use of specific targeted antigens or manipulated whole tumor cells. Targeted antigens are of a variety of categories, the most studied including the melanoma differentiation antigens and a number of oncofetal proteins. Several of these targets have epitopes restricted to HLA-A2 and therefore limit patient participation to those patients who possess that haplotype. Whole cell-based vaccines can employ allogeneic vaccines prepared from established cell lines or autologous vaccines. These vaccines include cell lysates or genetically modified cells. A few vaccination strategies that have demonstrated promise in phase I/II trials for stage IV patients are currently being tested in the adjuvant setting for patients at high risk for recurrence. These advances permit translational research to be applied not only for diagnosis of melanoma but also for development of novel therapeutic strategies.

MISCELLANEOUS SKIN CANCERS

Cutaneous T-cell lymphomas (CTCL) are malignancies of the skin derived from peripheral T-lymphocytes. Mycosis fungoides is the most common type, characterized by a scaly eruption that progresses to plaques, tumors and ulcers. Its name derives from Alibert's observation in 1835 of mushroom-shaped tumors in the late stages of the disease. Sézary syndrome describes those CTCL patients who present with chronic leukemia (i.e. Sézary cells above 1000/mm³), infiltrative erythroderma or 'red man' syndrome, severe pruritus, palmoplantar keratoderma with marked scaling and fissuring and lymphadenopathy. Histologically, many tumor cells, or convoluted T-cells, are seen in the dermis. Characteristically, these cells have the capacity to enter the epidermal compartment and form nests called Pautrier's microabscesses. Regional lymph node involvement and visceral dissemination occur in advanced disease. A TNM system is used for staging CTCL. Early disease consists of limited (T1) or generalized (T2) cutaneous plaques. Development of tumors larger than 1 cm constitutes T3 disease; generalized erythroderma marks T4 disease. Five-year survival rates decrease with advancing stages of disease (from 80% to 40%).

Kaposi's sarcoma (KS) is a malignancy of the vascular endothelium that occurs in elderly men (classic KS), African natives, renal transplantation patients and; more recently, in AIDS patients. The disease exhibits diverse clinical and histopathologic manifestations, but the typical cutaneous lesions are reddish to purplish-brown nodules of the extremities. The florid and infiltrative forms often invade bone, whereas the lymphadenopathic form, which is usually disseminated, involves superficial and deep nodes, as well as the mucosa of the GI tract, tracheobronchial tree and lung parenchyma. In all forms except the nodular form, the overall prognosis is poor.

Merkel cell tumors are rare malignancies of the skin. Merkel cells are non-dendritic, non-keratinocytic epithelial clear cells. The tumor cells contain peripheral, membrane-bound neurosecretory-type granules. Although Merkel cell carcinomas have a high local recurrence rate, most patients die from disseminated disease. Morphologically, the tumor can be difficult to distinguish from small cell (oat cell) carcinoma of the lung or from other small, blue cell malignancies of neuroendocrine origin.

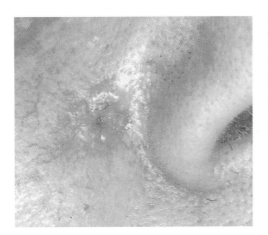

Fig. 11.24 Basal cell carcinoma. This early lesion is beginning to show the translucent, pearly appearance typical of these nodules as they begin to undergo central ulceration.

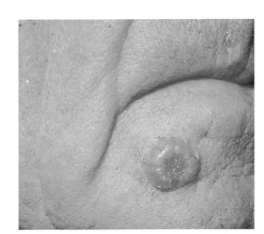

Fig. 11.25 Basal cell carcinoma. A typical lesion, with a rolled edge, appears on this patient's chin. Small vessels sweep over the edge and the center is ulcerated.

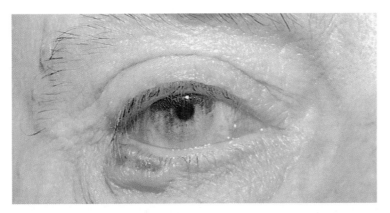

Fig. 11.26 Basal cell carcinoma. This is the most common malignant tumor of the eyelid and usually occurs either on the lower eyelid or at the medial canthus. This is an example of a relatively benign type of basal cell carcinoma with a classic pearly margin laced with blood vessels and a shallow ulcerated base at the center.

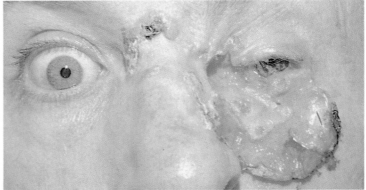

Fig. 11.27 Basal cell carcinoma. These tumors spread by direct extension and may be highly invasive, although they rarely metastasize. In this example, an extensive basal cell carcinoma has spread to involve surrounding structures.

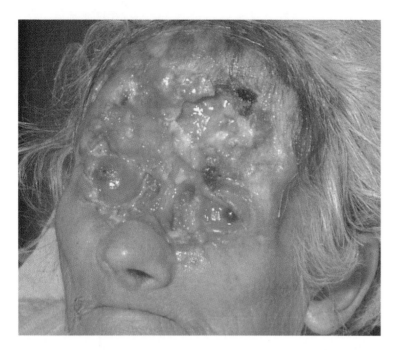

Fig. 11.28 Basal cell carcinoma. If neglected, the tumor grows inexorably, causing marked destruction of normal structures. (Courtesy of Dr D.E. Sharvill, Canterbury, UK.)

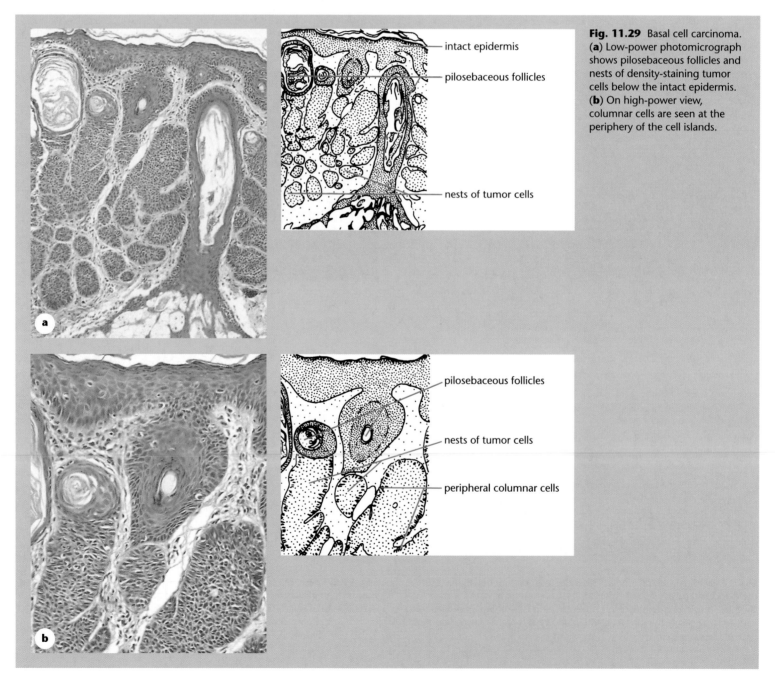

intact epidermis

pilosebaceous follicles

nests of tumor cells

pilosebaceous follicles

nests of tumor cells

peripheral columnar cells

Fig. 11.29 Basal cell carcinoma. (**a**) Low-power photomicrograph shows pilosebaceous follicles and nests of density-staining tumor cells below the intact epidermis. (**b**) On high-power view, columnar cells are seen at the periphery of the cell islands.

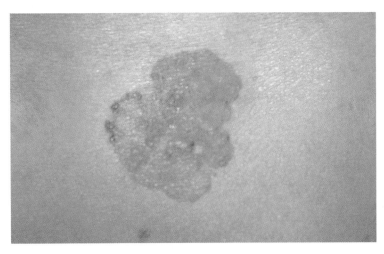

Fig. 11.30 Superficial basal cell carcinoma. This variant of basal cell carcinoma presents as a plaque with a rolled, pearly margin. It is a less aggressive version of the ulcerative type of basal cell tumor.

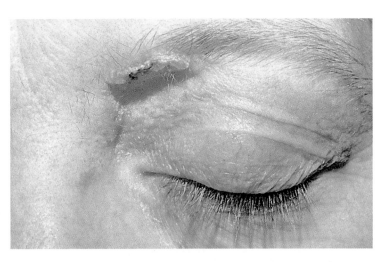

Fig. 11.31 Morpheic (sclerosing) basal cell carcinoma. This more malignant type of basal cell carcinoma receives its name from the degree of fibrous tissue present. It has a less clearly defined margin than the nodular-ulcerative variant. For this reason, a wider surgical excision is required to prevent recurrence.

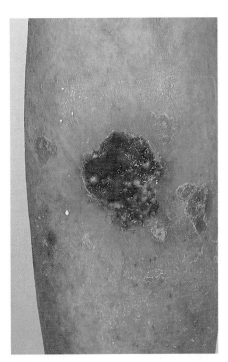

Fig. 11.32 Pigmented basal cell carcinoma. This subtype of basal cell tumor is similar in presentation to the nodular-ulcerative type except that the margin of the ulcer is rolled and pigmented. The clinical significance of this variant is that it may be mistaken for malignant melanoma. This lesion occurred on the leg, an unusual site.

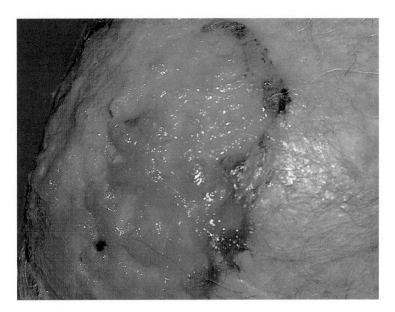

Fig. 11.33 Radiation-induced basal cell carcinoma. A tumor developed on this patient's scalp 60 years after she underwent irradiation for tinea capitis as a child. She had chronic alopecia following the over-irradiation. The lesion was successfully excised. (Courtesy of J.P. Bennett.)

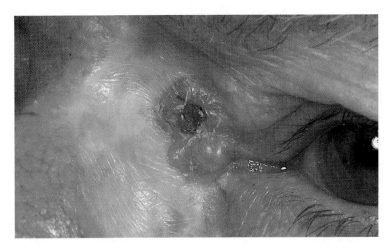

Fig. 11.34 Basal cell carcinoma. If improperly managed, basal cell tumors may recur, as shown here in a skin graft used to repair the site of an excised lesion.

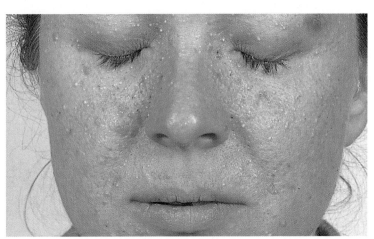

Fig. 11.35 Basal cell–nevus syndrome. In this autosomal dominant disorder, multiple basal cell carcinomas develop from childhood onward, as shown in this patient. (Courtesy of Dr A.C. Pembroke.)

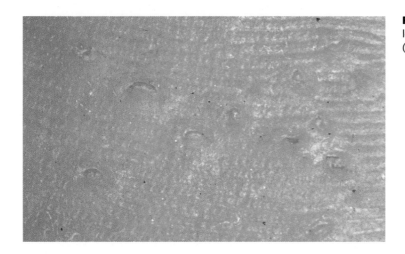

Fig. 11.36 Basal cell–nevus syndrome. Tiny pits on the palms, as shown in this low-power magnified view, are characteristic features of the condition. (Courtesy of Dr Eugene van Scott, Skin and Cancer Hospital, Philadelphia, PA.)

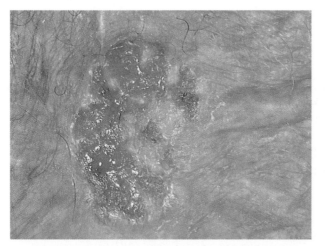

Fig. 11.37 Squamous cell carcinoma. The back of the hand is a common site for squamous cell carcinoma. This ulcerated lesion consists of a purulent base surrounded by a firm, everted and irregular margin. Note the surrounding atrophic, sun-damaged skin.

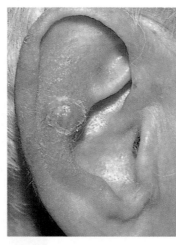

Fig. 11.38 Squamous cell carcinoma. This lesion, which arose within a preceding solar keratosis, presents as a firm, indurated nodule. The ear is a common site.

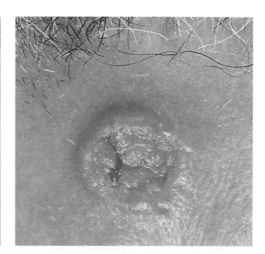

Fig. 11.39 Squamous cell carcinoma. The lesion may also present as an ulcer having a raised, firm, indurated margin.

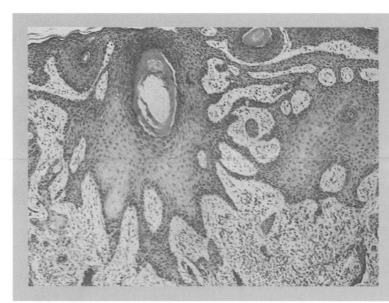

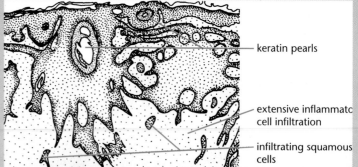

keratin pearls

extensive inflammato cell infiltration

infiltrating squamous cells

Fig. 11.40 Squamous cell carcinoma. Photomicrograph of a well-differentiated tumor shows proliferating squamous cell epithelium that is extensively infiltrating the underlying stroma. Keratin pearls and extensive inflammatory changes in the underlying stroma are common.

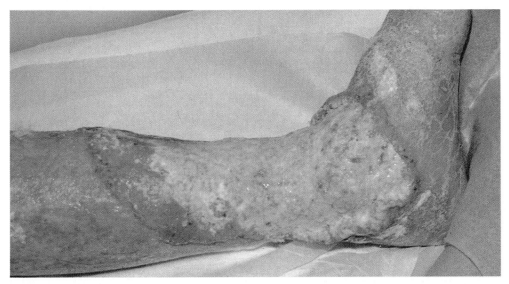

Fig. 11.41 Squamous cell carcinoma. Arising in an area of chronic ulceration, this large lesion, exhibiting a purulent base and indurated margin, had been misdiagnosed as a benign varicose ulcer.

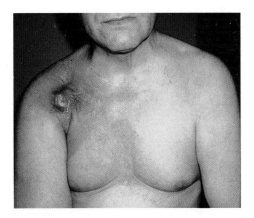

Fig. 11.42 Squamous cell carcinoma. Spread of metastases to the right anterior shoulder from a primary squamous cell carcinoma of the hand. There is extensive involvement of the axilla causing lymphatic obstruction and arm edema. Note ulceration of the tumor. Skin hyperemia is secondary to radiation therapy. In some patients, metastases can develop in the lung, bone, liver and other sites.

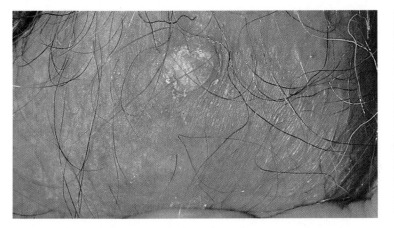

Fig. 11.43 Treatment-induced squamous cell carcinoma. This early stage lesion of the scrotum developed after a decade of nitrogen mustard therapy for mycosis fungoides. Topical nitrogen mustard and PUVA therapy for this disorder are known cutaneous carcinogens. (Courtesy of Dr Eugene van Scott, Skin and Cancer Hospital, Philadelphia, PA.)

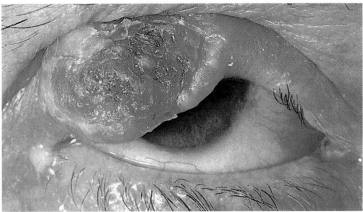

Fig. 11.44 Squamous cell carcinoma in xeroderma pigmentosum. Development of a squamous cell cancer in the rare syndrome of xeroderma pigmentosum is especially common. The lesion may arise *de novo* or from a pre-existing senile keratosis or keratoacanthoma and is relatively more common in sun-exposed areas. Characteristically, this lesion has an everted edge and is irregular in shape.

Fig. 11.45 Biology of melanoma. (Courtesy of Dr M. Herlyn, 1993.)

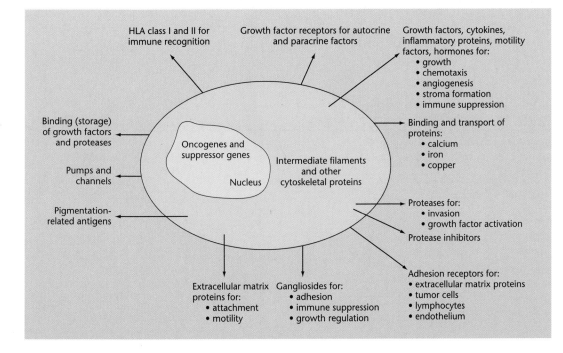

MAGE, BAGE and GAGE gene families
Several members to each family; resemble oncofetal proteins; found normally in testis and placenta
Melanocyte lineage proteins/normal differentiation antigens
Abundant proteins function in melanin production   Tyrosinase   gp75   gp100   Melan-A/MART1   Tyrosinase-related protein 2 (TRP2)
Tumor-specific antigens
Subtle mutations of normal cellular proteins: examples of coding region mutations   Cyclin-dependent kinase-4   β-catenin
Other mutated peptides
Activated as a result of cellular transformation   Mutated introns   p15
Candidate antigens identified by monocolonal antibodies
Melanoma gangliosides (GM2, GD2, GM3 and GD3)

Fig. 11.46 Examples of identified melanoma antigens. Melanoma rejection antigens have been identified as target T-cells. This list continues to expand both in numbers within groups as well as new categories of antigenic targets.

Table 11.1 Genetic alterations in malignant melanoma. Recent advances in molecular biology and understanding of genetics have localized several genes to the pathogenesis of melanoma. The most important is p16 or CDKN2A on chromosome 9p21 which encodes a cyclin-dependent kinase inhibitor that halts progression through the cell cycle. (Adapted from Haluska and Hodi, 1998.)

Gene	Chromosome	Frequency
CDKN2A/p16	9p21	80% cell lines 40% heredity cases 10–40% sporadic cases
CDK4	12p13	Rare in hereditary and sporadic cases
RB1	13q14	Rare in sporadic cases
CDKN2A/p19ARF	9p21	Altered concomitant to p16
p53	17p13	Overexpression
PTEN/NMAC1	10q24	40% cell lines
ras	1p (N-ras) 11p (Ha-ras) 12p (Ki-ras)	10–25% (10% of ras mutations) Rare (10% of ras mutations) Very rare

Table 11.2 Malignant melanoma: Differential features of major types.

	Superficial spreading	Lentigo maligna	Nodular
Percentage of all melanomas	70–75	5–10	10–15
Mean age at presentation (years)	47	69	50
Common location	Increased frequency on backs of both sexes Increased frequency on lower legs of females	Head, neck, back of hands (90%)	Any site
Duration of radial-growth phase	Months (up to a few	1–7 years (up to 14 years) years)	5–30 years (up to 50 years) Direct tumor invasion postulated, without radial phase
Border of lesion Histology of surrounding area	Raised Pagetoid distribution of melanocytes in epidermis	Flat Atypical melanocytic hyperplasia at dermal-epidermal junction	Raised No surrounding area Dermal invasion

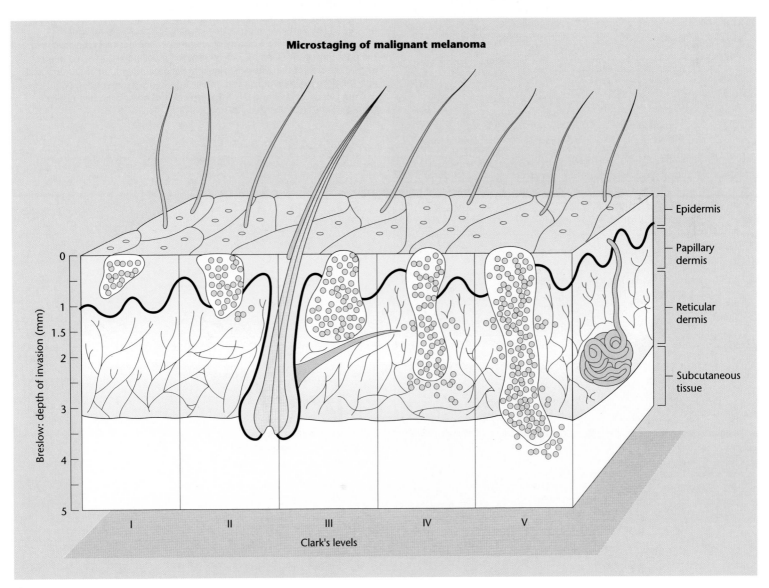

Microstaging of malignant melanoma

Fig. 11.47 Malignant melanoma. This diagram represents the combined microstaging techniques of Clark and Breslow. The Clark system of levels of invasion is based on anatomy, whereas the Breslow technique relies on the depth of invasion (in millimeters) from the granular layer of epidermis to the deepest tumor cell. (Adapted from Goldsmith, 1979.)

Table 11.3 Malignant melanoma: Clark levels of invasion, thickness of lesion, and survival.

Clark level	Thickness of lesion (mm)	Five-year survival rate (%)
I	–(in situ)	100 (theoretical)
II	<0.65	95
III	0.65–1.50 (overall)	75–85
	0.65–0.75	90
	0.75–1.50	70
IV	>1.50	45
V	>3.0 (subcutaneous)	25–35

Tumor

T1a	<1.00 mm	No ulceration
T1b		Ulceration or level IV/V
T2a	1.01-2.00 mm	No ulceration
T2b		Ulceration
T3a	2.01-4.00 mm	No ulceration
T3b		Ulceration
T4a	>4.00 mm	No ulceration
T4b		Ulceration

Nodes

N1	1 lymph node	Micrometasasis
N1b		Macrometasasis
N2a	2-3 lymph nodes	Micrometastasis
N2b		In-transit metastasis(es)/satellite Metastasis(es) without lymph Node involvement
N3	4 or more lymph nodes, or In-transit metastasis(es) or Ulceration with metastatic Lymph node involvement	

Metastases

M0	None	
M1	Distant skin, subcutaneous, or lymph nodes	Normal LDH
M2	Lung	Normal LDH
M3	Other distant sites	Normal or elevated LDH

Stage

0	Tis; N0; M0
IA	T1a; N0; M0
IB	T1b; T2a; N0; M0
IIA	T2b; T3a; N0; M0
IIB	T3b; T4a; N0; M0
IIC	T4b; N0; M0
IIIA	T1-4a; N1a; M0
IIIB	T1-4a; N1b; N2a;M0
IIIC	Any T; N2b; N2c; N3; M0
IV	Any T; Any N; Any M

a

Fig. 11.48 (**a**) Final new AJCC staging system for malignant melanoma. The new AJCC staging system demonstrates the importance of ulceration in determining prognosis, principally upstaging patients with evidence for ulceration. The number of lymph nodes involved for stage III patients and LDH and sites of metastatic disease for stage IV patients are also recognized as significant prognostic factors. Micrometastatic versus macrometastatic disease is recognized in the lymph node classification as sentinel lymph node mapping with biopsy has become more widely used (Adapted from Balch *et al.*, 2001.) (**b**) Sentinel lymph node mapping for staging in malignant melanoma. Patient with a history of an intermediate thickness melanoma of the right upper arm. One mCi of Tc-99m sulfur colloid was injected in the immediate area of the patient's known melanoma. Migration of radiotracer into the right axilla demonstrates uptake into two separate nodes. (Courtesy of Greg Lefeur, CNMT, and Drs Milos Janicek and Annick van den Abbeele, Dana-Farber Cancer Institute, Boston, MA.)

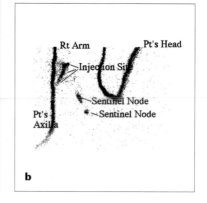

b

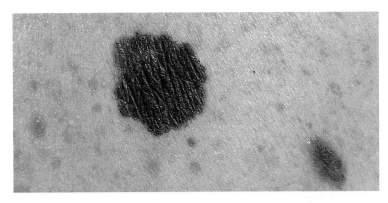

Fig. 11.49 Superficial spreading malignant melanoma. The lesion is almost totally black except for a brown area at the upper left edge. Note the surrounding lentigines from sun damage. The other mole is benign.

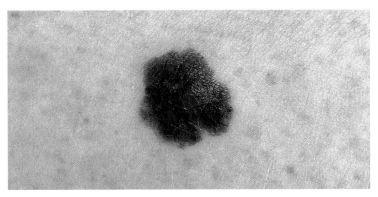

Fig. 11.50 Superficial spreading malignant melanoma. This lesion appears as a slightly raised plaque with a characteristic irregular outline. It is black and brown in color.

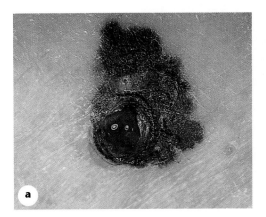

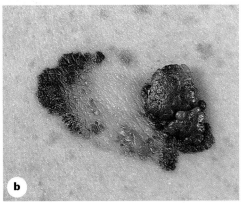

Fig. 11.51 Superficial spreading malignant melanoma. (**a**) The horizontal spreading phase of a lesion is ultimately followed by (**b**) vertical growth and deep invasion, together with formation of a nodule.

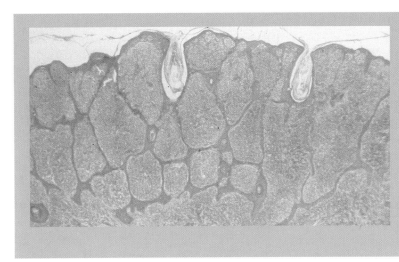

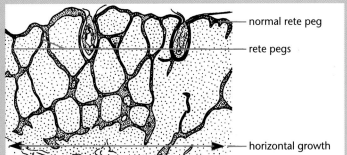

Fig. 11.52 Superficial spreading malignant melanoma. Low-power microscopic section shows horizontal dermal infiltration by melanoma cells. (Courtesy of Pathology Department, Brigham and Women's Hospital, Boston, MA.)

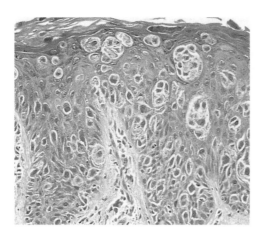

Fig. 11.53 Superficial spreading malignant melanoma. Clusters of 'Pagetoid' melanocytes are present at all layers of the epidermis. Note the widely distributed melanin pigment (so-called 'buckshot scatter').

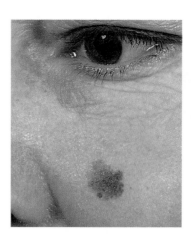

Fig. 11.54 Lentigo maligna. Initially, the lesion appears as a flat, pigmented area with an irregular outline. As it enlarges during its radial growth phase, abnormal melanocytes spread centrifugally in the epidermis, with minimal invasion of the papillary dermis. Its pigmentation varies from light tan to brown or black; red, blue, gray and white areas may also be present.

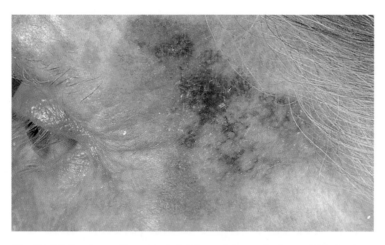

Fig. 11.55 Lentigo maligna. Typical of the radial growth phase, this lesion is made up of various colors and has an irregular, indented margin. Like many such tumors, it grew slowly and attained a large size before presentation.

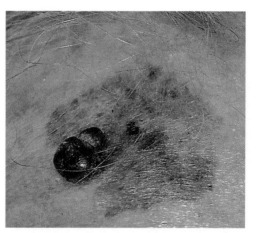

Fig. 11.56 Lentigo maligna melanoma. This lesion has begun to grow vertically and invade the dermis; at this stage it thickens and becomes nodular.

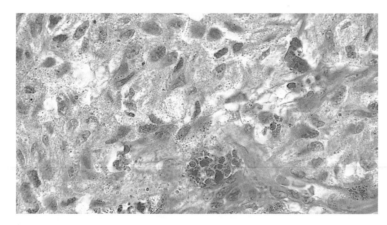

Fig. 11.57 Malignant melanoma. Tumor tissue is characterized by increased numbers of atypical melanocytes showing pleomorphism and prominent chromatin clumping. Fine particles of melanin can be seen throughout the cytoplasm.

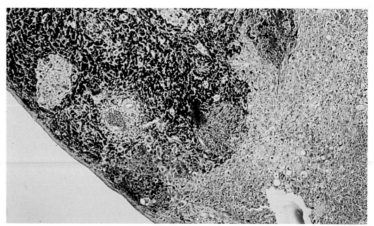

Fig. 11.58 Malignant melanoma. Low-power view of lymph node metastasis shows numerous heavily pigmented tumor cells as well as areas of amelanotic poorly differentiated malignant cells.

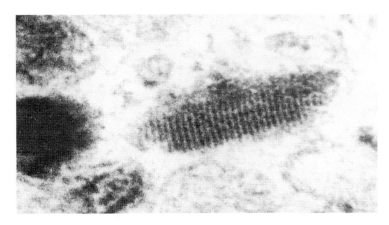

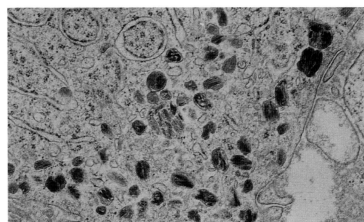

Fig. 11.59 Malignant melanoma. Electron micrograph of a melanosome in a case of malignant melanoma shows the typical oval structure of these tyrosinase-containing granules. This partially developed melanosome demonstrates the lamellated internal structure which is obscured by pigment production in mature granules.

Fig. 11.60 Malignant melanoma. Electron micrograph shows prominent, diagnostic dense-core granules. In some patients with amelanotic melanoma presenting with metastases from an unknown primary site, the presence of these granules will confirm a diagnosis of malignant melanoma.

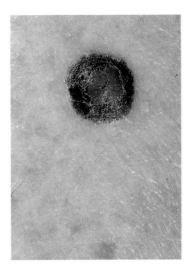

Fig. 11.61 Nodular malignant melanoma. This variant of malignant melanoma lacks a horizontal growth phase. The lesion grows vertically from the beginning and invasion produces a nodule. Note the surrounding lentigines.

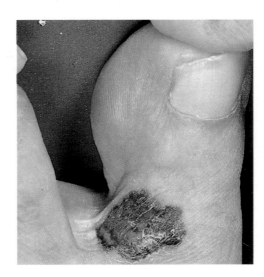

Fig. 11.62 Nodular malignant melanoma. This black nodule represents the classic conception of a malignant melanoma. The prognosis for these lesions is poor, yet diagnosis of less obvious lesions at an earlier stage may be life saving.

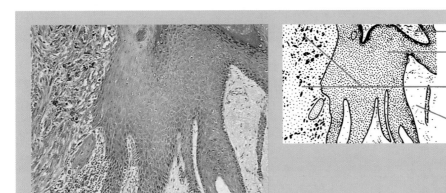

cornified layer

epidermis (free of tumor)

malignant melanoma

solar elastosis

Fig. 11.63 Nodular malignant melanoma. Histologically, the nodular type of malignant melanoma is marked by the absence of any *in situ* melanocytic lesion in the adjacent epithelium. Note the presence of solar elastosis at right.

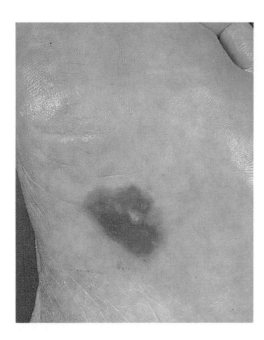

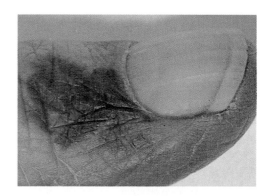

Fig. 11.64 Amelanotic malignant melanoma. Rarely, a lesion presents with no apparent visible pigmentation, as in the case of this plum-colored nodule on the sole of a foot. These lesions show aggressive behavior, evolving quickly and penetrating deeply.

Fig. 11.65 Acral lentiginous malignant melanoma. Clinically, this lesion appears similar to lentigo maligna, but it exhibits much more aggressive biologic behavior. It grows quickly, becoming raised and subsequently nodular, an indication of a vertical growth phase. (Courtesy of Dr A.C. Pembroke.)

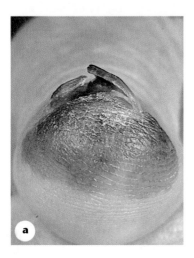
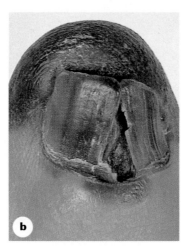
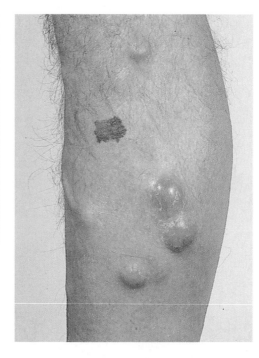

Fig. 11.67 Metastatic malignant melanoma. Hard flesh- and plum-colored tumors have spread from this man's neglected primary lesion. The leg is a common site for malignant melanoma.

Fig. 11.66 Acral lentiginous malignant melanoma. (**a, b**) This lesion arising from the nailbed has an irregular outline; its colors vary from black to gray and blue. As it invades, the lesion distorts and splits the nailplate. (Courtesy of Dr A.C. Pembroke.)

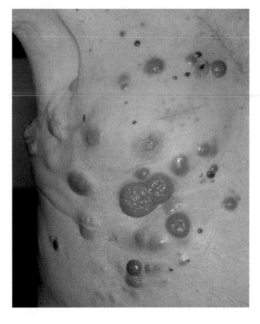
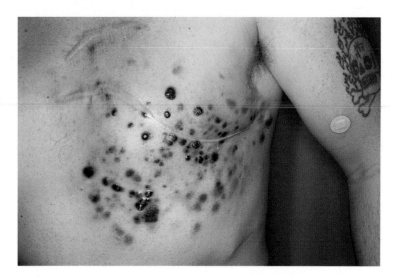

Fig. 11.68 Metastatic melanoma. Regional chest lesions in an 85-year-old man that developed several years after removal of the primary. Note lesions of variable size, age and depth of extension. Visceral metastases eventually occurred.

Fig. 11.69 Thirty-year-old man with numerous regional cutaneous metastases. In some patients, localized areas of metastases cluster together. Eventually, however, distant sites occur.

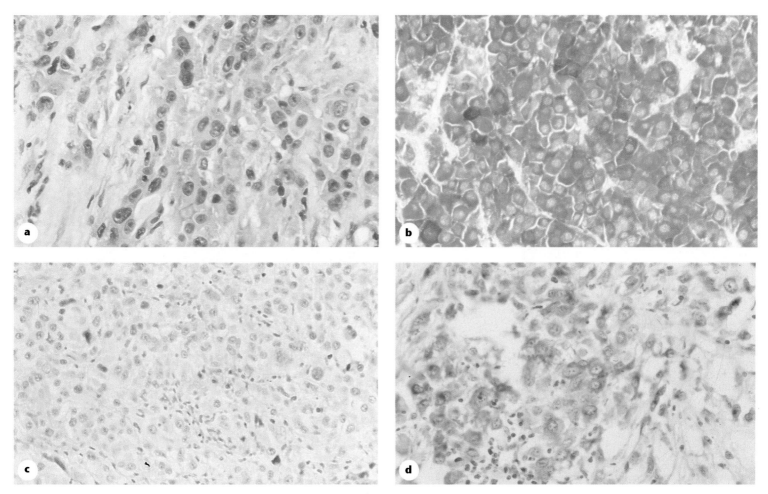

Fig. 11.70 Metastatic amelanotic melanoma. A 60-year-old man, who 6 years previously had a level III amelanotic malignant melanoma removed from his back, presented with cervical adenopathy. (**a**) Microscopic section of a lymph node biopsy specimen shows an undifferentiated malignancy. (**b**) Positive S-100 immunoperoxidase stain is consistent with malignant melanoma; a negative keratin stain (**c**) rules out an epithelium-derived carcinoma. (**d**) Positive immunoperoxidase staining with E-Mel (HMB-45) is diagnostic of melanoma. Electron microscopy, which may show dense-core granules, is also useful in confirming a diagnosis of malignant melanoma in patients who present with an undifferentiated malignancy.

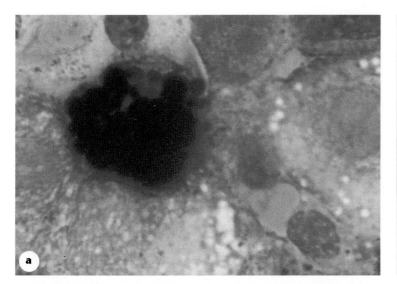
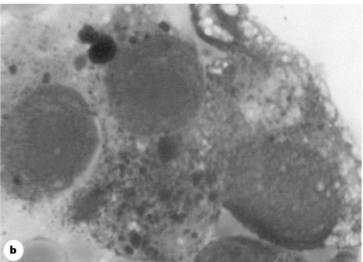

Fig. 11.71 Metastatic melanoma to the bone marrow. A 26-year-old man presented with level IV cutaneous melanoma involving the mid-back. He also had mild anemia. Bone marrow shows infiltration by clumps of large malignant cells with abundant basophilic cytoplasm, immature nuclei and very prominent nucleoli. Large clumps of extracellular melanin are noted (**a**). In addition, melanin granules (dark bluish-green in color) are noted in the cytoplasm of many individual melanoma cells (**b**) (× 1000, Wright-Giemsa stain.)

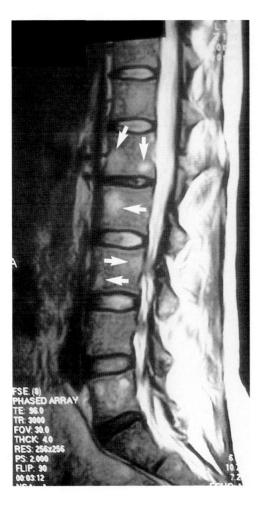

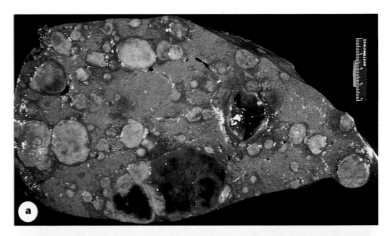

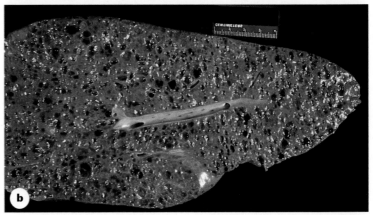

Fig. 11.72 Metastatic malignant melanoma to the bone. A 38-year-old woman with previous resection of a level III cutaneous melanoma developed subsequent metastases to the brain and liver. Because of mild back pain, MRI of the spine was carried out. Sagittal T2-weighted image of the lumbar spine reveals multiple foci of increased signal (arrows) consistent with metastases.

Fig. 11.73 Metastatic malignant melanoma to the liver. Metastases frequently occur to the liver. Two major patterns are noted, including large nodular deposits with hemorrhage, as well as pigment production (**a**) and a diffuse process with smaller size metastases (**b**). In the the latter case, the liver weighed 4060 g and contained numerous small, cystic metastases which were filled with blood.

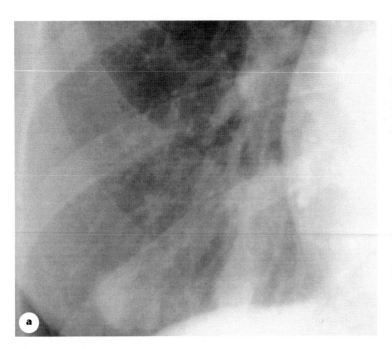

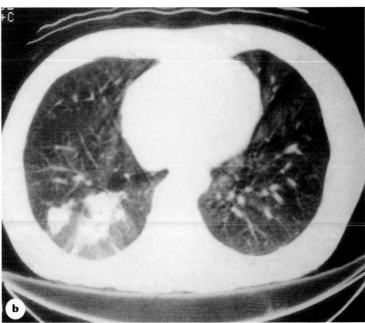

Fig. 11.74 Metastatic malignant melanoma to the lung. In some patients, metastatic disease to the lung may stimulate primary lung cancer. (**a**) Plain radiograph of the right lower lung of this 40-year-old patient, with previous resection of a cutaneous melanoma, reveals nodular infiltrate. (**b**) CT scan reveals the prominent localized metastases in the right lower lung.

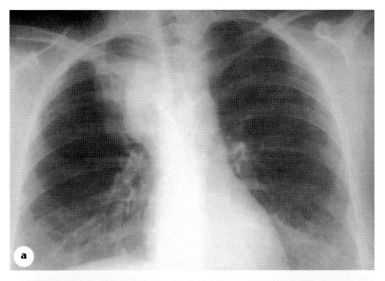

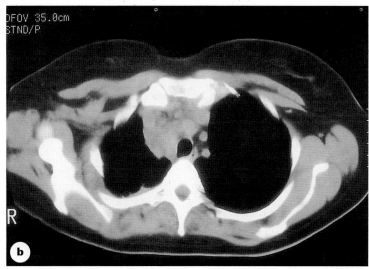

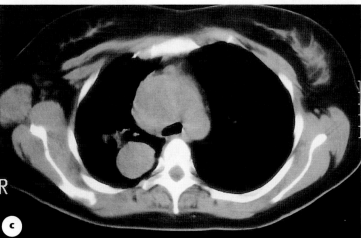

Fig. 11.75 Metastatic malignant melanoma to the lung. A 35-year-old woman with a previous resection of a cutaneous level IV melanoma presented with increasing cough and weight loss. (**a**) PA chest radiograph shows a large paratracheal mass in the right upper lung. (**b**) CT scan reveals multiple mediastinal metastases (**c**) Lower cut shows a prominent round, metastatic deposit. In some patients pulmonary features suggest a diagnosis of lung cancer particularly when the original cutaneous melanoma was resected many years earlier and no other sites of metastases are initially identified. The diagnosis is further confounded when the late metastases. are amelanotic (*see* Fig. 11.70).

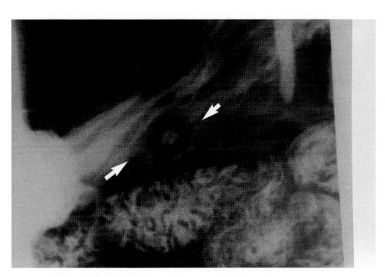

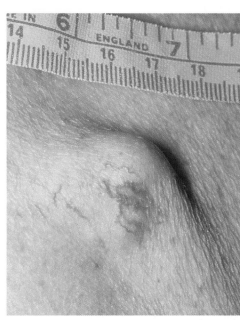

Fig. 11.77 Metastatic melanoma to subcutaneous tissues. In this 60-year-old man, the first evidence of metastatic malignant melanoma was the rapid growth of a subcutaneous nodule on his mid-back.

Fig. 11.76 Metastatic melanoma. Typical 'target lesion' noted in the stomach wall of this 50-year-old man with prior resection of a level IV cutaneous lesion, who recently presented with anemia due to gastric bleeding. The 'target' appearance is due to central necrosis and ulceration of the metastatic tumor masses.

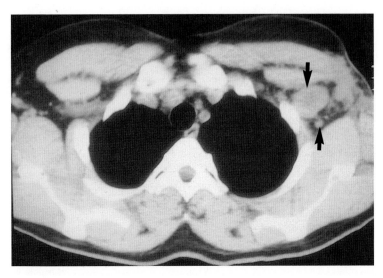

Fig. 11.78 Metastatic melanoma to lymph node. In this 40-year-old man with metastatic malignant melanoma, CT scan of the chest shows an enlarged left axillary lymph node (arrows).

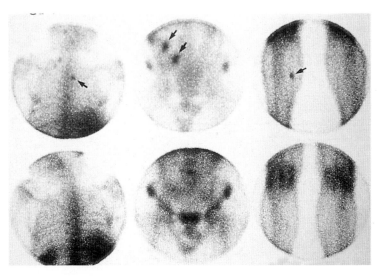

Fig. 11.79 Metastatic melanoma to soft tissues. Gallium-67 scanning will often reveal palpable as well as non-palpable early metastases to soft tissues as illustrated in this 60-year-old patient. The scan at 72 hours shows increased uptake in paraspinal tissues (upper left), iliac lymph nodes (upper center) and medial calf (upper right). Following scan repeated 6 weeks later, after multidrug chemotherapy, shows no significant uptake, corresponding to a clinical remission. The hot spots in the lower middle view represent normal marrow, bladder and rectal sites due to a higher count rate which accentuates the images.

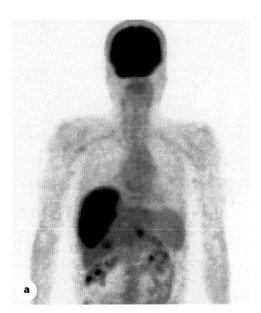

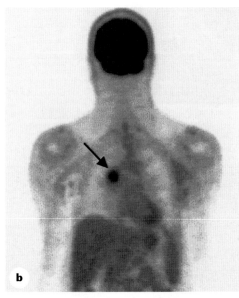

Fig. 11.80 PET scanning in melanoma. (**a**) Seventy-year-old patient with a history of ocular melanoma demonstrates FDG-glucose uptake in multiple liver metastases, including a dominant right hepatic lobe mass. (**b**) Fifty-six-year-old patient with a history of stage III malignant melanoma demonstrates uptake in a hilar mass (arrow) that was not significant on CT scan. (**c**) Same patient demonstrates an asymptomatic mass in the brain (arrow) that was subsequently confirmed by head MRI. (Courtesy of Drs Milos Janicek and Annick van den Abbeele, Dana-Farber Cancer Institute, Boston, MA.)

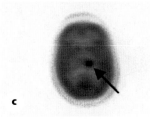

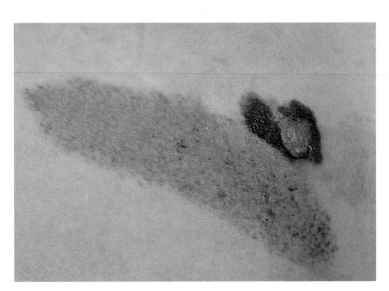

Fig. 11.81 Malignant melanoma. In the exceptional case, as shown here, malignant melanoma develops in a large melanocytic nevus that has been present from birth.

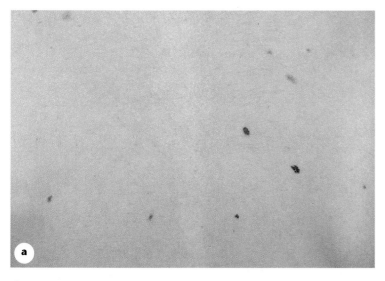

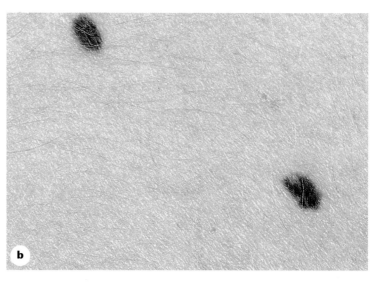

Fig. 11.82 Dysplastic nevus syndrome. (**a**) Photograph of the back of a 15-year-old girl who had a family history of malignant melanoma shows numerous atypical nevi. (**b**) Of the two moles shown on this close-up view, the one on the right with an irregular margin proved to be malignant.

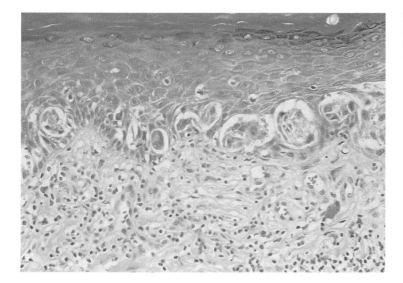

Fig. 11.83 Dysplastic nevus syndrome. Histologically, a dysplastic nevus is characterized by nests of basally localized melanocytes with abundant eosinophilic cytoplasm, vesicular nuclei and prominent nucleoli. There is dermal fibrosis, marked pigmentary incontinence and a lymphocytic infiltrate.

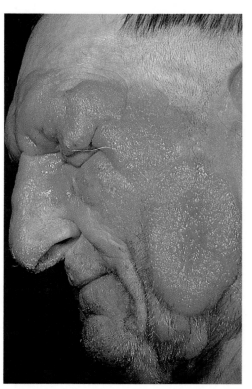

Fig. 11.84 Mycosis fungoides. In a late stage of the disease, lesions develop into mushroom-like tumors on the skin.

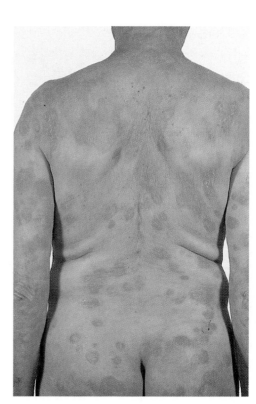

Fig. 11.85 Mycosis fungoides. Although these widespread lesions mimic psoriasis in their patch or premycotic stage, they are asymmetric, an unusual finding in psoriasis. Skin biopsy confirmed the diagnosis of mycosis fungoides. (Courtesy of Dr A.C. Pembroke.)

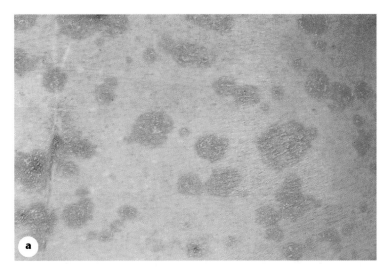

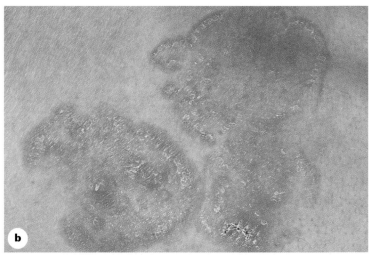

Fig. 11.86 Mycosis fungoides. (**a**) The pink, scaly patches may exhibit various shapes and sizes. This early stage disease is sometimes called 'parapsoriasis en plaque' (**b**) The borders of the eruptions may be quite bizarre.

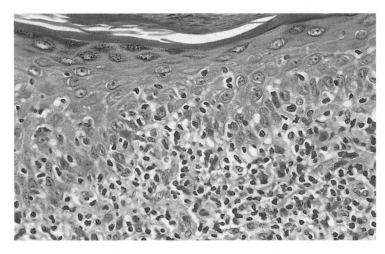

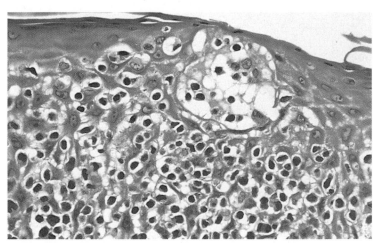

Fig. 11.87 Mycosis fungoides. This more advanced patch-stage lesion shows parakeratosis, orthohyperkeratosis and acanthosis. The epidermis and dermis are diffusely infiltrated by large numbers of cells with highly irregular cerebriform and dark-staining nuclei (mycosis cells).

Fig. 11.88 Mycosis fungoides. Photomicrograph of a plaque-stage lesion shows a characteristic Pautrier's microabscess situated just below the stratum corneum.

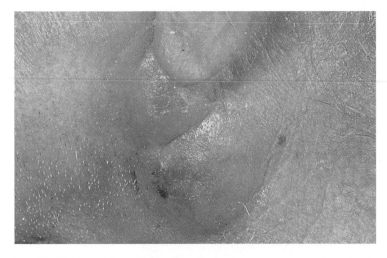

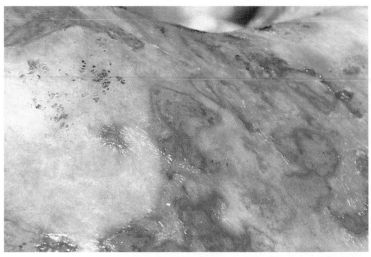

Fig. 11.89 Mycosis fungoides. As the disease progresses, plaques develop into tumorous masses, as seen in this large nodular lesion. This patient had widespread infiltrated plaques elsewhere. (Courtesy of Dr A.C. Pembroke.)

Fig. 11.90 Mycosis fungoides. Very occasionally, ulcerative lesions develop in the late stage of disease.

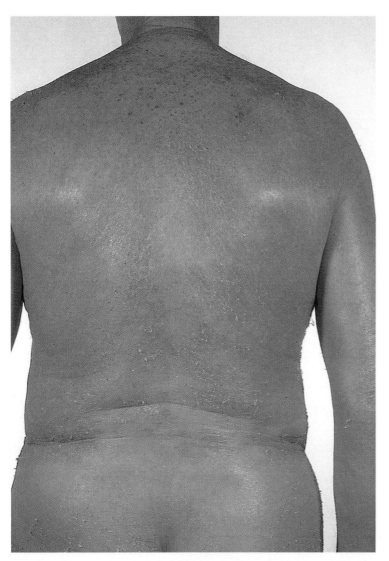

Fig. 11.91 Sézary syndrome. Clinically, this condition is an erythroderma or exfoliative dermatitis marked by a universal redness of the skin with associated scaling. This patient had a WBC of 90 000/mm³ with 70% Sézary cells (see Fig. 11.87).

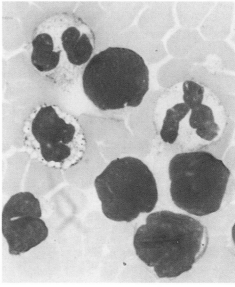

Fig. 11.92 Sézary syndrome/mycosis fungoides. The cerebriform, hyperchromatic nuclei of mycosis/Sézary cells are evident in this peripheral blood smear. Such cells are present in abundance in the peripheral blood in Sézary syndrome, but they are seen in smaller numbers in some patients with mycosis fungoides.

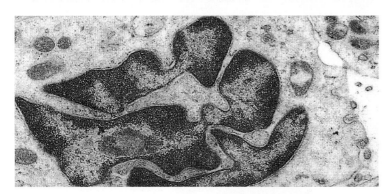

Fig. 11.93 Sézary syndrome/mycosis fungoides. Electron micrograph shows the characteristic appearance of the nucleus of a mycosis/Sézary cell. The T-lymphocyte exhibits abundant cytoplasm and a centrally located, irregular, highly convoluted nucleus with a peripheral chromatin distribution.

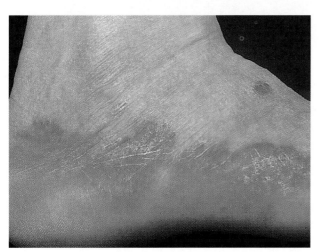

Fig. 11.94 Kaposi's sarcoma. Purple plaques and nodules, particularly on the lower legs and feet, are characteristic of this vascular malignancy. (Courtesy of Dr Neil Smith, Institute of Dermatology, London, UK.)

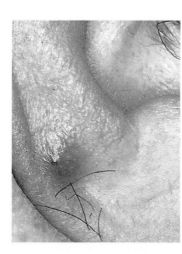

Fig. 11.95 Kaposi's sarcoma. The purplish-red nodule arising on the lateral surface of this patient's pinna is a Kaposi's sarcoma.

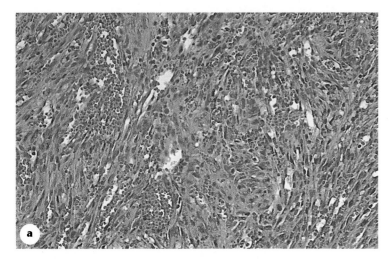

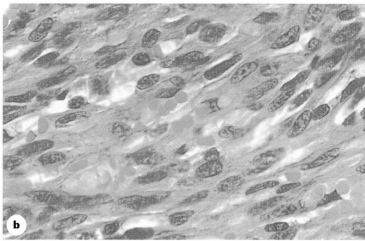

Fig. 11.96 Kaposi's sarcoma. (**a**) Histologically, this sarcoma of vascular endothelium exhibits numerous spindle cell formations, which contain small vascular slits. Hemorrhage and hemosiderin deposition are also evident. (**b**) Higher magnification shows the immature spindle cells more clearly.

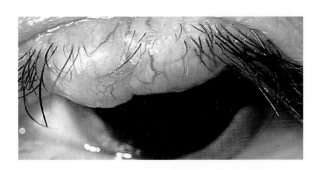

Fig. 11.97 Sebaceous sarcoma. The clinical appearance of this lesion simulates that of a large chalazion. It presents as a steadily enlarging, non-ulcerated nodule of the upper eyelid. Note the characteristic loss of hair over the lesion.

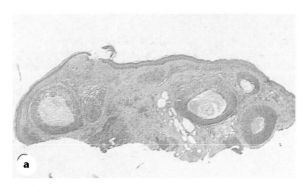

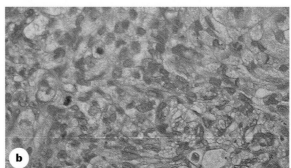

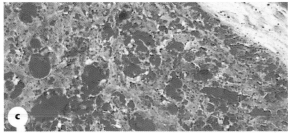

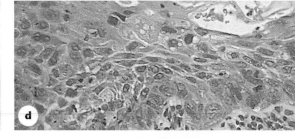

Fig. 11.98 Sebaceous carcinoma. (**a**) Whole-mount section of a lesion shows large tumor nodules in the dermis; most nodules exhibit central necrosis. (**b**) Increased magnification shows that numerous cells resemble sebaceous gland cells. A number of mitotic figures are present. (**c**) Many cells stain positively for fat (oil red-O). (**d**) In another case, large tumor cells are scattered throughout the epithelium in a condition called 'Pagetoid' change. Invasion of the epithelium by tumor can cause a chronic non-granulomatous blepharoconjunctivitis.

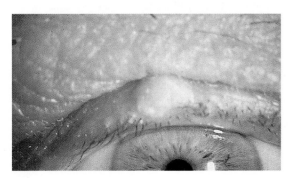

Fig. 11.99 Merkel cell tumor. Clinically, the lesion presents as a firm, raised, painless nodule, as shown here in the middle portion of the upper eyelid. The slowly enlarging tumor may be violaceous; ulceration is rare.

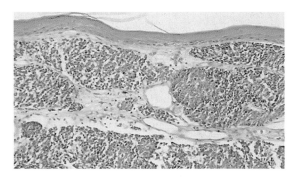

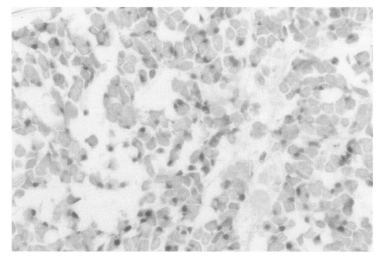

Fig. 11.100 Merkel cell tumor. Histologic section shows nests of dark, poorly differentiated cells in the dermis, as well as mitotic figures. Markers that are positive in Merkel cell tumors (MCT) but usually negative in small cell lung cancer (SCLC), include CK20 and NFP (neurofilament protein) while those negative in MCT but positive in SCLC include CK7 and TFF-1 (thyroid transcription factor).(Courtesy of Dr D.A. Morris.)

Fig. 11.101 Merkel cell tumor. Immunoperoxidase stain for keratin is positive in this section. The dot-like pattern of cytoplasmic staining is characteristic.

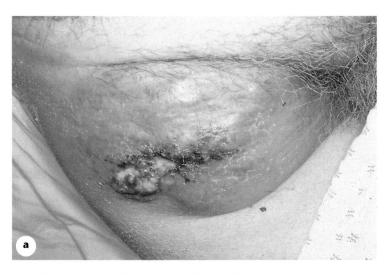

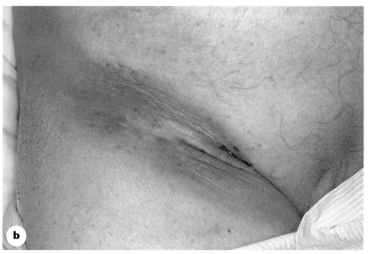

Fig. 11.102 Merkel cell tumor. (**a**) A 65-year-old man presented with a large, ulcerative skin lesion in the right groin. Biopsy showed a Merkel cell tumor. (**b**) Combination chemotherapy has resulted in a dramatic regression of the malignancy. Followup surgical resection and postoperative radiotherapy were carried out and the patient remained disease free 4 years later. Merkel cell tumors may be confused with other 'small blue cell' tumors such as small cell (oat cell) lung cancer. Widespread dissemination may occur in all of these highly malignant tumors, including metastases to the brain, skin, bone and bone marrow.

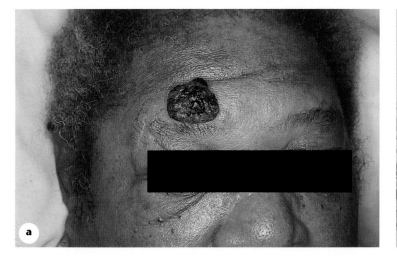

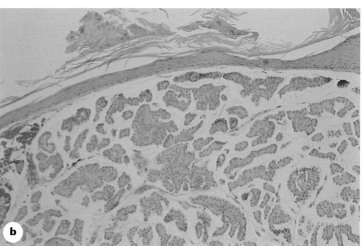

Fig. 11.103 Primary mucinous carcinoma of the skin. (**a**) Note pigmented, protuberant localized lesion in a 69-year-old black male, of about 1 year's duration. (**b**) Low-power view shows a pseudoglandular pattern with islands of solid tumor. This uncommon tumor is a histologic subtype of sweat gland (eccrine) carcinoma. It may be confused with metastatic adenocarcinoma to the skin. It has a low malignant potential with a long indolent clinical course (*see* Bellezza *et al.*, 2000).

REFERENCES

Alam M, Katner D: Cutaneous squamous-cell carcinoma. N Engl J Med 2001; 344(13):975–983.

Armstrong BK, English DR: Epidemiologic studies. In: Balch CM, Houghton AN, Milton GW, Sober AJ, Soong S-J, eds: Cutaneous Melanoma, 2nd edn. 166–17 Lippincott, Philadelphia, 1992.

Balch CM, Buzaid AC, Atkins MB, et al., A new American Joint Committee on Cancer Staging system for cutaneous melanoma. Cancer 2000; 88 : 1484–1491.

Balch CM, Buzaid AC, Soong SJ, et al., Final Version of the American Joint Committee on Cancer Staging system for cutaneous melanoma. J Clin Oncol 19: 3635–3648, 2001.

Bellezza G, Sidoni A, Bucciarelli A: Primary mucinous carcinoma of the skin. Am J Dermatopathol 2000; 22(2):166–170.

Boon T, van der Bruggen P: Human tumor antigens recognized by T lymphocytes. J Exp Med 1996; 183: 725–729.

Breslow A: Tumor thickness, level of invasion, and node dissection in stage I cutaneous melanoma. Ann Surg 1975; 182 : 572–575.

Buzaid AC, Ross MI, Balch, CM, et al.: Critical analysis of the current American Joint Committee on Cancer Staging System for cutaneous melanoma and proposal of a new staging system. J Clin Oncol 1997; 15: 1039–1051.

Ceballos P, Maldonado R, Mihm M: Melanoma in children. N Engl J Med 1995; 332 : 656–662.

Clark WH, Mihm MC: Moles and malignant melanoma. In: Fitzpatrick TB, Arndt KA, Clark WH, et al.: eds: Dermatology in General Medicine, McGraw-Hill, New York, 1971; 491–511.

Dhawan M, Kirkwood JM: Melanoma therapy: a report. Contemp Oncol 1994; Sept: 40–60.

Gershenwald JE, Thompson W, Mansfiedl PF, et al.: Multi-institutional melanoma lymphatic mapping experience: the prognostic value of sentinel lymph status in 612 stage I and II melanoma patients. J Clin Oncol 1999; 17 : 976–983.

Goessling W, McKee PH, Mayer R. Merkel Cell Carcinoma. J Clin Oncol 2002; 20:588–598.

Goldsmith HS: Melanoma: an overview. CA 1979; 29 : 194–215.

Greene MH, Clark WH, Tucker MA, et al.: High risk of malignant melanoma in melanoma-prone families with dysplastic nevi. Ann Intern Med 1985; 102 : 458–465.

Greenlee RT, Murray T, Bolden S, Wingo PA: Cancer statistics, 2000; CA Cancer J Clin 2000; 50 : 7–33.

Grin-Jorgensen CM, Rigel DS, Friedman RJ: The worldwide incidence of malignant melanoma. In: Balch CM, Houghton AN, Milton GW, Sober AJ, Soong S-J, eds: Cutaneous Melanoma, 2nd edn. Lippincott, Philadelphia, 1992.

Haluska FG, Hodi FS. Molecular genetics of familial cutaneous melanoma. J Clin Oncol 1998; 16 : 670–682.

Helm F, (ed): Cancer Dermatology. Lea & Febiger, Philadelphia, 1979.

Herlyn M: molecular biology of the melanoma cell surface – translational opportunities. Hem/Oncol Ann 1993; 1(4):251–255.

Karakousis C, Balch CM, Urist M, et al.: Local recurrence of malignant melanoma: long term results of a surgical trial. Ann Surg Oncol 1996; 3 : 446–452.

Koh MK, Miller DR, Geeler AC: Screening for melanoma and other skin cancers. Clinics in Dermatology 1992; 10(1):97–103.

Kraehn G, Schartl M, Peter R: Human malignant melanoma. A genetic disease? Cancer 1995; 75 : 1228–1237.

Loggie BW, Eddy JA: Solar considerations in the development of cutaneous melanoma. Semin Oncol 1988; 15 : 494–499.

Marghoob AA, Koenig K, Bittencourt FV, Kopf AW, Bart RS: Breslow thickness and Clark level in melanoma: support for including level in pathology reports and in American Joint Committee on Cancer Staging. Cancer 2000; 88 : 589–595.

Mihm MC, Clark WH, Reed RJ: The clinical diagnosis of malignant melanoma. Semin Oncol 1975; 2 : 105–118.

Odajnyk C, Muggia FM: Treatment of Kaposi's sarcoma: overview and analysis by clinical setting. J Clin Oncol 1985; 3 : 1277–1285.

Ottinger LW: Basal cell–nevus syndrome: clinicopathological exercises. N Engl J Med 1986; 314 : 700–706.

Palazzo J, Duray PH: Typical, dysplastic, congenital and Spitz nevi: a comparative immunohistochemical study. Hum Pathol 1989; 20 : 341–346.

Rivers JK, Kopf AW, Vinokur AF, et al.: Clinical characteristics of malignant melanomas developing in persons with dysplastic nevi. Cancer 1990; 65 : 1232–1236.

Ronan SG, Han MC, Dan Gupta TK: Histologic prognostic indicators in cutaneous malignant melanoma. Semin Oncol 1988; 15 : 558–565.

Rosenberg SA: The immunotherapy of solid cancers based on cloning the genes encoding tumor-rejection antigens. Ann Rev Med 1996; 47 : 481–491.

Sausville EA, Eddy JL, Makuch RW, et al.: Histopathologic staging at initial diagnosis of mycosis fungoides and the Sézary syndrome: definition of three distinctive prognostic groups. Ann Intern Med 1988; 109 : 372–382.

Trent JM, Meyskens FL, Salmon SE, et al.: Relation of cytogenetic abnormalities and clinical outcome in metastatic melanoma. N Engl J Med 1990; 322 : 1508–1511.

Tyler DS, Onaitis M, Kherani A, et al.: Positron emission tomography scanning in malignant melanoma. Cancer 2000; 89 : 1019–1025.

Walker MJ: The role of hormones and growth factors in melanoma. Semin Oncol 1988; 15 : 512.

Wick MM, Sober AJ, Fitzpatrick TB, et al.: Clinical characteristics of early cutaneous melanoma. Cancer 1980; 45: 2684–2686.

FIGURE CREDITS

The following books published by Gower Medical Publishing are sources of figures in the present chapter. The figure numbers given in the listing are those of the figures in the present chapter. The page numbers given in parentheses are those of the original publication.

Cawson RA, Eveson JW: Oral Pathology and Diagnosis. Heinemann Medical Books/Gower Medical Publishing, London, 1987; Figs 11.24 (p 13.16), 11.29 (p. 13.16).

du Vivier A: Atlas of Clinical Dermatology Churchill Livingstone/Gower Medical Publishing, Edinburgh/London, 1986; Figs 11.7 (p. 5.18), 11.8 (p. 5.18), 11.9 (p. 5.18), 11.12 (p. 6.16), 11.14 (p. 7.4), 11.15 (p. 7.5), 11.18 (p. 7.23), 11.19 (p. 7.34), 11.20 (p. 7.34), 11.23 (p. 7.9), 11.28 (p. 7.20), 11.30 (p. 7.22), 11.32 (p. 7.21), 11.33 (p. 7.35), 11.34 (p. 7.36), 11.35 (p. 7.24), 11.36 (p. 7.24), 11.37 (p. 7.15), 11.38 (p. 7.14), 11.39 (p. 7.14), 11.41 (p. 19.8) 11.43 (p.8.11), 11.49 (p. 7.29), 11.50 (p. 7.29), 11.51 (p. 7.30), 11.53 (p. 7.30), 11.54 (p. 7.28), 11.55 (p. 7.28), 11.56 (p. 7.28), 11.59 (p. 1.5), 11.61 (p. 7.32), 11.62 (p. 7.32), 11.63 (p. 7.33), 11.64 (p. 7.32), 11.65 (p. 7.31), 11.66 (p. 7.31), 11.67 (p. 7.30), 11.81 (p. 7.26), 11.82 (p. 7.27), 11.83 P. 7.27), 11.84 (p. 8.2), 11.85 (p. 8.2), 11.86 (p. 8.3), 11.87 (p. 8.8), 11.88 (p. 8.9), 11.89 (p. 8.6), 11.90 (p. 8.6), 11.91 (p. 8.12), 11.92 (p. 8.12), 11.93 (8.7)

Hawke M, Jahn AF: Diseases of the Ear: Clinical and Pathologic Aspects. Lea & Febiger/Gower Medical Publishing, Philadelphia/New York, 1987: Figs 11.1 (p. 1.45), 11.2 (p. 1.45), 11.3 (p. 1.44), 11.6 (p. 1.47), 11.17 (p. 1.47) 11.51 (p. 1.57), 11.95 (p. 1.58), 11.96 (p. 1.59).

Sharvill DE: Skin Diseases (Pocket Picture Guides to Clinical Medicine). Williams and Wilkins/Gower Medical Publishing, Baltimore/New York, 1984; Figs 11.4 (p. 54), 11.21 (p. 52), 11.22 (p. 53), 11.25 (p. 57).

Spalton DJ, Hitchings RA, Hunter PA: Atlas of Clinical Ophthalmology. Lippincott/Gower Medical Publishing, Philadelphia/London, 1984; Figs 11.5 (p. 2.9), 11.26 (p. 2.12), 11.29 (p. 2.13), 11.31 (p. 2.13), 11.40 (p. 2.14), 11.44 (p. 2.14).

Yanoff M, Fine BS: Ocular Pathology. Lippincott/Gower Medical Publishing, Philadelphia/New York, 1988: Figs 11.97 (p. 67), 11.98 (p. 67), 11.99 (p. 68), 11.100 (p. 68).

Zitelli BJ, Davis HW, eds: Atlas of Pediatric Physical Diagnosis. CV Mosby/Gower Medical Publishing, St Louis New York, 1987; Figs 11.6 (p. 8.22), 11.10 (p. 8.22).

Neoplasms of the central nervous system

12

Elizabeth A. Maher, Ann C. McKee

The incidence of primary central nervous system (CNS) cancers (intracranial and spinal axis) varies with age between two and 19 cases in every 100 000 people each year. An early peak in incidence starts at birth and extends to 4 years of age; after age 24, a gradual rise in incidence occurs, leading to a second peak at 50–79 years. In the United States, CNS tumors represent approximately 1% of all cancers and 2.5% of cancer deaths annually. Males are affected more often than females, in a ratio approaching 3 : 2. In children, CNS tumors are the most common solid neoplasms and are the second leading cause of cancer death in patients younger than 15 years of age.

The World Health Organization classification of primary brain tumors (Kleinues and Cavenee, 2000) is presented in Figure 12.1. All but the least common primary and secondary neoplasms of the CNS are reviewed in this chapter. Glioblastomas constitute 30% of all intracranial brain tumors, astrocytomas 20%, meningiomas 18% and other tumors, including ependymomas, oligodendrogliomas and medulloblastomas, 9%. Spinal cord neoplasms account for less than 15% of CNS tumors and 10% of these represent spinal metastases from a primary intracranial tumor. Of all primary tumors of the spinal cord, schwannomas and meningiomas each account for 30%, ependymomas 13%, sarcomas 12%, astrocytomas 7% and chrodomas 4%. The distribution of CNS tumors varies with age: 90% of adult brain tumors are supratentorial, whereas 70% of childhood brain tumors arise in the posterior fossa. The distribution and differential diagnoses of CNS tumors are given in Figure 12.2 and Table 12.1. Pituitary tumors, which represent between 5% and 15% of all brain tumors, are discussed in Chapter 7.

The biologic potential of CNS neoplasms depends largely on three factors: (1) the histology and degree of malignancy (grade) of the tumor; (2) the anatomic compartments involved (cerebral hemisphere, basal ganglia, posterior fossa, brainstem, third ventricle, visual system, spinal cord, etc.); and (3) the spatial delimitation of the tumor (e.g. diffuse, circumscribed, multifocal). CNS tumors of low histologic grade may have as poor a prognosis as high-grade malignancies if they are considered surgically unresectable – because they exhibit a diffusely infiltrating growth pattern, because they involve a critical anatomic structure or because they are technically unapproachable by surgery.

There has been an increase in the incidence of primary malignant brain tumors over the past 25 years with rates increasing at approximately 1.2% per year, particularly among the elderly. This increase does not appear to be related to an increase in lifespan over this same period of analysis. Although there have been significant improvements in diagnostic capabilities over the past 29 years, there is growing concern that the increase in incidence reflects exposure to an unrecognized, environmental toxin. The only known environmental risk for malignant brain tumors is radiation to the brain in childhood, usually as part of treatment for leukemia or fungal infection of the scalp. Large epidemiological studies have not identified absolute environmental risks but there have been trends toward increased risks from vinyl chloride, pesticides or fungicides, chemicals used in the rubber industry and electronic and electrical equipment. Despite the recent heightened concern that the low-level radiation associated with cellular telephone use poses an increased risk for the development of brain tumors, recent epidemiological data argue against such a risk.

There are well-recognized associations between malignant brain tumors and familial syndromes of germline mutations although these account for only a small proportion of total cases. Patients with Li–Fraumeni syndrome carry a germline mutation in p53 and develop a variety of tumors, including those of bone, breast, blood, adrenal cortex and brain. The majority of brain tumors are gliomas, predominantly low grade and occasional glioblastomas. Less common familial syndromes include neurofibromatosis type I (NFI), linked to a gene on chromosome 17, which is associated with nerve sheath tumors, astrocytomas and meningiomas in 5–10% of patients. Patients with neurofibromatosis type II (NFII) carry a genetic mutation on chromosome 22 which predisposes to schwannomas and meningiomas of the cranial nerves and spinal nerve roots, as well as astrocytomas in rare cases (Louis *et al.*, 1995). Tuberous sclerosis, associated with two distinct inherited loci, 9q34 (TSC1) and 16p13 (TSC2), predisposes to subependymal giant cell astrocytomas, subcortical glioneuronal hamartomas in addition to a wide variety of non-CNS tumors. Turcot's syndrome, familial intestinal polyposis, results from a mutation of 5q21 (APC) and predisposes to medulloblastoma. Other patients with this syndrome have lesions in 3p21 (hMLH1) or 7p22 (hPSM2), both associated with glioblastoma at low frequency. Medulloblastoma is also associated with Gorlin's syndrome, resulting from a mutation of 9q31 (PTCH). In some instances, primary brain neoplasms constitute an essential feature of the familial syndrome, as for example cerebellar hemangioblastoma in von Hippel–Lindau syndrome which results from a lesion in the VHL gene (3p25).

Sporadic mutations appear to play a major role in the genesis and maintenance of brain tumors although how the genetic pathways govern the biological behavior of the tumors is largely unknown. The data are perhaps strongest for gliomas where mutations in cell cycle control and receptor tyrosine kinase pathways are common (see below).

Primary and metastatic CNS neoplasms primary tumors

Tumors of neuroepithelial tissue

Astrocytic Tumors
Diffuse astrocytoma
    Variants: Fibrillary
                Protoplasmic
                Gemistocytic
Anaplastic astrocytoma
Glioblastoma
    Variants: Giant cell glioblastoma
                Gliosarcoma
Pilocytic astrocytoma
Pleomorphic xanthoastrocytome
Subependymal giant cell astrocytoma

Oligodendroglial Tumors
Oligodendroglioma
Anaplastic oligodendroglioma

Ependymal Tumors
Ependymoma
    Variants: Cellular
                Papillary
                Clear cell
                Tanycytic
Anaplastic ependymoma
Myxopapillary ependymoma
Subependymoma

Mixed gliomas
Oligo-astrocytoma
Anaplastic oligoastrocytoma

Choroid plexus tumors
Choroid plexus papilloma
Choroid plexus carcinoma

Glial tumors of uncertain origin
Astroblastoma
Choroid glioma of 3rd ventricle
Gliomatosis cerebri

Neuronal and mixed neuronal-glial tumors
Gangliocytoma
Ganglioglioma
Anaplastic ganglioglioma
Central neurocytoma
Dysplastic gangliocytoma of cerebellum
    (Lhermitte-Duclos)
Desmoplastic infantile ganglioglioma/astrocytoma
Dysembryoplastic neuroepithelial tumor
Paraganglioma of the filum terminale

Neuroblastic tumors
Olfactory neuroblastoma (Aesthesioneuroblastoma)
Olfactory neuroepithelioma
Neuroblastomas of adrenal gland and sympathetic
    nervous system

Pineal parenchymal tumors
Pineocytoma
Pineoblastoma
Pineal parenchymal tumor of intermediate
    differentiation

Embryonal tumors
Medulloepithelioma
    Variants: Neuroblastoma
                Ganglioneuroblastoma
Ependymoblastoma
Primitive neuroectodermal tumors (PNETs)
Medulloblastoma
    Variants: Medullomyoblastoma and
                Melanotic medulloblastoma
                Large cell medulloblastoma
Desmoplastic medulloblastoma

Tumors of cranial and spinal nerves

Schwannoma (Neurilemmoma, Neurinoma)
Neurofibroma
    Plexiform
Perineuroma
    Intra neural perineuroma
    Soft tissue perinuroma

Malignant peripheral nerve sheath tumor (MPSNT)
(Neurogenic sarcoma,
Anaplastic neurofibroma, 'Malignant schwannoma')
    Variants: Epithelioid MPSNT with divergent
                mesenchymal and/or epithelial
                differentiation
                Melanotic
                Melanotic psamamatuos

Tumors of the meninges

Tumors of meningothelial cells
Meningioma
    Variants: Meningothelial
                Fibrous (fibroblastic)
                Transitional
                Psammomatous
                Angiomatous
                Microcystic
                Secretory
                Clear cell
                Choroid
                Lymphoplasmacyte-rich
                Metaplastic
                Atypical meningioma
                Papillary meningioma
                Anaplastic meningioma
                Rhaboid

Mesenchymal, non-menigothelial tumors
Benign neoplasms
Osteocartilagenous tumors
Lipoma
Fibrous histiocytoma
Others

Malignant neoplasms
Hemangiopericytoma
Chondrosarcoma
    Variant: Mesenchymal chondrosarcoma
Malignant fibrous histiocytoma
Rhabomyosarcoma
Meningeal sarcomatosis
Others

Primary melanocytic lesions
Diffuse melanocytosis
Melanocytoma
Malignant melanoma
Meningeal melanomatosis

Tumors of uncertain histogenesis
Hemangioblastoma (Capillary hemangioblastoma)

Lymphomas and hemopoetic neoplasms

Malignant Lymphomas
Plasmacytoma
Granulocytic sarcoma

Germ cell tumors

Germinoma
Embryonal Carcinoma
Yolk sac tumor (Endodermal Sinus tumor)
Choriocarcinoma
Teratoma
    Variants: Immature
                Mature
                Teratoma with malignant
                    transformation
Mixed germ cell tumors

Cysts and tumor-like lesions

Rathke cleft cyst
Epidermoid cyst
Dermoid cyst
Colloid cyst of the third ventricle
Enterogenous cyst
Neuroglial cyst
Granular cell tumor (Choristoma, Pituicytoma)
Hypothalamic neuronal hamartoma
Nasal glial heterotopia
Plasma cell granuloma

Tumors of the sellar region

Pituitary Adenoma
Pituitary Carcinoma
Craniopharyngioma
    Variants: Adamantinomatous
                Papillary

Local extensions from regional tumors

Paraganglioma
Chordoma
Chondroma
Chondrosarcoma
Carcinoma

Unclassified tumors
Metastatic tumors

To Skull and Vertebral Column:
Carcinomas: Lung
            Breast
            Kidney
            Skin (malignant melanoma)
            Thyroid
            Nasopharynx and Nasal Sinuses
            Prostate
Neuroblastoma (children)
Multiple myeloma
Sarcomas
Lymphoma

To Meninges:
Lymphoma
Leukemias
Carcinomas of the: Breast
                    Lung
                    Stomach
                    Other
Malignant melanoma

To Brain and Spinal Cord:
Carcinomas of the: Lung (35%)
                    Breast (20%)
                    Skin (melanoma) (10%)
                    Kidney (renal cell carcinoma) (10%)
                    Gastrointestinal tract (5%)
                    Thyroid
                    Choriocarcinoma
             Rarely: Prostate
                    Ovary
                    Bladder
                    Thymus
Sarcomas (rare)

Partially adapted from Kleihues & Cavenee (2000) and Burger et al. (1991).

Fig. 12.1 Primary and metastatic neoplasms of the central nervous system.

Table 12.1 Distribution and differential diagnosis of tumors of the central nervous system.

Region	Adult tumors		Childhood and adolescent tumors	
Cerebral hemisphere	Astrocytoma Anaplastic astrocytoma Glioblastoma Meningioma	Metastatic carcinoma Oligodendroglioma Ependymoma Lymphoma Sarcoma	Astrocytoma Anaplastic astrocytoma Ependymoma	Oligodendroglioma Embryonal tumor Ganglion cell tumor
Lateral ventricle	Ependymoma Meningioma Subependymoma	Choroid plexus papilloma	Ependymoma Choroid plexus	Subependymal giant cell atrocytoma papilloma
Third ventricle	Colloid cyst	Ependymoma	Ependymoma	Choroid plexus papilloma
Peri-third ventricular region	Astrocytoma Anaplastic astrocytoma	Oligodrendroglioma Ependymoma Pilocytic Glioblastoma	Pilocytic astrocytoma Astrocytoma	
Pineal region	Germ cell tumor Pineal parenchymal tumor	Glioma	Germ cell tumor	Pineal parenchymal tumor
Optic chiasm and nerve	Meningioma	Astrocytoma	Astrocytoma	
Pituitary and sellar region	Pituitary adenoma Craniopharyngioma	Meningioma Germ cell neoplasms	Craniopharyngioma Germ cell neoplasms	Pitultary adenoma
Corpus callosum	Astrocytoma Anaplastic astrocytoma	Glioblastoma Oligodendroglioma Lipoma	Astrocytoma Anaplastic astrocytoma	Oligodendroglioma Lipoma
Brainstem	Astrocytoma Anaplastic astrocytoma	Glioblastoma	Astrocytoma Anaplastic astrocytoma	Glioblastoma
Cerebellopontine angle	Schwannoma Meningioma Epidermoid cyst	Choroid plexus papilloma	Ependymoma	
Cerebellum	Hemangioblastoma Metastatic carcinomas	Astrocytoma Medulloblastoma	Medulloblastoma	Dermoid cyst Astrocytoma
Fourth ventricle	Ependymoma Subependymoma	Choroid plexus papilloma	Ependymoma	Choroid plexus papilloma
Region of foramen magnum	Meningioma	Schwannoma		
Spinal region	Ependymoma Astrocytoma Hemangioblastoma Meningioma	Schwannoma Neurofibroma Paraganglioma	Ependymoma	Astrocytoma

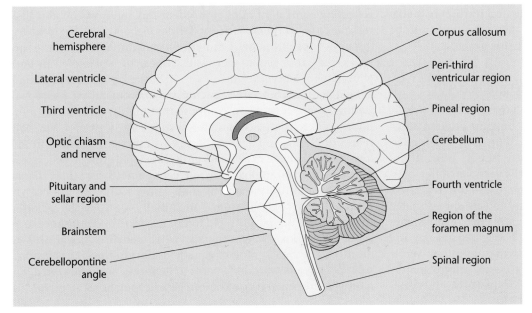

Fig. 12.2 Distribution and differential diagnosis of tumors of the CNS.

PRIMARY NEOPLASMS OF THE CENTRAL NERVOUS SYSTEM

TUMORS OF NEUROEPITHELIAL TISSUE

In the adult, over 60% of all primary central nervous system tumors are gliomas. In children, gliomas constitute 80–90% of all CNS neoplasms. Gliomas have been defined pathologically as tumors that display histological, immunohistochemical and ultrastructural evidence of glial differentiation. They are classified according to their differentiation lineage, i.e. astrocytic, oligodendroglial or ependymal cells, and further subdivided by tumor grade (Kleihues and Cavenee, 2000) as discussed below.

ASTROCYTIC TUMORS

Astrocytoma

Astrocytomas range in incidence from 5–7 new cases per 100 000 per year and are predominantly diffusely infiltrating tumors. Although they can arise anywhere in the CNS, they preferentially develop in the cerebral hemispheres. Three histologic types are recognized: fibrillary, gemistocytic and protoplasmic. Of these, fibrillary astrocytoma is by far the most common and protoplasmic astrocytoma the most unusual. Astrocytomas are graded on a scale of I–IV according to their degree of malignancy as judged by various histological features (see below). Unlike other solid tumors, gliomas do not metastasize outside the CNS and thus tumor grade is the primary determinant of clinical outcome. Grade I tumors are biologically benign and can be surgically cured if deemed resectable at the time of diagnosis; grade II tumors are low-grade malignancies which may follow long clinical courses but are not curable by surgery; grade III tumors are malignant and lead to death within a few years; grade IV tumors are highly malignant, usually recalcitrant to chemotherapy, and lethal within 9–12 months. Seventy percent of grade II gliomas transform into grade III and IV tumors within 5–10 years of diagnosis and then behave clinically like the higher-grade tumors.

The diffuse gliomas are classified histologically as astrocytomas, oligodendrogliomas or tumors with morphological features of both astrocytes and oligodendrocytes, termed oligoastrocytomas. Astrocytic tumors are subsequently graded as pilocytic astrocytoma, grade I; astrocytoma, grade II; anaplastic astrocytoma, grade III; and glioblastoma, grade IV. Oligodendrogliomas and oligoastrocytomas are subsequently graded as grade II or anaplastic, grade III. Such grading is related to the presence of histological features of malignancy, such as high cellularity, cellular pleomorphism, mitotic activity, microvascular proliferation and necrosis (Fig. 12.3).

Diffuse, low-grade astrocytoma (WHO grade II/IV)

The clinical hallmarks of low-grade astrocytomas are low mitotic rate, ability to migrate long distances away from the original site of tumor development and high propensity to progress to a higher-grade tumor after a long latency. These are tumors primarily of young adults, with peak age of incidence at 34 years, and often present initially with seizures. The tumor cells are well differentiated, exhibit robust glial marker immunoreactivity and are not associated with neovascularization or cellular necrosis. MRI often demonstrates a diffuse large mass that is hypointense on T1-weighted imaging and does not enhance following administration of gadolinium. While the reported median survival approaches 10 years, approximately 70% of patients transform to high-grade astrocytomas within 5 years

of initial diagnosis (see Figs 12.5a and b), the remaining 30% die of infiltrating low-grade tumor. Treatment is primarily surgical although radiation therapy is utilized as soon as there is any evidence of tumor progression. Mutational analysis of these tumors has identified two common genetic lesions: p53 loss-of-function mutations (Chung et al., 1991; von Deimling et al., 1992) and PDGF ligand and receptor overexpression (Heldin and Westermark, 1990; Claesson-Welsh, 1994). The molecular genetics governing the transition to high-grade astrocytoma have not been identified.

Anaplastic astrocytoma (WHO grade III/IV)

Anaplastic astrocytomas, also referred to as intermediate-grade astrocytomas, may arise *de novo* or develop from low-grade lesions. They are characterized primarily by a dramatic increase in mitotic rate over that seen in low-grade lesions without induction of neovascularization. MRI demonstrates enhancement of tumor following administration of gadolinium (Fig. 12.8). The median age at diagnosis is 41 years, patients presenting with symptoms similar to those described above for patients with low-grade astrocytomas. Survival is significantly shorter than for low-grade astrocytomas, ranging from 2 to 3 years. Treatment consists of surgery, external beam radiation and chemotherapy. Standard chemotherapy consists of the three-drug combination procarbazine, CCNU and vincristine. Genetic mutations associated with anaplastic astrocytomas include allelic losses on chromosomes 9p, 13q and, less frequently, by 12q amplification. Notably, these mutations are mutually exclusive events Ueki et al., 1996) and are now known to be key components of the retinoblastoma pathway governing cell cycle progression.

Glioblastoma multiforme (WHO grade IV/IV)

Two glioblastoma subtypes have been identified clinically (Kleihues and Cavenee, 2000) (Fig. 12.11). 'Primary glioblastoma' typically presents in older patients as an aggressive, highly invasive tumor, usually without any evidence of prior clinical disease. 'Secondary glioblastoma' has a very different clinical history. It is usually observed in younger patients who initially present with a low-grade astrocytoma that transforms into glioblastoma within 5–10 years of the initial diagnosis, regardless of prior therapy. There are striking similarities between these clinical subtypes. First, primary and secondary glioblastomas behave in a clinically indistinguishable fashion. The median survival from the time that glioblastoma is established does not statistically differ between these two subtypes, reflecting equivalent rates of proliferation and invasion as well as resistance to all therapeutic modalities. Second, although the frequency of specific genetic mutations may differ between the subtypes, the same genetic pathways appear to be targeted in both glioblastoma subtypes. Third, once established, primary and secondary glioblastoma both show microvascular proliferation, pseudopalisading necrosis and are composed of highly infiltrative, more poorly differentiated cells than low-grade astrocytomas. The hallmarks of glioblastoma, regardless of whether it originated from a low-grade glioma or as a *de novo* entity, are rapid growth, widespread invasion, marked angiogenesis and cellular necrosis. MRI is characterized by a diffuse enhancing mass, often with areas of necrosis. Although 95% of glioblastomas are initially controlled by radiation therapy, there is typically rapid tumor regrowth and resistance to all types of cytotoxic chemotherapy with median survival of 9–12 months. The cataloguing of genetic lesions in these glioblastoma subtypes has identified differences in their genetic profiles, predominantly in the penetrance of various genetic mutations. However, loss of the tumor suppressor genes, PTEN and IN4a/ARF, is prominent and often accompanied by activation of overexpression of the epidermal growth factor receptor (EGFR). While PTEN and INK4a/ARF mutations can be found in anaplastic astrocytomas, overexpression of EGFR occurs almost exclusively in glioblastoma, suggesting that this is a key pathway in the transition to glioblastoma and may be involved in mediating the aggressive biological phenotype.

Gliosarcoma

Gliosarcoma is a variant of glioblastoma characterized by the presence of both glial and sarcomatous elements. The origins of this tumor are unknown although it has been speculated that it represents malignant transformation of a neural stem cell or glial progenitor which retained the ability to differentiate into both glial and mesenchymal lineages. Gliosarcomas carry the same prognosis as glioblastomas and the general approach to treatment is the same as that described above for glioblastoma.

Pilocytic astrocytoma (WHO grade I/IV)

These tumors of childhood and adolescence differ from the diffuse astrocytomas previously discussed in that they are relatively well circumscribed and of low grade with little potential for malignant transformation. They are uncommon in the cerebral hemispheres and exhibit geographic preferences for the region of the third ventricle, optic chiasm and thalamus. Surgical resection is associated with long-term survival. Pilocytic astrocytomas are not associated with p53 mutations, suggesting a different genetic basis for these low-grade tumors.

Pleomorphic xanthoastrocytoma

These rare tumors occur most often in the temporal or parietal lobe of young people (third or fourth decade) with a history of epilepsy. Usually there is prominent leptomeningeal involvement; underlying cyst formation with mural nodules is also typical. These tumors are typically densely cellular and cytologically pleomorphic. However, mitoses are rare and necrosis is absent. The tumor is notable because it has a favorable prognosis yet bears superficial resemblance to a giant cell glioblastoma or malignant fibrous histiocytoma. Some tumors may eventually develop malignant transformation.

Subependymal giant cell astrocytoma

Although characteristically associated with tuberous sclerosis, subependymal giant cell astrocytoma occasionally occurs in the absence of the disease. It usually arises from the wall of the lateral ventricle and presents as an intraventricular mass obstructing the foramen of Monro. The clinical signs are commonly those of obstructive hydrocephalus. Subependymal astrocytomas are low-grade tumors, with essentially no tendency for malignant transformation.

Astrocytoma: sites of preference

OPTIC NERVE AND CHIASMAL ASTROCYTOMA Representing 1% of intracranial neoplasms in adults and 5% of intracranial tumors in children less than 10 years old, optic nerve and chiasmal astrocytomas most commonly (approximately 70%) arise in the first decade. The most frequent symptom is visual loss, which may be pronounced. Bilateral optic astrocytomas may arise in association with von Recklinghausen's neurofibromatosis, more often affecting the chiasm than the optic nerves. Although malignant transformation is rare, it occurs more frequently in adults with chiasmal lesions. Treatment is surgical; however, 20% of optic nerve tumors and 33% of optic chiasm tumors recur. The 20-year survival rate for optic nerve astrocytomas is 85%, as compared with 50% for optic chiasm tumors. The tumor grows by local extension and chiasmal tumors frequently extend into the third ventricle or the optic tract. The histology is that of a pilocytic astrocytoma.

ASTROCYTOMA OF THE THIRD VENTRICULAR REGION Both pilocytic astrocytomas and diffuse astrocytomas may be found in this site, most commonly in children. Although such tumors are benign and slow growing, their deep location limits surgical resection. The clinical signs are usually those of obstructive hydrocephalus.

BRAINSTEM ASTROCYTOMA Most commonly occurring in children, this tumor usually presents as a diffuse astrocytoma originating in the pons. As with astrocytomas of the third ventricle, surgical resection is hindered by the deep location and infiltrating character of this tumor. Malignant transformation is frequent and may occur early in the disease course. The clinical signs include symptoms of brainstem dysfunction and cranial nerve palsies. Obstructive hydrocephalus occurs late in the course owing to obstruction of the fourth ventricle. The prognosis depends on tumor grade; 30% of patients with well-differentiated astrocytoma survive for 15 years. Patients with high-grade astrocytomas have a typical survival time of less than 1 year. Occasionally brainstem astrocytomas are of the discrete pilocytic type, which is associated with prolonged survival.

CEREBELLAR ASTROCYTOMA Accounting for 5% of all brain gliomas and 15% of all intracranial tumors of children and adolescents, cerebellar astrocytomas may be either diffuse (15%) or, more commonly, pilocytic (85%). The presenting signs are usually those of cerebellar dysfunction and hydrocephalus owing to obstruction of the fourth ventricle. Surgical resection, even if partial, is associated with long-term survival. Malignant transformation and cerebrospinal dissemination are rare.

SPINAL CORD ASTROCYTOMA Representing approximately 13% of all neoplasms affecting the spinal cord, these tumors commonly appear as fusiform enlargements affecting the thoracic and cervical segments. Diffuse low-grade fibrillary astrocytoma is the usual histologic type, although high-grade astrocytomas may occur. As many as 40% of these tumors are associated with proximal or distal syringomyelia. The prognosis is related to tumor grade. Mean survival time for patients with well-differentiated tumors may be as long as 8 years, whereas with high-grade lesions it may be as short as 6 months. Death is usually the result of intercurrent infection or medullary extension of the tumor.

OLIGODENDROGLIAL TUMORS
Oligodendroglioma

Constituting 4% of all CNS neoplasms and 5–19% of all gliomas, oligodendroglioma is predominantly a tumor of the middle decades, with a peak incidence between 35 and 40 years, although they occasionally arise in younger persons. Considered to be tumors of the white matter, they have geographic predilections based largely on the amount of white matter in a given location. Sites of preference include the frontal, parietal and temporal lobes of the cerebral hemispheres, as well as the thalamus, particularly in the younger age groups. They occur rarely in the spinal cord and extremely rarely in the cerebellum. The clinical evolution may be prolonged and is frequently characterized by a long history of seizures. Calcification in these tumors is common, detectable radiographically in 40% of cases and histologically in 90%. Although previously graded like astrocytomas, the most recent WHO classification no longer recognizes glioblastoma as a grade of oliogodendrogliomas. Thus, these tumors are grade II or maximum III, even when necrosis and neovascularization are present. This change reflects the clear difference in biological behavior of the highest grade tumor when compared to glioblastomas of astrocytic origin. The high-grade oligodendrogliomas are often exquisitely sensitive to the standard glioma treatments, PCV or temozolamide (see response demonstrated in Fig. 12.21 after five cycles of chemotherapy) and median survival is often significantly longer than patients with anaplastic astrocytomas. Genetic analysis of these tumors demonstrates a high incidence of mutations in 1p and 19q. Although the specific genes mutated in these tumors have not yet been identified, they are likely to be involved in conferring the chemosensitivity of these tumors.

MIXED GLIOMA (OLIGOASTROCYTOMA)

Mixed gliomas refer to tumors that clearly demonstrate both malignant oligodendrocytes and astrocytes. Similar to gliosarcoma, the origin of these tumors is unknown although may represent malignant transformation of a neural stem cell or early glial progenitor. The molecular genetics are less clear that for pure oligodendrocytes, some having the characteristic 1p and 19q deletions while most have a genetic profile similar to anaplastic astrocytomas. Treatment is similar to anaplastic astrocytomas although prognosis may vary depending on the genetic profile of the tumor.

EPENDYMAL TUMORS
Ependymoma

Ependymomas represent approximately 3–9% of all neuroepithelial tumors. They are primarily tumors of childhood and adolescence with peak incidence occurring between 10 and 15 years. They represent 6–12% of all intracranial tumors in childhood and a striking 30% in children under 3 years of age. The tumors can occur at any site along the ventricular system and spinal canal but are predominantly found in the fourth ventricle and spinal cord. Embryologically, the ependyma is related to astrocytes and oligodendroglia, a glial heritage that is often expressed when the cells are neoplastically transformed. Characteristically, ependymomas are benign, slow-growing neoplasms; anaplastic transformation may occur, especially focally, but transformation to overt glioblastoma is rare. Due to its predominantly intraventricular location, symptoms are most often secondary to obstruction of CSF flow and resultant hydrocephalus. Tumors of the spinal cord are associated with symptoms related to the site of disease occurrence. The prognosis of ependymoma depends largely on the anatomic site of origin and the histologic grade. Long-term survivals tend to be the exception. Even benign-appearing tumors show a tendency to recur locally and metastasize via the subarachnoid space. Treatment is surgical resection, most often only partial, and radiotherapy.

Myxopapillary ependymoma

These tumors represent a special variant of ependymoma found almost exclusively in the region of the filum terminale, although occasionally they have been found higher in the spinal cord or,

rarely, in the brain. They may occur at any age, but most arise in the fourth decade. Myxopapillary ependymomas characteristically form a sausage-shaped mass in the lumbosacral region, displacing spinal nerve roots of the cauda equina. Their biologic behavior is usually benign, but because of their location they are often associated with significant compression-induced paralysis. Treatment consists of local excision, which must often be only partial because of the tumor's location; approximately 20% recur even after complete initial resection. Metastases infiltrating the CSF and extradural space may occur but transformation to anaplastic variants is extremely rare.

Subependymoma

This slow-growing, benign variant of ependymoma consists of proliferating ependyma and astrocytes. Seventy-five percent of these tumors are infratentorial, arising on ependymal surfaces. They are commonly found along the fourth ventricle, the walls of the lateral ventricles, the septum pellucidum and the cerebellopontine angle. They are often an incidental finding at autopsy, particularly in the middle-aged and elderly. Symptomatic tumors may arise at any age, most commonly in the fourth decade, and exhibit a male predominance. The clinical signs are usually those of hydrocephalus resulting from blockage of CSF flow through the ventricles. Treatment is surgical and the prognosis depends entirely on the tumor's location and resectability.

CHOROID PLEXUS TUMORS
Choroid plexus papilloma

Choroid plexus papillomas occur most frequently in the first decade of life, accounting for 10–20% of intracranial neoplasms in children; they are occasionally congenital. The lateral ventricle and third ventricle are the favored sites in children; the rare adult neoplasm favors the fourth ventricle. Symptoms are usually caused by hydrocephalus, which may result from mechanical obstruction to CSF flow or overproduction of CSF by the tumor. Although they are benign neoplasms and can be cured by surgery, they have a tendency to disseminate widely via the CSF, particularly after surgical intervention.

Choroid plexus carcinoma

This malignant tumor is distinguishable from choroid plexus papilloma on the basis of local brain invasion, a solid pattern of growth and cytologic features of anaplasia, including necrosis and mitoses. Choroid plexus carcinoma almost always occurs in patients under the age of 10, grows more rapidly than choroid plexus papillomas and has a 5-year survival rate of approximately 40%. In older individuals, it should be distinguished from the much more common metastatic papillary adenocarcinoma.

NEUROEPITHELIAL TUMORS OF UNCERTAIN ORIGIN
Gliomatosis cerebri

This extreme form of diffuse astrocytoma in adults is characterized by widely infiltrating anaplastic glia, although the cell of origin is unknown. It typically presents in the second or third decade and diffusely enlarges the cerebral hemispheres, brainstem and/or cerebellum. There is often expansion of compact fiber pathways, such as the optic nerves, corpus callosum, fornices or cerebral peduncles. Its distinct clinical behavior is likely related to the overall very poor prognosis.

NEURONAL AND MIXED NEURONAL – GLIAL TUMORS
Gangliocytoma and ganglioglioma

Gangliogliomas are distinguished from gangliocytomas (ganglioneuromas) by the presence of glial elements in gangliogliomas. Both tumors show a geographic predilection for the temporal lobes in children and young adults and thus seizures are the most common presenting symptoms. However, these tumors occur in all brain regions, including the frontal lobes, third ventricle and hypothalamus. They carry an excellent prognosis following surgical resection although transformation of the glial elements in gangliogliomas can occur which then carry a less favorable prognosis.

Central neurocytoma

The central neurocytoma is a tumor of young adults typically, in whom a discrete, often partially calcified mass intrudes into the lateral ventricle near the foramen of Monro. Symptoms are often related to increased intracranial pressure rather than focal neurological deficits. Surgery may be curative if complete resection is achieved.

Paraganglioma

Paragangliomas are tumors derived from neural crest cells, the most common type of which is the pheochromocytoma. The designation also includes tumors of the carotid body, glomus jugulare, glomus tympanicum, filum terminale, vagus nerve, orbit and duodenum. Certain of these tumors show a predilection for middle-aged women, such as the jugulotympanic paraganglioma, which usually arises from the lateral portion of the temporal bone, and the vagal body paraganglioma, which often presents as a mass in the neck or at the skull base beneath the jugular foramen. Clinically, these tumors manifest with signs of cranial nerve palsies. In the case of paragangliomas involving the cauda equina, which tend to be sausage-shaped intradural tumors, symptoms include lower back pain, sensorimotor deficits and incontinence. Carotid body tumors present as painless masses of the skull base where they may produce cranial nerve palsies, a palpable thrill and an audible bruit. The incidence of carotid body tumors is markedly increased in regions of high altitude, possibly as a result of hypoxia-induced hyperplasia. An autosomal dominant pattern of inheritance for these tumors has been recognized and familial tumors may be bilateral. Most paragangliomas are benign and carry a favorable postoperative prognosis, although recurrences are not uncommon. Approximately 5% of these tumors are malignant and may invade tissue locally or metastasize to lymph nodes, lung or bone marrow.

Olfactory neuroblastoma (esthesioneuroblastoma)

This rare neoplasm arises high in the nasal cavity from neurosensory receptor cells or basilar cells in the olfactory mucosa. The age distribution is bimodal, one peak occurring in adolescence and young adulthood, the second peak occurring in late middle age. Olfactory neuroblastomas are slow growing but aggressive, locally invasive tumors that may invade nasal sinuses, nasopharynx, palate, orbit, cribiform plate and brain. Metastases to the CSF, lymph nodes and viscera may occur. There appear to be several types of esthesioneuroblastoma, one with classic features of neuroblastoma, the type most likely to occur in young patients, the other with characteristics of neuroendocrine carcinoma, more common in older patients. The importance of initial gross total surgical excision has been emphasized. As the tumor is highly radiosensitive, radiotherapy is often indicated. The 10-year survival rate has been reported as 77% for patients with neuroendocrine carcinoma and 67% for those with neuroblastoma.

PINEAL PARENCHYMAL TUMORS
Pineocytoma and pineoblastoma

These uncommon tumors, derived from pineal parenchymal cells, are divided into two types: the pineocytoma, originating from mature cells, and the pineoblastoma, derived from more primitive pineal cells. Pineocytoma, which may occur at any age, is typically well circumscribed, slow growing and non-invasive and it rarely metastasizes via the CSF. Its highly malignant anaplastic counterpart, the pineoblastoma, occurs primarily in children and frequently metastasizes via the CSF. Because pineocytomas tend to be less radiosensitive than pineoblastomas, their treatment usually includes surgical resection. Mean survival time is approximately 5 years for pineocytoma, whereas it is less than 2 years for pineoblastoma.

EMBRYONAL TUMORS
Medulloepithelioma

Believed to arise from the primitive medullary plate and neural tube, these rare, highly malignant tumors occur early in life, most frequently between the ages of 6 months and 5 years. The preferred geographic location is periventricular in the cerebral hemispheres; tumors are often deeply situated and lie near the midline. These tumors can also arise in the cauda equina, presacral area, outside the CNS along nerve trunks and in the eye. Radical surgical removal, followed by extensive neuraxial radiation, is the treatment of choice, given the highly primitive and malignant character of these tumors. Mortality is high and extracranial metastases may occur.

Neuroblastoma (cerebral)

Derived from ganglion cell precursors, central neuroblastomas are rare tumors, occurring most frequently in children in the first decade of life. They are frequently situated deep in the cerebrum, forming a well-defined mass. Approximately 50% disseminate via CSF pathways and distant metastases may occur. Treatment consists of radical surgical excision followed by radiation, as the primitive character of these lesions suggests some degree of sensitivity to radiotherapy. The 5-year postoperative survival rate is approximately 30%.

Ependymoblastoma

Although their histologic designation is somewhat controversial, ependymoblastomas are distinguished from ependymomas by their highly malignant biologic behavior and the frequency of focal microscopic invasion and leptomeningeal involvement. They are rare tumors affecting predominantly the cerebral hemispheres of neonates and young children. They are generally large and supratentorial, closely approximated to the ventricles. They have a propensity for CSF seeding, rapid local growth and extraneural and extracranial metastases.

PRIMITIVE NEUROECTODERMAL TUMORS (PNET)
Medulloblastoma

These embryonic cerebellar tumors are believed to originate from remnants of the fetal external granular cell layer of the cerebellum. Overall, they account for less than 0.5% of intracranial PNET, but in children they represent 25% of intracranial tumors. Most arise in patients younger than 25 years of age, although occasionally they occur as late as the fifth decade, and have a male predominance (65%).

Medulloblastomas arise in the cerebellum, particularly favoring the midline in early life, whereas later cases tend to arise in the lateral hemispheres. The clinical signs are usually those of cerebellar dysfunction and increased intracranial pressure owing to obstruction of the fourth ventricle. Medulloblastomas frequently infiltrate the subarachnoid space early and extensively and metastasize widely via CSF pathways. Systemic metastases to bone and lymph nodes may occur, although the lung characteristically remains free of metastatic deposits. As these tumors are extremely radiosensitive, the treatment of choice is radiotherapy of the entire neuraxis, usually in combination with surgical extirpation. The 5-year survival rate ranges from 40% to 80%. Variants of medulloblastoma include medullomyoblastoma, containing myoblasts or myocytes, and melanotic medulloblastoma containing melanosomes and premelanosomes.

Grade I/IV:

Pilocytic astrocytoma

Elongated, bipolar astrocytes
Rosenthal fibers

Grade II/IV:

Well-differentiated, low grade astrocytoma

Mild hypercellularity
One histologic criterion:
    nuclear atypia
No mitoses
No vascular proliferation
No necrosis

Grade III/IV:

Anaplastic astrocytoma

Increased cellularity
Two histologic criteria:
    usually nuclear atypia and
    mitotic activity

Grade IV/IV:

Glioblastoma multiforme

Densely cellular tumor with at least three criteria:
    nuclear atypia
    endothelial proliferation and/or
    necrosis

Fig. 12.3 Histologic grading of astrocytomas.

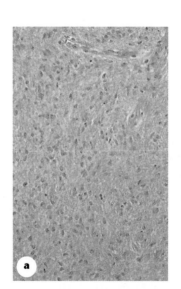
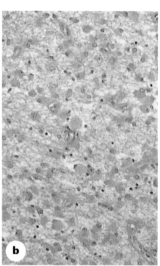
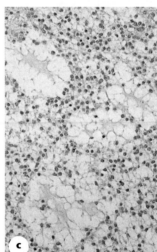

Fig. 12.4 Diffuse astrocytoma. The three common types of diffuse astrocytoma are: (**a**) fibrillary, composed of tightly interlacing bundles of small, spindle-shaped cells amid a predominantly fibrillar matrix; (**b**) gemistocytic, containing plump cells with distinct, round, pink cytoplasm arranged on a more delicately interlacing fibrillar matrix; and (**c**) protoplasmic, composed of small, round, regular cells with indistinct cytoplasmic boundaries arranged on a loosely fibrillar stroma.

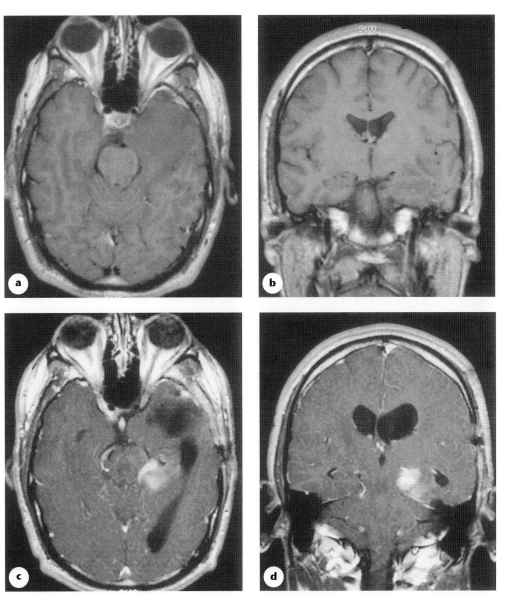

Fig. 12.5 Diffuse low-grade astrocytoma. (**a**) Axial T1-weighted MR image after gadolinium administration. A large left temporal tumor is present (arrows) without any abnormal enhancement. The tumor is evident through its obliteration of normal sulci and gyri. (**b**) Coronal T1-weighted MR image after gadolinium enhancement. The tumor is slightly heterogeneous signal (arrows) but shows no abnormal enhancement. It extends into the deep temporal structures. (**c**) Axial T1-weighted MR image after gadolinium enhancement. Recurrent tumor is seen in the deep temporal region abutting the brainstem (arrows). The temporal and occipital horns of the left lateral ventrical (v) are dilated due to *ex vacuuo* changes related to intervening treatment. (**d**) Coronal T1-weighted MR image after gadolinium administration. Enhancing tumor extends into the deep temporal structures just above the tentorium (arrows). Dilatation of the left lateral ventricle (v) is present.

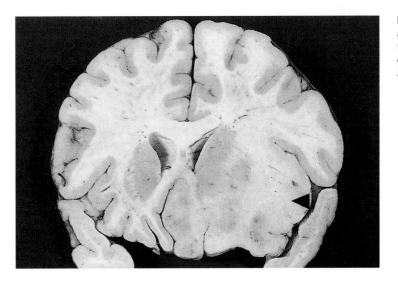

Fig. 12.6 Diffuse, low-grade astrocytoma (grade II/IV). Coronal section shows a tumor diffusely infiltrating the right frontal lobe. Gross determination of the tumor's boundaries is almost impossible, but the tumor is evident as an ill-defined area of enlargement (arrow), with loss of distinction between the gray and white matter.

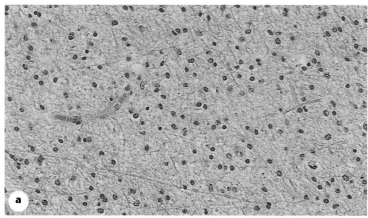 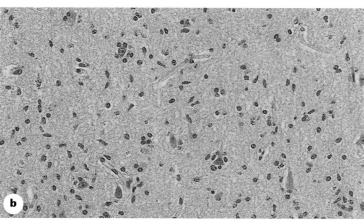

Fig. 12.7 Diffuse, low-grade astrocytoma (grade II/IV). In the (**a**) white and (**b**) gray matter, there is a subtle infiltration of astrocytes with only slightly irregular features. In the gray matter, the neoplastic astrocytes cluster around neurons. This feature, termed satellitosis, is not seen in reactive astrocytes.

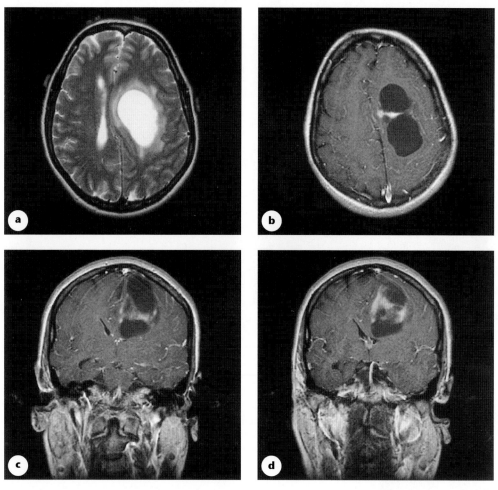

Fig. 12.8 Anaplastic astrocytoma (grade III/IV). (**a**) Axial T2-weighted image at the level of the upper portion of the lateral ventricles. A large cystic tumor (C) is present on the left with relatively little surrounding edema (white arrows). The tumor shifts the midline to the right (black arrow). (**b**) Axial T1-weighted image after gadolinium administration at a level just above the lateral ventricles. Two adjacent cystic components are present (C) along with some nodular enhancing solid tumor (arrow). (**c**) Coronal T1-weighted image after gadolinium administration. A focal linear area of enhancing tumor is present between adjacent cystic components (arrows). (**d**) Coronal T1-weighted MR image after gadolinium administration just posterior to the level shown in (c). Solid tumor is again seen (white arrows) adjacent to cystic components. The tumor compresses and displaces the left lateral ventricle downward (black arrow).

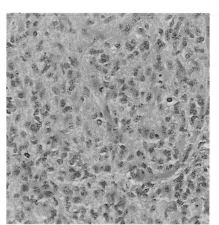

Fig. 12.9 Anaplastic astrocytoma (grade III/IV). Microscopy reveals a densely cellular tumor with a high degree of cellular pleomorphism and increased mitotic activity. This tumor is distinguished from glioblastoma multiforme by the conspicuous absence of two other criteria of malignancy: necrosis and endothelial proliferation. However, its high cellularity and pleomorphism raise suspicion that a larger sample size might have included areas exhibiting features of greater malignancy.

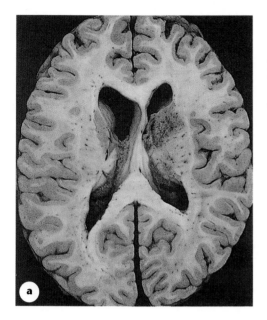

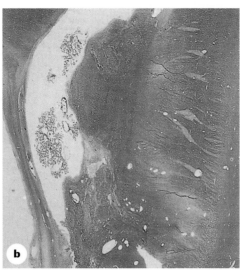

Fig. 12.10 Anaplastic astrocytoma (grade III/IV). (**a**) Arising in the right basal ganglia, this tumor has caused enlargement of the caudate nucleus with hemorrhage, disruption of the ventricular ependyma and extension into the ventricular space. (**b**) These features are further emphasized in this histologic section taken from the involved area. Note the high cellularity of the tumor.

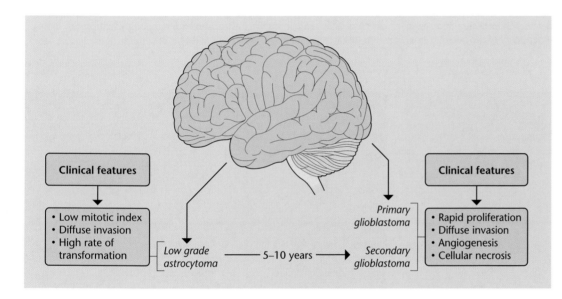

Fig. 12.11 Two pathways to glioblastoma. Glioblastoma can develop over 5–10 years from a low-grade astrocytoma (secondary glioblastoma) or it can be the initial pathology at diagnosis (primary glioblastoma). The clinical features of glioblastoma are the same regardless of clinical route. (Reproduced with permission from *Genes and Development* 2001.)

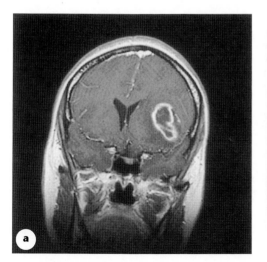

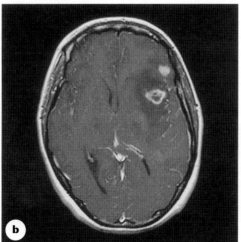

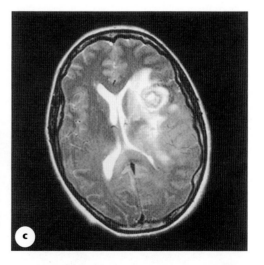

Fig. 12.12 Glioblastoma multiforme (grade IV/IV). (**a**) Coronal T1-weighted MR image after gadolinium administration. An irregular mass is present in the left frontal region with central necrosis (n) and surrounding rim of abnormal enhancement. The mass compresses and displaces the left lateral ventricle (arrow). (**b**) Axial T1-weighted MR image after gadolinium administration. The mass is seen in the left frontal region with a solid nodular component (arrow) as well as a larger necrotic mass. (**c**) Axial T2-weighted MR image. The rounded tumor mass in the left frontal region is seen (arrows) with extensive surrounding vasogenic edema extending along white matter tracts.

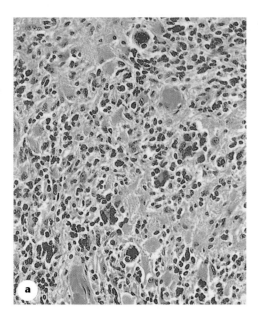
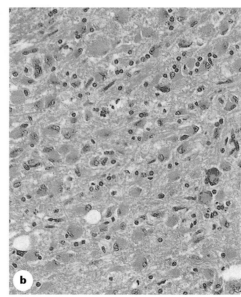
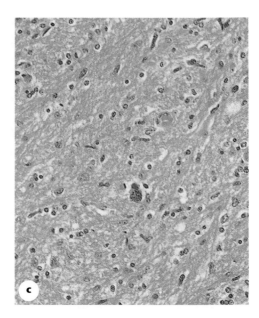

Fig. 12.13 Glioblastoma (grade IV/IV). Variations in tumor sampling may dramatically bias the histologic determination of tumor grade. (**a**) The center of the tumor is densely populated with highly pleomorphic neoplastic cells, including giant cells, gemistocytic astrocytes and small anaplastic cells. Also typical are mitotic activity, proliferation of blood vessel endothelium and zones of necrosis. The cell nuclei tend to line up at the periphery of the necrotic area, a feature termed 'pseudopalisading'. A biopsy from this area would result in the diagnosis of glioblastoma multiforme. (**b**) Other areas are characterized by gemistocytic astrocytes only. Sampling from this area would be interpreted as gemistocytic astrocytoma, grade II. (**c**) At the periphery of the tumor, there is only a mild increase in fibrillary astrocytes with rare, bizarre astrocytes. Biopsy from this area would also yield a diagnosis of astrocytoma, grade II.

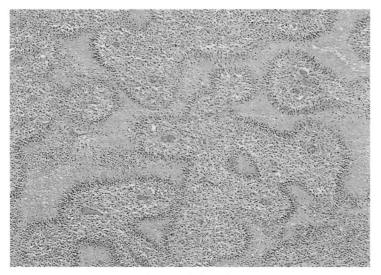

Fig. 12.14 Glioblastoma multiforme. Pseudopalisading around areas of necrosis may be a dominant feature. Zones of necrosis appear as serpiginous, cell-free, pink areas.

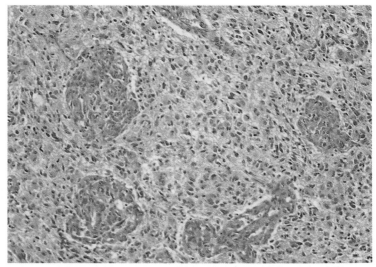

Fig. 12.15 Glioblastoma multiforme. Endothelial proliferation may reach dramatic proportions with the formation of tangled clusters of neovascular channels, occasionally referred to as 'glomeruloid' blood vessels because of their resemblance to renal glomeruli.

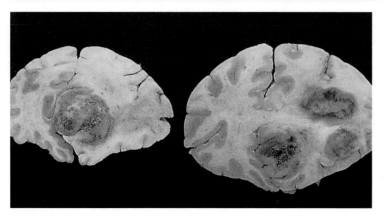

Fig. 12.16 Astrocytoma. Multifocal malignant transformation occurring within an astrocytoma may simulate a metastatic neoplasm, as illustrated here, with three apparently discrete tumor masses within the right frontal lobe.

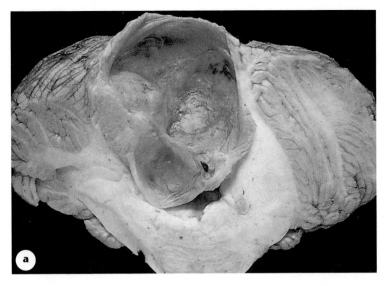

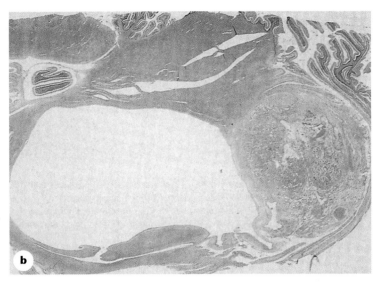

Fig. 12.17 Pilocytic astrocytoma. (**a**) This specimen from a 37-year-old male who presented with gait ataxia and limb dysmetria shows a large midline cyst-tumor nodule of the cerebellum. (**b**) The cyst-nodule relationship is well illustrated by a whole-mount section in which it can be seen that the cyst wall is composed of compressed white matter, not tumor.

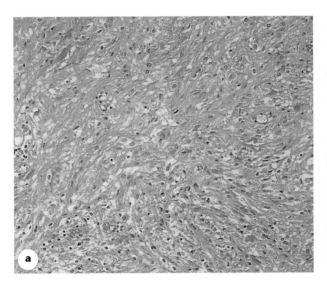

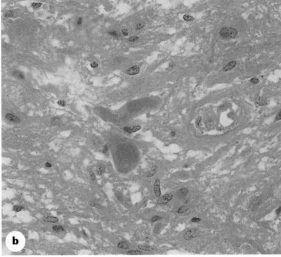

Fig. 12.18 Pilocytic astrocytoma. (**a**) Low-power microscopic view discloses elongated, bipolar cells aligned in intersecting bundles. (**b**) Sausage-shaped, brightly eosinophilic fibers, known as Rosenthal fibers, are very characteristic of pilocytic astrocytomas and other low-grade, slowly progressing gliomas.

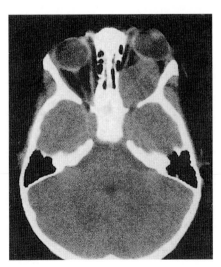

Fig. 12.19 Optic nerve astrocytoma. CT scan of a 2-year-old girl with proptosis shows a large pilocytic tumor surrounding and involving the right optic nerve.

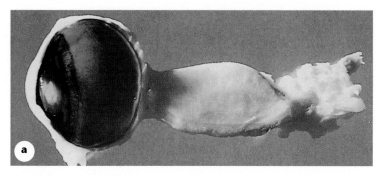

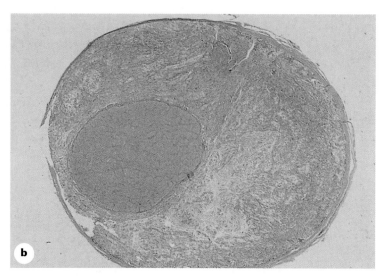

Fig. 12.20 Optic nerve astrocytoma. (**a**) Surgical specimen consisting of the globe and optic nerve from a 5-year-old girl with neurofibromatosis shows the tumor as a fusiform enlargement of the nerve. (**b**) On cross-sectional view, this optic nerve exhibits only modest enlargement but there is marked infiltration of the surrounding subarachnoid space by tumor.

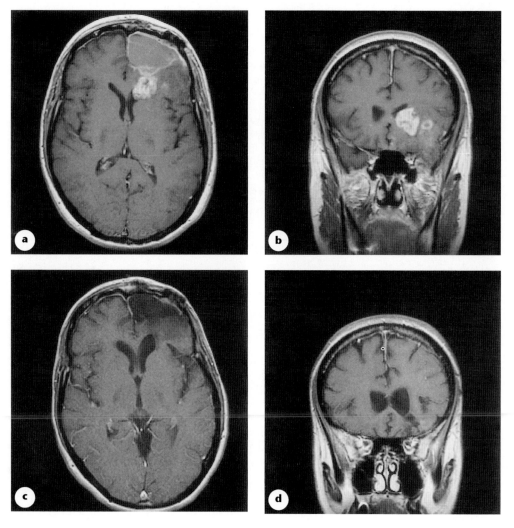

Fig. 12.21 Anaplastic oligodendroglioma. (**a**) Axial T1-weighted MR image after gadolinium enhancement. The patient has undergone a left craniotomy with a postoperative cavity (C) with some peripheral rim enhancement likely representing surgical change. There is also nodular enhancement abutting the left lateral ventricle (arrow) compatible with residual tumor. (**b**) Coronal T1-weighted MR image after gadolinium enhancement. Multifocal tumor is evident (arrows) which encroaches on and displaces the left lateral ventricle. (**c**) Axial T1-weighted MR image after gadolinium enhancement. This study after treatment shows complete resolution of the prior enhancing periventricular mass. There is *ex vacuuo* dilatation of the frontal horn of the left lateral ventricle (v). (**d**) Coronal T1-weighted MR image after gadolinium enhancement. No residual enhancing tumor is visible and there are now only low signal areas likely representing fluid as well as mild dilatation of the frontal horn of the left lateral ventricle (v).

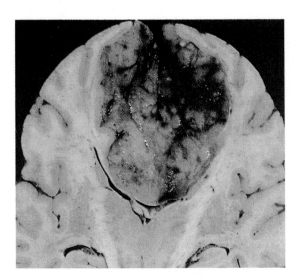

Fig. 12.22 Oligodendroglioma. This specimen from a 42-year-old man shows a massive bifrontal, relatively circumscribed tumor.

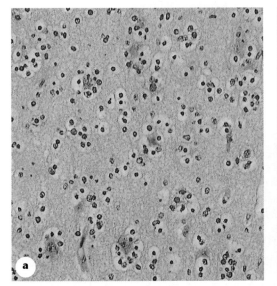

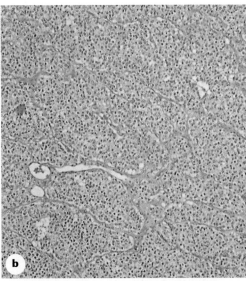

Fig. 12.23 Oligodendroglioma.
(**a**) Microscopic section from the periphery of the tumor shown in Figure 12.22 reveals the neoplastic oligodendrocytes as uniform cells with small, round nuclei and a characteristic perinuclear halo ('fried egg' cells). Satellitosis of the neoplastic cells around neurons is also a characteristic feature of this tumor.
(**b**) A section from the center of the tumor demonstrates a monotonous cellular pattern and delicate vasculature. Blood vessels often form fine, straight lines that intersect each other at right angles.

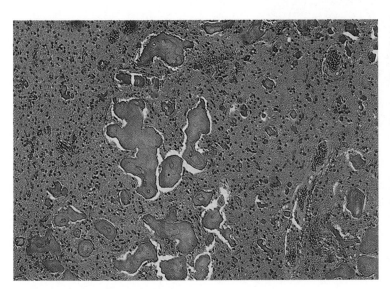

Fig. 12.24 Oligodendroglioma. Calcifications are very characteristic of this tumor and are often most pronounced at the periphery of the neoplasm.

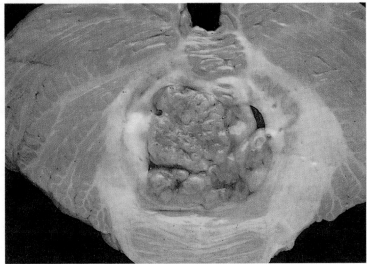

Fig. 12.25 Ependymoma. This specimen from a 42-year-old woman shows a tumor arising from the floor of the fourth ventricle, filling and expanding the ventricle and compressing the underlying pons. The lobulated gross appearance of the tumor is characteristic.

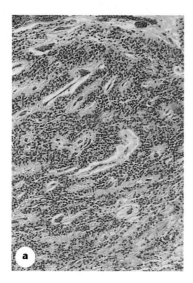

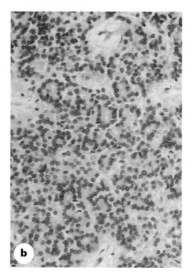

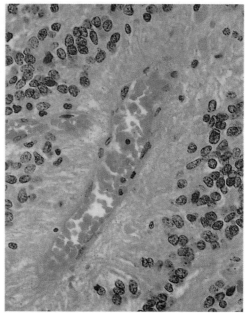

Fig. 12.27
Ependymoma. High-power photomicrograph of a pseudorosette shows that it is composed of cells aligned around a blood vessel with their processes toward the lumen of the vessel.

Fig. 12.26 Ependymoma. (**a**) The low-power microscopic pattern of this tumor is often quite characteristic. Note the striking pattern of pseudorosettes and tubules. The perivascular pseudorosettes appear as a maze of tubules when sectioned longitudinally to the blood vessel. (**b**) A typically cellular tumor is composed of uniform cells with regular, round nuclei arranged in pseudorosettes.

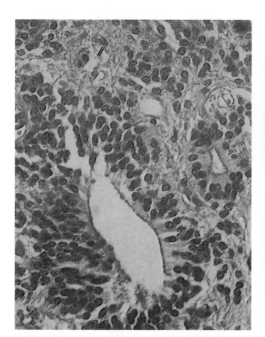

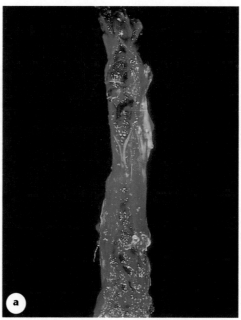

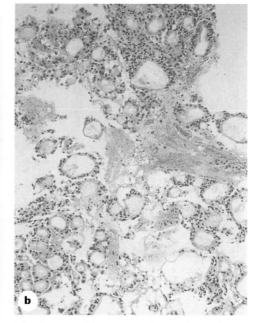

Fig. 12.28 Ependymoma. True rosettes are also a feature of ependymomas, although less common than pseudorosettes. A true rosette consists of cells aligned around a central lumen that does not contain a blood vessel.

Fig. 12.29 Myxopapillary ependymoma. (**a**) This spinal cord specimen was resected from a 15-year-old boy who experienced rapid onset of lower-limb paraplegia and incontinence. The red-brown tumor appears deeply vascular. (**b**) Microscopically, it is composed of cuboidal or columnar cells arranged in a papillary fashion around a fibrovascular stalk. Abundant mucin accumulation may be present, either in the neoplastic cells or in the associated connective tissue.

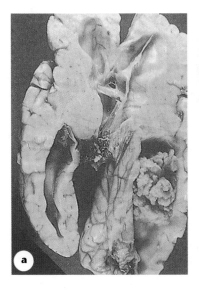
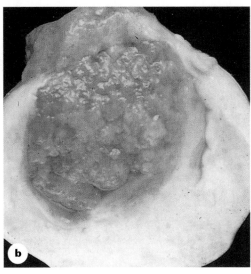

Fig. 12.30 Choroid plexus papilloma. (**a**) In this specimen from a 10-year-old boy, a discrete, irregular papillary mass is confined to the left posterior horn. There is massive dilatation of the entire ventricular system, with marked compression of the surrounding cerebral tissue. (**b**) A tumor involving the fourth ventricle has expanded and severely compressed the medulla. Although this pattern of growth may compromise surgical resection, it should not be confused with parenchymal invasion. Note the vascular nature of the tumor; these tumors have a tendency toward spontaneous hemorrhage.

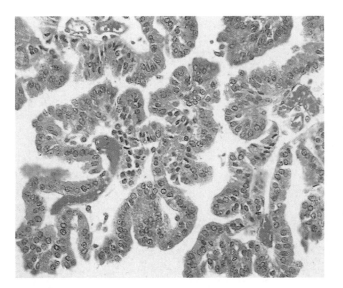

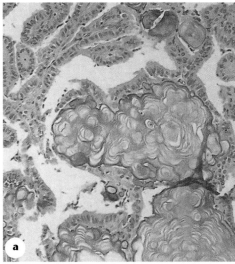
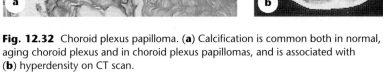

Fig. 12.31 Choroid plexus papilloma. The microscopic appearance of this tumor closely resembles that of normal choroid plexus.

Fig. 12.32 Choroid plexus papilloma. (**a**) Calcification is common both in normal, aging choroid plexus and in choroid plexus papillomas, and is associated with (**b**) hyperdensity on CT scan.

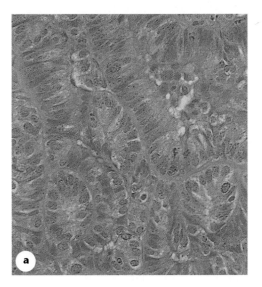
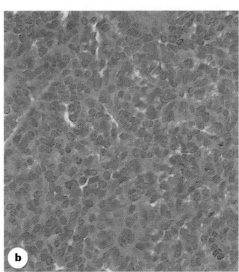

Fig. 12.33 Choroid plexus carcinoma. A spectrum of morphologic atypia links choroid plexus papilloma with the rare choroid plexus carcinoma. (**a**) A low grade malignancy is characterized by piling up of epithelium and mitotic activity. (**b**) At the farther end of the spectrum, this anaplastic example demonstrates an absence of the orderly architectural features of a papilloma.

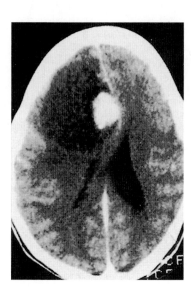

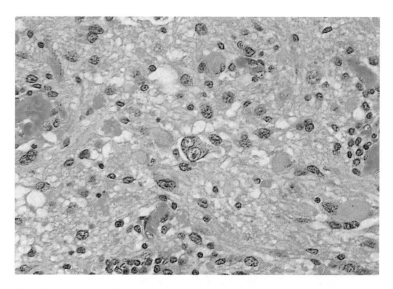

Fig. 12.34 Ganglioglioma. The CT appearance of gangliogliomas and ganglioneuromas is characteristic; foci of calcification and small cysts are common. Occasionally, the tumor consists of a single, large cyst with a single, calcified mural nodule, as illustrated here.

Fig. 12.35 Ganglioglioma. The key histologic feature is the presence of neoplastic ganglion cells like the binucleate cell in the center of this field. The primary differential distinction is from infiltrative glioma with entrapment of normal neuron.

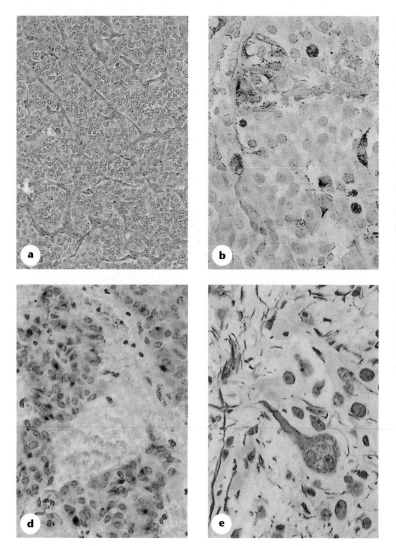

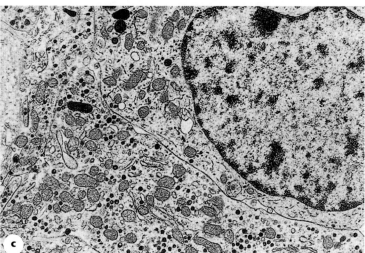

Fig. 12.36 Paraganglioma. (**a**) The tumor is composed of well-defined lobules (Zellballen) of regular, round, clear cells intersected by thin-walled capillaries. A diffuse pattern may also be seen. (**b**)Tumor cells are argyrophilic (Grimelius). (**c**) Electron microscopy reveals cytoplasmic neurosecretory granules. Immunostaining techniques are positive for both (**d**) neurofilament protein and (not shown) neuron-specific enolase. (**e**) Approximately half of tumors of the filum terminale show ganglionic differentiation (Bodian method).

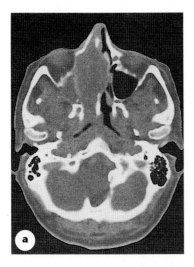
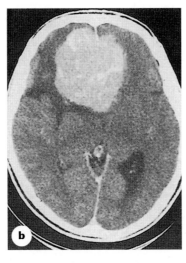
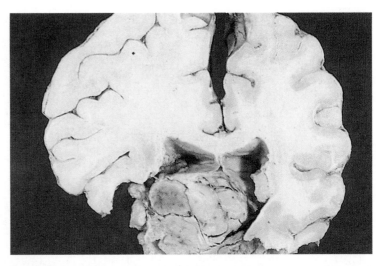

Fig. 12.37 Olfactory neuroblastoma (esthesioneuroblastoma). (**a**) CT scan in a 19-year-old boy shows a mass filling the left nasal cavity. (**b**) In the case of a 15-year-old girl, a large tumor mass is apparent at the base of the left frontal lobe; it extends across the midline and is associated with surrounding edema. These tumors may grow either downward to fill the nasal cavity or upward through the the cribriform plate to enter the cranial vault.

Fig. 12.38 Olfactory neuroblastoma (esthesioneuroblastoma). Autopsy specimen shows a tumor mass that has destroyed and replaced a large proportion of the base of the anterior brain.

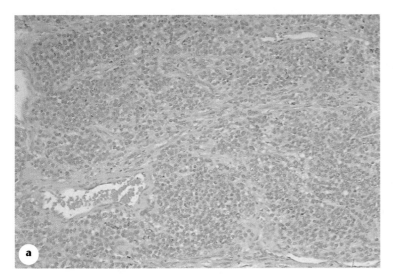
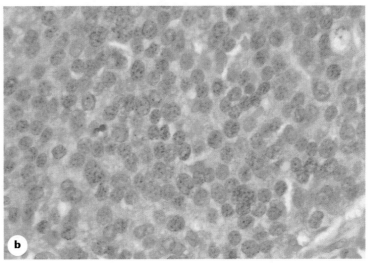

Fig. 12.39 Olfactory neuroblastoma (esthesioneuroblastoma). (**a**) In a typical neuroendocrine-type esthesioneuroblastoma, low-power microscopy reveals rather monotonous-looking cells arranged in lobules on a delicate fibrovascular stroma. (**b**) With high magnification, there may be no particular pattern. Some esthesioneuroblastomas contain true Homer–Wright rosettes and axons may be demonstrable with special stains. Electron microscopy may be required to identify this tumor and to distinguish it from other small, round cell tumors.

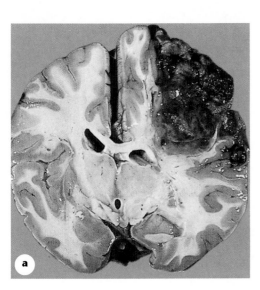
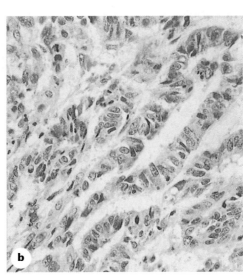

Fig. 12.40 Medulloepithelioma. (**a**) Like most embryonal tumors, this left frontal neoplasm arising in a 5-year-old girl is solid and discrete, with a soft, grayish-pink, highly necrotic appearance. (**b**) The distinctive microscopic features consist of a papillary or tubular arrangement of columnar cells.

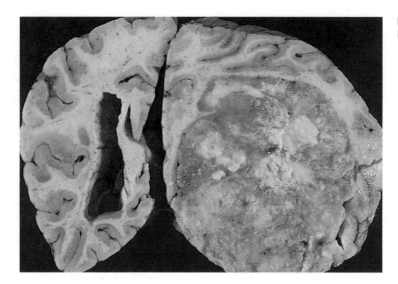

Fig. 12.41 Cerebral neuroblastoma. This large central tumor in a 10-year-old boy is commonly well demarcated from the surrounding tissue.

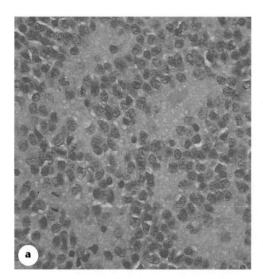

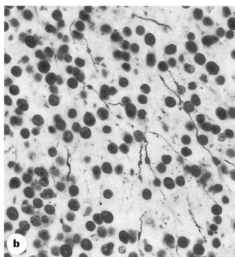

Fig. 12.42 Cerebral neuroblastoma. (**a**) Neuroblastomas consist of a fairly uniform population of cells frequently arranged in Homer–Wright rosettes. Desmoplasia may also be a feature. (**b**) Special stain for neuritic processes highlights the immature axons (frozen Bielschowky). Neuroblastomas in tissue culture form similar neuritic processes. Occasionally, tumors show the formation of mature neurons (not shown).

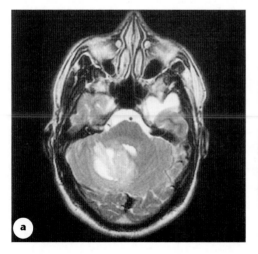

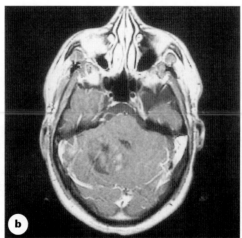

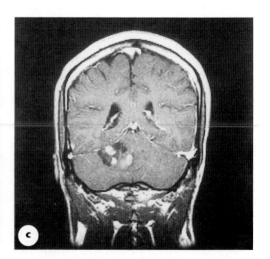

Fig. 12.43 Medulloblastoma. (**a**) Axial T2-weighted MR image at the level of the fourth ventricle. A large heterogeneous mass is present in the right cerebellum which compresses and displaces the fourth ventricles (arrow). (**b**) Axial T1-weighted MR image after gadolinium administration at the same level, showing some nodular enhancement of the tumor (arrows). (**c**) Coronal T1-weighted MR image after gadolinium administration at a level posterior to the brainstem. The tumor abuts the tentorium (arrows) and again shows heterogeneous enhancement.

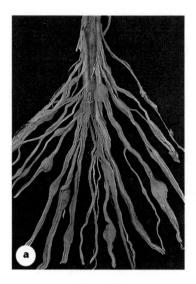

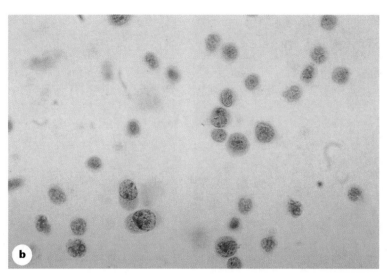

Fig. 12.44 Medulloblastoma. Spinal arachnoid spread of tumor may entirely encase and deform the cord and produce (**a**) studding of the caudal nerve roots. (**b**) Malignant cells are often readily identified on CSF examination.

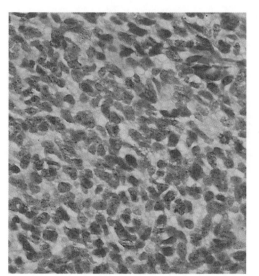

Fig. 12.45 Medulloblastoma. The tumor is highly cellular and composed of dark-staining, ovoid cells with hyperchromatic nuclei and ill-defined cytoplasmic outlines; there is no definite architectural arrangement.

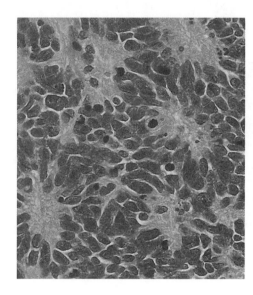

Fig. 12.46 Medulloblastoma. In approximately one-third of case, characteristic Homer–Wright rosettes are found, with nuclei arranged radially around a delicately fibrillated, eosinophilic center. Pseudorosettes, marked by a perivascular arrangement of tumor cells, may also occur.

415

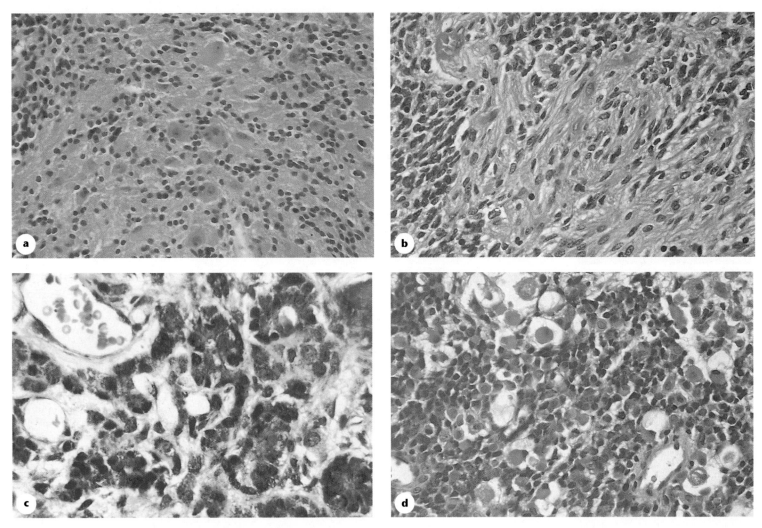

Fig. 12.47 Medulloblastoma. This tumor is marked by a capacity for differentiation in a variety of forms, as can be seen by the presence of (**a**) neurons, (**b**) glial cells, (**c**) pigmented neuroepithelium and, in rare cases, (**d**) striated muscle.

TUMORS OF CRANIAL AND SPINAL NERVES

SCHWANNOMA

Constituting 5–10% of all intracranial tumors, schwannomas are usually solitary tumors discovered in the middle and later decades of life. Schwannomas presenting at an early age and/or bilaterally are seen in association with neurofibromatosis. The lesions are firm, encapsulated, slow growing and benign. Schwannomas show a marked predilection for sensory nerves. In the cranial cavity, they principally involve cranial nerve VIII (particularly the vestibular component) and, far less commonly, cranial nerves V, IX and X. Clinical symptoms of auditory and/or cerebellar dysfunction are common. Intraspinal schwannomas, representing 30% of these tumors, most often involve the lumbar segment and give rise to signs of local root irritation and spinal cord compression. Both intra and extradural growth is observed and large lesions may traverse and expand the intervertebral foraminae, resulting in a dumbell-shaped lesion. Schwannomas are treated surgically and may recur if resection is not complete. Malignant transformation is rare.

NEUROFIBROMA
Variants: circumscribed (solitary) and plexiform

Like schwannomas, neurofibromas are tumors of Schwann cells and can be distinguished by their morphology. Intraneural neurofibromas diffusely transform a nerve segment and its branches (the 'plexiform' variant) and only infrequently produce an isolated lesion involving one nerve fascicle (the 'circumscribed' or 'solitary' variant). It is the plexiform variety that is pathognomic of neurofibromatosis, whereas solitary neurofibromas infrequently share this association. Neurofibromas may be found along cranial or spinal nerve roots and ganglia, major nerves of the trunk and limbs, including the sympathetic system and subcutaneous branches, and along visceral sympathetic plexuses. Symptoms are related to compression of surrounding structures by tumor. Treatment is surgical, but resection almost invariably sacrifices the involved nerve because neurofibromas infiltrate the nerve directly. Partial resection may result in recurrence.

As discussed above, patients with neurofibromatosis type II (NFII) are predisposed to schwannomas and meningiomas of the cranial nerves and spinal nerve roots, whereas patients with neurofibromatosis type I (NFI) are susceptible to peripheral neurofibromas. The NFI gene has been mapped to chromosome 17 and recently the NFII gene was mapped to chromosome 22. Alterations in the NFI gene may also be associated with pilocytic astrocytomas.

Malignant peripheral nerve sheath tumors (MPNST)

Malignant peripheral nerve sheath tumors arise by malignant transformation of a neurofibroma, usually plexiform, or arise *de novo* in a normal nerve sheath. MPNST are highly malignant tumors that infiltrate locally and commonly metastasize to distant sites. The tumors occur primarily in adults, in whom they present as painful, rapidly enlarging masses that favor the trunk, neck and proximal limbs, and only rarely affect cranial nerves. Treatment is usually surgical; the prognosis is directly related to tumor size. Fewer than 20% of patients survive 5 years.

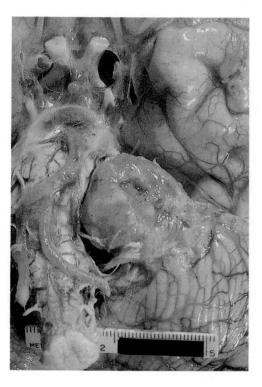

Fig. 12.48
Schwannoma (acoustic neuroma). A large, discrete tumor nodule, arising from the left eighth cranial nerve, obscures the underlying seventh and eighth cranial nerves and causes lateral compression of the pons and medulla.

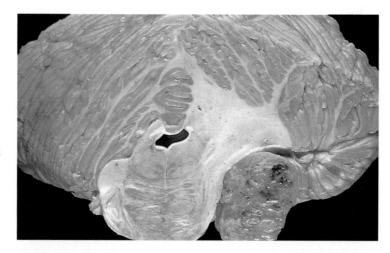

Fig. 12.49 Schwannoma (acoustic neuroma). This horizontal section through the pons and cerebellum demonstrates the usual gross appearance of a schwannoma. The tumor is well circumscribed, mottled red-yellow in color and most commonly originates on the vestibular portion of the eighth cranial nerve.

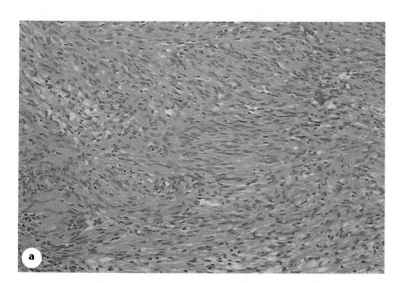

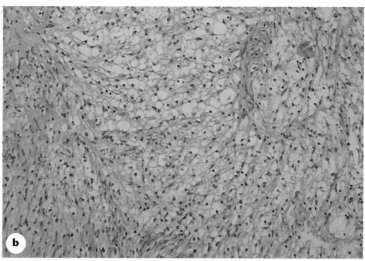

Fig. 12.50 Schwannoma (acoustic neuroma). Microscopic features include (**a**) compact areas composed of densely interlacing bundles of spindle-shaped cells (Antoni A pattern) and (**b**) more loosely arranged round-to-ovoid cells with pale cytoplasm (Antoni B pattern).

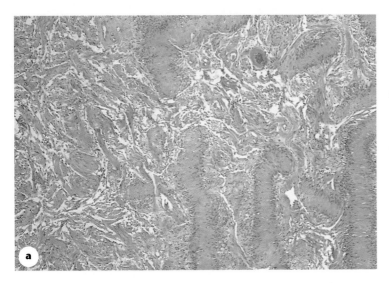 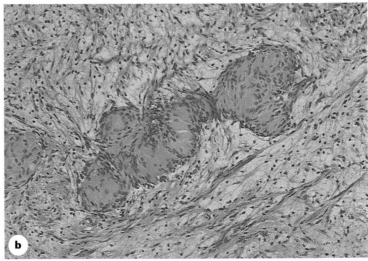

Fig. 12.51 Schwannoma (**a**). Palisading, or lining up of nuclei, may be a striking feature, particularly in spinal schwannomas. (**b**) If the palisading forms are pronounced, the term 'Verocay body' is commonly applied.

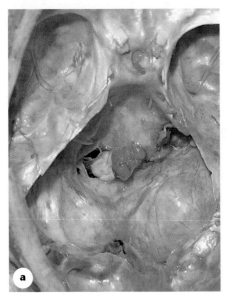 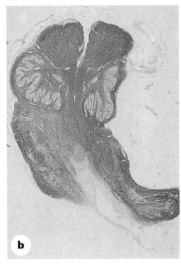 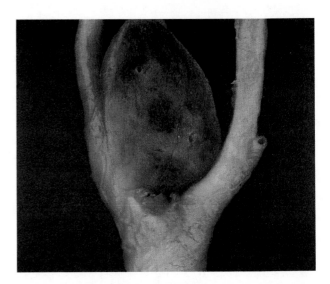

Fig. 12.52 Glomus jugulare tumor. (**a**) A tumor of the skull base compresses the high cervical spinal cord and medulla (seen in cross-section). (**b**) This whole-mount transverse section reveals the degree of medullary deformity.

Fig. 12.53 Carotid body tumor. A globoid, encapsulated carotid body ganglioglioma overlies the bifurcation of the common carotid artery.

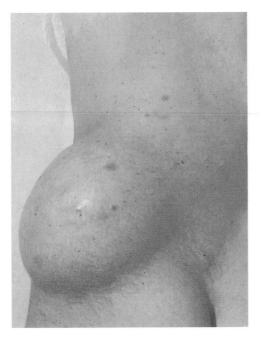

Fig. 12.54 Malignant peripheral nerve sheath tumor. A large tumor has arisen in the left flank of a 28-year-old woman with neurofibromatosis. Note the extensive café-au-lait patch surrounding the tumor.

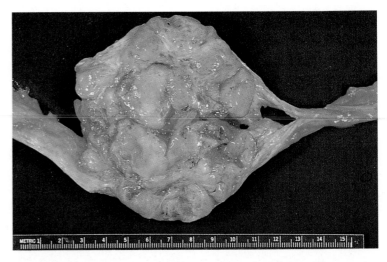

Fig. 12.55 Malignant peripheral nerve sheath tumor. In this cross-section of a tumor arising in the sciatic nerve, its origin from the nerve can clearly be seen, a helpful feature in the diagnosis. The tumor is typically encapsulated and on cross-section appears more vascular and variegated than a benign neurofibroma.

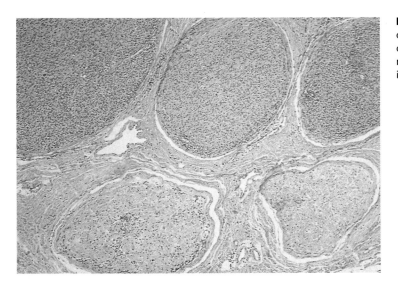

Fig. 12.56 Malignant peripheral nerve sheath tumor. Tumor involves three of the five nerve fascicles shown here, as evidenced by their increased cellularity; there is no obvious deformity of the nerve structure. Surgical resection margins must be evaluated with great care because of such insidious intraneural growth.

TUMORS OF THE MENINGES

TUMORS OF MENINGOTHELIAL CELLS
Meningioma

Meningiomas constitute 15% of intracranial and 25–32% of intraspinal tumors in adults; they are uncommon in children. There is a striking female preponderance, especially among intraspinal tumors, believed to be related to a stimulatory effect of female hormones. Approximately 90% of meningiomas are supratentorial, favoring such sites as the parasagittal region, falx cerebri, cerebral convexities, olfactory groove, sphenoid ridge and tuberculum sellae. Infratentorial meningiomas frequently are attached to the tentorium cerebelli or the foramen magnum. Meningiomas are commonly divided into descriptive subtypes on the basis of their histologic appearance: meningothelial, fibrous (fibroblastic), transitional (mixed), psammomatous, angiomatous, microcystic, secretory, clear cell, chordoid, lymphoplasmacyte rich and metaplastic meningioma. With rare exceptions, the biologic behavior does not vary among these subtypes. All are slow-growing neoplasms that usually only displace normal structures. Occasionally, they invade the cerebral parenchyma by finger-like processes and they commonly invade dura, bone and soft tissues. In rare instances, penetration of the facial sinuses presents as a nasal polyp. Hyperostosis of overlying bone is a frequently encountered radiologic sign, whose presence does not necessarily indicate bone invasion.

Atypical and anaplastic (malignant) meningioma

Atypical and malignant tumors are associated with a high recurrence rate. Atypical features in meningiomas include high cellularity, lack of lobularity or a 'sheeting' pattern of growth, prominent nucleoli, mitotic figures and focal necrosis. The necrosis may be accompanied by pseudopalisading. Invasion of brain and/or metastases, either to the CNS or extracranially, signify frank malignancy.

Papillary meningioma

This subtype of meningioma is of special interest because of its locally aggressive nature, its tendency for late distant metastases and its occurrence in children and young adults.

MESENCHYMAL, NON-MENINGOTHELIAL TUMORS
Malignant neoplasms

HEMANGIOPERICYTOMA ('ANGIOBLASTIC MENINGIOMA') Although this tumor was previously considered an usual and highly malignant form of meningioma, the 'angioblastic meningioma', the WHO classification clearly designates this entity as a mesenchymal tumor of non-meningeal origin. Intracranial meningeal hemangiopericytomas, like their somatic soft tissue counterpart, are highly vascular tumors with the capability of rapid growth and all have a marked tendency for systemic metastasis. Meningeal hemangiopericytomas may occur at any age, but there is a marked increase in incidence in the fourth to sixth decades. Their geographic sites of origin are similar to those of meningiomas. Treatment consists of surgical resection and adjuvant radiotherapy, but in 75% of cases tumors recur despite therapy. The diagnosis is often suspected angiographically.

Sarcomas

A wide variety of sarcomas affect the CNS; most are highly malignant and all are unusual. Fibrosarcomas and malignant fibrous histiocytomas (fibrous histiocytic sarcomas) grow both inside and outside the dura, but despite their fairly circumscribed appearance, they tend to infiltrate the brain parenchyma. Some of these tumors arise as complications of high-dose radiotherapy after a long latent interval. They must be distinguished from anaplastic meningiomas and gliosarcomas. Meningeal sarcomatosis, a rapidly fatal disorder, is a diffuse sarcoma of the leptomeninges, occurring in young or middle-aged patients. Rhabdomyosarcomas may occur as the dominant feature of teratomas or in conjunction with medulloblastomas; they may also arise *de novo* in the leptomeninges. Chondrosarcomas may affect the clivus, sella, nasopharynx or vertebrae. Patients range in age from 20 to 60 years and the tumors are seen more commonly in males. Osteosarcomas very rarely occur in the skull and only exceptionally is the skull the site of metastases from osteosarcomas elsewhere in the skeleton.

TUMORS OF UNCERTAIN HISTOGENESIS
Hemangioblastoma (capillary hemangioblastoma)

Hemangioblastomas constitute 1.2% of all intracranial neoplasms. Most arise in the third to fifth decade with a twofold male preponderance. Sites of preference, in descending order of frequency, are the cerebellar vermis and hemispheres, the roof of the fourth ventri-cle (area postrema), the spinal cord and occasionally the cerebral hemispheres, where they tend to be meningeal rather than intra-parenchymal. This tumor has a tendency to form large cysts and multiplicity is common. The clinical signs are frequently those of cerebellar dysfunction and obstructive hydrocephalus. Approximately 10% of hemangioblastomas occur in association with von Hippel–Lindau disease, a term reserved for hereditary forms of cerebellar hemangioblastoma in combination with angiomas of the retina, hypernephromas and cysts of the pancreas and kidney. Hemangioblastomas are benign brain tumors, although they may infiltrate the brain parenchyma. Malignant transforma-tion and metastasis have not been recorded. Treatment is surgical resection, which usually results in cure unless a second tumor has been overlooked or the cyst is opened at surgery. Approximately 10–20% secrete erythropoietin and thus give rise to polycythemia.

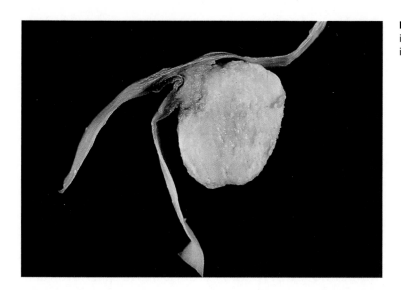

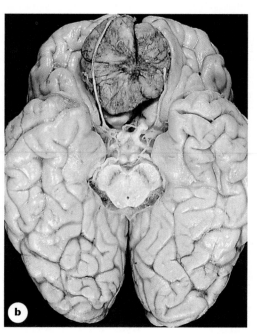

Fig. 12.57 Meningioma. In this parasagittal tumor, the sagittal sinus is involved, a feature that affects respectability and results in increased incidence of recurrence of meningiomas at this site.

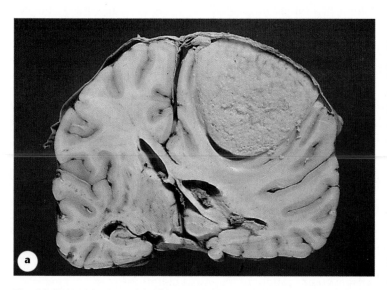

Fig. 12.58 Meningioma. (**a**) A large convexity meningioma severely displaces the underlying tissue downward and laterally, creating a midline shift and marked ventricular compression. (**b**) An olfactory groove meningioma bows the olfactory nerves and splays the frontal lobes.

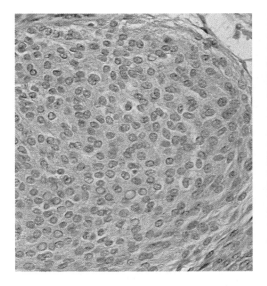

Fig. 12.59 Meningiotheliomatous meningioma. These tumors are characterized by lobules of uniform, oval epithelioid cells with typical intranuclear haloes.

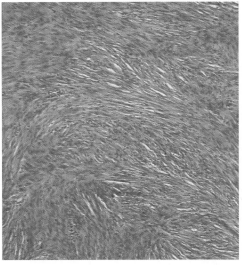

Fig. 12.60 Fibrous (fibroblastic) meningioma. This variant of meningioma is marked by collections of spindle-shaped cells (bearing some resemblance to fibroblasts) arranged in a dense network of intersecting bundles.

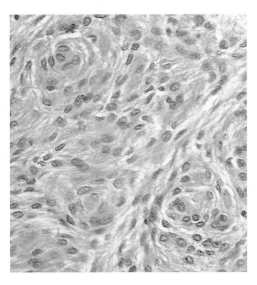

Fig. 12.61 Transitional (mixed) meningioma. Meningotheliomatous and fibrous features intermix in this histologic subtype of meningioma. The whorled architecture is a common finding.

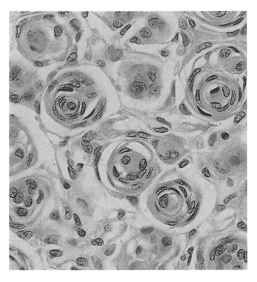

Fig. 12.62 Meningioma. Whorl formation is often a valuable diagnostic feature. The whorls may be quite prominent, with cells tightly wrapping around one another in an 'onion-skin' pattern.

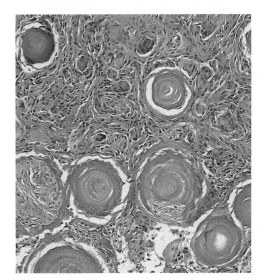

Fig. 12.63 Psammomatous meningioma. These tumors contain rounded microcalcifications that often center on the meningeal whorls. The psammoma bodies arise extracellularly, originating within the matrix produced by the tumor cells.

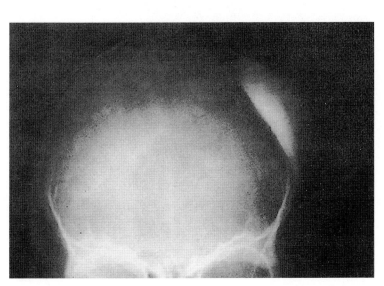

Fig. 12.64 Meningioma. Focal hypertrophy of the overlying skull is frequently a valuable radiologic sign, suggesting the presence of a meningioma. Usually a reactive process, osseous hypertrophy may also be caused by meningiomatous invasion of bone, as demonstrated in this radiograph.

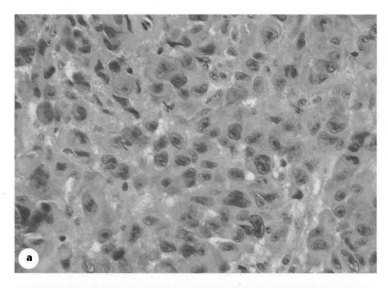

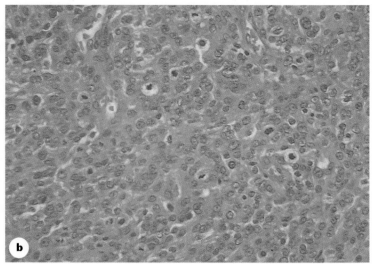

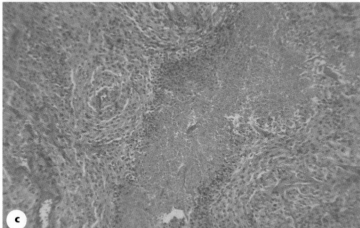

Fig. 12.65 Atypical meningioma. Features indicating atypicality and potential malignant behavior are: (**a**) prominence of nucleoli, (**b**) mitotic figures with high cell density and a sheet-like growth pattern, and (**c**) necrosis, occasionally with pseudopalisading.

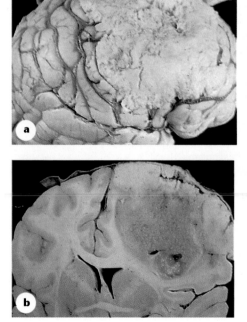

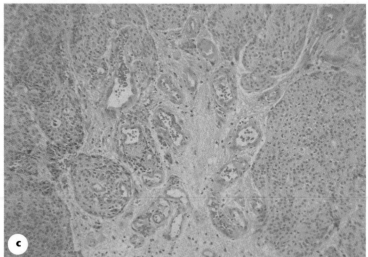

Fig. 12.66 Malignant meningioma. The determination of frank malignancy rests on demonstration of invasion into adjacent brain parenchyma, a feature that can be identified grossly (**a,b**) as well as microscopically (**c**).

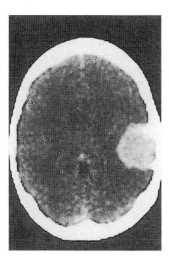

Fig. 12.67 Malignant fibrous histiocytoma. CT scan in a 16-year-old girl shows a discrete, enhancing tumor based in the dura.

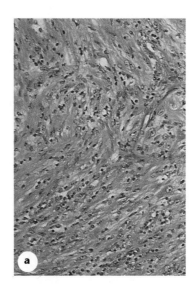 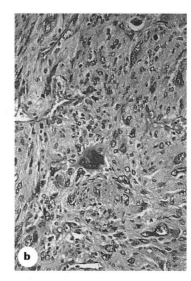

Fig. 12.68 Malignant fibrous histiocytoma. (**a**) Its microscopic appearance is marked by spindle-shaped and plump cells arranged in fascicles. Inflammatory cells are occasionally present. (**b**) In rare instances, giant cells and mitoses are observed in addition to bizarre, spindle-shaped cells. Such lesions must be distinguished from giant cell astrocytoma secondarily involving the meninges.

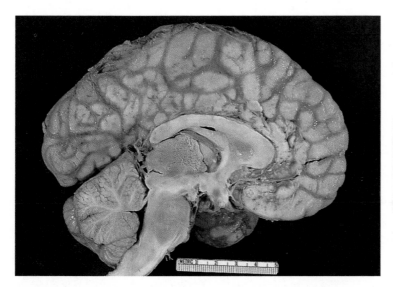

Fig. 12.69 Rhabdomyosarcoma. In this specimen from a child, the tumor involves the pineal region and is associated with diffuse leptomeningeal seeding.

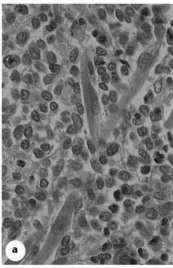

Fig. 12.70 Rhabdomyosarcoma. (**a**) The tumor is composed of small, poorly differentiated, round cells intermingled with elongated, eosinophilic muscle fibers. (**b**) On PTAH stain, the myoblasts show cytoplasmic cross-striations. Microscopic sampling of such neoplasms is necessary to exclude the presence of coexisting germ cell tumor components.

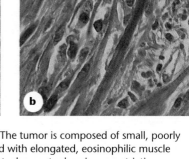

Fig. 12.71 Hemangioblastoma. (**a**) CT scan of a 35-year-old male reveals an enhancing cystic lesion of the cerebellum with a central tumor nodule, features characteristic of hemangioblastoma. (**b**) Gross specimen confirms a central, vascular tumor nodule surrounded by cystic, gliotic and darkly discolored cerebellar white matter.

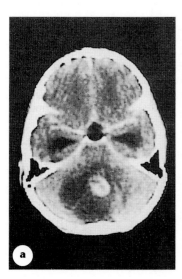 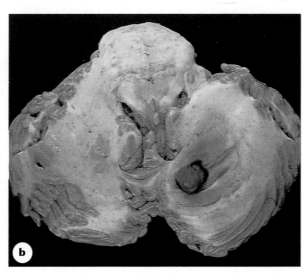

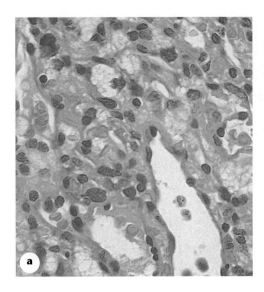

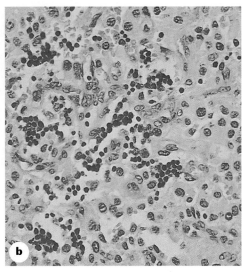

Fig. 12.72 Hemangioblastoma. (**a**) Its histologic appearance is marked by large, oval, often foamy cells amid a dense network of thin-walled, closely packed blood vessels. (**b**) Occasionally, clusters of immature red blood cells are seen, indirect evidence of the known capacity of hemangioblastomas to secrete erythropoietin (extramedullary erythropoiesis).

LYMPHOMAS AND HEMOPOIETIC NEOPLASMS

Malignant lymphoma

Primary CNS non-Hodgkin's lymphomas have become increasingly common over the last 10 years with the advent of the AIDS epidemic. They represent approximately 2% of all intracranial tumors and show a marked male predominance. All immunosuppressed patients, including post-transplantation and AIDS patients, are particularly vulnerable. The tumors tend to be supratentorial, most commonly deeply situated and midline. The majority is B-cell neoplasms, although T-cell forms have been reported. The tumors may be multiple; they may form a discrete mass or they may infiltrate diffusely by expanding existing structures without destroying their gross architecture. Although cerebral lymphomas are extremely sensitive to radiotherapy and steroids, overall median survival time is between 2 and 4 years with the addition of high-dose methotrexate. In the setting of immunosuppression, the survival time is considerably shorter.

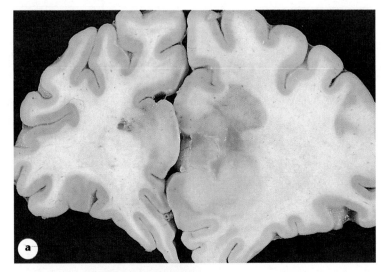

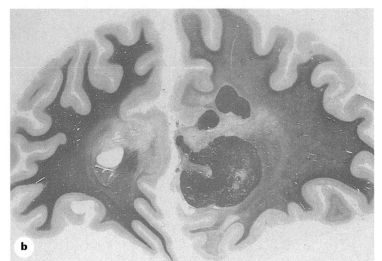

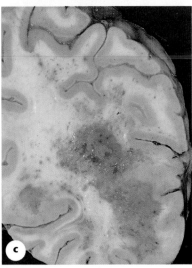

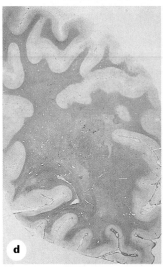

Fig. 12.73 Primary cerebral lymphoma. (**a**) A reasonably circumscribed mass of white tumor tissue lies within the paramedian right frontal lobe. The deeply staining lymphomatous masses are more easily visualized on the corresponding whole-mount section (**b**). The pale areas surrounding the tumor nodules represent edema. (**c,d**) The lesion may be more diffuse, like that shown here in the right posterior temporoparietal lobe; no discrete mass is evident.

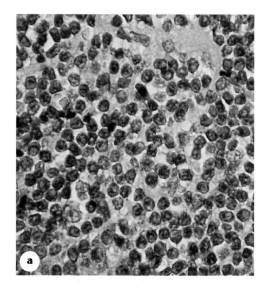

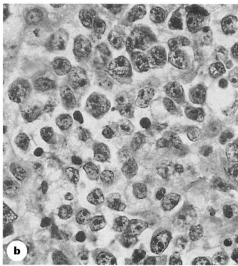

Fig. 12.74 Primary cerebral lymphoma. The histologic appearance is variable, ranging from (**a**) small cell tumors to (**b**) the more common large cell, immunoblastic type. Monotypic immunoreactivity for immunoglobulin components is typical of B-cell lymphoma. (*See also* Chapter 17: AIDS-Associated Malignancies and Chapter 14: Hodgkin's Disease and Non-Hodgkin's Lymphomas.)

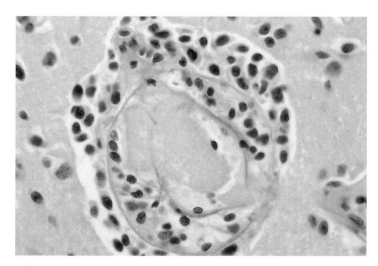

Fig. 12.75 Primary cerebral lymphoma. The growth pattern is typically perivascular. Neoplastic lymphocytes not only surround small blood vessels but also penetrate the vascular wall.

GERM CELL TUMORS

Germinoma

Germinomas, which are derived from developmental germ cell rests, represent 0.5–0.7% of brain tumors, with a slightly higher incidence among Asian peoples. The pineal region is the most common site of occurrence and men represent 70–90% of cases, as is true of most tumors of the pineal region. Germinomas may exhibit a circumscribed or an infiltrative growth pattern. They may disseminate via the CSF and occasionally via the bloodstream to extracranial sites, including lungs, lymph nodes and liver. These tumors are extremely radiosensitive; the 5-year survival rate following surgery and postoperative radiation may be as high as 80%.

Teratoma

Accounting for 0.2–0.9% of all brain tumors, teratomas show a marked male preponderance and a tendency to occur in the first two decades. They are most typically found in the pineal and sellar regions. Classically, they are composed of three germinal layers. The majority are benign and slow growing, although instances of malignant change and CSF seeding have been described. Teratomas tend to be well circumscribed and surgical resection is often associated with an excellent prognosis.

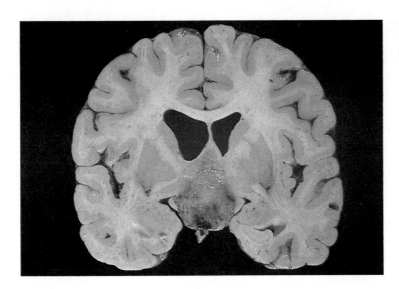

Fig. 12.76 Germinoma. This coronal section shows a lesion of the hypothalamic region which, together with the pineal region, are the primary site of occurrence.

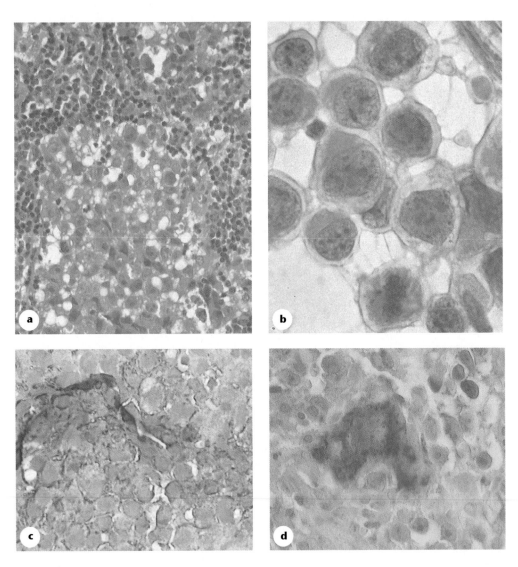

Fig. 12.77 Germinoma. (**a**) Two distinct cell populations are present: one is a population of small lymphocytes and the other of large, spheroidal cells, each with a prominent central nucleus containing distinct nucleoli and vesiculated nucleoplasm. Granuloma formation is infrequent, unlike the situation with gonadal tumors. (**b**) Touch preparation demonstrates common cytologic features of tumor cells, including a high nucleus-to-cytoplasm ratio, round nuclei and somewhat elongated nucleoli. Immunostaining techniques reveal the presence of (**c**) placental alkaline phosphatase within tumor cells, as well as (**d**) occasional syncytiotrophoblastic giant cells reactive for HCG. Carrying no prognostic significance, the latter finding may be associated with elevated levels of HCG in CSF and blood.

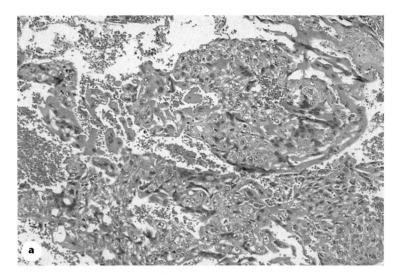

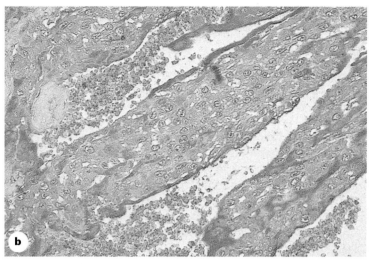

Fig. 12.78 Choriocarcinoma. (**a**) This rare form of germ cell tumor shows a tendency to hemorrhage, as seen microscopically in this tumor arising in the pineal region in a 12-year-old girl, who had a sudden intracranial hemorrhage and died on the same day. The tumor consists of multinucleate syncytiotrophoblastic and cytotrophoblastic cells arranged in a bilayer fashion, often surrounding vascular spaces. (**b**) Immunostaining reveals HCG reactivity in the syncytiotrophoblasts.

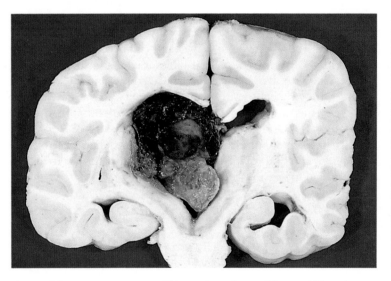

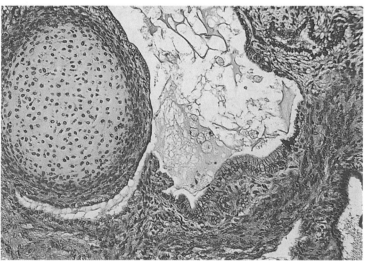

Fig. 12.79 Immature teratoma. This specimen from a 12-year-old boy shows a tumor projecting anteriorly from the pineal region. Intraventricular hemorrhage occurred postoperatively.

Fig. 12.80 Immature teratoma. Resembling fetal tissue, the constituents of this tumor include cartilage on the left and mucin-producing columnar epithelium in the center, together with a spindle cell stroma.

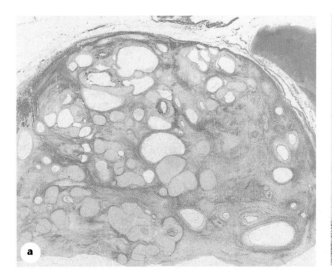

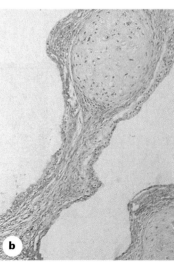

Fig. 12.81 Mature teratoma. (**a, b**) Unlike its immature counterpart, this tumor resembles benign adult tissue, exhibiting mature hyaline cartilage, respiratory epithelium and a loose, fibrous stroma. Mature teratomas are far less common than immature teratomas.

TUMORS OF THE SELLAR REGION

Craniopharyngioma

Craniopharyngiomas are tumors of children and adolescents in whom they constitute 2–3% of all intracranial neoplasms. Two distinct varieties exist: the classic adamantinomatous craniopharyngioma and a less common form, the papillary craniopharyngioma. The majority of these tumors of maldevelopmental origin are found above the sella, although a few arise in the sella itself. They grow slowly, compressing neighboring tissue and frequently affecting the pituitary, optic chiasm and their ventricle. The adamantinomatous craniopharyngioma usually presents with disturbances of the hypothalamic–pituitary axis, visual symptoms and hydrocephalus as a result of obstructed CSF flow. Most adamantinomatous craniopharyngiomas are sufficiently calcified to be visualized on skull radiographs. Combined radiotherapy and surgical resection is the recommended treatment; however, recurrences are frequent (up to 40% of cases), particularly in the pediatric age group. The papillary craniopharyngioma, on the other hand, is often solid rather than cystic and infrequently calcified. In addition, the tumor appears to arise in the third ventricle and usually does not affect the sella. The prognosis of patients with the papillary craniopharyngioma is better than with the adamantinomatous tumor, as the papillary variety is more discrete and less infiltrative.

LOCAL EXTENSION FROM REGIONAL TUMORS

Chordoma

Representing approximately 0.2% of all brain tumors, chordomas are most commonly encountered in the fourth to sixth decades; there is a slight male preponderance. Derived from notochordal rests, they tend to be midline tumors of the skull base. The sella and clivus are the predominant cranial sites, from which these tumors may expand into the foramen magnum, nasopharynx or optic chiasm, with considerable bone erosion and destruction. Spinal column tumors favor the dens of the axis and the sacrococcygeal region. Complete surgical resection is usually not feasible and metastases to lungs, lymph nodes, bone and skin may occur, particularly in sacrococcygeal chordomas. The survival time for cranial chordomas averages from 2 to 3 years and from 6 to 7 years for sacrococcygeal tumors.

Chondroma

Chondromas constitute less than 1% of all brain tumors. They commonly arise in the dura of the skull base, but may arise in dura over the cerebral convexities or spinal cord, in the sinuses or, rarely, in the choroid plexus. They are typically benign and slow growing. Treatment is surgical, which may be difficult because of the tumors' tendency to invade bone, a typical feature not considered a sign of malignant potential. Metastatic deposits represent 40% of all CNS tumors; they are commonly multiple. The most common carcinomas metastasizing to the CNS are those of the lung, breast, skin (melanoma), kidney (renal cell carcinoma), gastrointestinal tract and thyroid. Perhaps as a result of prolonged survival, the incidence of cerebral metastases in patients with sarcomas has increased in the past decade.

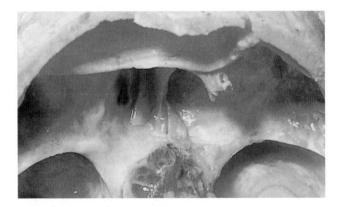

Fig. 12.82 Cystic craniopharyngioma. Usually partially solid and partially cystic, these tumors often contain a dark, oily fluid which has been likened to machine oil. This specimen shows a small cystic lesion in the suprasellar region.

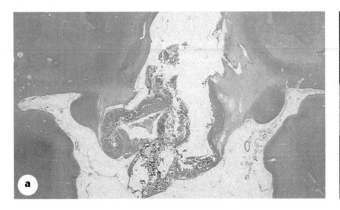

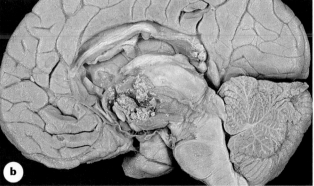

Fig. 12.83 Cystic craniopharyngioma. The tumor may grow, extending into the third ventricle, as seen (**a**) in this coronal-section photomicrograph and (**b**) in this midsagittal section, where a massive tumor fills the third ventricle.

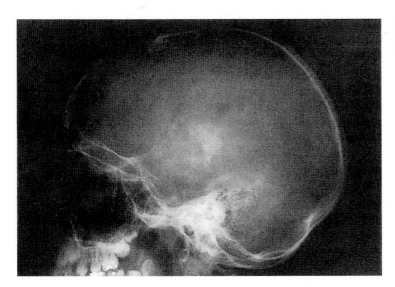

Fig. 12.84 Cystic craniopharyngioma. Lateral skull radiograph demonstrates the radial calcifications of a large, suprasellar tumor.

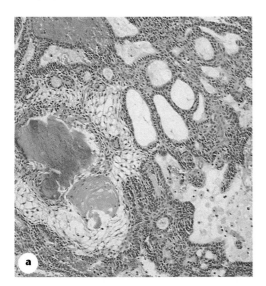

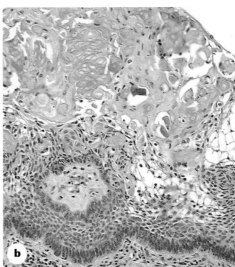

Fig. 12.85 Craniopharyngioma. (**a**) The tumor is composed of a complex arrangement of columnar epithelium and prominent cystic spaces. (**b**) In many areas, the epithelium is squamous and arranged in whorls with keratin pearl formation. Craniopharyngiomas have irregular contours and often show finger-like extensions into the surrounding brain, thus evoking intense gliosis.

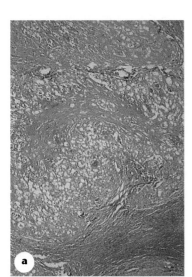

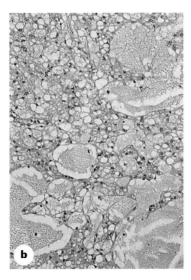

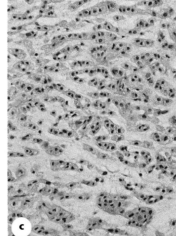

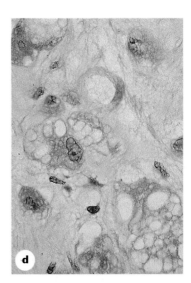

Fig. 12.86 Chordoma. The spectrum of microscopic features of this tumor include: (**a**) a lobular growth pattern, (**b**) pools of mucin among cells with abundant, foamy vacuoles, (**c**) elongated cords of pale, eosinophilic cells with regular cytologic features, and (**d**) large, physaliphorous ('bubbly') cells. Partial cartilaginous differentiation marks a 'chondroid' chordoma (not shown), a variant associated with a more favorable prognosis.

METASTATIC TUMORS

SITES OF PREFERENCE
Skull and epidura

Metastatic tumor deposits in the skull and vertebrae may penetrate and destroy bone and dura. They may extend into the epidural or subarachnoid space, compressing adjacent neural tissue.

Dural tumors

Tumors with a tendency toward dural metastasis include those of the breast and prostate, as well as lymphomas and peripheral neuroblastoma. Prostatic carcinoma is unusual in that it favors dural metastasis to the exclusion of parenchymal invasion. Dural metastases often evoke an intense desmoplastic reaction, which may give the false impression of a meningioma on radiographic studies. Dural metastases may form either discrete, nodular masses or a thick lining of tumor on the inner aspect of the dura.

Leptomeninges

Leptomeningeal metastasis or meningeal carcinomatosis refers to diffuse involvement of the subarachnoid space by metastatic tumor and is often accompanied by perivascular infiltration of adjacent brain. Clinical signs include cranial and spinal nerve dysfunction, meningismus and headache. Diagnosis is made by demonstration of tumor cells in the CSF. Adenocarcinomas of the lung, ovary and stomach are the tumors most frequently associated with leptomeningeal spread.

Parenchyma

Metastases to the brain and spinal cord are proportional to the volume of the structures. Parenchymal metastases tend to be multiple and well circumscribed. Metastases from small cell (oat cell) carcinoma of the lung, choriocarcinoma and melanoma have a tendency to spontaneous hemorrhage. Other tumor types, such as renal cell carcinoma, may undergo cystic degeneration.

SYSTEMIC LYMPHOMA INVOLVING THE CNS

Most systemic lymphomas that involve the CNS are hematogenous metastases or direct extensions of systemic tumors. Metastases may involve the dura, leptomeninges or parenchyma, often in combination.

NON-HODGKIN'S LYMPHOMA

Lymphomatous leptomeningitis, both cerebral and spinal, is the most common pattern of neoplastic infiltration in non-Hodgkin's lymphomas. Subarachnoid infiltration is often associated with perivascular and subependymal infiltration of the parenchyma, as well as the spinal and cranial nerve roots. The optic chiasm, tuber cinereum and hypothalamus are the regions most frequently involved. The incidence of subarachnoid and parenchymal invasion of the CNS in non-Hodgkin's lymphoma is relatively high, with reported frequency varying between 6% and 29%. Large cell lymphomas (diffuse and immunoblastic), followed closely by small cell lymphomas (undifferentiated and poorly differentiated lymphocytic), are the most common types of lymphoma that spread to the CNS. Nodular or follicular lymphomas do not involve the CNS, unless they have progressed to a diffuse pattern.

Dural infiltration by non-Hodgkin's lymphomas is also common. The spinal axis is affected more frequently than the cranial cavity. Clinical signs may result from direct spinal cord compression or ischemia secondary to involvement of the spinal radicular arteries. If the dural deposits remain relatively restricted, they may be amenable to surgical removal. Most spinal epidural lymphomas are of the diffuse, small cell type, which have a relatively favorable prognosis owing to their low grade of malignancy and their responsiveness to radiation.

HODGKIN'S DISEASE

Secondary intracranial Hodgkin's disease is a rare event, with an incidence of approximately 0.5%. Metastases may be dural, in which case they are usually associated with involvement of adjacent bone, or subdural, often forming lobulated masses simulating a meningioma. Leptomeningeal infiltration occurs infrequently and intracerebral parenchymal involvement is rare.

Intraspinal epidural masses arising as extensions of adjacent bony or soft tissue deposits are the most common form of metastatic disease. The thoracic segment is most frequently affected, followed by the lumbar and cervical regions.

LEUKEMIA

The incidence of leukemic involvement of the CNS has dropped dramatically over the past 10 years, largely due to more intensive modalities of treatment. Recent figures indicate that 20% show intraparenchymal involvement. Acute leukemias have a greater tendency to involve the CNS than chronic leukemias, with acute lymphoblastic leukemia having a greater propensity than acute myeloblastic disease. Both children and adults are prone to this complication. Leukemic involvement of the CNS usually takes two forms: (1) diffuse leptomeningeal infiltration, often in combination with cranial and spinal nerve root invasion, and focal intraparenchymal and microscopic dural infiltration; and (2) massive hemorrhagic stasis and impaction of leukemic cells in blood vessels with resultant destruction of the vessel wall, hemorrhage and infarction of the central white matter. Epidural, subdural or intracerebral solid tumor deposits (myeloblastomas or 'chloromas') originating from the skull or spine have become extremely rare in recent years. Intracranial hemorrhage, either intracerebral or subarachnoid, is a frequent terminal event, accounting for death in 20% of cases. Fatal intracerebral hemorrhages are associated with intracerebral leukostasis and the development of leukemic nodules; the critical leukocyte count is approximately 100 000/mm³. Fatal subarachnoid hemorrhages are not associated with blast crises and appear to be related to thrombocytopenia.

| Skull and epidura |
| Dura |
| Leptomeninges |
| Parenchyma |

Fig. 12.87 CNS sites of preference of metastatic tumors.

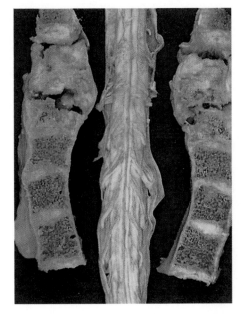

Fig. 12.88 Metastatic lung adenocarcinoma. Osseous metastases have expanded and destroyed several cervical vertebrae, with consequent flattening and distortion of the spinal cord. The subdural space was free of tumor.

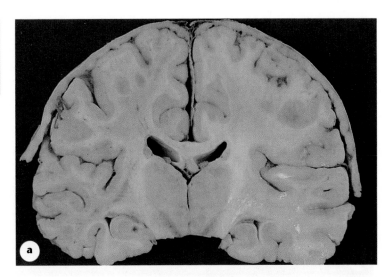

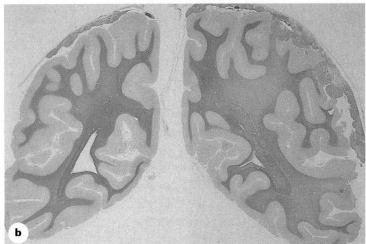

Fig. 12.89 Metastatic breast carcinoma. (**a**) Coronal section of a brain and dura shows diffuse subdural involvement by metastatic deposits. The dura is uniformly and symmetrically thickened. (**b**) Corresponding whole-mount section shows focal, direct extension of tumor into the right parietal cortex and subcortical white matter, with resultant edema evidenced by pallor of the white matter.

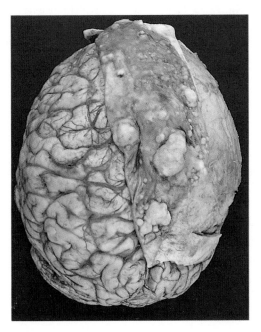

Fig. 12.90 Metastatic breast carcinoma. The dura of this specimen has been reflected to reveal multiple subdural metastatic deposits. Note the lack of discernible infiltration of the subjacent brain by tumor.

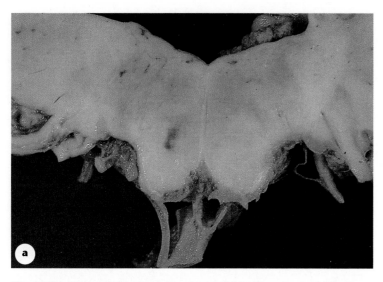

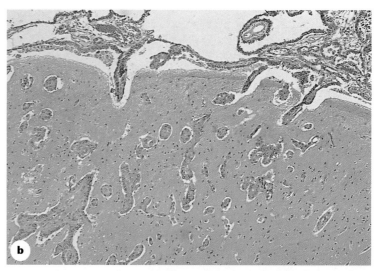

Fig. 12.91 Metastatic lung adenocarcinoma. (**a**) Leptomeningeal infiltration in this specimen is diffuse, appearing as a glassy coat. (**b**) Microscopically, in addition to infiltration of the leptomeninges, tumor extension into the cerebral cortex via perivascular (Virchow–Robin) spaces is evident.

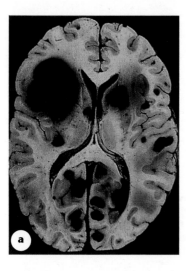

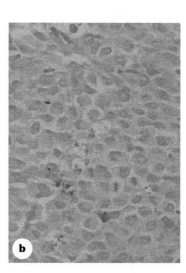

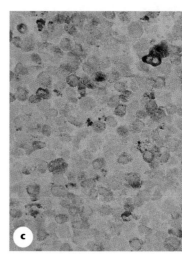

Fig. 12.92 Metastatic malignant melanoma. (**a**) Deeply pigmented, hemorrhagic metastases are characteristic. Melanin may be absent or (**b**) very sparse by H&E staining, but (**c**) is usually visible on special (Fontana) stain.

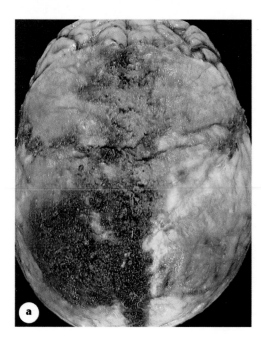

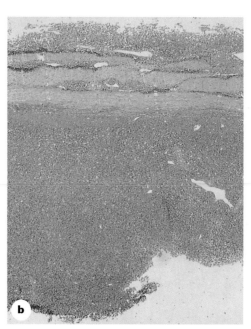

Fig. 12.93 Systemic non-Hodgkin's lymphoma involving the CNS. (**a**) This specimen shows diffuse, granular, hemorrhagic epidural and subdural tumor deposits. (**b**) On microscopy, there is extensive infiltration of the dura, together with a large, subdural accumulation of tumor. Morphologic and immunophenotypic studies were diagnostic of a B-large cell lymphoma.

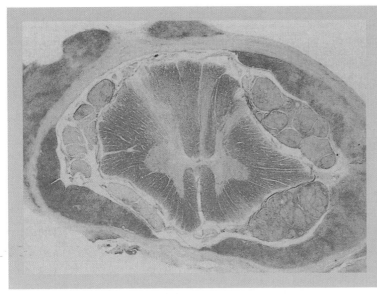

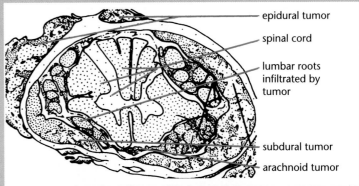

epidural tumor

spinal cord

lumbar roots infiltrated by tumor

subdural tumor

arachnoid tumor

Fig. 12.94 Systemic non-Hodgkin's lymphoma involving the CNS. Cross-sectional photomicrograph of lumbar spinal cord shows dense subdural and epidural tumor deposits and spinal root infiltration. There is also mild dorsolateral cord compression.

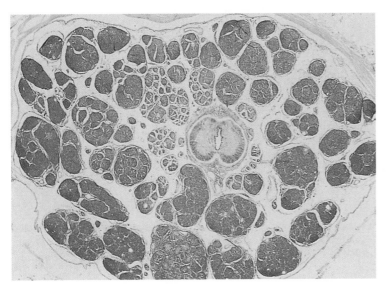

Fig. 12.95 Secondary leukemic involvement of CNS. Cross-sectional micrograph of the sacral spinal cord and cauda equina nerve roots in a 4-year-old girl with acute lymphoblastic leukemia shows dense infiltration of nerve roots by deep blue-staining leukemic cells.

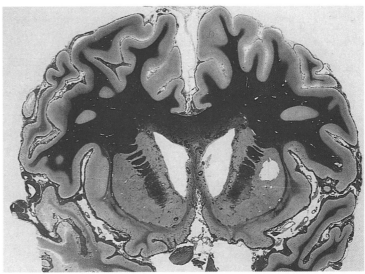

Fig. 12.96 Secondary leukemic involvement of CNS. Whole-mount coronal section from a 10-year-old boy with acute lymphoblastic leukemia demonstrate thick, subarachnoid accumulations of leukemic cells, which encase the entire neuraxis.

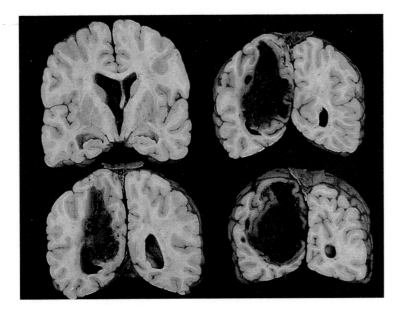

Fig. 12.97 Secondary leukemic involvement of CNS. These coronal sections of the brain of a 20-year-old man with acute myeloblastic leukemia show a large left posterior cerebral hemorrhage. Intracerebral hemorrhage is a frequent complication of non-lymphocytic forms of leukemia, perhaps secondary to associated thrombocytopenia.

REFERENCES

Alexander E, Moriarty T, Davis R, *et al.*: Stereotactic radiosurgery for the definitive noninvasive treatment of brain metastases. J Natl Cancer Inst 1995; 86:34–40.

Ashley Hill D, Pfeifer J, Marley E, *et al.*: WT1 staining reliably differentiates desmoplastic small round cell tumor from Ewing sarcoma/primitive neuroectodermal tumor: an immunohistochemical and molecular diagnostic study. Am J Clin Pathol 2000; 114:345–353.

Bondy M, Wiencke J, Wrensch M, Kyritis AP: Genetics of primary brain tumors; a review. J Neurooncol 1993; 18:69–81.

Bruner JM: Neuropathology of malignant gliomas. Semin Oncol 1994; 21:126–138.

Burger PC, Scheithauer BW, Vogel FS: Surgical Pathology of the Nervous System and Its Coverings, 3rd edn. Churchill Livingstone, New York, 1991.

Chung R, Whaley J, Kley N, *et al.*: TP53 gene mutations and 17p deletions in human astrocytomas. Genes Chromosomes Cancer 1991; 3(5):323–331.

Claesson-Welsh L: Platelet-derived growth factor receptor signals. J Biol Chem 1994; 269(51):32023–32026.

Ganju V, Jenkins RB, O'Fallon JR, *et al.*: Prognostic factors in gliomas. Cancer 1994; 74:920–927.

Greig NH, Ries LG, Yancik R, Rapoport SI: Increasing annual incidence of primary malignant brain tumors in the elderly. J Natl Cancer Inst 1990 82:1621–1624.

Harkin JC, Reed RJ: Tumors of the peripheral nervous system. In: Atlas of Tumor Pathology, 2nd ser., fasc. 3. Armed Forces Institute of Pathology, Washington, DC, 1969.

Heldin CH, Westermark B: Platelet-derived growth factor: mechanism of action and possible in vivo function. Cell Regul 1990; 1(8):555–566.

Henske EP, Ozelius L, Gusella JF, Haines JL, Kwiatkowski DJ: A high resolution linkage map of human 9q34.1. Genomics 1993; 17:587–591.

Inskip PD, Tarone RE, Hatch EE, *et al.*: Cellular telephone use and brain tumors. N Engl J Med 2001; 344:79–86.

Keeps JJ: Pleomorphic xanthoastrocytoma: the birth of a diagnosis and concept. Br Pathol 1993; 3:269–274.

Kleihues P, Cavenee WK: World Health Organization Classification of Tumours of the Nervous System. IARC/WHO, Lyon, 2000.

Kurpad SN, Wikstrand CJ, Bigner DD: Immunobiology of malignant astrocytomas. Semin Oncol 1994; 21:149–161.

LeBihan D, Jezzard P, Haxby J, *et al.*: Functional magnetic resonance imaging of the brain. Ann Intern Med 1995; 122:296–303.

Louis DN: The p53 gene and protein in human brain tumors. J Neuropathol Exp Neurol 1994; 53:11–21.

Louis DN, von Deimling A, Chung RY, *et al.*: Comparative study on p53 gene and protein alteration in human astrocytomas. J Neuropathol Exp Neurol 1993; 52:31–38.

Louis DN, Ramesh V, Gusella JF: Neuropathology and molecular genetics of neurofibromatosis 2 and related tumors. Brain Pathol 1995; 5(2):163–172.

Lucas DR, Bentley G, Dan ME, *et al.*: Ewing sarcoma vs lymphoblastic lymphoma: a comparative immunohistochemical study. Am J Clin Pathol 2001; 115:11–17.

Maher E, Fine HA: Primary CNS lymphoma. Semin Oncol 1999; 26(3):346–356.

Maher E, Furnari FB, Bachoo RM, *et al.*: Malignant glioma: genetics and biology of a grave matter. Genes and Development 2001; 15:1311–1333.

Mills SE, Frierson HF Jr: Olfactory neuroblastoma: a clinicopathological study of 21 cases. Am J Surg Pathol 1985; 9:317–327.

Neglia JP, Meadows AT, Robison LL, *et al.*: Second neoplasms after acute lymphoblastic leukemia in childhood. N Engl J Med 1991; 325:1330–1336.

Okazaki H, Scheithauer BW: Atlas of Neuropathology. Lippincott/Gower Medical Publishing, New York/Philadelphia, 1988.

Ron E, Modan B, Boice JD, *et al.*: Tumors of the brain and nervous system and radiotherapy in childhood. N Engl J Med 1988; 319:1033–1039.

Rubinstein LJ: Tumors of the central nervous system. In: Atlas of Tumor Pathology, 2nd ser., fasc. 6. Armed Forces Institute of Pathology, Washington, DC, 1972.

Russell DS, Rubinstein LJ: Pathology of Tumors of the Nervous System, 5th edn. Williams and Wilkins, Baltimore, MD, 1989.

Schochet SS Jr, Peters B, O'Neal J, McCormick WF: Intracranial esthesioneuroblastoma: a light and electron microscopic study. Act Neuropathol (Berlin) 1975: 31:181–189.

Smith J, Tachibana I, Passe S, *et al.*: PTEN mutation, EGFR amplification and outcome in patients with anaplastic astrocytoma and glioblastoma multiforme. J Natl Cancer Inst 2001; 93:1246–1256.

Stuart ET, Kioussi C, Aguzzi A, *et al.*: PAX5 expression correlates with increasing malignancy in human astrocytomas. Clin Cancer Res 1995; 1:207–214.

The European Chromosome 16 Tuberous Sclerosis Consortium: Identification and characterization of the tuberous sclerosis gene on chromosome 16. Cell 1993; 75:1305–1315.

Ueki K, Ono Y, Henson JW, Efird JT, von Deimling A, Louis DN: CDKN2/p16 or RB alterations occur in the majority of glioblastomas and are inversely correlated. Cancer Res 1996; 56(1):150–153.

von Deimling A, Eibl RH, Ohgaki H, Louis DN, von Ammon K, Petersen I, Kleihues P, Chung RY, Wiestler OD, Seizinger BR p53 mutations are associated with 17p allelic loss in grade II and grade III astrocytoma. Cancer Res 1992 May 15; 52(10):2987–90.

Watkins D, Rouleau GA: Genetics, prognosis and therapy of central nervous system tumors. Cancer Detection Prev 1994; 18:139–144.

Wong AJ, Zoltick PW, Moscatello DK: The molecular biology and molecular genetics of astrocytic neoplasms. Semin Oncol 1994; 21:139–148.

Zulch KJ: Brain Tumors, 3rd edn. Springer-Verlag, New York, 1986.

FIGURE CREDITS

The following books published by Gower Medical Publishing are sources of figures in the present chapter. The figure numbers given in the listing are those of the figures in the present chapter. The page numbers given in parentheses are those of the original publication.

Hawke M, Jahn AF: Diseases of the Ear: Clinical and Pathologic Aspects. Lea and Febiger/Gower Medical Publishing, New York/Philadelphia, 1987: Fig. 12.78 (p. 5.42).

Okazaki H, Scheithauer BW: Atlas of Neuropathology. Lippincott/Gower Medical Publishing, New York/Philadelphia, 1988: Figs 12.2 (p. 60), 12.3 (p. 62), 12.4 (p. 65), 12.6 (p. 65), 12.7 (p. 65), 12.9 (p. 75), 12.10 (p. 67), 12.13 (p. 69), 12.14 (p. 69), 12.15 (p. 70), 12.16 (p. 86), 12.17 (p. 77), 12.18 (p. 82), 12.19 (p. 82), 12.20 (p. 89), 12.22 (p. 90), 12.23 (p. 91), 12.24 (p. 93), 12.26 (p. 93), 12.27 (p. 94), 12.29 (p. 103), 12.30 (p. 103), 12.31 (p. 109), 12.32 (p. 113), 12.33 (p. 114), 12.34 (p. 110), 12.35 (p. 111), 12.36a,b (p. 111), 12.36c,d (p. 112), 12.37 (p. 114), 12.38 (p. 115), 12.39 (p. 116), 12.40 (p. 116), 12.41 (p. 116), 12.42 (p. 121), 12.44 (p. 126), 12.45 (p. 126), 12.46 (p. 130), 12.47 (p. 130), 12.48 (p. 131), 12.49 (p. 131), 12.50 (p. 131), 12.51 (p. 133), 12.52a,b (p. 134), 12.52c (p. 135), 12.53a–c (p. 135), 12.54 (p. 98), 12.55 (p. 99), 12.56 (p. 99), 12.57 (p. 99), 12.58 (p. 139), 12.59a (p. 140), 12.59b (p. 141), 12.60 (p. 148), 12.61 (p. 149), 12.63 (p. 142), 12.64 (p. 142), 12.65 (p. 143), 12.66 (p. 143), 12.67 (p. 146), 12.68 (p. 151), 12.69A,B (p. 151), 12.69c,d (p. 152), 12.70 (p. 154), 12.71 (p. 154), 12.72 (p. 155), 12.73 (p. 156), 12.74 (p. 157), 12.75 (p. 157), 12.76 (p. 157), 12.77 (p. 158), 12.79 (p. 183), 12.80 (p. 184), 12.81 (p. 184), 12.82 (p. 198), 12.83 (p. 199), 12.84a–d (p. 198), 12.84e (p. 199), 12.85 (p. 192), 10.86 (p. 192), 10.87 (p. 193), 10.89 (p. 165), 10.90 (p. 167), 10.91 (p. 167), 10.92 (p. 169), 10.93 (p. 171), 10.94 (p. 174), 10.95 (p. 177), 10.96 (p. 178), 10.97 (p. 178), 10.98 (p. 179).

Acute and chronic leukemias

David M. Dorfman, Arthur T. Skarin

13

ACUTE LEUKEMIAS

Acute leukemias are neoplastic disorders marked by uncontrolled proliferation of hematopoietic cells, with a predominance of immature lymphoid or myeloid cells, in the bone marrow and peripheral blood. Although leukemic cells do not divide more rapidly than normal marrow cells, they possess a growth advantage because the blasts fail to differentiate in response to normal hormonal signals and cellular interactions. The malignant cells eventually replace the marrow and invade other tissues and organs, leading to manifestations of the disease. Production of normal erythrocytes, granulocytes and megakaryocytes is diminished, resulting in anemia, infection and hemorrhage.

Approximately 13 000 cases of acute leukemia occur in the United States each year. The incidence increases with age. About 80% of leukemic children have acute lymphoblastic leukemia (ALL), the most common childhood malignant neoplasm, while 80% of adults with leukemia have acute non-lymphocytic leukemia (ANLL). The known etiologies include: chromosomal damage from ionizing radiation, chemicals (e.g. benzene and alkylating agents used in therapy), congenital disease (e.g. Down's syndrome), and chronic bone marrow diseases (e.g. myeloid metaplasia), congenital predisposition (e.g. identical twins with leukemia) and congenital immunodeficiency syndromes (e.g. ataxia-telangiectasia).

MORPHOLOGY AND BIOLOGY

Acute leukemias (defined as ≥20% blasts in blood/or bone marrow under the new World Health Organization (WHO) criteria) are classified according to the predominant neoplastic cell line, and thus may be designated as lymphoblastic or non-lymphoblastic (myeloblastic/monocytic). They are subclassified according to the French–American–British (FAB) study group by morphologic and histochemical criteria (*see* Table 13.1). Cytogenic findings are included in the new WHO classification. About 70–80% of cases can be classified on the basis of morphology alone, whereas an additional 10–15% of cases require histochemical determinations for specific diagnosis. In approximately 10% of cases, surface marker and cytogenetic studies are necessary for accurate classification, particularly in the 'undifferentiated' acute leukemias. Use of monoclonal antibodies has revealed that about 20% of cases of acute lymphoblastic leukemia are of T-cell origin; most of the remainder are of B-cell or pre-B cell origin (*see* Table 13.3).

Development of colony assays and new monoclonal antibodies has led to a clearer understanding of normal myeloid ontogeny. The patterns of expression of a variety of antigens during normal myeloid differentiation have been established. Immunophenotyping techniques have demonstrated that some cases of acute 'undifferentiated' leukemia, or those considered on the basis of morphology to be ALL, exhibit myeloid markers. Improvement of cytogenetic studies by the use of new banding techniques has revealed that almost all acute leukemias are characterized by chromosomal abnormalities, ranging from hypoploidy to polyploidy. Significant cytogenetic defects that have prognostic importance (e.g. are seen only with certain subgroups) have been identified, involving the acute lymphoblastic as well as the acute non-lymphocytic leukemias. Genetic abnormalities in the acute leukemias can affect genes for proteins involved in signal transduction, transcription regulation, cellular differentiation and apoptosis, as well as tumor suppression (antioncogenes).

In about 10% of adults with ALL, cytogenetic studies will show the presence of the Philadelphia chromosome (t (9;22) (q34; q11)). These Ph-positive patients tend to be older (median age 46 years vs 35 years), have a lower incidence of anemia and higher incidence of leukocytosis than Ph-negative patients (Preti *et al.*, 1994). Ph-positive ALL patients are also likely to have FAB-L2 morphology (*see* Table 13.1), to be CALLA (CD10) positive and CD34 positive, and have a worse prognosis than Ph-negative ALL cases. In a small number of patients with ALL and ANLL who are Ph negative, molecular studies (e.g. polymerase chain reaction) will reveal the presence of bcr-abl transcripts diagnostic of the Philadelphia chromosome abnormality not otherwise detected because of insufficient metaphases (Kantanjian *et al.*, 1994).

CLINICAL MANIFESTATIONS

Patients may present with a variety of clinical manifestations, which correlate with the degree of marrow and other organ involvement. Among the more common symptoms are fatigue, bruisability, oral lesions, fever and infection. Perirectal infections are particularly frequent in ANLL and skin and gum infiltrates are seen mainly in acute moncytic leukemias. Joint swelling and bone pain with rheumatic symptoms occur commonly in ALL, which may also present as a meningitis-like syndrome. Diffuse lymphadenopathy and hepatosplenomegaly are more common in ALL (about 50% of cases) than in ANLL.

In patients with ANLL, unusual masses in soft tissues, nodal sites or other areas may appear, representing collections of extramedullary immature myeloid cells. These lesions may precede overt marrow and peripheral blood invasion (and thus the diagnosis of ANLL) and may be mistaken for lymphoma or metastatic carcinoma. When they are localized, these extramedullary leukemic infiltrates have been called myeloblastomas; the older term, granulocytic sarcoma, is inappropriate. Another term, chloroma, has been used when the tumor appears green colored, owing to the presence in the leukemic cells of enzymes capable of metabolizing heme products; the green color rapidly disappears after oxidation on exposure to air. Myeloblastomas can occur anywhere, but the most common sites are soft tissues, skin, periosteum, bone and lymph nodes. Diagnosis can be rapidly established on a touch prep stained with Wright–Giemsa and examined for Auer rods or azurophilic granules. The latter are peroxidase and specific-esterase positive.

HEMATOLOGIC DISORDERS WITH A TENDENCY TO LEUKEMIC TRANSFORMATION

MYELODYSPLASTIC SYNDROMES

The myelodysplastic syndromes (MDS) are a group of disorders that primarily occur in the elderly, who present with an anemia that proves refractory to treatment, with progressive neutropenia and thrombocytopenia, or with various combinations of these. In the past these syndromes, particularly those with normal numbers of blasts (< 5%) in the marrow, have been referred to as 'preleukemia'. To varying degrees, there is a tendency to progression to acute leukemia, ranging from progression in approximately 10% of cases of refractory anemia and refractory anemia with ringed sideroblasts to progression in greater than 40% of cases of refractory anemia with excess blasts.

Classification and cytogenetics

The myelodysplastic syndromes have been classified into five subgroups (*see* Fig. 13.54). The blood film abnormalities in each subgroup are highly variable, although general features include macrocytic red cells, qualitative granulocytic and monocytic changes, and giant platelets. Whereas patients with refractory anemia may show no gross changes in blood morphology, patients with refractory anemia with ringed sideroblasts frequently exhibit a dimorphic red cell population. Leukoerythroblastic changes are common in patients with refractory anemia with excess blasts. 'Chronic myelomonocytic leukemia', a diagnostic entity often included with the myelodysplastic syndromes, is marked by abnormal myelomonocytic cells and monocytosis of greater than 1.0×10^9/l, with or without splenomegaly. A former category, RAEB-T, is no longer an entity under the WHO classification and is considered a progression to acute myeloid leukemia.

The bone marrow in the myelodysplastic syndromes is typically hypercellular and shows morphologic abnormalities, often in all three series of hematopoietic cells. Cytogenetic abnormalities are common, particularly in secondary MDS (related to prior radiotherapy or therapy with alkylating agents). They include –5 or –5q, –7 or –7q, –20 or –20q, +8 and –9q. Patients with complex cytogenetic abnormalities (the most common chromosomal abnormality observed) or –7 or –7q typically have an aggressive clinical course. There is usually evidence of dyserythropoiesis with nuclear atypia, some megaloblastosis and ringed sideroblasts. In some cases, reticulin is increased, while occasional cases are hypocellular. Granulocytic abnormalities include hypogranular or agranular myelocytes, metamyelocytes and neutrophils, pseudo Pelger–Huet cells and hypersegmented or polypoid neutrophils. Megakaryocyte abnormalities include small mononuclear or binuclear forms or large megakaryocytes with multiple, round nuclei and large granules in the cytoplasm. In the more advanced myelodysplastic syndromes, the blast cell population is also increased, but by definition these cells constitute less than 20% of the marrow cell total. When the level of blast cells exceeds this figure, it is assumed that a transformation to acute myeloblastic leukemia has occurred.

Clinical manifestations

Clinically, patients present with symptoms related to bone marrow failure, with frequent episodes of infection and with bleeding abnormalities. These complications of severe neutropenia or thrombocytopenia result in death in many patients, but in others the disease progresses to frank acute myeloblastic leukemia. Typically, the liver, spleen and lymph nodes are not enlarged. Gum hypertrophy and skin deposits do not usually occur.

POLYCYTHEMIA VERA AND MYELOFIBROSIS

Transformation is generally accepted as part of the natural history of the myeloproliferative syndrome. Polycythemia vera undergoes transformation to myelofibrosis in approximately 30% of cases and to acute leukemia, usually AML, in about half that number. There is a similar incidence of leukemia in patients treated with ^{32}P or chemotherapy. Myelofibrosis undergoes leukemic transformation in 20% of patients. Survival after the transition to leukemia in either condition is brief.

ACUTE MYELOFIBROSIS

Patients with this syndrome present acutely with symptoms due to anemia, neutropenia or thrombocytopenia. Peripheral blood examination reveals leukoerythroblastic changes and needle biopsy of bone marrow shows evidence of myelofibrosis; attempts at marrow aspiration are usually unsuccessful. In typical cases, the features of the blast cells indicate that a transformation to the megakaryoblastic variant (M7) or AML has occurred; transformation to lymphoma has also been reported. Other diagnostic possibilities include agnogenic myeloid metaplasia in acute transformation and AML other than M7 with fibrosis. The majority of patients do not have gross splenomegaly. This acute syndrome has a poor prognosis (see section on Chronic Leukemias).

Table 13.1 Morphologic classification of acute leukemias.

Proposed WHO classifications of acute myeloid leukemias	Acute non-lymphoblastic leukemias	
	Designation	Morphology
AMLs with recurrent cytogenetic translocations		
• AML with t(8,21)(q22;q22), AML1(CBF-α/ETO)	M0	Myelobalastic, without maturation, minimally differentiated
• Acute promyelocytic leukemia (AML with t(15;17)(q22;q11–12) and variants, PML/RAR-α)		
• AML with abnormal bone marrow eosinophils (inv(16)(p13q22)ort(16;16)(p13;q11), CBF/MYH11X)	M1	Myelobastic, without maturation
• AML with 11q23(MLL) abnormalities	M2	Myeloblastic, with maturation
AML with multilineage dysplasia	M3	Promyelocytic
• With prior myelodysplastic syndrome		
• Without prior myelodysplastic syndrome	M4	Myelomonocytic
AML and myelodysplastic syndromes, therapy related	M5	Monocytic
• Alkylating agent related		
• Topoisomerase II related	M6	Erythroleukemia
AML not otherwise categorized	M7	Megakaryoblastic
• AML minimally differentiated (MO)		
• AML without maturation (MI)		
• AML with maturation (M2)		
• Acute myelomonocytic leukemia (M4)		
• Acute monocytic leukemia (M5)		
• Acute erythroid leukemia (M6)		
• Acute megakaryocytic leukemia (M7)		
• Acute basophilic leukemia		
• Acute panmyelosis with myelofibrosis		
Acute biphenotypic leukemias		
Proposed WHO classification of acute lymphoid leukemias*		
• B-cell neoplasms		
Precursor B-cell lymphoblastic leukemia/lymphoma		
• T-cell neoplasms		
Precursor T-cell lymphoblastic leukemia/lymphoma		

*Adapted from Harris *et al.* (1999).

According to the French–American–British (FAB) classification, acute lymphoblastic leukemias (ALL) are divided into three morphologic types (L1–L3); the morphology of acute non-lymphoblastic (myeloblastic) leukemias (ANLL) comprises eight types (M0–M7). A number of acute leukemias may display both lymphoid and myeloid (biphenotypic) characteristics or may be composed of a heterogeneous population of both lymphoid and myeloid (biclonal) cells; both situations are classified as acute mixed lineage leukemia

Table 13.2 Morphologic criteria for lymphoblastic leukemic cells

Cytologic features	LI (small cell)	L2 (large and small cell)	L3 (Burkitt's cell type)
Cell size	Predominance of small cells	Large; heterogeneous in size	Medium; homogeneous
Nuclear chomatin	Homogeneous in any one case	Variable; heterogeneous in any one case	Finely stippled; homogeneous
Nuclear shape	Regular; occasional clefting or indentation	Irregular; clefting and indentation common	Regular; oval to round
Nucleoli	Not visible or small, inconspicuous	One or more present; often large	Prominent; one or more vesicular
Amount of cytoplasm	Scanty	Variable; often moderately abundant	Small to moderate
Basophilia of cytoplasm	Slight or moderate; rarely intense	Variable; deep in some cases	Very deep
Cytoplasmic vacuolation	Variable	Variable	Often prominent

Table 13.3 Immunologic classification of acute lymphoblastic leukemias (ALL).

Subtype/Translocation	Molecular alteration	Frequency (%)	FAB type	HLA-DR	CALLA	CD19/CD20	c	Sig	T cell	TdT
B-precursor ALL			L1,L2	+	+/−	+−/+	+	−	−	+
t(12;21)(p13;q22)	TEL-AML1	20–25								
t(1;19)(q23;p13.3)	E2A-PBX1	5–6								
t(17;19)(q22;p13.3)	E2A-HLF	<1								
t(9;22)(q34;q11)	BCR-ABL	4								
t(4;11)(q21;q23)	MLL-AF4	4								
Other 11q23	Other MLL fusions	1								
t(5;14(q31;q32)	IL-3 dysregulation	<1								
B-cell ALL		2	L3	+	+	+/+	−	+	−	−
t(8;14)(q24;q32)	MYC dysregulation									
t(2;8)(q12;q24)										
t(8;22)(q24;q11)										
T-cell ALL		8	L1,L2	−	−/−	−/−	−	−	+	+
t(1;14)(p32;q11)	TAL1 dysregulation									
t(1;7)(p32;q35)	TAL1 dysregulation									
t(7;9)(q34;q32)	TAL2 dysregulation									
t(7;19)(q34;p13)	LYL1 dysregulation									
t(10;14)(q24;q11)	HOX11 dysregulation									
t(7;10)(q35;q24)	HOX11 dysregulation									
t(11;14)(p15;q11)	LMO1 dysregulation									
t(7;11)(q35;p13)	LMO2 dysregulation									
t(11;14)(p13;q11)	LMO2 dysregulation									
t(1;7)(p34;q34)	LCK dysregulation									
t(7;9)(q34;q34)	TAN1 dysregulation									

*In children (Data from Pui *et al.*, 1993)

**Additional cytogenic abnormalities include hyperdiploidy with >50 chromosomes (favorable prognostic factor), hyperdiploidy with 47–50 chromosomes, and hypodiploidy (unfavorable prognostic factor). The presence of t(9; 22) or T(4; 11) is associated with poor prognosis as well.

Key: HLA-DR, also Ia antigen; CALLA, common ALL antigen (CD10); CD19, B4 antigen; CD20, BI antigen; Sig, surface immunologlobulin (IgM); T cell, Markers include CD7 and CD2; TdT, terminal deoxynucleotidyl transferase.

About 80% of children have non-I cell ALL (early pre-B and pre-B cell types) derived from early B-cell progeny. In adults, 20% of leukemias are pre-B cell ALL, expressing HLA-DR (Ia), CD19 (B4), CD10 (CALLA=common ALL angtigen) and CD20 (B1) antigens; expression of surface immunoglobulin (sIg) marks B-cell acute leukemia (FAB type L3), which is also called Burkitt's type. T-cell acute leukemias are heterogeneous, but most express early stage I thymocyte markers. Terminal deoxynucleotidyl transferase (TdT) is also positive in T-cell ALL, as well as in some non-B cell types. Cytogenetic abnormalities include the Ph chromosome in some cases of undifferentiated or common ALL and t(8;14) and t(8;22) in B-cell ALL. Compared with other types, B- and T-cell ALLs are high-risk leukemias, although modern intensive therapy has improved the prognosis.

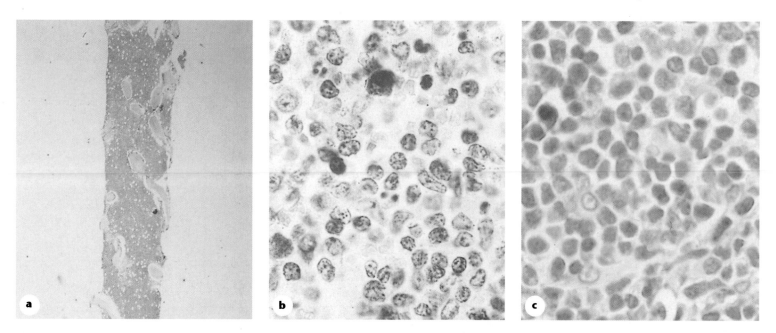

Fig. 13.1 Acute lymphoblastic leukemia (L1, T-cell subtype). (**a**) Low magnification of a bone marrow core biopsy shows a markedly hypercellular marrow (Giemsa stain). (**b**) At high magnification, convoluted lymphoblasts can be seen; the small to intermediate-sized cells exhibit a characteristic irregular or cerebriform nuclear outline, finely dispersed chromatin and scant cytoplasm. The nucleolus is typically indistinct (Giemsa stain). (**c**) Lymphoblasts stain positively with hematoxylin and eosin. Immunophenotyping showed positivity for CD5 (T1), CD4 (T4), CD8 (T8) and CD2 (T11).

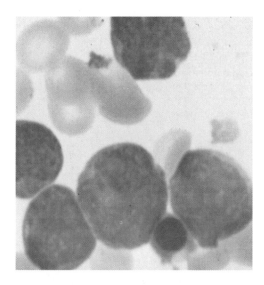

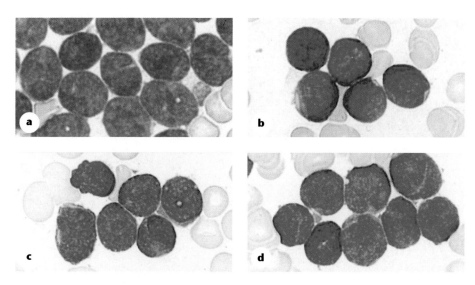

Fig. 13.2 Acute lymphoblastic leukemia (L1, T-cell subtype). High-power view of a bone marrow aspirate reveals small lymphoblasts with scanty cytoplasm and indistinct nucleoli. The nuclear contours in many of the cells are convoluted or cerebriform.

Fig. 13.3 Acute lymphoblastic leukemia (L1, CALLA (CD10) positive pre-B subtype). (**a–d**) Lymphoblasts are rather small and uniform, with scanty cytoplasm and rounded or cleft nuclei, which may have one, indistinct nucleolus.

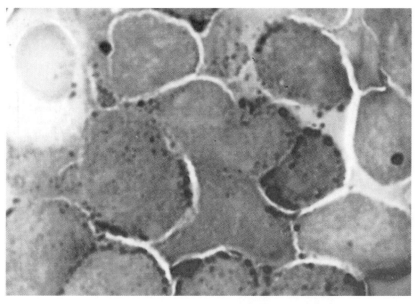

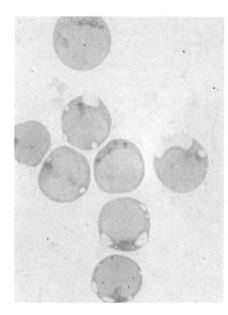

Fig. 13.5 Acute lymphoblastic leukemia (L1, T-cell subtype). Red staining of the cytoplasm in this bone marrow aspirate, with marked coloration of the Golgi zone adjacent to or indented into the nucleus, supports a diagnosis of T-cell ALL. However, this occurs in only 50–75% of cases (acid phosphatase stain).

Fig. 13.4 Acute lymphoblastic leukemia (L1, CALLA (CD10) positive pre-B cell subtype). This bone marrow aspirate shows cells with numerous coarse cytoplasmic granules or blocks staining positive with PAS. Seen in about 80% of cases, these findings are diagnostic of ALL. By contrast, myeloblasts may have small, fine-staining granules.

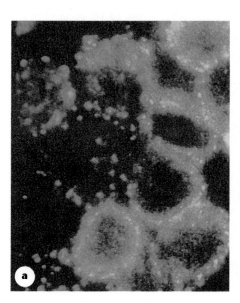

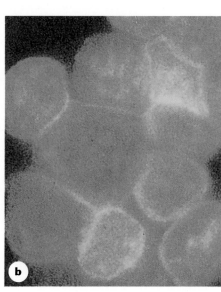

Fig. 13.6 Acute lymphoblastic leukemia (L1, T-cell subtype). Indirect immunofluorescence microscopy of bone marrow aspirates demonstrates (**a**) red staining cell membrane T antigen and (**b**) green staining nuclear TdT. (Courtesy of Prof. G. Janossy.)

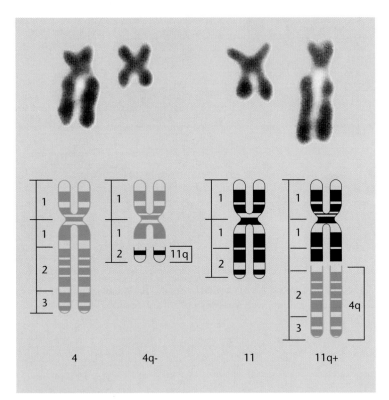

Fig. 13.7 Acute lymphoblastic leukemia (L1 subtype). This partial karyotype of G-banded chromosomes 4 and 11 (above) was obtained from a patient with blasts of 'null' phenotype (TdT positive, CALLA (CD10) negative). The translocated chromosomes are on the right in each pair. The corresponding diagrams (below) represent a systematized description of the structural aberration. (Courtesy of Dr L.M. Secker-Walker.)

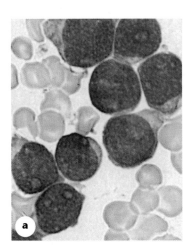
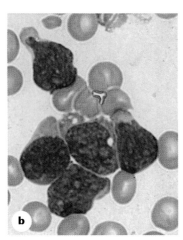
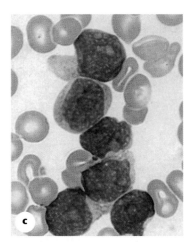

Fig. 13.8 Acute lymphoblastic leukemia (L2 subtype). (**a–c**) Blast cells in these peripheral blood smears vary considerably in size and amount of cytoplasm; the nucleus-to-cytoplasm ratio is rarely as high as in the L1 subtype. The nuclei are of various shapes and often contain multiple nucleoli.

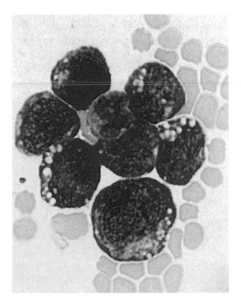

Fig. 13.9 Acute lymphoblastic leukemia (L3 subtype). The deeply staining, blue cytoplasm of these blast cells contains many small, perinuclear vacuoles; prominent nucleoli are commonly seen. This appearance is associated with B-cell ALL. Identical cells are seen in Burkitt's small non-cleaved cell leukemia/lymphoma.

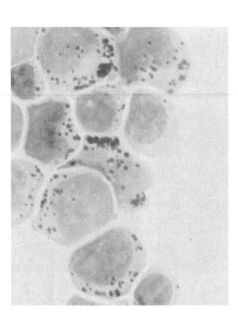

Fig. 13.10 Acute lymphoblastic leukemia (L3 subtype). Bone marrow aspirate stained with oil red-O shows prominent cytoplasmic lipid collections corresponding to some of the vacuoles shown by Romanowsky staining (*see* Fig. 13.9).

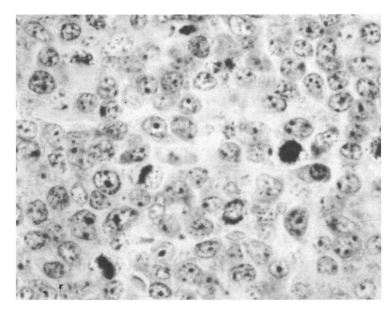

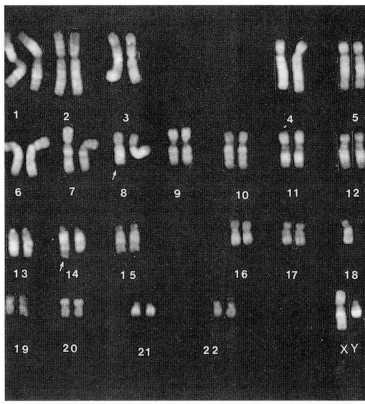

Fig. 13.11 Acute lymphoblastic leukemia (L3 subtype). Bone marrow core biopsy of a markedly hypercellular marrow containing small to intermediate-size cells with one or more distinct nucleoli. Multiple mitotic figures are seen (Giemsa stain).

Fig. 13.12 Acute lymphoblastic leukemia (L3, Burkitt's leukemia/lymphoma). This Q-banded karyotype shows 46;XY, t(8;14) (q24;q23). (Courtesy of Ramana Tantravahi PhD, Dana-Farber Cancer Institute, Boston, MA.)

Table 13.4 Proposed risk classification of ALL			
Risk group	**Features**	**Patients affected (%)**	**Recommended therapy (1998)**
Low risk	1. Hyperdiploid (DI>1.16)	20	Conventional anti-metabolite based
	2. *TEL-AML1* fusion	20	
Intermediate risk	Standard-risk[a] age/leukocyte count without genetic risk features	15	Intensified anti-metabolite based
High-risk	1. *E2A-PBX1* fusion	6	
	2. T-cell ALL	15	Intensive chemotherapy
	3. High-risk[a] age/leukocyte count without genetic risk features	15	
Very high risk	1. *BCR-ABL* fusion with high WBC	3	
	2. *MLL* rearrangement	4	Allogeneic bone marrow transplantation in first remission
	3. Induction failures	2	

ALL, acute lymphoblastic leukemia; DI, DNA Index; WBC, white blood cell count.

[a]Standard- and high-risk refer to National Cancer Institute criteria.

Adapted from Rubnitz and Look, 1998.

Table 13.5 Classification of acute non-lymphoblastic (myeloblastic) leukemias (ANLL)

Subtype	FAB type	Frequency (%)[b]	Morphology	MP	SE	NSE	Immune markers	Cytogenetic abnormalities[c]	Genes involved
Acute myeloblastic leukemia with minimal differentiation	MO	3	Rare granules no Auer rodes	–	–	–	CD 11, CD13, CD33 HLA-DR	inv (3q26), t(3;3)	EVII
Acute myeloblastic leukemia (AML) without maturation	M1	15–20	A few azurophilic granules or Auer rods	+[g]	+/–	–	CD11, CD13, CD33 HLA-DR	t(9;22) +8 t(v;11)[f] –7e –5 or 5q	
AML with maturation	M2	25–30	Some maturation beyond promyelocytes; Auer rods	++	++	–	CD11, CD13, CD33 HLA-DR	t(8;21)[d] t(9;22),t(6;9) +8 –7e –5 or–5q	AMLI-ETO DEK-CAN
Acute promyelocytic leukemia (APL)	M3	5–10	Hypergranular promyelocytes; multiple Auer rods	+++	+++	–	CD11, CD13, CD33	t(915;17) t(11;17) t(5;17)	PML-RAR PLZF-RAR NPM-RAR
Acute myelomonocytic leukemia (AMML)	M4	20	≥20% monocytes; monocytoid cells in blood; Auer rods	++	++	++	CD11, CD13, CD14, CD 33 HLA-DR	11q23 inv (3q26), t(3;3)EVI t(6;9) +8 –7 –5 or 5q	MLL DEK-CAN
	*M4E	5–10	Eosinophilia; early eosinophils with large purple granules	++	++	++	CD2, CD13, CD14, CD33 HLA-DR	inv(16)[d], del(16)(q22) t(16;16)d	CBF-MYHII
Acute monocytic leukemia (AMOL)	M5	2–9	Monoblastic (M5A) Promonocytic (M5B), no Auer rods	–	–	+++	CD11, CD13, CD14, CD33 HLA-DR	11q23 t(8;16) +8	
Erythroleukemia	M6	3–5	Predominance of erythroblasts; dyserythropoiesis; Auer rods in myeloblasts	+	–	–	CD33, Glycophorin A	+8 –7e –5 or 5q	MLL MOZ-CBP
Acute megakaryoblastic leukemia	M7	3–12	'Dry' aspirate; biopsy with blasts and dysplastic megakaryocytes; no Auer rods	–	–	–	CD33, CD41, CD61 HLA-DR	t(1;22) –7e –5or 5q	

[a] Findings may be somewhat variable

[b] In adults (data from Cowenberg et al., 1999)

[c] Complex chromosome defects may be seen in M0, M1, M2, M4–M7

[d] Associated with a more favorable prognosis

[e] Associated with a less favorable prognosis

[g] More than 3% blasts positive

* Eosinophilic variant of M4

Key: MP, myeloperoxidase; SE, specific esterase (chloracetate); NSE, non-specific esterase (naphthylbutyrate);-, negative; +/–, equivocal;+, positive; ++, moderately positive +++, very positive.

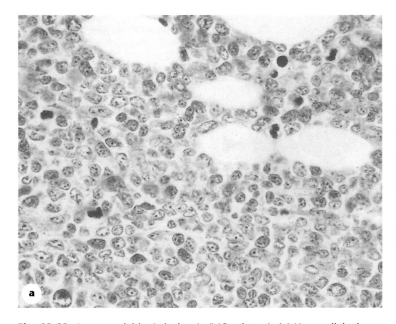

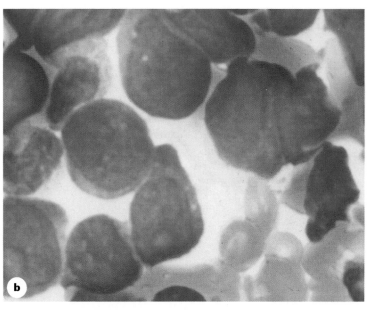

Fig. 13.13 Acute myeloblastic leukemia (MO subtype). (**a**) Hypercellular bone marrow biopsy composed of myeloblasts with minimal differentiation. The blasts were negative for Auer rods and histochemical markers of AML, but were positive for myeloid differentiation markers (CD13, CD33) by flow cytometric examination (Giemsa stain). (**b**) Bone marrow aspiration smear from same case showing blasts with prominent nucleoli and basophilic cytoplasm without any granules (×1000; Wright–Giemsa stain).

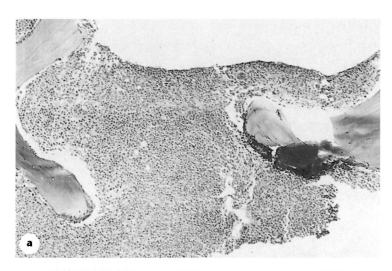

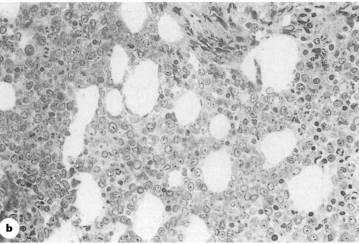

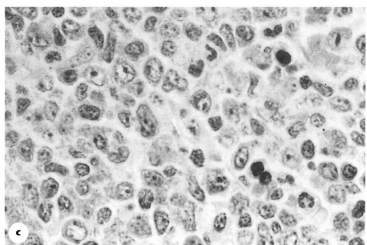

Fig. 13.14 Acute myeloblastic leukemia (M1 subtype). (**a**) Acute leukemia is marked by replacement of the normal bone marrow by blasts. In this instance, the cellularity is 99%, whereas normal cellularity is about 50%, with fat representing the remaining 50%. Rare cases of 'hypocellular' ANLL have been described in which the background fat is normal or increased. (**b,c**) At higher magnification, characteristic myeloblasts can be seen exhibiting predominantly round nuclear outlines, distinct nucleoli (often centrally located) and a moderate amount of cytoplasm). Distinct red-pink cytoplasmic granules are occasionally noted (Giemsa stain).

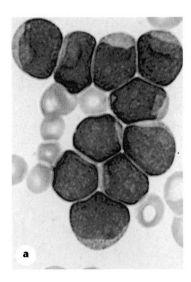
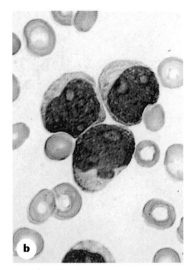
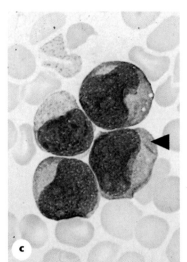

Fig. 13.15 Acute myeloblastic leukemia (M1 subtype). These bone marrow aspirates show blasts with large, often irregular nuclei having one or more nucleoli. (**a,b**) Typical type 1 blasts contain loose, open chromatin with distinct nucleoli and immature cytoplasm without granules. (**c**) Type II blasts are similar but contain up to 15 delicate cytoplasmic azurophilic granules and an occasional Auer rod (arrow). At least 3% of cells stain by Sudan black or myeloperoxidase.

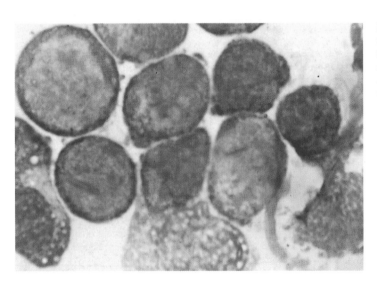

Fig. 13.16 Acute myeloblastic leukemia (M1 subtype). Peroxidase staining (Kaplan method) of a bone marrow aspirate shows many Auer rods and early azurophilic granules (golden color) in myeloblasts.

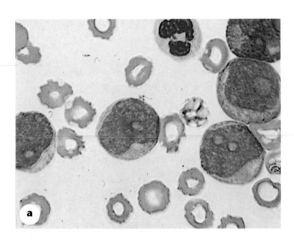
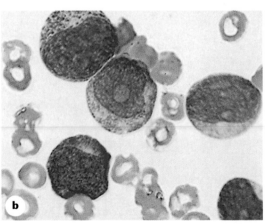

Fig. 13.17 Acute myeloblastic leukemia with maturation (M2 subtype). (**a,b**) Type III blasts, which predominate in this subtype, have relatively numerous azurophilic granules but still lack a Golgi area. Auer rods may be present. A characteristic t(8;21) chromosomal abnormality is usually present (see Fig. 13.18).

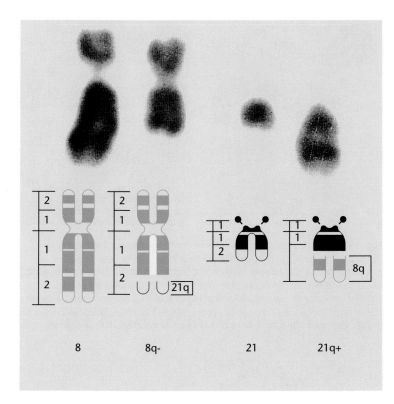

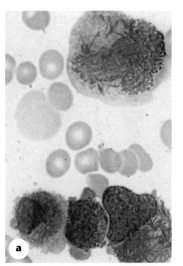

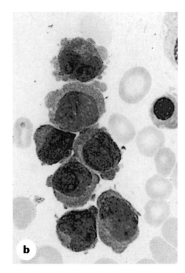

Fig. 13.18 Acute myeloblastic leukemia with maturation (M2 subtype). A partial karyotype of G-banded chromosomes 8 and 21 is shown above. The translocated chromosomes are on the right in each pair. The corresponding diagrams below represent a systematized description of the structural aberration. (Courtesy of Dr L.M. Secker-Walker.)

Fig. 13.19 Acute promyelocytic leukemia (M3 subtype). (**a,b**) Promyelocytes contain coarse, azurophilic granules and Auer rods, which stain similarly to the granules. The nuclei have one or two nucleoli. A prominent Golgi area is noted in most cells. This subtype is associated with chromosomal rearrangement t(15;17) (*see* Fig. 13.22). A serious complication of M3 ANLL is bleeding due in part to release of tissue factors from the blasts, leading to disseminated intravascular coagulation.

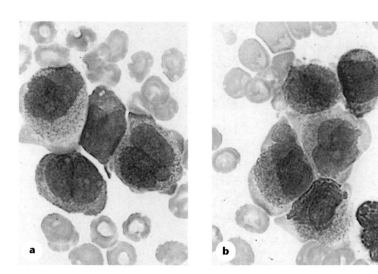

Fig. 13.20 Acute promyelocytic leukemia (M3 subtype, microgranular variant). The usually bilobar cells contain many small, azurophilic granules. In some cases, the cells resemble monocytes ('pseudomonocytic leukemia'), but peroxidase and specific esterase stains are strongly positive, confirming a diagnosis of M3 ANLL. Non-specific esterase is negative.

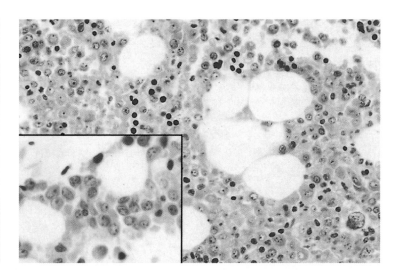

Fig. 13.21 Acute promyelocytic leukemia (M3 subtype). High-power photomicrograph of a bone marrow core biopsy shows abundant promyelocytes intermixed with occasional erythroid elements and megakaryocytes. (Inset) Characteristically, promyelocytes exhibit abundant pink cytoplasm and an eccentric nucleus. Diagnostic Auer rods may occasionally be seen.

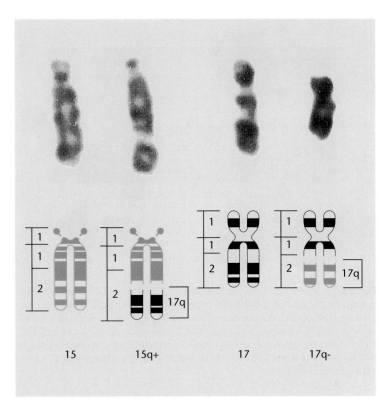

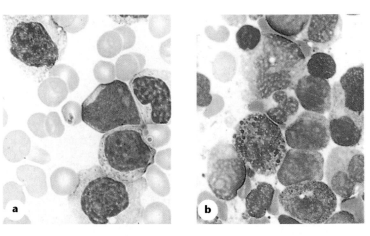

Fig. 13.23 Acute myelomonocytic leukemia (M4 subtype). (**a**) Blast cells contain cytoplasmic granules (myeloblasts and promyelocytes) or pale cytoplasm with occasional vacuoles and granules, as well as folded or rounded nuclei (monoblasts). (**b**) Eosinophils with basophilic granules are present. Specific cytogenetic abnormalities (inv(16) or t(16;16)) are associated with the presence of abnormal or dysplastic eosinophils in M4 ANLL. Eosinophils may be greatly increased. (**a**: Courtesy of Dr M. Bilter; **b**: courtesy of Prof. J. Rowley.)

Fig. 13.22 Acute promyelocytic leukemia (M3 subtype). A partial karyotype of G-banded chromosomes 15 and 17 is shown (above). The translocated chromosomes are on the right in each pair. The corresponding diagrams (below) represent a systematized description of the structural aberration which fuses the PML gene on chromosome 15 with the retinoic acid receptor-a on chromosome 17, resulting in a fusion protein involved in leukemogenesis. (Courtesy of Dr L.M. Secker-Walker.)

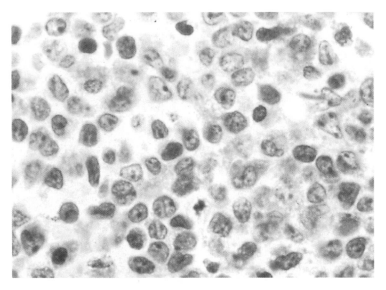

Fig. 13.24 Acute myelomonocytic leukemia (M4 subtype). High magnification of a bone marrow core biopsy shows many blasts with irregular, folded nuclear outlines and some with pink-red cytoplasmic granules. Histochemical staining is necessary for definitive diagnosis.

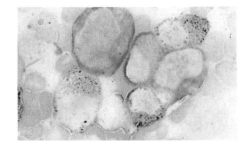

Fig. 13.25 Acute myelomonocytic leukemia (M4 subtype). Histochemical staining of a bone marrow aspirate shows a deep red-orange staining of monoblast cytoplasm by non-specific esterase and blue staining of myeloblast cytoplasm by chloracetate (specific esterase).

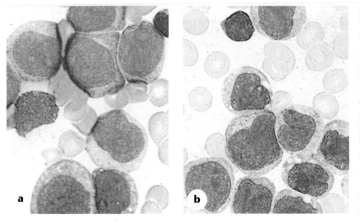

Fig. 13.26 Acute monocytic leukemia (M5A and M5B subtypes). (**a**) Blast cells of the M5A (monoblastic) variant have pale blue cytoplasm or perinuclear 'haloes', prominent nucleoli and cytoplasmic vacuoles, but only occasional granules. (**b**) The usually centrally placed nuclei are folded, rounded or kidney-shaped in the M5B (promonocytic) type, which is marked by more differentiated promonocytes that often contain fine granules.

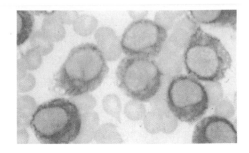

Fig. 13.27 Acute monocytic leukemia (M5A subtype). Histochemical staining of a bone marrow aspirate shows deep red-orange monoblast cytoplasm by non-specific esterase.

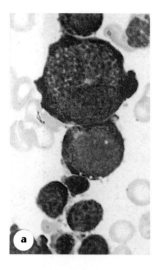
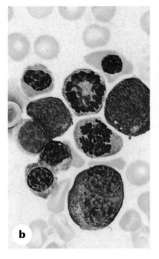
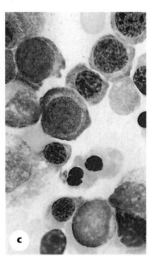

Fig. 13.28 Erythroleukemia (M6 subtype). (**a–c**) Erythroblasts predominate in these high-power views of a bone marrow aspirate and many dyserythropoietic features are evident, such as multinucleate cells, vacuolated cytoplasm, abnormal mitoses and megaloblastic nuclei. Myeloblasts are often present and may predominate in end-stage disease. Di Guglielmo's syndrome refers to different phases of this disease: erythroleukemia, erythremic myelosis and acute myeloblastic leukemia.

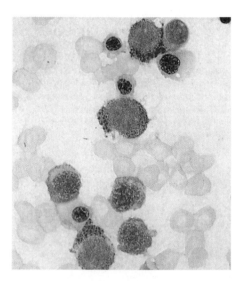

Fig. 13.29 Erythroleukemia (M6 subtype). The cytoplasm of some erythroblasts in this bone marrow aspirate shows block-positive red staining by PAS.

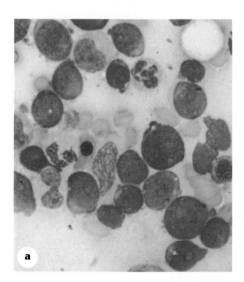
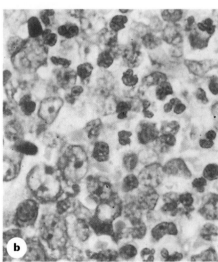
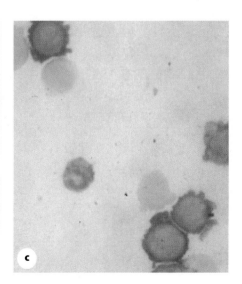

Fig. 13.30 Acute megakaryocytic leukemia (M7 subtype). (**a**) The blasts are large to medium sized and many cells have distinct nucleoli. The cytoplasm shows pseudopod-like margins, an appearance associated with but not confined to this subtype. (**b**) Appearance of bone marrow biopsy from a patient with acute megakaryocytic leukemia with numerous blast forms present in the marrow (Giemsa stain). (**c**) The blasts are PAS positive but peroxidase-stain negative. Immunohistochemical stain for glycoprotein IIIa (CD61) is diagnostically positive in this case.

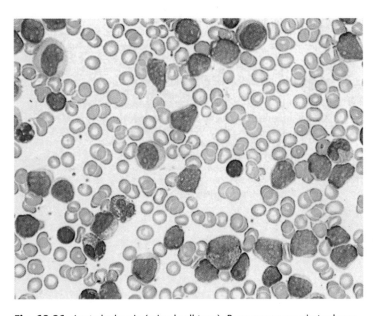

Fig. 13.31 Acute leukemia (mixed cell type). Bone marrow aspirate shows blasts of various sizes and morphology. Some possess scanty cytoplasm without granules (lymphoblastic), whereas others, usually large blasts, show eccentric nuclei, substantial cytoplasm and granules (myeloblastic). Histochemical stains and cell surface markers will clarify the diagnosis (*see* Table 13.3, Fig. 13.2). Very rarely, the blasts may express both lymphoid and myeloid markers, e.g. CALLA (CD10), CD19 (B4), MY7 (CD13) and MY9 (CD33).

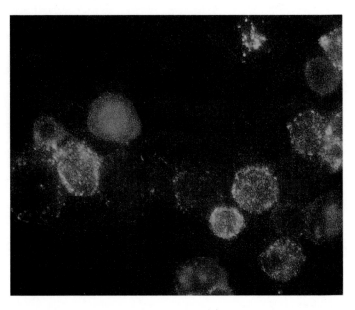

Fig. 13.32 Acute leukemia (mixed cell type). Indirect immunofluorescence microscopy of a bone marrow aspirate shows one population of cells (lymphoblasts) to have nuclear TdT (green), while another population (myeloblasts) has myeloid surface antigen (yellow-orange). Mixed lineage leukemias (biphenotypic) are unusual, but recent studies using monoclonal antibodies directed toward myeloid-associated cell surface antigens have demonstrated two populations of blasts in up to 20% of cases. This has been confirmed by immunoglobulin and T-cell receptor gene rearrangement studies. The choice of therapy may be affected by the finding of biphenotypic acute leukemia. (Courtesy of Prof. G. Janossy.)

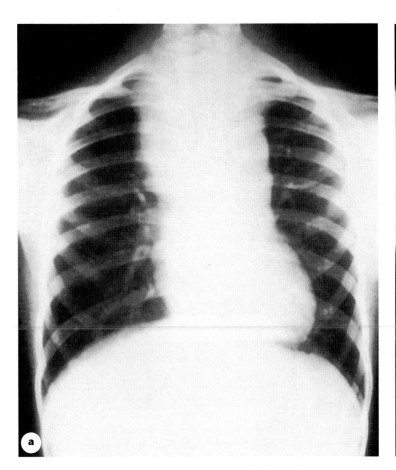

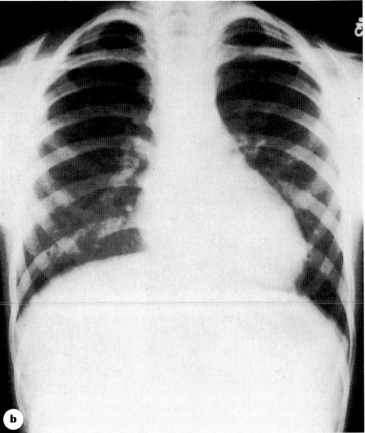

Fig. 13.33 Mediastinal involvement. (**a**) A mediastinal mass is clearly seen on this chest radiograph in a case of T-cell ALL. (**b**) Repeat film after 2 weeks of therapy with vincristine and prednisolone shows rapid response, with shrinkage of the mass. Further intensive therapy is required, including CNS prophylaxis.

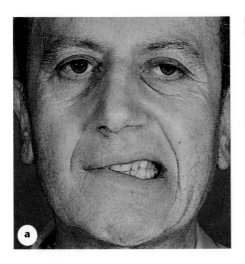

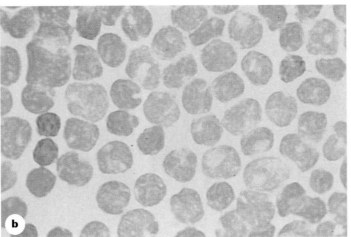

Fig. 13.34 Meningeal infiltration. (**a**) This 59-year-old man with ALL has facial asymmetry because of a right lower motor neuron VII nerve palsy resulting from leukemic infiltration of the CNS. (**b**) Stained centrifuge sample of cerebrospinal fluid shows L1-type lymphoid blast cells in a case of meningeal leukemia. CNS leukemia is uncommon in ANLL. (**a**: Courtesy of Dr H.G. Prentice.)

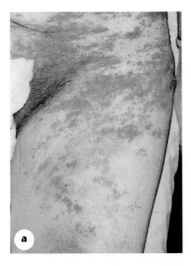

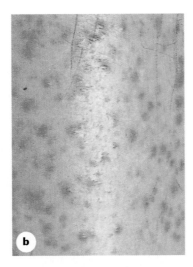

Fig. 13.35 Cutaneous manifestations. (**a**) Marked ecchymoses, petechial hemorrhages and bruises involve the groin and thigh in this patient with AML. (**b**) Petechial hemorrhages, seen here covering the leg, represent the most common cutaneous presentation of acute leukemia; they are due to severe thrombocytopenia.

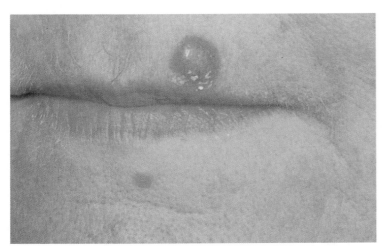

Fig. 13.36 Leukemia cutis. Firm, red-purple papules or nodules occasionally occur in ANLL, especially on the face. Skin involvement is rare in ALL.

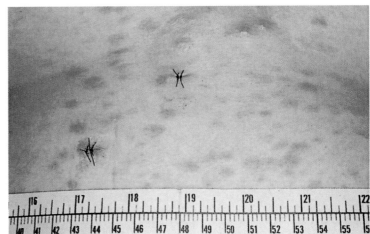

Fig. 13.37 Cutaneous manifestations. A 35-year-old woman with previous AMOL developed extensive skin lesions on the anterior chest as the first evidence of relapse. Biopsy showed infiltration of the dermis by monoblasts. Leukemic skin infiltrates can occur in any type of ANLL but are especially common in the M4 and M5 subtypes. They may be flat or raised, solitary or multiple.

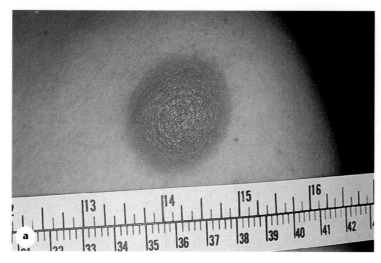

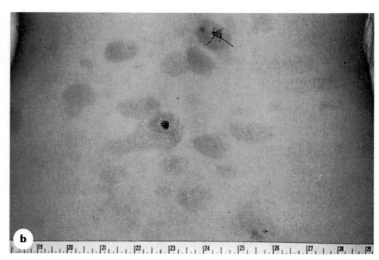

Fig. 13.38 Cutaneous manifestations. A 23-year-old woman with AMOL developed skin lesions on (**a**) the right shoulder and (**b**) lower back. The lesions regressed after 2 weeks' chemotherapy.

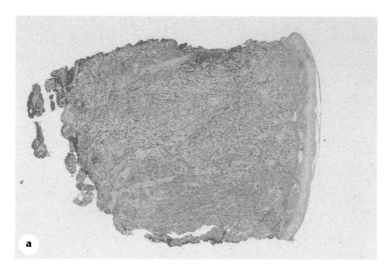

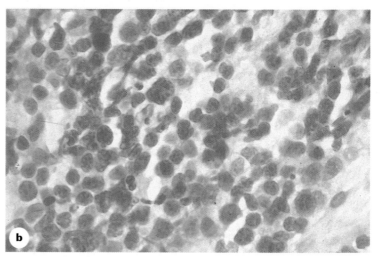

Fig. 13.39 (**a**) Histologic section (low power) from a patient with leukemia cutis, showing diffuse infiltration of the dermis and subcutaneous tissue. (**b**) High-power view shows immature myeloid cells, including numerous blast forms (hematoxylin and eosin). (Courtesy of Dr S. Granter.)

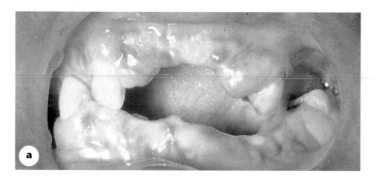

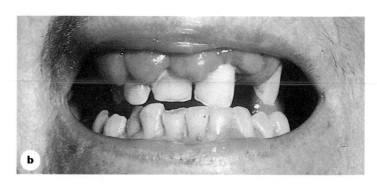

Fig. 13.40 Intraoral manifestations. (**a, b**) Leukemic infiltration of the gums in these patients with AMOL results in severe tissue hypertrophy and partial covering of the teeth.

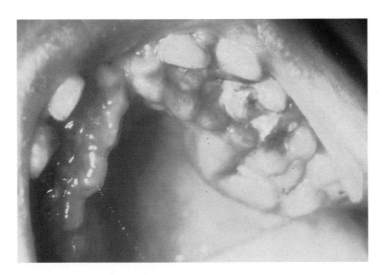

Fig. 13.41 Intraoral manifestations. Gingival hypertrophy most often occurs when there is a monoblastic element in ANLL. It is not seen in edentulous patients. This patient had AMOL.

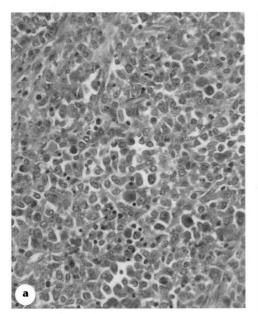

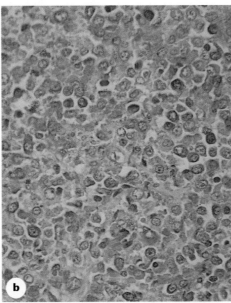

Fig. 13.42 Myeloblastoma (granulocytic sarcoma). A destructive maxillary tumor was the presenting symptom in an apparently healthy 20-year-old man. (**a**) The cellular picture is pleomorphic, but the eosinophilia of the myeloblasts is conspicuous even at low magnification. (**b**) Positive eosinophilic staining of myeloid cells is confirmed by the naphthol AS-D-chloracetate esterase reaction. Other confirmatory studies include a positive lysozyme stain and a positive myeloperoxidase stain of a touch prep.

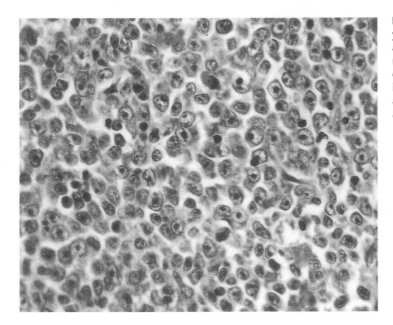

Fig. 13.43 Myeloblastoma presenting in a lymph node. In this 30-year-old man who presented with cervical lymphadenopathy, nodal architecture was effaced by homogeneous myeloblasts with large, round nuclei with prominent central nucleoli. The differential diagnosis includes non-Hodgkin's lymphoma, large cell, immunoblastic type. The infiltrate was reactive for myeloperoxidase and chloracetate esterase, confirming a diagnosis of extramedullary acute myeloblastic leukemia.

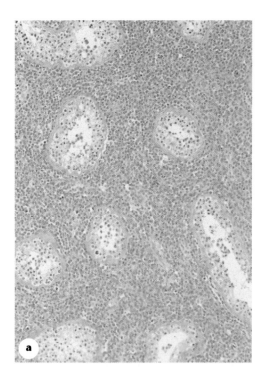
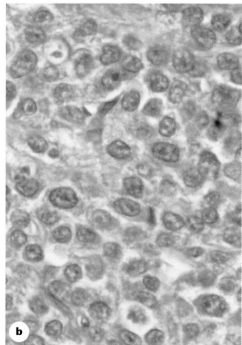
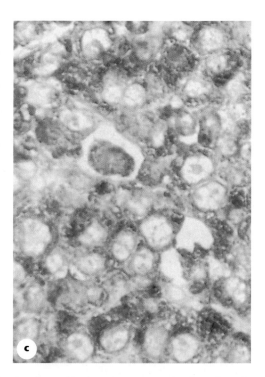

Fig. 13.44 Myeloblastoma (granulocytic sarcoma). A 37-year-old man underwent orchidectomy for a testicular mass believed to represent primary testicular carcinoma. (**a**) Histologic examination, however, reveals AML, as evidenced by the dense leukemic infiltrate enveloping the intact seminiferous tubules. (**b**) High magnification shows that the tumor is composed of cells with predominantly round nuclear outlines and distinct nucleoli. (**c**) Immunoperoxidase staining for lysozyme is strongly reactive.

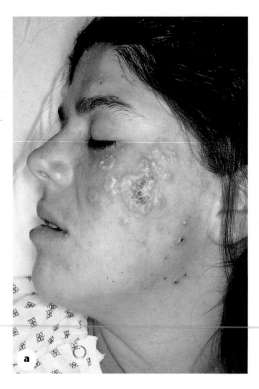
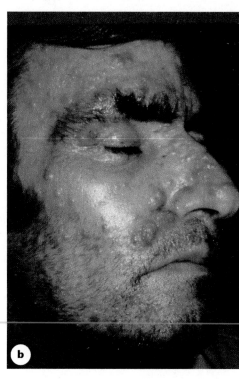

Fig. 13.45 Acute febrile neutrophilic dermatosis (Sweet's syndrome). (**a, b**) These patients with ANLL developed fever and multiple cutaneous, tender, red plaque-like lesions on the face, arms and hands. Skin biopsy showed a dense nodular and patchy dermal infiltrate composed primarily of mature neutrophils. There was marked edema of the papillary dermis, but the epidermis was essentially normal. There was eventual total resolution of the lesions following corticosteroid treatment. Sweet's syndrome occurs in association with AML or AMOL and may predate the diagnosis of acute leukemia. It is also associated with chronic myeloproliferative disorders and miscellaneous malignancies, or it may be idiopathic. The differential diagnosis includes pyoderma. The lesions may involve the mucous membranes or cause pulmonary infiltrates; systemic symptoms may also occur. The etiology remains obscure.

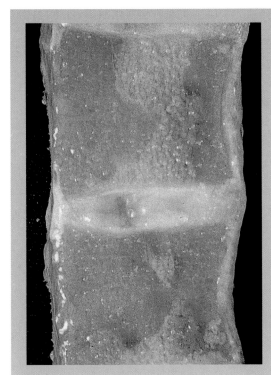

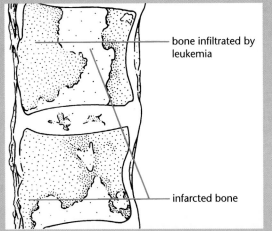

Fig. 13.46 Vertebral infiltration. This sagittal section through the spine is from a child who died of acute leukemia. Areas of necrosis within the vertebral bodies are marked by yellow opacification of the bone and marrow, which are surrounded by a thin rim of hyperemic tissue. Viable bone marrow has a fleshy tan color, reflecting leukemic infiltration.

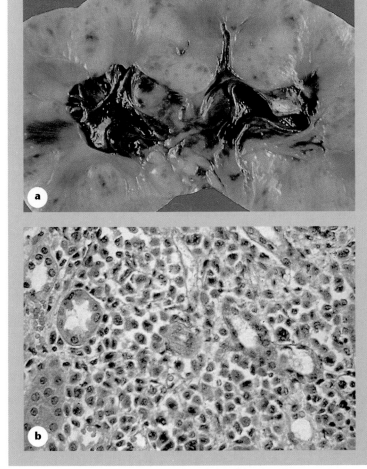

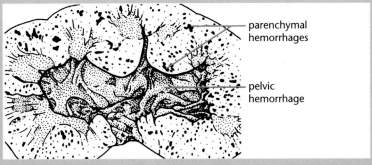

Fig. 13.47 Kidney involvement. (**a**) Leukemic infiltrates in this case of AML are diffusely present throughout the cortex of the kidney. Parenchymal and pelvic mucosal hemorrhages are secondary to severe thrombocytopenia. (**b**) Microscopically, many myeloblasts are seen in the interstitial infiltrates.

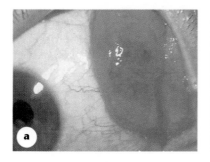
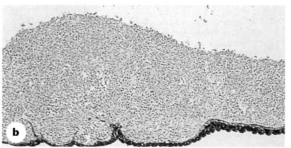

Fig. 13.48 Ophthalmic involvement. (**a**) This patient with AML presented with a large infiltrate of leukemic cells positioned nasally within the conjunctiva of the right eye; this clinical picture is characteristic. Lesions such as this appear quite similar to those caused by benign lymphoid hyperplasia or amyloidosis. (**b**) Biopsy of the lesion reveals myeloblasts.

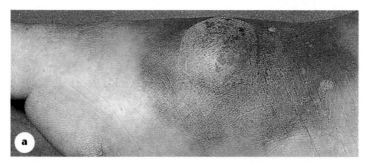
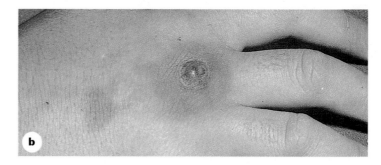

Fig. 13.49 Complications of acute leukemia. (**a**) A purplish-black bullous lesion with surrounding erythema in this patient with AML is caused by

Pseudomonas pyocyanea infection of the foot. (**b**) A similar but less marked infection is present on the back of the hand.

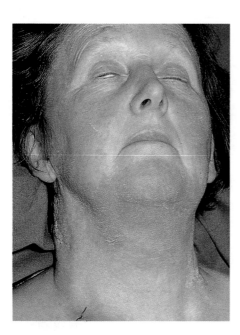

Fig. 13.50 Complications of acute leukemia. Spreading cellulitis of the neck and chin in this woman with AML results from mixed streptococcal and candidal infection, previous chemotherapy and prolonged periods of neutropenia.

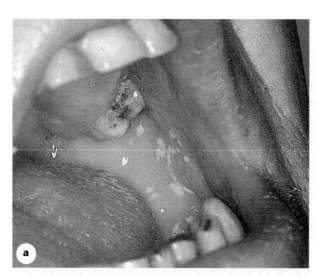

Fig. 13.51 Complications of acute leukemia. Plaques of *Candida albicans* are present on (**a**) the buccal mucosa and (**b**) the soft palate in a patient with AML.

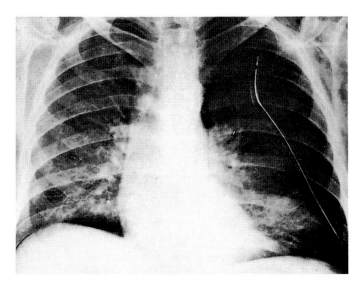

Fig. 13.52 Complications of acute leukemia. Chest radiograph of a patient with ALL shows consolidation spreading bilaterally from the hilar regions ('bat-wing' shadowing) due to infection with *Pneumocystis carinii*.

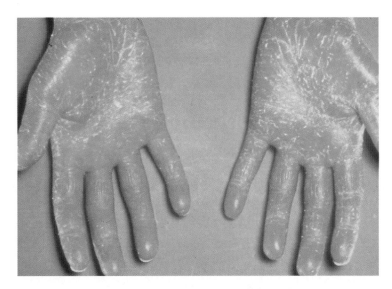

Fig. 13.53 Complications of therapy of acute leukemia. Graft versus host disease is a major cause of morbidity and mortality following allogenic bone marrow transplantation. It manifests as abnormalities of the skin, liver and gut. Skin involvement ranges from mild erythema to papulosquamous eruptions and desquamation and is often most marked on the palms and soles.

FAB Classification	WHO Classification
Refractory anemia (RA) Cytopenia of one peripheral blood cell (PBC) line Normo- or gypercellular marrow with dysplasias <1% PBC blasts and <5% bone marrow (BM) blasts	**RA** <5% blasts

RA with ringed sideroblasts (RARS)
Cytopenia, dysplasia, and same % blasts involvement
   as in RA
Ringed sideroblasts account for >15% of nucleated
   cells in marrow
	RARS
	<5% blasts
	
	Refractory Cytopenia with Multilineage Dysplasia (RCMD)
	<5% BM blasts
	Dysplasia of >2 PBC lines

Refactory anemia with excess blasts (RAEB) Cytopenia of two PBC lines Dysplasia involving all three lineages >5% PB blasts and 5-20% BM blasts	**RAEB 1** 5-10% blasts **RAEB 2** 11-20% blasts
RAEB in transformation (RAEB-T) Hematologic features of RAEB >5% PB blasts and 5-20% BM blasts	**Sq-Syndrome** **Unclassifiable**
Chronic myelomonocytic leukemia (CMML) Monocytosis in PB (>1x109/L) <5% PBC blasts 20% BM blasts	**Myelodysplastic/Myeloproliferative Disease** CMML Atypical Chronic Myelogenous Leukemia (aCML)

Fig. 13.54 French–American–British (FAB) and WHO classifications of the myelodysplastic syndromes.

Table 13.6 Common cytogenic abnormalities in MDS

Abnormality	Incidence (%)
Loss of all or part of chromosome 5	13
Loss of all or part of chromosome 7	5
Trisomy 8	5
del17p	<1
del20q	2
Loss of X or Y	2

Adapted from Greenberg *et al.*, 1997.

Table 13.7 International prognostic scoring system for MDS

Overall score*	Median survival (years)
Low (0)	5.7

Intermediate
   1 (0.5 or 1.0)
   2 (1.5 or 2.0)
	
	3.5
	1.2

High (≥2.5)	0.4

*The overall score is the sum of the scores for bone marrow blasts, karyotype and cytopenias. The percentage of blasts is scored as follows: <5%, 0; 5–10%, 0.5; 11–20%, 1.5; and 21–30%, 2.0. Cytogenetic features associated with a good prognosis (normal karyotype, Y-, 5q-, or 20q-) are scored as 0; those associated with a poor prognosis (abnormal chromosome 7 or three or more abnormalities) are scored as 1.0; and all other cytogenetic abnormalities, which are associated with an intermediate prognosis, are scored as 0.5. A score of 0 is assigned if the patient has no cytopenia or only one type and a score of 0.5 is assigned if the patient has two or three types of cytopenia. The various types of cytopenia are defined as follows: hemoglobin, <10 per deciliter, absolute neutrophil count, <1500 per cubic millimeter, and platelet count, <100 000 per cubic millimeter. (Adapted from Greenberg *et al.*, 1997.)

(Rosenfeld, 2000)

Pre-myelodysplastic syndrome (MDS)

MDS is initated by enviromental, occupational and/or toxic exposure in genetically predisposed individuals. Targeted injury or mutation within heatopoietic stem cell may be followed by an immunologic response adversely affecting progenitor survival.

Early MDS

Characterized by <10% blasts. Progenitor cell damage elicits an immune response.

Late MDS

Characterized by >10% blasts. Establishment of an abnormal clone associated with telomere shortening.

MDS-related AML

Disease progession is associated with loss of tumor supressor activity.

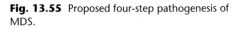

Fig. 13.55 Proposed four-step pathogenesis of MDS.

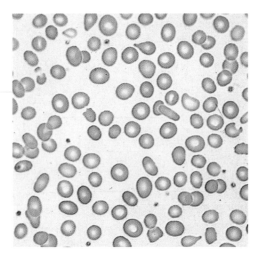

Fig. 13.56 Refractory anemia (MDS type I). Peripheral blood film shows marked anisocytosis and poikilocytosis.

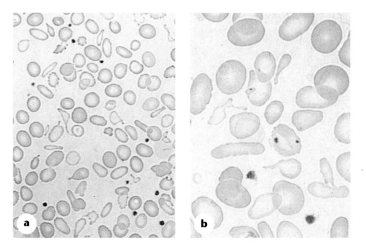

Fig. 13.57 Acquired sideroblastic anemia (MDS type II). (**a**) Peripheral blood film shows marked red cell anisocytosis and poikilocytosis. Although the majority of cells are markedly hypochromic, a second population of cells is normochromic. (**b**) At higher magnification, the central red cell shows two small basophilic inclusions (Pappenheimer bodies). Perls' staining demonstrated that similar inclusions were Prussian-blue positive (siderotic granules). These granules are far more numerous after splenectomy.

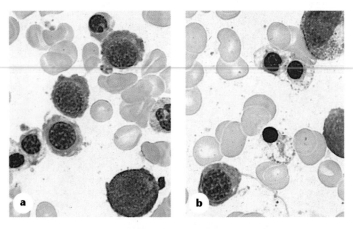

Fig. 13.58 Acquired sideroblastic anemia (MDS type II). Bone marrow aspiration smear shows marked, defective hemoglobinization and vacuolation in later stage polychromatic and pyknotic erythroblasts.

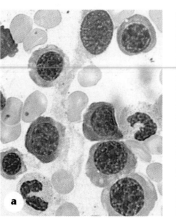
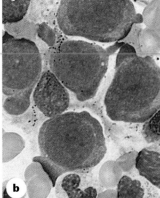

Fig. 13.59 Acquired sideroblastic anemia (MDS type II). Bone marrow aspiration smear shows erythroblasts with (**a**) vacuolation of cytoplasm in later cells, mild megaloblastic features and (**b**) a prominent group of proerythroblasts.

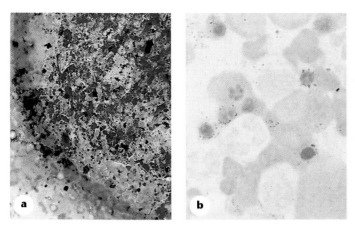

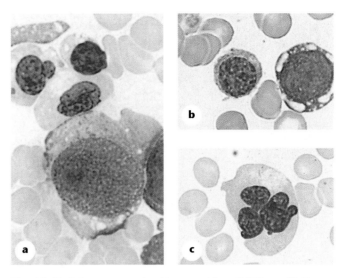

Fig. 13.60 Acquired sideroblastic anemia (MDS type II). Bone marrow fragment shows (**a**) increased iron stores and (**b**) pathologic ring sideroblasts at higher magnification (Perls' stain).

Fig. 13.61 Refractory anemia with excess blasts (MDS type II). Bone marrow aspirate shows (**a**) abnormal proerythroblasts and megaloblast-like changes and (**b**) prominent cytoplasmic vacuolation in the basophilic erythroblasts, evidence of dyserythropoiesis.

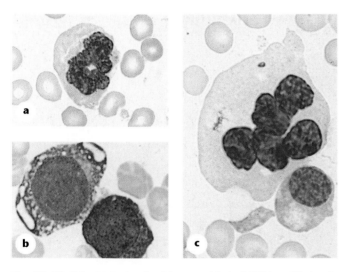

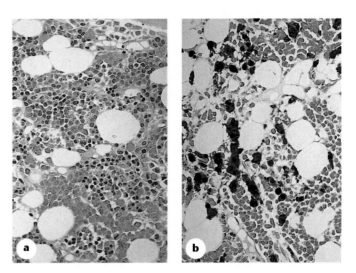

Fig. 13.62 Refractory anemia with excess blasts (MDS type III). (**a–c**) Bone marrow aspirate shows three examples of polypoid multinucleate polychromatic erythroblasts, further evidence of gross dyserythropoiesis.

Fig. 13.63 Refractory anemia with excess blasts (MDS type III). Needle biopsies show (**a**) clusters of blast forms and prominent hemosiderin-laden macrophages and (**b**) a gross increase in reticuloendothelial iron stores, confirmed by Perls' staining.

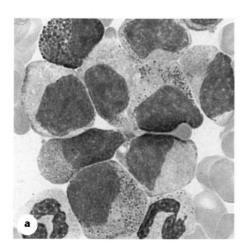

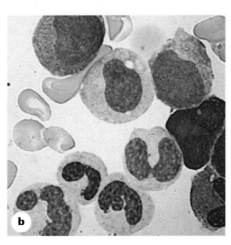

Fig. 13.64 Refractory anemia with excess blasts (MDS type III). Bone marrow aspirates shows disturbed granulopoiesis with (**a**) agranular promyelocytes and (**b**) agranular neutrophils and abnormal myelomonocytic cells. Some cells ('paramyeloid' cells) are difficult to classify as monocytic or granulocytic.

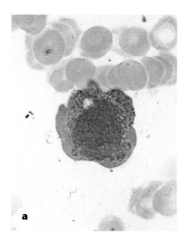
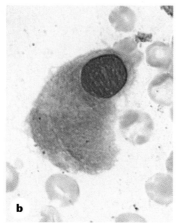
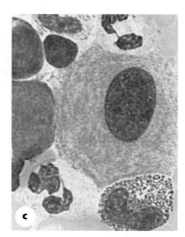

Fig. 13.65 Refractory anemia with excess blasts (MDS type III). Bone marrow aspirates show (**a**) an atypical megakaryoblast and (**b, c**) atypical mononuclear megakaryocytes, all of which exhibit evidence of cytoplasmic maturation and granulation.

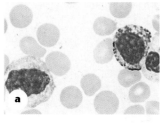
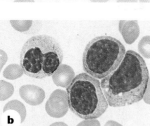
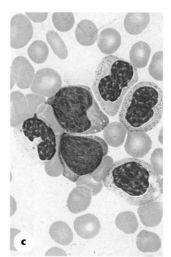
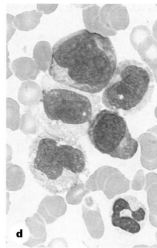

Fig. 13.66 Chronic myelomonocytic leukemia (MDS type IV). (**a–c**) In these peripheral blood films showing white cells, there are many atypical myelomonocytic cells and pseudo-Pelger neutrophils, some of which are agranular. (**d**) The majority of cells shown here are more monocytoid; the neutrophil is agranular.

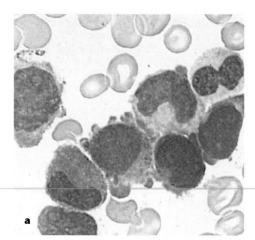
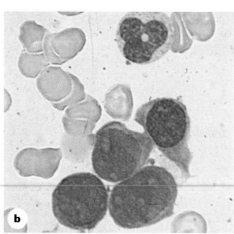

Fig. 13.67 Refractory anemia with excess blasts in transformation (MDS type V). Bone marrow aspirates show increased numbers of blast cells, some of which have atypical features. Blast cells constituted 23% of total marrow cells. Agranular neutrophils and myelomonocytic cells are also evident.

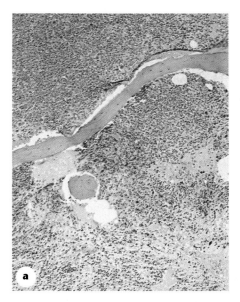

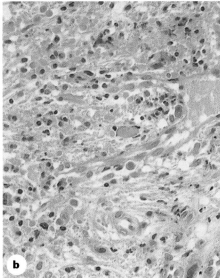

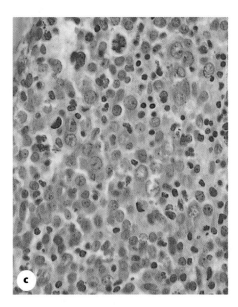

Fig. 13.68 Myelofibrosis transformed to acute leukemia. (**a**) Low magnification of needle biopsy shows areas in the lower portion of the field that are consistent with myelofibrosis, but the intertrabecular space in the upper part of the field contains sheets of closely packed mononuclear cells without obvious stromal connective tissue. (**b**) High-power view of the lower area shows isolated hematopoietic cells surrounded by a loose, fibrous connective tissue. (**c**) Primitive myeloid blast cells and promyelocytes predominate in this high-magnification view of the upper area. After a 9-year history of myelofibrosis, this patient presented with fever and bronchopneumonia. About 10% of patients with myelofibrosis (agnogenic or postpolycythemia) eventually develop acute myeloblastic leukemia.

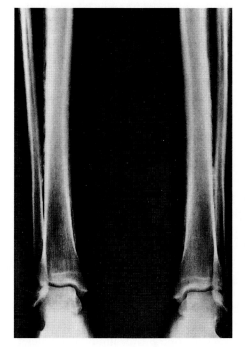

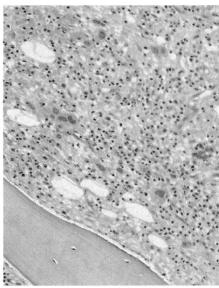

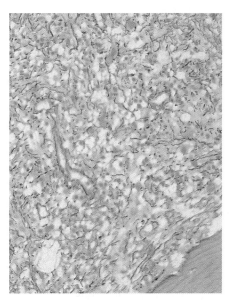

Fig. 13.69 Myelofibrosis transformed to acute leukemia. Radiograph of the lower legs of a middle-aged man shows extensive periosteal elevation due to infiltration by myeloid blast cells from underlying medullary bone. Although the medullary cavities of these bones in adults usually contain only fat, there may be extension of hemopoietic tissue to distal skeletal tissues in long-standing myeloproliferative disease.

Fig. 13.70 Acute myelofibrosis. Bone needle biopsy shows abnormal hemopoietic tissue with predominant mononuclear cells, isolated megakaroycytes and abundant fibrous stroma.

Fig. 13.71 Acute myelofibrosis. Bone needle biopsy with silver staining shows a marked increase in reticulin fiber density.

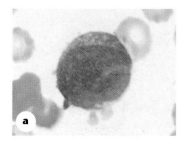

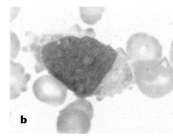

Fig. 13.72 Acute myelofibrosis. (**a, b**) Peripheral blood films show blast cells that are somewhat larger than classic myeloblasts and have irregular cytoplasmic borders. Electron microscopic studies and detection of factor VIIIR:AG in their cytoplasm, using monoclonal antibodies, confirmed that they were megakaryoblasts. A diagnosis of M7 ANLL requires >30% blasts in the peripheral blood and/or bone marrow.

CHRONIC LEUKEMIAS

CHRONIC LYMPHOCYTIC LEUKEMIA

Chronic lymphocytic leukemia (CLL) is a malignant hematologic disorder characterized by a persistent absolute increase in mature-appearing lymphocytes in the peripheral blood and bone marrow. In the majority of cases, surface marker studies have shown that the cells are a monoclonal population of immature B-lymphocytes possessing low-density surface immunoglobulin (*see* Table 13.10); in about 5–10% of patients, CLL is of T-cell origin. The disease is rare in individuals less than 30 years of age, increasing in incidence with each decade. The average patient age is about 65 years of age and CLL is more common in men than in women. About 6000 new cases occur in the United States each year, with an annual incidence of 2.6 cases per 100 000 people.

Staging of CLL is carried out by the Rai or International Workshop system, based on blood counts, lymphadenopathy and splenomegaly (*see* Tables 13.8 and 13.9). The survival time varies widely, ranging from less than 2 years to more than 10 years.

In about 20% of patients, CLL is an incidental finding on routine blood counts, at which time the physical examination may be otherwise normal. A small number of patients have a prolonged, asymptomatic course, without significant change in the lymphocytosis. Cytogenetic studies have demonstrated trisomy 12 as well as structural abnormalities of 13q, 14q, 6q and 11 in a significant number of CLL patients, with an associated poor prognosis. As the disease progresses, symmetrical lymphadenopathy develops, accompanied by hepatosplenomegaly and variable degrees of anemia and thrombocytopenia. Symptoms include weight loss, fatigue, fever and recurrent infections. Immunologic abnormalities appear, such as hypogammaglobulinemia, development of monoclonal proteins, 'warm' autoimmune hemolytic anemia (10% of cases) and, in a small number of cases, autoimmune thrombocytopenia.

From 1% to 10% of patients develop transition to a DLCL or immunoblastic sarcoma (Richter's syndrome) during the clinical course of CLL. The patients usually have active or advanced CLL, although some have been in remission (Robertson *et al.*, 1993). The transition is heralded by sudden clinical deterioration, with increasing adenopathy, extranodal disease, systemic symptoms, elevated LDH and a monoclonal gammopathy. Ig gene rearrangement and light chain isotype analysis support a common origin for the malignant cells of both diseases in most cases. Prognosis is poor with Richter's syndrome; median survival is only 5 months, despite multidrug therapy. Recently Gleevac (formerly STIs71), a tyrosine kinase inhibitor, was developed for gene product-targeted therapy for CML. In clinical studies it has induced cytogenetic and hematologic responses in CML patients at a high rate, emerging as a significant new treatment option for CML.

Prolymphocytic leukemia

This variant of chronic lymphocytic leukemia usually occurs in the elderly and is associated with marked splenomegaly, absolute lymphocytosis (usually $> 100 \times 10^9/l$), and minimal lymph node enlargement. Peripheral blood films reveal larger lymphocytes than are found in classic CLL. In the majority of patients, surface marker studies indicate a B-cell origin of prolymphocytes, but occasionally patients have a T-cell variant of this disease and concomitantly a less predictable prognosis.

LGL leukemia

Clonal diseases of large granular lymphocytes (LGL) are either of T-cell origin (T-LGL leukemia) or of NK cell origin (NK-LGL leukemia). T-LGL leukemia is associated with neutropenia and consequent recurrent bacterial infections and may also be associated with rheumatoid arthritis, resembling Felty's syndrome, with the triad of arthritis, neutropenia and splenomegaly. The majority of patients have a chronic disease course, with major complications secondary to neutropenia. Neoplastic cells are typically CD3, CD8, CD16 and CD57 positive and exhibit T-cell receptor gene rearrangements. NK-LGL leukemia typically has an acute clinical course, with pancytopenia, massive hepatosplenomegaly and systemic illness. Neoplastic cells are typically CD3, CD8 and CD57 negative and CD16 and CD56 positive, without T-cell receptor gene rearrangements. In both types of LGL leukemia the cause is unknown.

Hairy cell leukemia

This rare disorder, also known as leukemic reticuloendotheliosis, is characterized by pancytopenia, massive splenomegaly and accumulation in peripheral blood of lymphoid-appearing cells with 'hairy' cytoplasmic projections. In many patients, the marrow is difficult to aspirate ('dry tap') owing to myelofibrosis and infiltration by hairy cells. The characteristic cells are almost always of B-cell origin, and coexpress CD11c, CD25 and CD103. New purine analogs are extremely effective for the treatment of hairy cell leukemias.

CHRONIC MYELOGENOUS LEUKEMIA

Chronic myelogenous leukemia (CML), also called chronic granulocytic leukemia, is a clonal myeloproliferative disorder arising from neoplastic proliferation at the level of the pleuripotential stem cell. In most patients (90%), normal marrow is replaced by cells with an abnormal G group chromosome, the Philadelphia (Ph) chromosome. About 4000–5000 new cases are diagnosed in the United States each year. Although CML can occur at any age, it is rare in childhood and peaks in the mid-fifth decade.

The Ph chromosome abnormality results from a reciprocal translocation involving the long arm of chromosome 9 band q34 and chromosome 22 band q11 (*see* Fig. 13.101). The cellular oncogene c-abl, which codes for a tyrosine protein kinase, is translocated to a specific breakpoint cluster region (bcr) of chromosome 22. Part of the bcr gene (the 5′ end) remains on chromosome 22, the 3′ end moving to chromosome 9 together with the oncogene c-sis (which codes for a protein with close homology to one of the two subunits of platelet-derived growth factor). As a result of the translocation onto chromosome 22, a chimeric oncogene is formed that produces a bcr/c-*abl* messenger RNA (mRNA) encoding a 210 kDa fusion protein that transforms normal hematopoietic cells (*see* Fig. 13.102). Clonal proliferation of these abnormal cells leads to progressive expansion of the total burden of granulocytes. The Ph chromosome is present in granulocytic, erythroid and megakaryocytic precursor cells, but not in fibroblasts. It has also been demonstrated in B- and T-lymphocytes (e.g. in leukemic transformation) and has also been observed in cases of *de novo* acute lymphoblastic leukemia. From 10% to 30% of patients with typical CML are Ph negative as defined by cytogenic analysis but exhibit bcr rearrangement by molecular analyses. These patients have clinical characteristics, response to therapy and prognosis similar to those with Ph-positive CML.

CML in some patients is diagnosed incidentally after a routine blood count. The WBC count progressively rises, reaching levels of $50-500 \times 10^9/l$, and a complete spectrum of granulocytic cells is seen in the blood smear. The bone marrow is hypercellular, with a predominating granulocyte population.

The symptoms of CML are related to hypermetabolism and include anorexia, lassitude, weight loss and night sweats. Splenomegaly, often massive, is common. As the spleen enlarges symptoms of compression may develop, such as early satiety and peripheral leg edema. Splenic infarcts may occur, causing splenic pain referred to the left shoulder.

An accelerated phase known as 'CML crisis' is characterized by the appearance of new symptoms, similar to those mentioned above, with a rapid rise in white blood cell count. Approximately 70–80% of patients undergo blastic transformation, with the presence of 30% blasts in the peripheral blood or bone marrow, which is associated with rapid clinical deterioration and progressive bone marrow failure.

Infiltration of the skin and other non-hematopoietic tissues may occur. The transformation may be myeloblastic, lymphoblastic, mixed or, rarely, monoblastic or erythroblastic.

About 5–10% of patients have a variant of CML (Ph negative) that is associated with fewer myelocytes, more monocytoid cells and atypical neutrophils in the peripheral blood. Severe anemia and thrombocytopenia are more frequent than in classic CML. Although the Ph chromosome is not found in these patients, in one-third of cases the chimeric bcr/c-*abl* mRNA is produced and can be demonstrated with molecular diagnostic methods. As a group, patients with true Ph-negative CML are elderly, have an less favorable prognosis and present with leukocytosis and multilineage dysplasia that evolves into acute leukemia in 30–40% of patients. Another Ph-negative variant occurs in children, referred to as juvenile myelomonocytic leukemia, and is often accompanied by marked lymphadenopathy and eczematoid rashes. As in the adult form, there are morphologic differences from classic CML.

World Health Organisation classification of neoplastic disease of the chronic lymphoid leukemias (proposed)
B-cell neoplasms
B-cell chronic lymphocytic leukemia/small lymphocytic lymphoma
B-cell prolymphocytic leukemia
Hairy cell leukemia
T-cell neoplasms
T-cell prolymphocytic leukemia
T-cell large granular lymphocytic leukemia
(Adapted from Harris et al. 1999)

Fig. 13.73 WHO classification of neoplastic diseases of the chronic lymphoid leukemias (proposed).

Table 13.8 The Rai staging system for chronic lymphocytic leukemia

Stage	Features	Median survival (years)
0	Lymphocytosis in blood and marrow	12.5
I	Lymphocytosis with lymphadenopathy	8.4
II	Lymphocytosis with splenomegaly	5.9
III	Lymphocytosis with anemia	1.6
IV	Lymphocytosis with thrombocytopenia	1.6

Table 13.9 International workshop staging classification of chronic lymphocytic leukemia

Stage	Features	Median survival (years)
A	Lymphocytosis with clinical involvement of <3 lymph node groups* No anemia or thrombocytopenia	>10
B	>3 Lymph node groups involved	5
C	Anemia or thrombocytopenia regardless of number of lymph node groups involved	2

*International workshop staging classification of chronic lymphocytic leukemia.

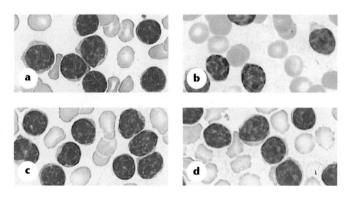

Fig. 13.74 Chronic lymphocytic leukemia. (**a–d**) Lymphocytes in the peripheral blood of four different patients show a thin rim of cytoplasm, condensed coarse chromatin and only rare nucleoli.

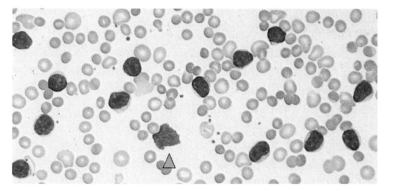

Fig. 13.75 Chronic lymphocytic leukemia with autoimmune hemolytic anemia. Peripheral blood film shows increased numbers of lymphocytes, red cell spherocytosis and polychromasia. The direct Coombs' test was strongly positive with IgG on the cell surfaces. Note the 'smudge' cell (arrow), which is often seen in CLL.

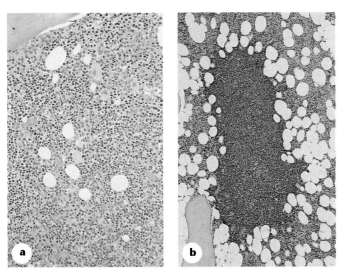

Fig. 13.76 Chronic lymphocytic leukemia. Bone needle biopsies show (**a**) a marked, diffuse increase in marrow lymphocytes, which are closely packed and have small dense nuclei. (**b**) In a different patient, there is a nodular pattern of lymphocyte accumulation.

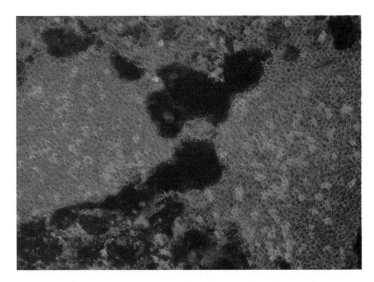

Fig. 13.77 Chronic lymphocyte leukemia. Two neoplastic lymphoid nodules in this bone marrow biopsy contain predominantly B-cells that react positively for IgM (green fluorescein staining). Many reactive T-cells are identified by a monoclonal antibody to the CD5 (T1) antigen (red rhodamine staining). (Courtesy of Dr G. Pizzolo and Dr M. Chilosi.)

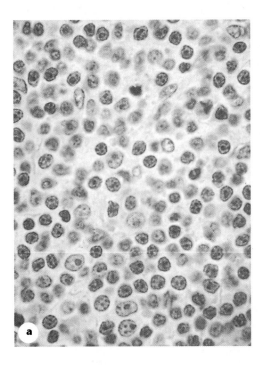

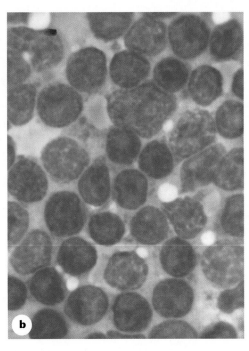

Fig. 13.78 Lymph node involvement. (**a**) High magnification of a lymph node biopsy specimen from a patient with CLL shows small, well-differentiated lymphocytes with scanty cytoplasm. (**b**) Touch prep reveals typical small lymphocytes with condensed nuclear chromatin and a rim of cytoplasm (Wright–Giemsa stain). Immunoperoxidase staining (not shown) for IgM was weakly positive; it was also positive for both CD20 (B1) and CD5 (T1), which is characteristic for CLL.

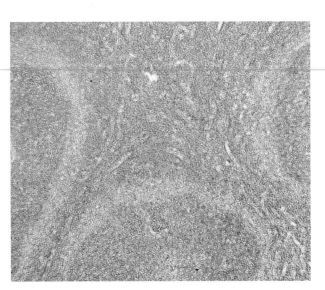

Fig. 13.79 Splenic involvement. Histologic section of spleen from a patient with CLL and secondary autoimmune hemolytic anemia shows expansion of lymphoid tissue in the periarterial sheaths of the white pulp and obvious red cell entrapment in the reticuloendothelial cords and splenic sinuses.

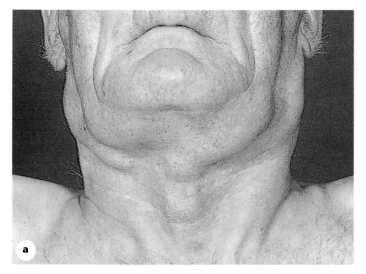

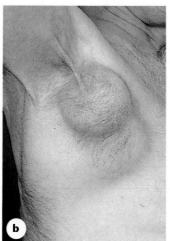

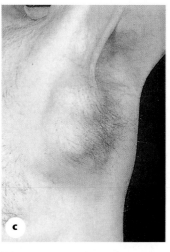

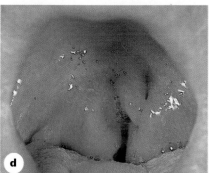

Fig. 13.80
Lymphadenopathy. This 65-year-old man with CLL presented with bilateral (**a**) cervical and (**b, c**) axillary lymphadenopathy, as well as (**d**) massive enlargement of the pharyngeal tonsils.

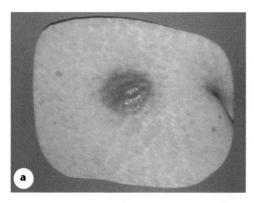

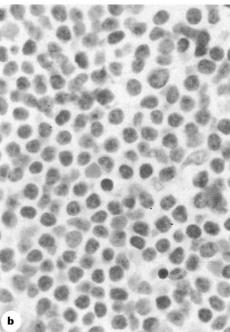

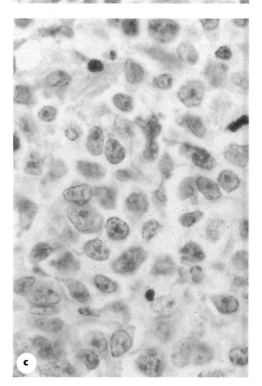

Fig. 13.81
Transformation to large cell lymphoma (Richter's syndrome). A 78-year-old woman who had stable CLL of 3 years' duration developed new subcutaneous masses on the trunk along with generalized adenopathy, weight loss and fatigue. (**a**) This 3 × 3 cm abdominal wall tumor mass appears fixed, raised and reddish-tan. Biopsy showed a B immunoblastic-type, diffuse large cell lymphoma (DLCL). (**b**) The small cells of CLL contrast sharply with (**c**) the large, irregular, malignant lymphoid cells of DLCL. Richter's syndrome, originally described in 1928, was thought to represent a new malignancy (reticulum cell sarcoma) arising in a patient with CLL. Immunophenotyping and gene arrangement studies, however, typically reveal identical lineage consistent with clonal progression to an activated, aggressive lymphoma cell line.

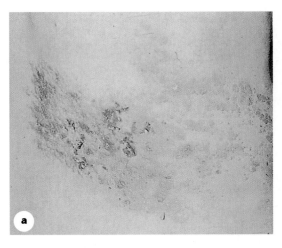

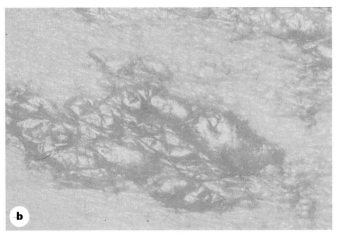

Fig. 13.82 Complications of chronic lymphocytic leukemia. (**a**) The posterior right lateral flank of this 68-year-old woman with CLL is extensively affected with a herpes zoster infection. (**b**) The eruption is typically vesicular with an erythematous base.

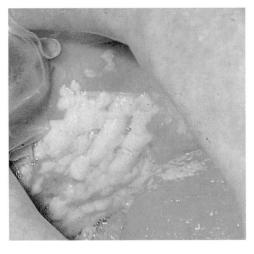

Fig. 13.83 Complications of chronic lymphocytic leukemia. Extensive *Candida albicans* infection involves the buccal mucosa of a 73-year-old woman.

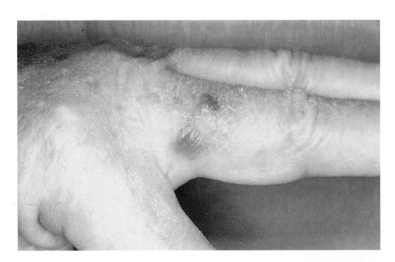

Fig. 13.84 Complications of chronic lymphocytic leukemia. Hypersensitivity to insect bites occasionally occurs, as noted on the middle finger of this 66-year-old man 10 days after mosquito bites. The hemorrhagic lesions are generally quite painful and may become infected. The hypersensitivity reaction, which is poorly understood, is related in part to underlying immune abnormalities.

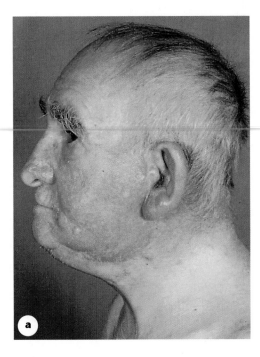

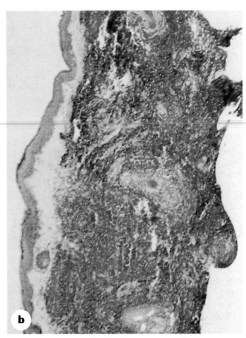

Fig. 13.85 Cutaneous involvement. (**a**) This 75-year-old man with T-cell CLL developed edema of the face and ears, along with generalized adenopathy and edema. Note the marked erythema and thickening of the ears. (**b**) Skin biopsy revealed infiltration of the dermis by small, well-differentiated lymphocytes. Although skin lesions may be seen in patients with B-cell CLL, they are more common in the T-cell type, which usually has a more aggressive clinical course.

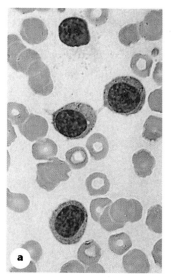

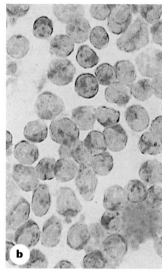

Fig. 13.86 Chronic lymphocytic leukemia (T-cell type). Peripheral blood films show (**a**) abnormal lymphocytes in which nuclear 'convolutions' are occasionally seen and (**b**) characteristic 'clump' positivity in the Golgi zone on acid-phosphatase staining. The clinical course is usually more rapid, compared with B-cell CLL.

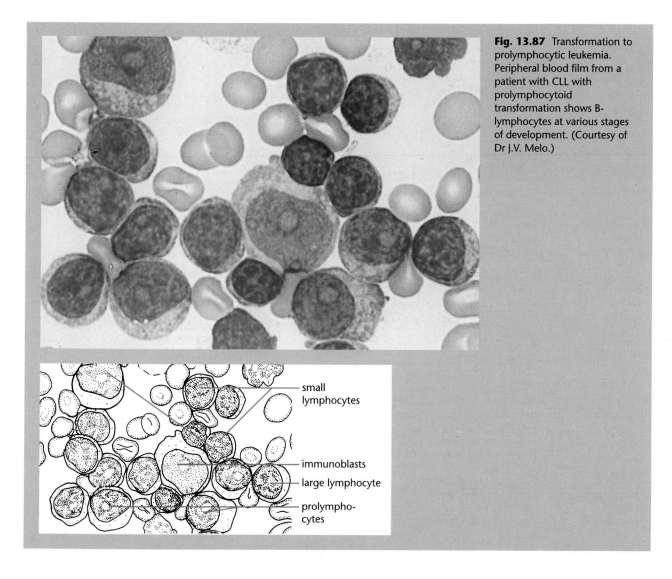

Fig. 13.87 Transformation to prolymphocytic leukemia. Peripheral blood film from a patient with CLL with prolymphocytoid transformation shows B-lymphocytes at various stages of development. (Courtesy of Dr J.V. Melo.)

small lymphocytes

immunoblasts

large lymphocyte

prolympho-cytes

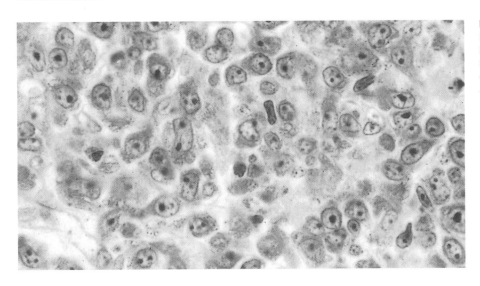

Fig. 13.88 Prolymphocytic leukemia. Bone marrow biopsy shows a diffuse infiltrate composed predominantly of lymphoid cells larger than those seen in CLL, with round nuclei and prominent central nucleoli (Giemsa stain).

Table 13.10 Immunologic classification of chronic lymphocytic leukemias

	Study	B cell (CLL)	B cell (PLL)	Hairy cell leukemia	T cell CLL/PLL
Surface antigens	SIg	±(IgM±IgD)	++(IgM±IgD)	+(IgM or IgG or IgA)	–
	MRBC Rosettes	++	±	±	–
	SRBC Rosettes	–	–	–	+
	HLA-DR (Ia)	+	+	+	–
	CD19	+	+	+	–
	CD20	+	+	+	–
	CD5	+	–/+	–	–
	CD2	–	–	–	+
	CD3	–	–	–	+
	FMC7	–	+	±	–
	DBA.44 & CD103	–	–	+	–
Gene rearrangement	IgH	+	+	+	–
	TCR	–	–	–	+

CLL, chronic lymphocytic leukemia; PLL, prolymphocytic leukemia; sIg, surface immunoglobulin; MRBC, mouse red blood cell; SRBC, sheep red blood cell; FMC7, a cell membrane antigen occurring on late B-lymphocytes; DBA.44, a monoclonal antibody highly sensitive for neoplastic cells of hairy cell leukemia; IgH, immunoglobulin heavy chain; TCRβ, T-cell receptor β-chain; ++, strongly postive; ±, equivocal; –, negative.

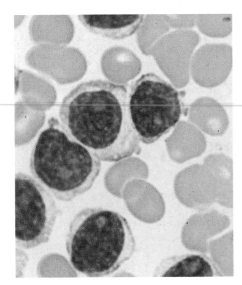

Fig. 13.89 Prolymphocytic leukemia (B-cell type). Peripheral blood film shows prolymphocytes with prominent, central nucleoli and an abundance of pale cytoplasm. A high density of surface immunoglobulin confirmed their B-cell nature. (Courtesy of Dr D. Catovsky.)

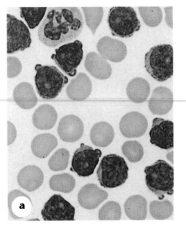
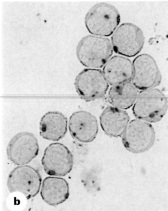

Fig. 13.90 Prolymphocytic leukemia (T-cell type). (**a**) Peripheral blood film shows prolymphocytes and a single neutrophil. Cell marker studies revealed positive reactions with anti-T cell antisera and an absence of surface immunoglobulin. The majority of cases of T-PLL exhibit structural abnormalities of chromosome 14, most commonly inv(14). (**b**) The cells show 'clump' positivity with acid-phosphatase staining. (Courtesy of Dr D. Catovsky.)

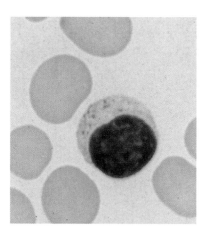

Fig. 13.91 LGL leukemia. Peripheral blood film shows a large lymphocyte with many coarse, azurophilic cytoplasmic granules (LGL). Immunologic marker studies demonstrated that the cells were positive for surface antigens CD8 (T8) and CD3 (T3), as well as for natural killer (NK) cell markers. The patient had rheumatoid arthritis, splenomegaly, chronic neutropenia and lymphocytosis. LGL leukemias represent a heterogeneous group of lymphoproliferative disorders including at least three distinct clinical syndromes that can present with acute or chronic manifestations (Loughran, 1993).

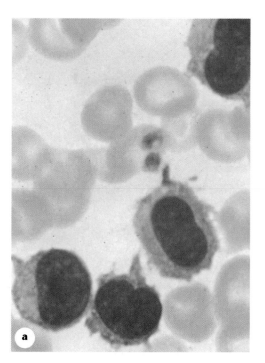

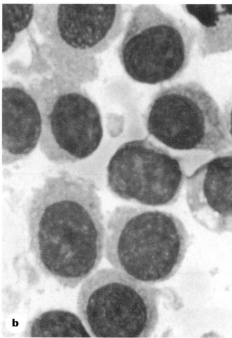

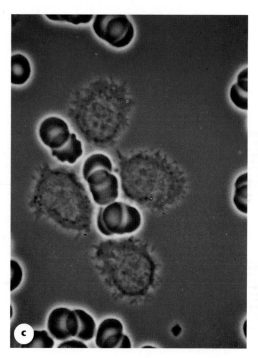

Fig. 13.92 Hairy cell leukemia. A 58-year-old man presented with fatigue, weight loss and abdominal distension. Evaluation shows pancytopenia and (**a**) this peripheral blood film demonstrates characteristic lymphoid cells with fine hair-like cytoplasmic projections. Some cells have an ovoid or kidney-shaped nucleus and small nucleoli may be seen. Bone marrow aspiration was 'dry,' but (**b**) marrow biopsy shows infiltration by hairy cells, some with abundant cytoplasm (Wright–Giemsa stain). (**c**) Phase-contrast microscopy of a drop of peripheral blood diluted with saline dramatically demonstrates the cells' hairy projections. Immunophenotyping in this case showed positivity for IgM, HLA-DR (Ia), CD20 (B1), CD19 (B4), CD22 (B3), CD11c, CD25 (IL2R) and PCA-1.

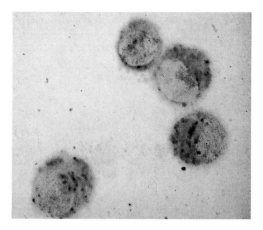

Fig. 13.93 Hairy cell leukemia. Typically, hairy cells show a strongly positive cytochemical reaction to tartaric acid-resistant acid phosphatase. Alphanaphthyl butyrate esterase staining (not shown) is also positive in these cells, which often exhibit a fine, granular, crescentic positive accumulation at one side of the nucleus.

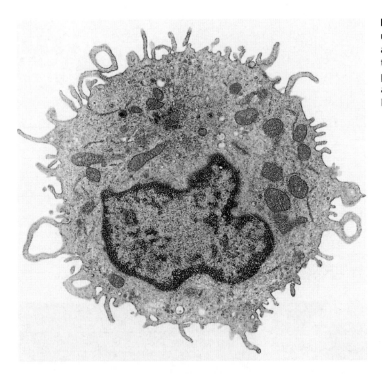

Fig. 13.94 Hairy cell leukemia. Typical ultrastructural features of the hairy cell are its abundant cytoplasm, low nucleus-to-cytoplasm ratio and the cytoplasmic projections or villi giving it a 'hairy' appearance (× 9200). (Courtesy of Mrs D. Robinson and Dr D. Catovsky.)

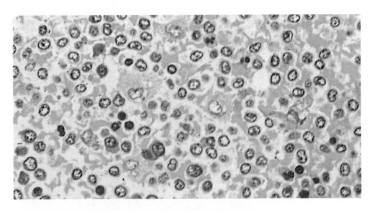

Fig. 13.95 Hairy cell leukemia. Needle biopsy of bone marrow shows extensive replacement of normal hematopoietic tissue by discrete mononuclear hairy cells. The nuclei are typically surrounded by a clear zone of cytoplasm (methacrylate section).

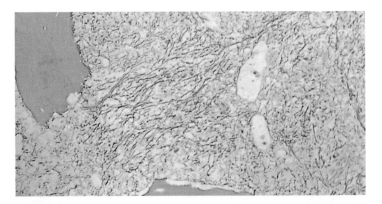

Fig. 13.96 Hairy cell leukemia. Needle biopsy of bone marrow shows increased fiber density and thickness in the reticulin fiber pattern (silver impregnation technique).

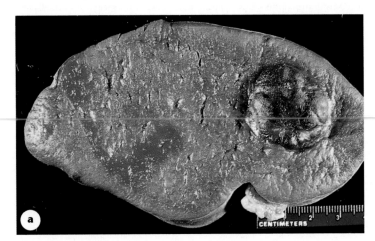

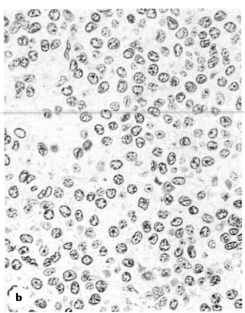

Fig. 13.97 Splenic involvement in HCL. (**a**) Localized intrasplenic hemorrhage has resulted in formation of a large 'blood lake'. (**b**) Microscopic section of spleen reveals the characteristic spacing of individual, uniform mononuclear cells with reniform nuclei, indistinct nucleoli, finely stippled chromatin and abundant, pale cytoplasm.

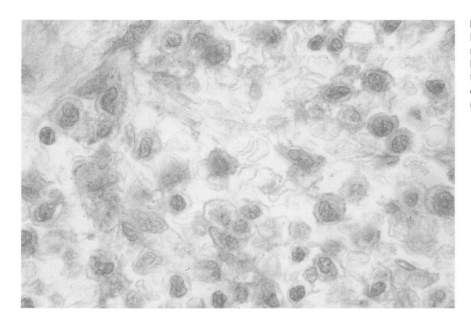

Fig. 13.98 Hairy cell leukemia. Neoplastic cells are reactive with monoclonal antibody DBA.44, which is highly sensitive for hairy cells, outlines their cytoplasmic projections and is capable of detecting minimal bone marrow involvement.

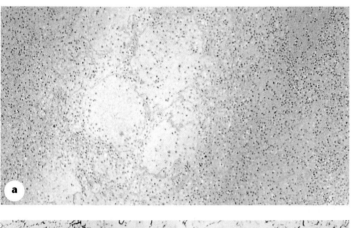

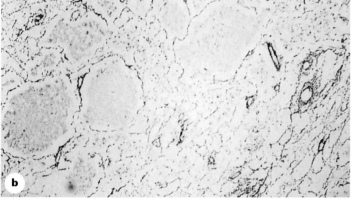

Fig. 13.99 Splenic involvement in HCL. (**a**) Hairy cells have infiltrated the reticuloendothelial cords and sinuses. Many blood 'lakes' are seen in the center of the field. (**b**) Silver impregnation technique shows more clearly the reticulin fiber pattern outlining the abnormal venous 'lakes'. The presence of these structures may explain the extensive splenic red cell pooling that occurs in this disease.

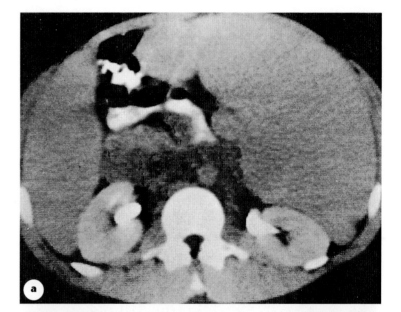

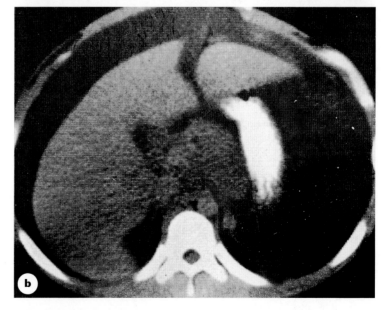

Fig. 13.100 Splenic involvement in HCL. (**a**) Abdominal CT scan shows massive splenomegaly displacing the stomach and bowel medially. No retroperitoneal lymphadenopathy is present. (**b**) Followup scan 2 years after splenectomy reveals ascites and enlarged retroperitoneal nodes. The ascitic fluid was positive for hairy cells, which is an unusual feature.

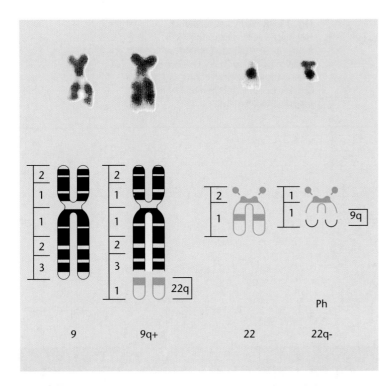

Fig. 13.101 Chronic myelogenous leukemia. The translocated chromosomes are on the right in each pair shown in this partial karyotype of G-banded chromosomes 9 and 22 (above). The corresponding diagrams (below) represent a systematized description of the structural aberration (Ph = Philadelphia chromosome). (Courtesy of Dr L.M. Secker-Walker.)

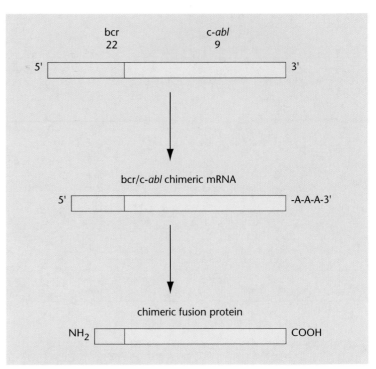

Fig. 13.102 Chronic myelogenous leukemia. Chimeric bcr/c-*abl* mRNA is coded for partly by the breakpoint cluster region (bcr) of chromosome 22 and partly by the c-*abl* oncogene translocated from chromosome 9 to 22.

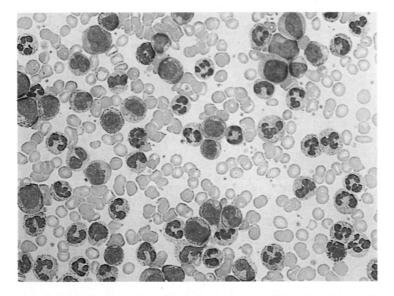

Fig. 13.103 Chronic myelogenous leukemia. Peripheral blood film shows cells at all stages of granulopoietic development.

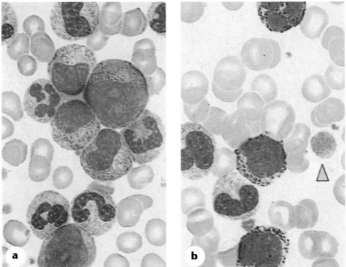

Fig. 13.104 Chronic myelogenous leukemia. Peripheral blood films show (**a**) a myeloblast, promyelocytes, myelocytes, metamyelocytes and band and segmented neutrophils, as well as (**b**) basophils and a giant platelet (arrow).

Proposed WHO classificatio of myeloproliferative and myelodysplastic/myeloprolifenative disease

Myeloproliferative diseases

Chronic myelogenous leukemia, Philadelphia chromosome positive (t(9;22)(qq34;q11),*BCR/ABL*
    Chronic neutrophilic leukemia
    Chronic eosinophilic leukemia/hypereosinophilic syndrome
    Chronic idiopathic myelofibrosis
    Polycythemia vera
    Essential thrombocythemia
    Myeloproliferative disease, unclassifiable

Myelodysplastic/myeloproliferative disease

    Chronic myelomonocytic leukemia
    Atypical chronic myelogenous leukemia
    Juvenile myelomonocytic leukemia

(Adapted from Harris *et al.* 1999)

Fig. 13.105 Proposed WHO classification of myeloproliferative and myelodysplastic/myeloproliferative diseases.

Clinical findings*

Fatigue, anorexia, weight loss
Splenomegaly
Hepatomegaly

Peripheral blood findings

Eldvated white-cell count (usually greater than 25,000/mm3)
Elevated platelet count in 30-50% of cases
Basophilia
Reduced leukocyte alkaline phosphatase activity
All stages of granulocyte differentiation visible on peripheral smear

Bone marrow findings

Hypercellularity, reduced fat content
Increased ratio of myeloid cells to erythroid cells
Increased numbers of megakaryocytes
Blasts and promyelocytes constitute less than 10% of all cells

*Approximately 40% of patients are asymptomatic (Adapted from Sawyers, 1999)

Fig. 13.106 Characteristics of patients with chronic myeloid leukemia at presentation.

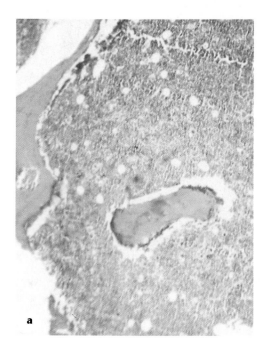
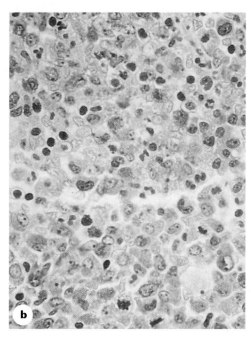
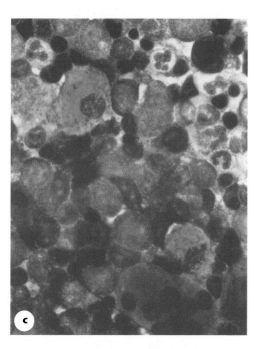

Fig. 13.107 Chronic myelogenous leukemia. (**a**) Bone marrow biopsy shows hypercellularity with about 10% residual fat. (**b**) At higher magnification, packed marrow exhibits increased myeloid elements ranging from blasts to mature forms. There are increased numbers of eosinophilic myeloid forms (Giemsa stain). (**c**) Occasional 'sea-blue' histocytes are noted with Wright–Giemsa stain; these represent benign reactive storage cells attracted by the increased cellular debris.

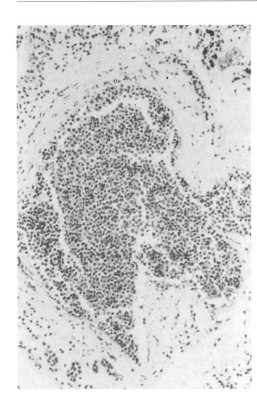

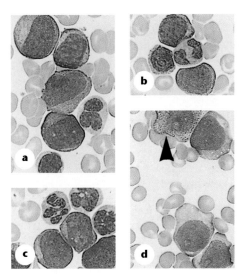

Fig. 13.108 Pulmonary involvement (leukostasis). In some patients with accelerated CML or blastic transformation, dyspnea may occur as a result of pulmonary leukostasis, as noted in this vessel obstructed by excess myeloid cells. Chest radiograph often reveals bilateral infiltrates. Leukostasis may also occur in cerebral vessels, yielding a clinical picture resembling a stroke. Some patients with ANLL, especially M4 and M5 subtypes, also develop leukostasis with or without hemorrhage, particularly when the WBC count is >100 000/μl. The syndrome is very rare in ALL and CLL.

Fig. 13.109 Blast cell transformation (accelerated CML). (**a–d**) Peripheral blood films at high magnification show many myeloblasts, atypical neutrophils and an abnormal promyelocyte (arrow).

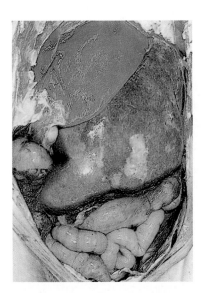

Fig. 13.110 Splenic involvement. The abdominal contents at autopsy of a 54-year-old man are dominated by a grossly enlarged spleen that extends toward the right iliac fossa. The central, pale area covered by fibrinous exudate overlays an extensive splenic infarct. The liver is moderately enlarged.

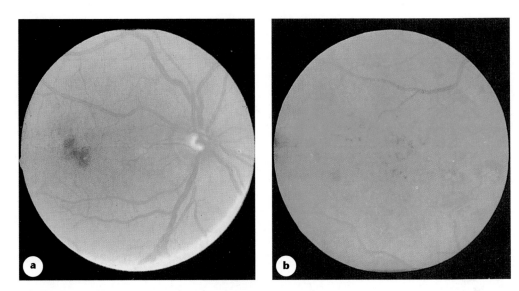

Fig. 13.111 Ophthalmic involvement (hyperviscosity syndrome). (**a**) The ocular fundus shows distended retinal veins and deep retinal hemorrhages at the macula. (**b**) There are also prominent leukemic infiltrates fringed by areas of retinal hemorrhage.

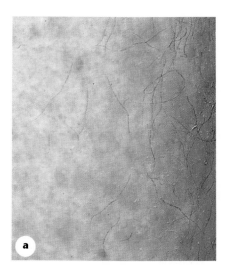
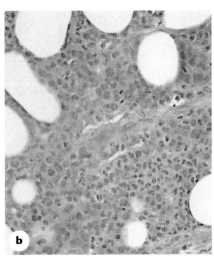

Fig. 13.112 Cutaneous involvement. (**a**) Nodular leukemic infiltrates are present in the skin over the anterior surface of the tibia in a 48-year-old woman with blast cell transformation. (**b**) Histologic section of skin reveals infiltration by myeloblasts and other early myeloid cells.

REFERENCES

Anderson KC, Boyd AW, Fisher DC, *et al.*: Hairy cell leukemia: a tumor of pre-plasma cells. Blood 1985; 65 : 620–629.

Bennett JM, Catovsky D, Daniel MT, *et al.*: Proposed revised criteria for the classification of acute myeloid leukemia. Ann Intern Med 1985; 103 : 626–629.

Brunning RD, McKenna RW: Tumors of the bone marrow. In: Brunning RD, McKenna RW Atlas of Tumor Pathology, 3rd ser., fasc. 9. Armed Forces Institute of Pathology, Washington, DC, 1994.

Canellos GP: Diagnosis and treatment of chronic granulocytic leukemia. In: Wiernik PH, Canellos GP, Kyle RA, Schiffer CA, eds: Neoplastic Diseases of the Blood, vol 1. Churchill Livingstone, New York, 1985; pp. 81–103.

Cannistra SA: Chronic myelogenous leukemia as a model for genetic basis of cancer. Hematol Oncol Clin North Am 1990; 4 : 337–357.

Carey JL, Hanson CA. Flow cytometric analysis of leukemia and lymphoma. In: Keren DF, Hanson CA, Hurtubise PE (eds). Flow Cytometry and Clinical Diagnosis. American Society of Clinical Pathologists, Chicago, 1994; p:197–308.

Chang KL, Stroup R, Weiss LM: Hairy cell leukemia: current status. Am J Clin Pathol 1992; 97 : 719–738.

Cheson BD, Cassileth PA, Head DR, *et al.*: Report of the National Cancer Institute – sponsored workshop on definitions of diagnosis and response in acute myeloid leukemia. J Clin Oncol 1990; 8 : 813–819.

Cline MJ: The molecular basis of leukemia. N Engl J Med 1994; 330 : 328–336.

Cooper PH, Innes DJ, Greer KE: Acute febrile neutrophilic dermatosis (Sweet's syndrome) and myeloproliferative disorders. Cancer 1983; 51 : 1518–1526.

Copelan E, McGuire: The biology and treatment of acute lymphoblastic leukemia in adults. Blood 1995; 85 : 1151–1168.

Creutzig U, Ritter J-Budde M, *et al.*: Early deaths due to hemorrhage and leukostasis in childhood acute myelogenous leukemia. Cancer 1987; 60 : 3071–3079.

Davey FR, Abraham N, Brunetto VL, *et al.*: Morphologic characteristics of erythro-leukemia (acute myeloid leukemia: FAB-M6). Am J Hematol 1995; 49 : 29–38.

Faderl S, Talpaz M, Estrov Z, *et al.*: The biology of chronic myeloid leukemia. N Engl J Med 1999; 341 : 164–172.

Foon KA, Rai KR, Gale RP: Chronic lymphocytic leukemia: new insights into biology and therapy. Ann Intern Med 1990; 113 : 525–539.

Freedman AS, Boyd AW, Bieber FR: Normal cellular counterparts of B cell chronic lymphocytic leukemia. Blood 1987; 70 : 418–427.

Goldman JM, Druker BJ: Chronic myeloid leakemia; current treatment options. Blood 2001; 98 : 2039–2042.

Greenberg P, Cox C, LeBeau MM, *et al.*: International scoring system for evaluating prognosis in myelodysplastic syndromes. Blood 1997; 89 : 2079–2088.

Griffin JD, Nadler LM: Immunobiology of chronic leukemias. In: Wiernik PH, Canellos GP, Kyle RA, Schiffer CA, eds: Neoplastic Diseases of the

Blood, 2nd edn. Churchill Livingstone, New York, 1991; p. 39–60.

Harris NL, Jaffe ES, Diebold J, *et al.*: World Health Organization classification of neoplastic diseases of the hematopoietic and lymphoid tissues: report of the clinical advisory committee meeting – Airlie House, Virginia, November 1997. J Clin Oncol 1999; 17 : 3835–3849.

Hounieu H, Chittal SM, Al Saati T: Hairy cell leukemia: diagnosis of bone marrow involvement in paraffin-embedded sections with monoclonal antibody DBA.44. Am J Clin Pathol 1992; 98 : 26–33.

Kantarjian HM, Dixon D, Keating MJ, *et al.*: Characteristics of accelerated disease in chronic myelogenous leukemia. Cancer 1988; 61 : 1441–1446.

Kantarjian HM, Hirsch-Ginsberg C, Yee G, *et al.*: Mixed lineage leukemia revisited: acute lymphocytic leukemia with myeloperoxidase-positive blasts by electron microscopy. Blood 1990; 76 : 808–813.

Kantarjian HM, Deisseroth A, Kurzock R, *et al.*: Chronic myelogenous leukemia: a concise update. Blood 1993; 82 : 691–703.

Kantarjian H, Talpaz M, Estey E, *et al.*: What is the contribution of molecular studies to the diagnosis of BCR-ABL-positive disease in adult acute leukemia? Am J Med 1994; 96 : 133–138.

Larson RA, Williams SF, LeBeau MM, *et al.*: Acute myelomonocytic leukemia with abnormal eosinophils and onv (16) or t (16;16) has a favorable prognosis. Blood 1986; 68 : 1242–1249.

Loughran TP: Clonal diseases of large granular lymphocytes. Blood 1993; 82 : 1–14.

Lowenberg B, Downing JR, Burnett A: Acute myeloid leukemia. N Engl J Med 1999; 341 : 1051–1062.

Myers TJ, Cole SR, Klatsky AU, *et al.*: Respiratory failure due to pulmonary leukostasis following chemotherapy of acute nonlymphocytic leukemia. Cancer 1983; 51 : 1808–1813.

O'Brien S, del Giglio A, Keating M: Advances in the biology and treatment of B-cell chronic lymphocytic leukemia. Blood 1995; 85 : 307–318.

O'Dwyer ME, Mauro MJ, Druker BJ: Recent advances in the treatment of chronic myelogenous leukemia. Ann Rev Med 2002; 53:369–38.

Paietta E, Wiernik PH, Anderson J, *et al.*: Acute myeloid leukemia M4 with inv(16) (p 13q22) exhibits a specific immunophenotype with CD2 expression. Blood 1993; 82 : 2595.

Preti HA, O'Brien S, Giralt S, *et al.*: Philadelphia-chromosome-positive adult acute lymphocytic leukemia: characteristics, treatment results, and prognosis in 41 patients. Am J Med 1994; 97 : 60–65.

Pui C-H, Behm FG, Crist WM: Clinical and biologic relevance of immunologic marker studies in childhood acute lymphoblastic leukemia. Blood 1993; 82 : 343–362.

Robertson LE, Pugh W, O'Brien S, *et al.*: Richter's syndrome: a report of 39 patients. J Clin Oncol 1993; 11 : 1985–1989.

Rosenfeld C, Lista A: A hypothesis for the pathogenesis of myelodysplastic syndromes: implications for new techniques. Leukemia 2000; 14 : 2–8.

Rowley JD: Chromosome abnormalities in leukemia. J Clin Oncol 1988; 6 : 194–202.

Rozman C, Montserrat E: Chronic lymphocytic leukemia. N Engl J Med 1995; 333 : 1052–1057.

Rubnitz JE, Look AT: Molecular genetics of childhood leukemias. J Ped Hematol/Oncol 1998; 20 : 1–11.

Savin A, Piro L: Newer purine analogues for the treatment of hairy-cell leukemia. N Engl J Med 1994; 330 : 691–697.

Sawyers CL: Chronic myeloid leukemia. N Engl J Med 1999; 340 : 1330–1340.

Semenzato G, Zambello R, Starkebaum G, et al.: The lymphoproliferative disease of granular lymphocytes: updated criteria for diagnosis. Blood 1997; 89 : 256–260.

Skarin AT: Pathology and morphology of chronic leukemias and related disorders. In: Wiernik PH, Canellos GP, Kyle RA, Schiffer CA, eds: Neoplastic Diseases of the Blood, 2nd edn. Churchill Livingstone, New York, 1991; pp. 15–38.

Stasi R, Del Poeta G, Vendetti A, et al.: Analysis of treatment failure in patients with minimally differentiated acute myeloid leukemia (AML-MO). Blood 1994; 83(6):1619–1625.

Tefferi A: Myelofibrosis with myeloid metaplasia. N Engl J Med 2000; 342 : 1255–1265.

Traweek A:. Immunophenotypic analysis of acute leukemia. Am J Clin Pathol 1993; 99 : 504–512.

Waldmann T: Human T-cell lymphotropic virus Type I-associated adult T-cell leukemia. JAMA 1995; 273 : 735–737.

Warrell R, de Thé H, Wang Z, et al.: Acute promyelocytic leukemia. N Engl J Med 1993; 329 : 177–189.

FIGURE CREDITS

The following books published by Gower Medical Publishing are sources of figures in the present chapter. The figure numbers given in the listing are those of the figures in the present chapter. The page numbers given in parentheses are those of the original publication.

Bullough PG, Boachie-Adjei O: Atlas of Spinal Diseases. Lippincott/Gower Medical Publishing, Philadelphia/New York, 1988; Fig. 13.46 (p. 203).

Cawson RA, Eveson JW: Oral Pathology and Diagnosis. Heinemann Medical Books/Gower Medical Publishing, London, 1987: Fig. 13.42 (p. 18.8).

du Vivier A: Atlas of Clinical Dermatology. Churchill Livingstone/Gower Medical Publishing, Edinburgh/London, 1986: Fig. 13.36 (p. 8.16).

Hewitt PE: Blood Diseases (Pocket Picture Guides). Gower Medical Publishing, London, 1985: Figs 13.33 (p. 21), 13.34b (p. 22), 13.53 (p. 27), 13.82b (p. 39).

Hoffbrand AV, Pettit JE: Clinical Haematology Illustrated. Churchill Livingstone/Gower Medical Publishing, Edinburgh/London, 1987: Figs 13.3 (p. 8.9), 13.4 (p. 8.11), 13.5 (p. 8.11), 13.6 (p. 8.12), 13.7 (p. 8.16), 13.8 (p. 8.9), 13.9 (p. 8.10), 13.10 (p. 8.11), 13.15 (p. 8.7), 13.17 (p. 8.7), 13.18 (p. 8.16), 13.19 (p. 8.8), 13.20 (p. 8.8), 13.21 (p. 8.16), 13.23 (p. 8.8), 13.25 (p. 8.11), 13.26 (p. 8.8), 13.27 (p. 8.11), 13.28 (p. 8.9), 13.29 (p. 8.11), 13.30 (p. 8.9), 13.31 (p. 8.13), 13.32 (p. 8.13), 13.34 (p. 8.6), 13.35 (p. 8.5), 13.40 (p. 8.5), 13.49 (p. 8.2), 13.50 (p. 8.3), 13.51 (p. 8.5), 13.52 (p. 8.5), 13.56 (p. 9.12), 13.57 (p. 9.12), 13.58 (p. 9.13), 13.59 (p. 9.13), 13.60 (p. 9.13), 13.61 (p. 9.13), 13.62 (p. 9.13), 13.63 (p. 9.13), 13.64 (p. 9.14), 13.65 (p. 9.14), 13.66 (p. 9.12), 13.67 (p. 9.14), 13.68 (p. 12.11), 13.69 (p. 12.11), 13.70 (p. 12.11), 13.71 (p. 12.11), 13.72 (p. 12.12), 13.74 (p. 9.3), 13.75 (p. 9.3), 13.76 (p. 9.4), 13.77 (p. 9.4), 13.79 (p. 9.4), 13.80 (p. 9.2), 13.82a (p. 9.3), 13.83 (p. 9.3), 13.86 (p. 9.5), 13.87 (p. 1.24), 13.89 (p. 9.5), 13.90 (p. 9.5), 13.91 (p. 9.5), 13.93 (p. 9.6), 13.94 (p. x), 13.95 (p. 9.7), 13.96 (p. 9.7), 13.99 (p. 9.7), 13.101 (p. 9.8), 13.103 (p. 9.9), 13.104 (p. 9.9), 13.109 (p. 9.10), 13.110 (p. 9.8), 13.111 (p. 9.8), 13.112 (p. 9.10).

Weiss MA, Mills SE: Atlas of Genitourinary Tract Disorders. Lippincott/Gower Medical Publishing, Philadelphia/New York, 1988: Fig. 13.47 (p. 11.57).

Yanoff M, Fine BS: Ocular Pathology. Lippincott/Gower Medical Publishing, Philadelphia/New York, 1988: Fig. 13.48 (p. 116).

Hodgkin's disease and non-Hodgkin's lymphomas

David M. Dorfman, Arthur T. Skarin

14

HODGKIN'S DISEASE

About 7400 new cases of Hodgkin's disease are diagnosed in the United States each year, with a slightly higher incidence in men. A bimodal age distribution is observed in the Western world, with peaks at 30 and 70 years of age. In Japan, however, this disease is less common in young adults. A bimodal distribution is not seen in underdeveloped countries, suggesting that Hodgkin's disease is an uncommon, late complication of a common childhood infection. However, the cause is unknown.

CLASSIFICATION AND IMMUNOBIOLOGY

The histology features of Hodgkin's disease vary widely and may not exhibit the classic criteria for malignancy. Moreover, in about 10–15% of cases, recognition of the disorder and its distinction from benign and other malignant lymphoreticular disorders are difficult. In these cases, surface marker studies may be extremely important and accurate diagnosis may depend on the availability of fresh tissue for evaluation by an experienced hematopathologist.

The first histopathologic classification of Hodgkin's disease was established in 1966 by an international conference in Rye, New York, and consists of four subtypes. The subtypes are still included in the new World Health Organization (WHO) classification (*see* Fig. 14.1). The majority of cells comprising a tumor mass appear to be benign or reactive and include lymphocytes, eosinophils, granulocytes, plasma cells, fibroblasts and mononuclear cells. The pathognomonic finding for the diagnosis is the Reed–Sternberg cell in the appropriate immunoreactive background.

Molecular biological analysis of micromanipulated Reed–Sternberg cells supports the B-lymphocyte as the cell of origin. It is noteworthy that cells morphologically indistinguishable from Reed–Sternberg cells have been found in other hematologic disorders, both benign (e.g. infectious mononucleosis) and malignant (e.g. T-cell immunoblastic lymphoma). Surface marker studies are useful in the differential diagnosis. The immunophenotype of the typical Reed–Sternberg cell is positive for Ki-1 (CD30), CD15 (Leu-M1), HLA-DR and CD25 (IL-2 receptor); it is negative for leukocyte common antigen (LCA) (CD45) and is usually negative for T-cell and B-cell antigens, as well for most monocyte, macrophage and histiocyte antigens. An exception is lymphocyte-predominant Hodgkin's disease in which Reed–Sternberg cells have the immunophenotype of B-cells.

The Reed–Sternberg cell is known to secrete a number of cytokines, including interleukin-1 (IL-1), IL-5, IL-6, IL-9, tumor necrosis factor-α, macrophage colony stimulating factor and transforming growth factor-β. These cytokines may attract the mixed inflammatory cell infiltrate seen in Hodgkin's disease, result in the characteristic fibrosis seen in the nodular sclerosis subtype and contribute to the immunosuppression that may occur in Hodgkin's disease. Epstein–Barr virus has been associated with a significant percentage of cases of Hodgkin's disease, particularly the mixed cellularity type, by a number of investigational methods.

CLINICAL EVALUATION AND STAGING

Evaluation of a patient includes a detailed history and physical examination, complete blood cell (CBC) count with differential, blood chemistries, chest radiograph, CT scan of the chest, abdomen and pelvis and bone marrow aspiration and biopsy. Retroperitoneal nodes can accurately be assessed by lymphangiography, although the latter has been replaced by CT scanning at many medical centers. Lymphangiography should not be carried out when large obstructing nodes are present because collateral vessels may allow shunting of contrast agent into the lungs, resulting in dyspnea and other symptoms. A useful study is gallium-67 citrate scanning, utilizing a dose of 10 nCi, with delayed views up to 72 and 96 hours if necessary, for optimal imaging. Clinically inapparent sites may be gallium avid. In addition, gallium scans are useful in the differential diagnosis of residual masses and in following the response to therapy. In the absence of infection, persistent gallium uptake signifies active disease.

Staging laparotomy is often indicated when a choice must be made among several possible therapeutic approaches. This procedure requires a skilled surgeon who can adequately biopsy a variety of structures and nodal sites that may be difficult to reach. Because the spleen is involved in up to 50% of cases, splenectomy is necessary and should be followed by careful preparation of multiple thin sections for review by a hematopathologist. The extent of splenic involvement by Hodgkin's disease is an important factor in determining the prognosis and the choice of therapy. Extensive involvement, probably owing to hematogenous spread, is a poor prognostic feature.

In most cases, Hodgkin's disease tends to progress in an orderly fashion from one lymph node-bearing area to the next. The results of the staging workup are a part of the Ann Arbor staging system (*see* Fig. 14.13). The designation CS is used for clinical stage and PS is used for pathologic stage, the latter signifying histologic evidence of malignancy in tissue obtained at staging laparotomy. Treatment is then planned: radiotherapy for early disease (stages I, II and III$_1$), chemotherapy for advanced disease (stages III$_2$ and IV) or combination therapy for certain selected cases.

CLINICAL MANIFESTATIONS

Most patients present with early or localized disease. Lymph node enlargement may wax and wane for unknown reasons, although 'spontaneous' remissions are rare as compared with the non-Hodgkin's lymphomas. About 20–30% of cases have B symptoms; however, only 5–10% of patients present with extranodal sites of disease, including lung, liver and bone marrow. The latter presentation is more often seen in patients over 60 years of age.

Hodgkin's lymphoma (Hodgkin's Disease)
Nodular lymphocyte-predominant Hodgkin's lymphoma (5%)
Clasical Hodgkin's lymphoma (95%)
Hodgkin's lymphoma, nodular sclerosis (Grades 1 and 11)
Classical Hodgkin's lymphoma. Lymphocyte rich
Hodgkin's lymphoma. Mixed cellularity
Hodgkin's lymphoma. Lymphocytic depletion (includes most Hodgkin's-like anaplastic large-cell lymphoma)

Fig. 14.1 Histologic classification of Hodgkin's disease. The original classification developed by Jackson and Parker in 1944 was modified by Lukes and colleagues in 1966 into a clinically useful system and simplified in the same year by the Rye classification. This was later modified in the Revised European–American Classification of Lymphoid Neoplasms (REAL) and the current WHO classification listed here.

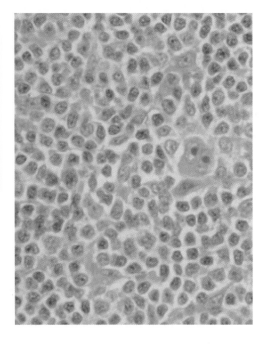

Fig. 14.2 Hodgkin's disease (lymphocyte-predominant type). A rare, diagnostic Reed–Sternberg cell is seen (center) in a 'sea' of lymphocytes. Optimal cytologic detail is obtained by use of B5 fixative, which also preserves cell antigens very well for subsequent immunoperoxidase studies utilizing monoclonal antibodies.

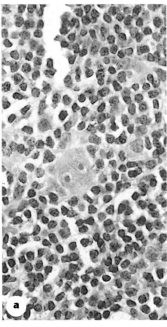

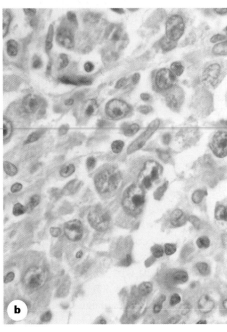

Fig. 14.3 Hodgkin's disease. (a) Lymph node biopsy specimen shows a single Reed–Sternberg cell surrounded by lymphocytes and other mononuclear cells in lymphocyte-predominant disease. (b) In lymphocyte-depleted disease, large numbers of Reed–Sternberg cells and mononuclear variants can typically be seen, but only small numbers of lymphocytes are present.

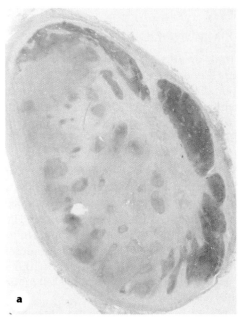

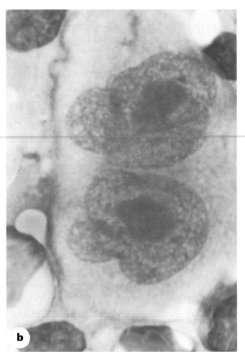

Fig. 14.4 Hodgkin's disease (nodular-sclerosis type). (a) Low magnification of a lymph node shows aggregates of tumor cells (blue areas) surrounded by sclerosing fibrous bands (eosinophilic or pink areas). (b) Lymph node touch prep reveals a classic Reed–Sternberg cell with a bilobed nucleus and large, round, inclusion-like nucleoli.

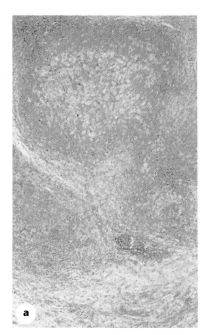

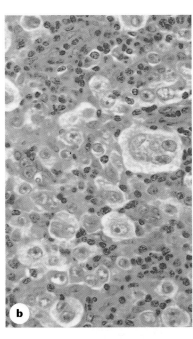

Fig. 14.5 Hodgkin's disease (nodular-sclerosis type). (**a**) Gross capsular thickening and fibrous tissue bands divide this lymph node into discrete nodules containing foci of pale 'lacunar' cells. (**b**) At high magnification, characteristic 'lacunar' cell variants of Reed–Sternberg cells exhibit haloes, representing shrinking of the cells' abundant, pale cytoplasm during fixation in formalin.

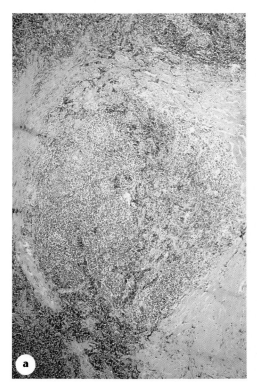

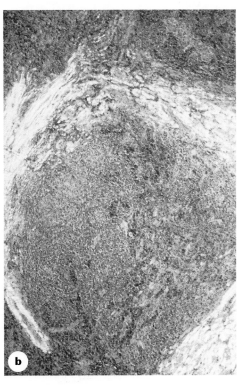

Fig. 14.6 Hodgkin's disease (nodular-sclerosis type). (**a**) This lymphoid tumor nodule is surrounded by characteristic sclerosing bands of collagen that are birefringent with polarized light (**b**). Nodular sclerosis Hodgkin's disease is the only type that is more common in women than men.

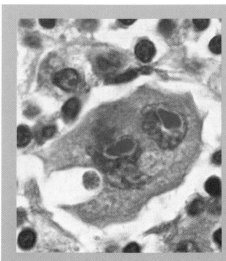

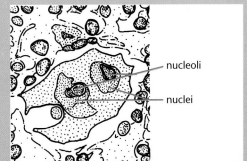

Fig. 14.7 Hodgkin's disease. High-power photomicrograph demonstrates a binucleate Reed–Sternberg cell exhibiting prominent inclusion-like eosinophilic nucleoli giving it an 'owl's eye' appearance.

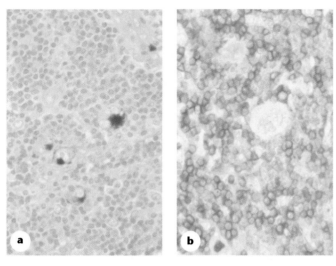

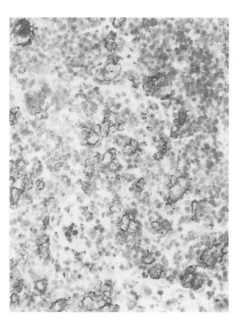

Fig. 14.8 Hodgkin's disease immunoperoxidase staining of Reed–Sternberg cells and variants reveals (**a**) their characteristic immunoreactivity for CD15 (Leu-M1) in a perinuclear localization pattern and (**b**) a lack of reactivity for LCA (CD45); note the strong reactivity of the surrounding lymphocytes. CD15 (Leu-M1) also stains some non-lymphoid tumors, for example, various adenocarcinomas and papillary thyroid cancer, as well as some non-Hodgkin's lymphomas.

Fig. 14.9 Hodgkin's disease. Lymph node biopsy specimen shows a positive reaction for the monoclonal antibody to Ki-1 (CD30), which reacts particularly, but not exclusively, with Reed–Sternberg cells (alkaline phosphatase-antialkaline phosphatase). (Courtesy of Prof. H. Stein.)

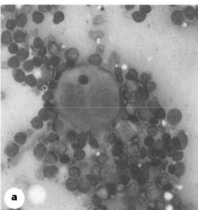

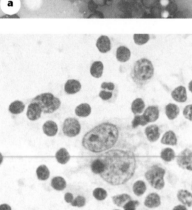

Fig. 14.10 Hodgkin's disease. Fine-needle aspiration biopsy specimens of involved lymph nodes demonstrate Reed–Sternberg cells stained (**a**) by May–Grünwald–Giemsa and (**b**) Papanicolaou techniques.

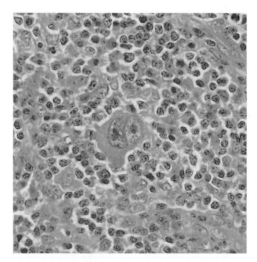

Fig. 14.11 Hodgkin's disease (mixed cellularity type). The histopathologic features characteristically seen in this type include abundant and readily identifiable Reed–Sternberg cells and variants, which are easily seen in most low-power microscope fields; in this instance, a conspicuous Reed–Sternberg cell is present, exhibiting mirror-image nuclei and prominent nucleoli. This type is also marked by a mixed cellular background, in this case containing sheets of lymphocytes, plasma cells and eosinophils, and the absence of sclerosing fibrosis.

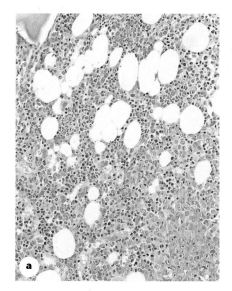
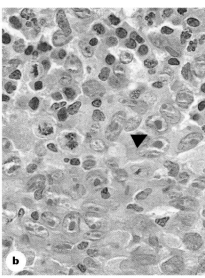

Fig. 14.12 Hodgkin's disease. Marrow biopsy specimen shows (**a**) Hodgkin's tissue replacing normal hematopoietic elements in the lower right field. (**b**) On higher power view, there is extensive replacement of hematopoietic tissue by atypical mononuclear cells in the center and lower fields. Note the Reed–Sternberg cell (arrow).

Ann arbor staging system for hodgkin's disease and non-hodgkin's lymphomas

Stage I

- involvement of single lymph node region
- or involvement of single extralymphatic site (stage I_E)

Stage II

- involvement of ≥ 2 lymph node regions on same side of diaphragm
- may include localized extralymphatic involvement on same side of diaphragm (stage II_E)

Stage III

- involvement of lymph node regions on both sides of diaphragm
- may include involvement of spleen (stage III_S) or localized extranodal disease (stage III_E) or both (III_{E+S})

For Hodgkin's Disease:
III_1
- disease limited to upper abdomen – spleen, splenic hilar, celiac, or porta hepatic nodes

III_2
- disease limited to lower abdomen – periaortic, pelvic, or inguinal nodes

Stage IV

- disseminated (multifocal) extralymphatic disease involving one or more organs (e.g., liver, bone marrow, lung, skin), +/- associated lymph node involvement
- or isolated extralymphatic disease with distant (non-regional) lymph node involvement

Note: Stage designation "B" indicates unexplained weight loss > 10% of body weight in preceding six months and/or fevers of > 38°C and/or night sweats. Stage designation "A" indicates the absence of the features characterizing "B".

Fig. 14.13 Ann Arbor staging of Hodgkin's disease and non-Hodgkin's lymphomas. Lymph node involvement in one area is designated as stage I disease. Involvement of two or more areas confined to one side of the diaphragm constitutes stage II disease. In stage III disease, lymph node areas above and below the diaphragm are affected. The spleen may be involved (stage IIIS) and this often precedes widespread hematogenous dissemination. In Hodgkin's disease, stage III is subdivided into stage III_1, for disease limited to the upper abdomen (spleen; and splenic hilar, celiac or porta hepatis nodes), and

III_2, for disease involving the lower abdomen (periaortic, pelvic or inguinal nodes). Stage IV is marked by diffuse extralymphatic disease that may affect, for example, the liver, bone marrow, lung and skin. A subscript E in stages I, II and III disease indicates localized extranodal extension from a nodal mass, and designation of a stage as either A or B indicates the absence (A) or presence (B) of unexplained weight loss greater than 10% of body weight in the preceding 6 months and/or fever of greater than 38°C and/or night sweats.

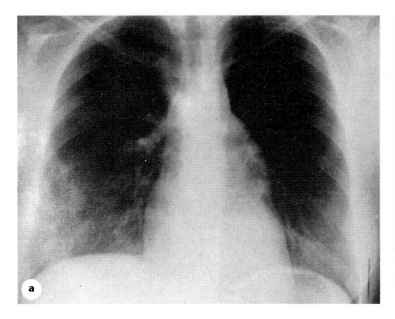

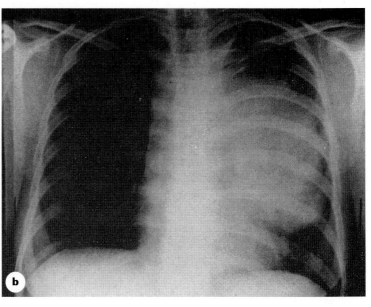

Fig. 14.14 Hodgkin's disease (stage IA$_E$). (**a**) Routine chest radiograph of a 24-year-old woman, which was originally read as normal, shows mediastinal widening in the left parahilar region. (**b**) Two years later a huge mass extends to the lateral chest wall, a classic example of the natural history of untreated Hodgkin's disease. The patient was cured with chemotherapy and radiotherapy.

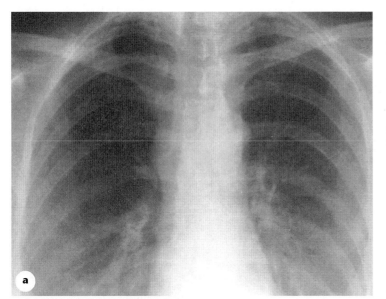

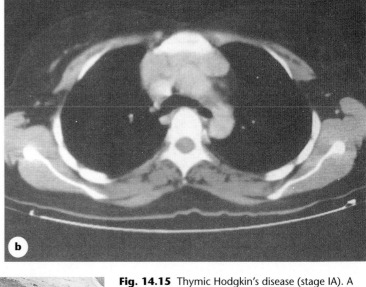

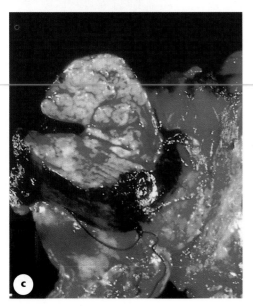

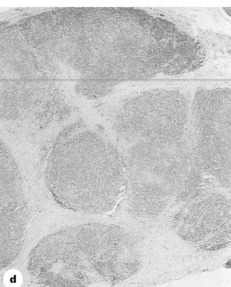

Fig. 14.15 Thymic Hodgkin's disease (stage IA). A 17-year-old woman was found to have asymptomatic mediastinal adenopathy. (**a**) Chest radiograph shows bilateral mediastinal widening, greater on the right than on the left. (**b**) CT scan at the carina reveals an anterior mediastinal mass in the region of the thymus. Thymectomy was performed for a probable thymoma. (**c**) On cut section, the tumor appears to be composed of nodular, fleshy aggregates. (**d**) Microscopically, these nodules comprise tumor cells surrounded by sclerotic bands of collagen, characteristic of nodular sclerosis type. High magnification (not shown) revealed Reed–Sternberg cells and variants.

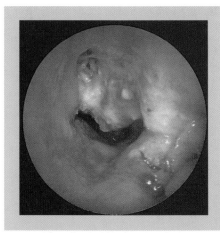

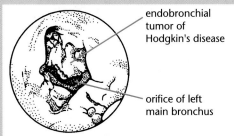

endobronchial
tumor of
Hodgkin's disease

orifice of left
main bronchus

Fig. 14.16 Hodgkin's disease (stage IIA_E). Endobronchial disease, shown here affecting the left lower bronchus (photographed through a rigid bronchoscope for clarity), is unusual and patients often present with hemoptysis. (This view is oriented for a bronchoscopist standing in front of the patient.) (Courtesy of Dr P Stradling.)

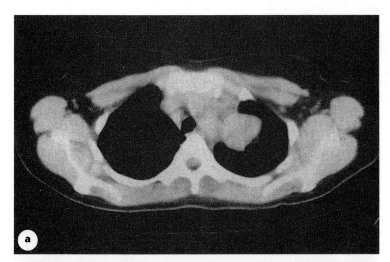

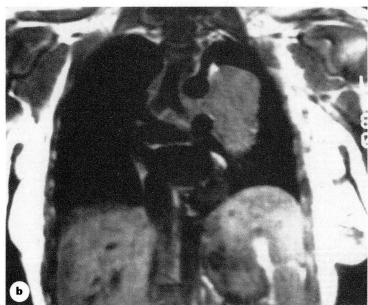

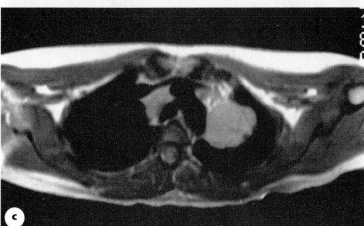

Fig. 14.17 Hodgkin's disease (stage IIA). A 19-year-old woman presented with cervical adenopathy. Chest radiography showed a predominantly left-sided mediastinal mass, which appears well delineated (**a**) on CT scan. There is no parenchymal extension. (**b**) T1-weighted MR scan clearly shows the extent of disease in the coronal plane. The mass has the same intensity as muscle. (**c**) T2-weighted image in the axial plane reveals the mass to be almost as intense as fat. This change from lower (muscle) to higher (fat) intensity in the shift from T1- to T2-weighted imaging indicates an active tumor.

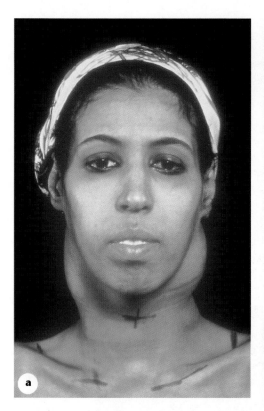
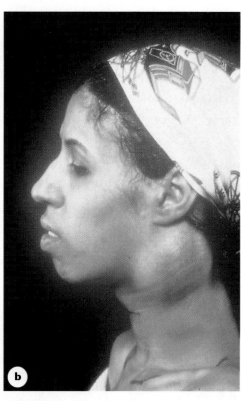

Fig. 14.18 Hodgkin's disease (stage IIA). (**a, b**) Marked enlargement of cervical lymph nodes is present in this patient. It is usually painless and may be confined to only one area or may affect two or more areas. A scar from a previous biopsy can be seen on the lateral view.

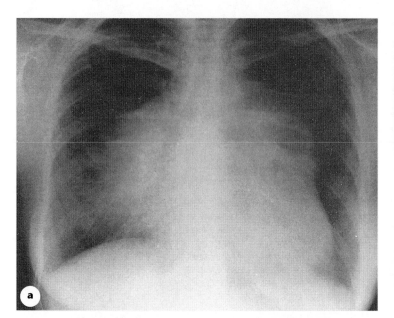
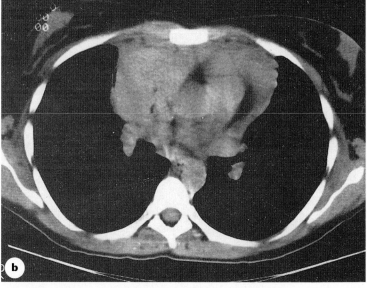
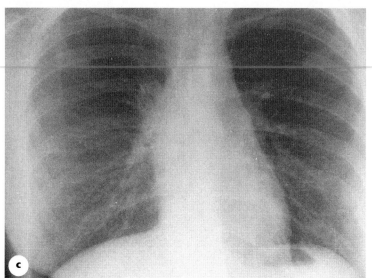

Fig. 14.19 Hodgkin's disease (stage IIA). A 21-year-old woman presented with cough and chest discomfort. (**a**) Chest film and (**b**) CT scan show bulky mediastinal adenopathy. (**c**) Chest film after treatment shows that the mediastinum is almost normal. Residual widening in the aortopulmonary window is a common finding after treatment and does not necessarily indicate residual tumor. Gallium-67 citrate scan is usually negative unless lymphoma persists.

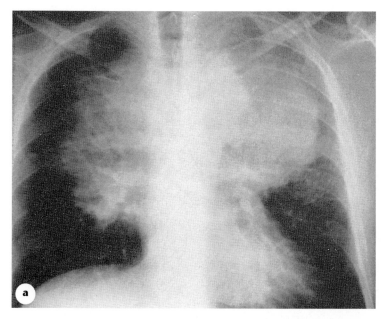

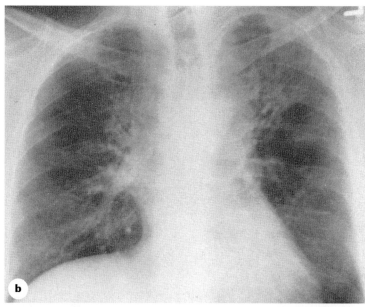

Fig. 14.20 Hodgkin's disease (stage II$_E$). (**a**) Chest radiograph of a 30-year-old man who presented with cough and dyspnea shows extensive bilateral, bulky, mediastinal adenopathy with extension into the pulmonary parenchyma of the right lung. (**b**) Marked reduction in tumor mass is noted after combined chemotherapy and radiotherapy.

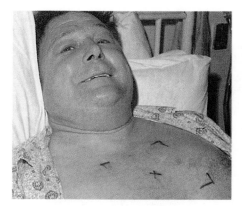

Fig. 14.21 Hodgkin's disease (stage II). Cyanosis and edema of the face, neck and upper trunk are due to superior vena cava obstruction caused by mediastinal node involvement (*see* Fig. 4.49). The skin markings over the anterior chest indicate the field of radiotherapy.

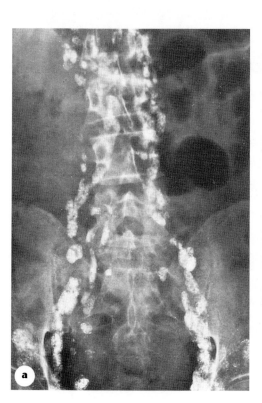

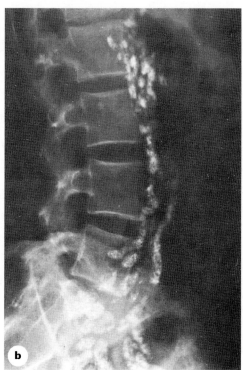

Fig. 14.22 Hodgkin's disease (stage IIIA$_2$). (**a, b**) Positive nodal-phase lymphangiogram of a 35-year-old man demonstrates enlargement of all the iliac and para-aortic nodes. More important is the alteration in the normal architecture of the nodes, with many small filling defects and a generalized 'foamy' appearance. These findings are typical of lymphomatous involvement, confirmed in this case at laparotomy. Lymphangiography has been essentially replaced by CT scanning and in many cases by Ga67 or PET scanning which require less time, are highly acurate and also useful for follow-up evaluation for residual disease even in normal sized nodes (see Chapter 2).

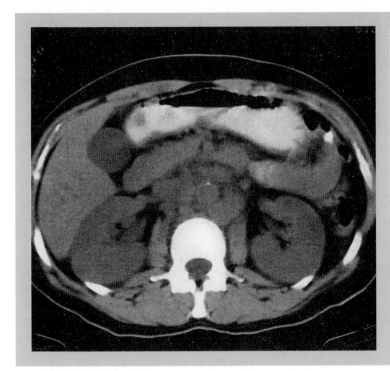

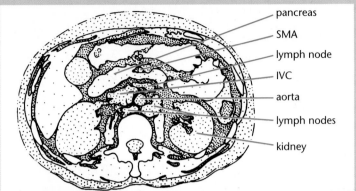

Fig. 14.23 Hodgkin's disease (stage IIIB$_2$). A 32-year-old woman presented with fever and night sweats and was found to have left cervical adenopathy. Biopsy showed nodular sclerosis-type Hodgkin's disease. This CT scan of the abdomen demonstrates retroperitoneal adenopathy at the level of the renal hilum. Calcification in the wall of the aorta can also be noted. Gallium-67 citrate scan of the abdomen (not shown) was positive in the retroperitoneum, correlating with the CT scan abnormalities.

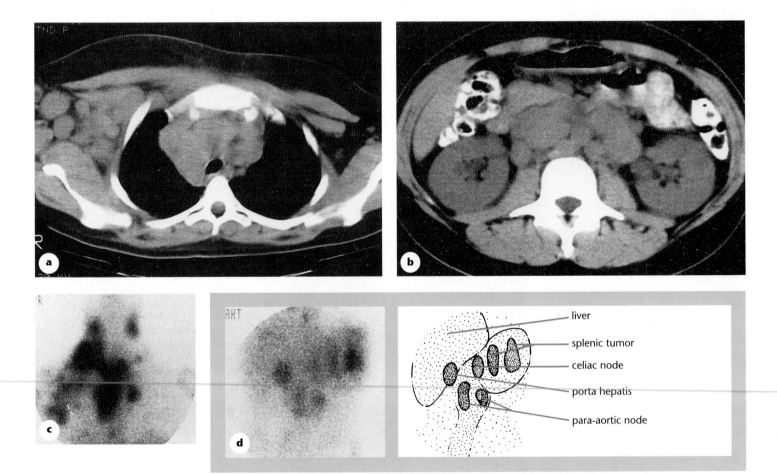

Fig. 14.24 Hodgkin's disease (stage IIIA$_2$). A 24-year-old woman presented with cervical and axillary adenopathy. (**a**) CT scan of the chest shows mediastinal disease hand also bulky right axillary adenopathy. (**b**) Retroperitoneal adenopathy and a mass at the porta hepatis were also present. An abdominal CT scan (not shown) revealed an enlarged spleen with a heterogeneous texture, consistent with involvement by Hodgkin's disease. Images from a gallium-67 citrate scan show uptake (**c**) in the neck bilaterally, right axilla and mediastinum, and (**d**) in the porta hepatis and spleen. Retroperitoneal and pelvic lymph nodes (not shown) also demonstrated increased uptake. Biopsy revealed the nodular-sclerosis type of Hodgkin's disease.

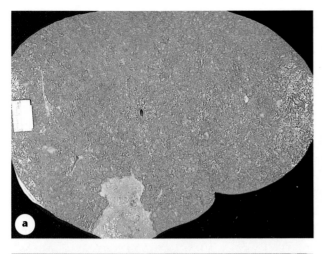

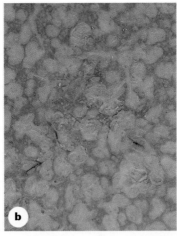

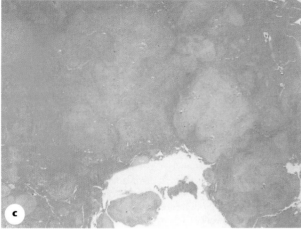

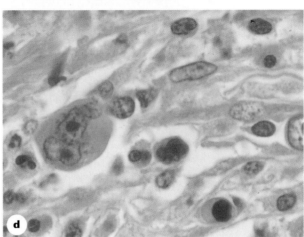

Fig. 14.25 Hodgkin's disease (stage III$_S$). (**a**) Cross-section of a spleen removed at laparotomy shows a single, large Hodgkin's deposit adjacent to the capsule. Many focal grayish-yellow areas, up to 4 mm in diameter, are also scattered throughout the tissue. (**b**) Higher magnification reveals the classic appearance of the spleen in Hodgkin's disease (so-called 'salami' spleen), although almost any macroscopic distribution may be seen, as in non-Hodgkin's lymphomas. (**c**) The white pulp is expanded and replaced by innumerable irregular, pale deposits of tumor. (**d**) These deposits contain a mixed inflammatory cell infiltrate as well as characteristic Reed–Sternberg cells and variants.

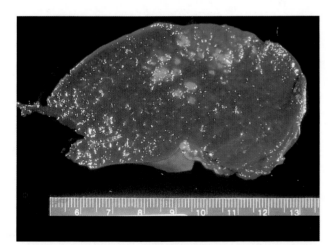

Fig. 14.26 Another example of a spleen involved by Hodgkin's disease, removed during a staging laparotomy. The scattered macroscopic nodules seen were not detected by a prior CT scan (not shown).

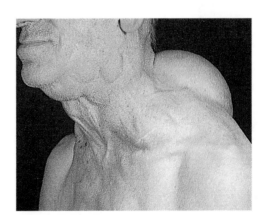

Fig. 14.27 Hodgkin's disease (stage IV). Massive cervical and suboccipital lymphadenopathy is seen in a 73-year-old man who presented with stage IV$_B$ disease.

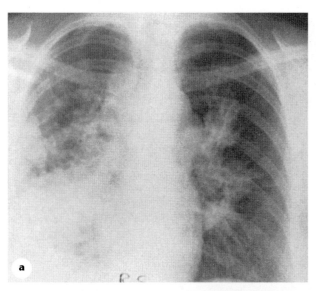

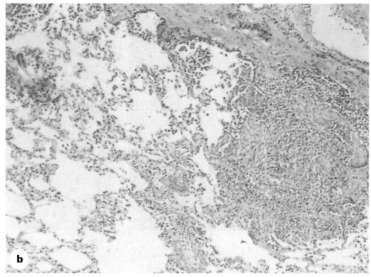

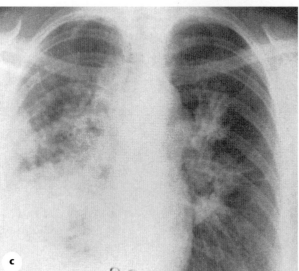

Fig. 14.28 Hodgkin's disease (stage IVB). A 25-year-old woman presented with weight loss, fever and night sweats and was found to have cervical and axillary adenopathy. (**a**) Chest radiograph shows bilateral pulmonary infiltrates, consistent with involvement with Hodgkin's disease. (**b**) Lung biopsy confirms earlier lymph node biopsy findings, which were positive for Hodgkin's disease, mixed cellularity type. CT scan (not shown) demonstrated hepatosplenomegaly. She was treated with chemotherapy and showed a clinically complete response. (**c**) Chest radiograph demonstrates residual pulmonary scarring 2 months later. A new mediastinal mass developed 3 years afterward and responded to radiotherapy. Seven years later, because of fever and anemia, a bone marrow biopsy was obtained, showing involvement by Hodgkin's disease. Once again she responded to chemotherapy, but died 6 years later from recurrent Hodgkin's disease. Although most relapses occur within 4 years of therapy, rare late relapses beyond 10 years have been reported, as in this patient who died 16 years after the initial diagnosis.

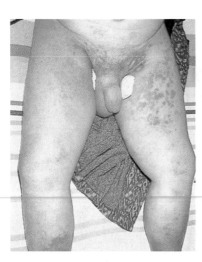

Fig. 14.29 Hodgkin's disease (stage IV). Gross edema of the legs, genitals and lower abdominal wall (with umbilical herniation) is due to lymphatic obstruction resulting from extensive involvement of the inguinal and pelvic lymph nodes. There is a staphylococcal infection in the skin folds of the groins.

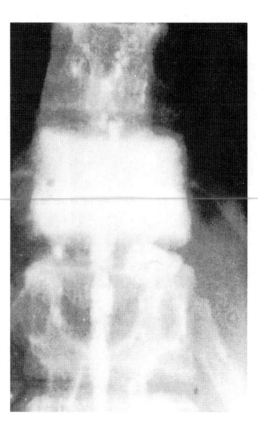

Fig. 14.30 Hodgkin's disease (stage IV). This radiograph of the thoracic spine in a 35-year-old man who presented with vague back pain shows a single, dense, sclerotic ('ivory') vertebra, which on biopsy proved to be involved by Hodgkin's disease. Bone involvement manifests with considerable marrow fibrosis and reactive bone formation, which may be extensive enough to obscure the lymphomatous tissue.

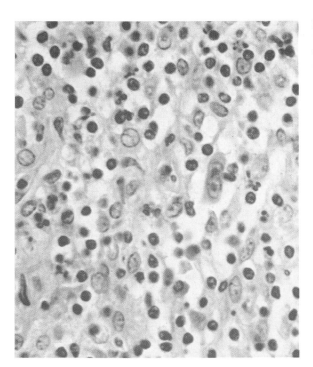

Fig. 14.31 Hodgkin's disease (stage IV). Photomicrograph of an area of Hodgkin's disease in bone shows a fibrous stroma with a mixed cellular infiltrate of small round cells, larger histiocytes and a diagnostic Reed–Sternberg cell near the center.

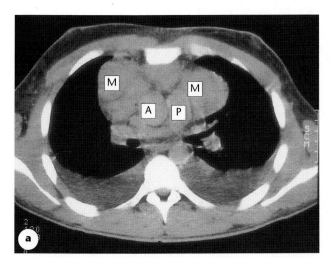

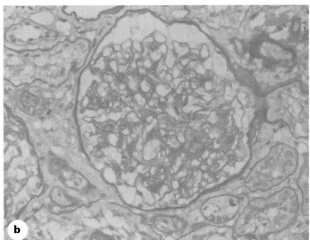

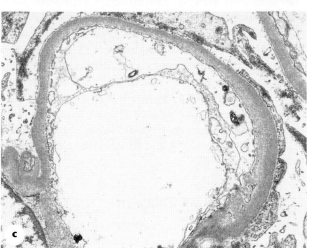

Fig. 14.32 Hodgkin's disease (nephrotic syndrome). An 18-year-old man presented with classic features of nephrotic syndrome including facial edema, ascites and peripheral edema. Cervical adenopathy was present and lymph node biopsy showed nodular sclerosis-type Hodgkin's disease. (**a**) Axial CT image at the level of the main pulmonary artery, without intravenous contrast, shows a large, lobular mass (M) extending to the right and left of the great vessels anteriorly. Bilateral pleural effusions (arrows) are present. A=ascending aorta; P=main pulmonary artery. (**b**) Renal biopsy shows glomeruli with open capillary loops and thin, delicate basement membranes (light microscopy, high power). (**c**) Electron microscopy reveals extensive effacement of podocyte foot processes diagnostic of minimal change disease (lipoid nephrosis). Nephrotic syndrome (NS) associated with Hodgkin's disease is rare, with under 50 reported cases. Pathogenesis of NS is unknown but includes immune complex deposition, abnormalities of T-cell function, viral antigens, tumor antigens and fetal antigen expression (Dabbs *et al.*, 1986). (**c**: Courtesy of Dr FS Lee and Dr A Krishnan.)

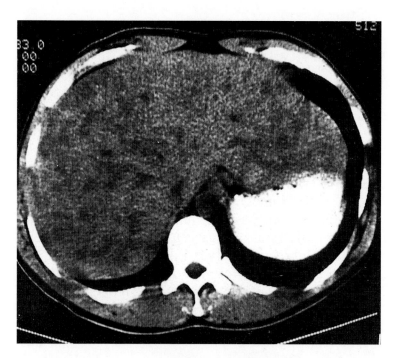

Fig. 14.33 Hodgkin's disease (relapse). A 26-year-old man presented with stage IA disease (mixed cellularity type) and was treated by radiotherapy. Relapse occurred at multiple nodal sites within 2 years, followed 3 years later by liver involvement, as seen in this non-contrast enhanced CT scan. The liver shows diffuse areas of low attenuation, consistent with infiltration by Hodgkin's disease.

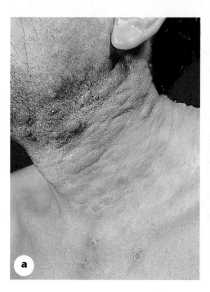

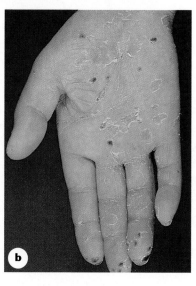

Fig. 14.34 Hodgkin's disease (relapse). Depressed cell-mediated immunity in Hodgkin's disease is associated with an increased incidence of infections, particularly herpes zoster, as seen here represented by (**a**) a vesicular cutaneous eruption of the neck and (**b**) an atypical herpetic eruption on the palmar surface of the hand in a patient who relapsed after primary radiotherapy. Lymphopenia, particularly with depression of the CD4:CD8 T-cell ratio secondary to radiotherapy, may further contribute to increased infections.

NON-HODGKIN'S LYMPHOMA

Non-Hodgkin's lymphomas are a diverse group of malignancies of the lymphoreticular system that have heterogeneous histopathologic, immunologic, cytogenetic and clinical characteristics. About 55 000 new cases are diagnosed in the United States each year and the incidence is rising, particularly in AIDS patients. Although the disease can appear at any age, the median age is 50 years and the incidence increases with age. Diffuse lymphomas are more common in men (2 : 1) compared with nodular (follicular) lymphomas (1 : 1). Nodular lymphomas are rare in children. Although the etiology is unknown, malignant lymphomas are more common in patients with immune deficiency syndromes (e.g. acquired hypogammaglobulinemia), autoimmune disorders (e.g. rheumatoid arthritis), immunosuppressive states (e.g. renal transplants) and acquired immunodeficiency syndrome (AIDS). In AIDS patients, for example, 5–10% develop intermediate- to high-grade

B-cell non-Hodgkin's lymphomas and these are included as part of the CDC AIDS diagnosis criteria. Epstein–Barr virus has been observed in a significant percentage of AIDS-associated lymphomas and appears to have an etiologic role in their pathogenesis (*see* Chapter 17). The African form of Burkitt's lymphoma is associated with Epstein–Barr virus infection as well. A form of aggressive T-cell leukemia-lymphoma associated with HTLV-1 infection has been reported in southern Japan, the Caribbean and the southeastern United States. Genetic factors may also predispose to lymphomas, as evidenced by cases in patients with chromosomal disorders (e.g. ataxia telangiectasia) and those with immunodeficiency disorders other than AIDS.

CLASSIFICATION AND IMMUNOBIOLOGY

Histopathologic classifications and frequency of non-Hodgkin's lymphoma subsets are shown in Figure 14.35 and Tables 14.1 and

14.8. The Working Formulation classification (see Fig. 14.35), devised by an international panel of clinicians and pathologists sponsored by the National Cancer Institute, retained the relevant features of the Rappaport system and divided lymphomas into 10 separate subgroups (A–J) and three major prognostic categories. The terminology is based mainly on the Lukes–Collins system and the Kiel (Lennert) system used in Europe, both of which recognize the immunologic origin of lymphomas from T, B or 'null' cells. Thus, the nodular (follicular) growth pattern represents lymphomas arising from follicular center cells (B-cells) of normal lymphoid follicles, whereas lymphomas of large cells, formerly believed to arise from 'histiocytes' of the monocyte–macrophage system, are in reality almost always derived from transformed B- or T-cells. These classification schemes have been replaced by the WHO classification of lymphoid neoplasms based on morphologic, immunophenotypic and cytogenetic features (Harris et al., 1999).

A considerable understanding of the immunology of lymphomas has been achieved by the availability of specific monoclonal antibodies directed against cell surface antigens (see Figs 14.37 and 14.38 and Table 14.5). It has been found that the malignant cells of most lymphomas have normal cell counterparts. By use of an extensive panel of monoclonal antibodies, about 80% of lymphomas can be identified as B-cell lymphomas and 20% as T-cell lymphomas: less than 1% are true 'histiocytic' lymphomas.

Most lymphomas express leukocyte common antigen (LCA) (CD45), which is detectable by immunoperoxidase staining using monoclonal antibodies against LCA, LCA staining is very useful because it is immunoreactive (positive) even in poorly differentiated lymphomas that might otherwise be mistaken for carcinoma, sarcoma or melanoma, all of which are LCA negative. Furthermore, LCA staining can be performed on formalin- and B5-fixed tissues. (The latter is preferred because of better histologic detail, particularly of the cell nucleus.) Cell lineage as determined by the use of monoclonal antibodies usually requires fresh tissue. The monoclonality of B-cell lymphomas can be confirmed by immunoperoxidase staining for one class of immunoglobulin light chain or by immunoglobulin gene rearrangement studies. T-cell lymphomas, on the other hand, do not express cell surface immunoglobulins but many exhibit clonal loss of expression of pan-T cell antigens, which can be tested using monoclonal antibodies. Gene rearrangement studies of the T-cell receptor may also be used to determine monoclonality. Lymphomas of T-cell lineage can also be identified by the formation of so-called 'rosettes' on reaction with sheep erythrocytes. T-cell phenotyping is carried out by reaction with available monoclonal antibodies (see Fig. 14.38).

Many chromosomal, molecular and genetic defects have been detected in various lymphomas. These are described in the section on lymphoma subsets (see below). A better understanding of the biology of lymphomas allows for clarification of the pathogenesis and also for future novel therapeutic approaches.

Amplification of DNA can now be performed on small amounts of tissue by the polymerase chain reaction (PCR) technique, thus allowing for detection of abnormal clones (i.e. monoclonal population of malignant cells). The method is extremely sensitive and may detect residual tumor or early disease relapse.

HISTOLOGIC SUBTYPES

Immunophenotypic and other classification markers are noted in Figs 14.37, 14.38, 14.39 and 14.40 and Table 14.5.

Small lymphocytic lymphoma (SLL)

This subtype of malignant is a low-grade lymphoma with a favorable prognosis characterized by a diffuse pattern with effacement of nodal architecture by round lymphocytes of small-to-medium size. Mitotic figures are rare. In a minority of cases there may be plasmacytic differentiation with associated macroglobulinemia. SLL and chronic lymphocytic leukemia (CLL) probably represent different clinical manifestations of the same disease process, the former marked mainly by adenopathy and the latter by lymphocytosis involving the bone marrow and peripheral blood.

Mantle cell lymphoma

This uncommon lymphoma subgroup is not easily placed in the NCI Working Formulation classification. It is composed of small lymphocytes having nuclei intermediate in size between those of WDLL and a small cleaved cell-type follicular center cell lymphoma, poorly differentiated lymphocytic (PDL) lymphoma. The lymphoma appears to arise from B-lymphocytes found in the mantle zone of lymphoid follicles. The histologic pattern of mantle cell lymphoma may be nodular, with neoplastic cells surrounding residual germinal centers (mantle zone pattern) or diffuse. Fifty percent or more of cases exhibit a t(11;14) chromosomal translocation involving the bcl-1 locus on chromosome 11, resulting in overexpression of the PRAD1 gene, the product of which, cyclin D1, is involved in cell cycle regulation. Mantle cell lymphoma typically pursues an aggressive course (median survival 3–4 years).

Follicular lymphoma

A mixed lymphoma is composed of both small lymphocytes and large lymphoid cells (formerly erroneously identified as histiocytes), the latter accounting for 25–50% of the total cell population. When the proportion of large cells falls below 25% of the cell population, the tumor is identified grade 1 lesion. On the other hand, if large lymphoid cells constitute more than 50% of the cell population, the tumor is classified as a grade 3 lesion. Follicular lymphomas may be predominantly follicular (>75%), follicular and diffuse (25–75% follicular), and predominantly diffuse (<25% follicular). These tumors have a prolonged to intermediate clinical course. Most cases of nodular follicular center cell lymphomas, including large cell lymphoma, exhibit a t(14;18) chromosomal translocation, which results in deregulation of expression of the bcl-2 proto-oncogene on chromosome 18. This gene blocks programmed cell death (apoptosis) and its overexpression results in prolongation of the lifespan of involved cells, contributing to the pathogenesis of lymphoma. Approximately 20% of diffuse non-Hodgkin's lymphomas of follicular center cell origin exhibit the t(14;18) translocation. Mixed lymphomas derived from T-cells, however, are characterized by aggressive disease and a shorter duration of survival, although modern treatment regimens have improved the prognosis.

Large cell lymphomas

Large cell lymphomas constitute a heterogeneous group of malignancies comprising several histologic subtypes (see Table 14.8). Most cases exhibit a diffuse pattern and are called diffuse large cell lymphomas (DLCL); they follow a clinically aggressive course. The few cases displaying a nodular pattern follow an intermediate clinical course. Approximately 75–80% of large cell lymphomas are of B-cell origin, whereas 20% are composed of large T-cells and the remaining few cases are of indeterminate or monocyte–macrophage origin. In the Rappaport classification, the term diffuse histiocytic lymphoma (DHL) was used to describe this malignancy, because it was believed that it was derived from histiocytes. Immunophenotyping, however, has revealed that most large cell lymphomas are derived from transformed B- or T-lymphocytes. It is noteworthy, though, that benign, reactive histiocytes are present in many cases of DLCL. Modern methods of treatment have dramatically improved the rate of survival of patients with these tumors, with approximately 50–60% of cases cured at present.

Large cell lymphoma, true histiocytic type

Diffuse large cell lymphomas of pure histiocytic (monocytic) origin are quite rare and are difficult to distinguish morphologically from other subtypes of DLCL. True histiocytic lymphomas exhibit a predominantly sinusoidal pattern similar to that observed in histiocytic medullary reticulosis and other primary histiocytic disorders, which usually occur in children and young adults.

Anaplastic large cell lymphoma (ALCL)

This distinct clinicopathologic entity, usually T-cell or null cell in phenotype, expresses CD30 (Ki-1) and, in the systemic form, is associated with a t(2;5) chromosome translocation and expression of the ALK protein. Cases of ALCL with a cutaneous presentation may be a different entity, in as much as they lack the t(2;5), ALK protein expression and have a clinically indolent course. It is of interest to note that the Ki-1 (CD30) antigen is also expressed on Reed–Sternberg cells in Hodgkin's disease, as well as on activated B- and T-cells. The classic type ALCL is characterized by a preferential perifollicular involvement of the lymph node, with sinusoidal and subcapsular infiltration. Two peaks in the age distribution have been observed, a large peak in the second to third decades and a smaller peak in the sixth to seventh decades. The disease is rapidly progressive and usually involves lymph nodes, skin and visceral sites. ALCL may be confused with metastatic carcinoma or Hodgkin's disease. The differential diagnosis, utilizing monoclonal antibodies, of several entities with similar clinical presentations is shown in Table 14.9.

Burkitt's lymphoma and Burkitt-like lymphoma

Small non-cleaved cell lymphomas have a characteristic cytogenetic finding, t(8;14), which occurs in about 80% of cases of Burkitt's type. The c-*myc* proto-oncogene on chromosome 8, thought to have a role in repressing differentiation and stimulating proliferation of cells, becomes constitutively expressed when it relocates to the immunoglobulin heavy chain locus on chromosome 14, with reciprocal relocation of the heavy chain gene locus to the c-*myc* locus on chromosome 8. Variant translocations t(2;8) and t(8;22) involving immunoglobulin light chain loci can be detected in the remaining 20% of cases. Classic Burkitt's lymphoma is marked by small- to medium-sized malignant cells exhibiting one to several distinct nucleoli, basophilic cytoplasm and characteristic vacuoles. It is most commonly seen in pediatric patients. In Africa, patients classically present with large tumor masses of the maxilla or mandible, whereas in the United States a rapidly expanding abdominal mass is the usual presentation, occasionally accompanied by central nervous system or bone marrow involvement.

Burkitt's lymphoma exhibits greater cell pleomorphism than Burkitt's lymphoma. It is composed of small- to intermediate-sized immature lymphoid cells with basophilic cytoplasm and several distinct nucleoli. In patients who have undergone treatment for Hodgkin's disease and in those with AIDS, this is the most common type of lymphoma occurring as a complicating factor. Unlike Burkitt's lymphomas, c-*myc* gene rearrangements usually do not occur in this subtype. Both Burkitt's lymphoma and Burkitt-like lymphoma have a proliferation fraction (e.g. based on Ki-67 staining) close to 100%.

Precursor B- and T-lymphoblastic leukemia/lymphoma

Common in children, particularly boys, and in young adults, lymphoblastic lymphoma is a high-grade, immature T-cell lymphoma that is usually associated with a prominent mediastinal mass and often with superior vena cava (SVC) syndrome. It is the counterpart of childhood T-cell acute lymphoblastic leukemia and patients in both groups are at high risk for CNS involvement. Skin lesions are also occasionally present. Its morphology is marked by malignant cells that are small and uniform in appearance, exhibiting scanty cytoplasm and indistinct nucleoli. Characteristic nuclear convolutions are usually present; mitoses are frequent.

Adult T-cell lymphoma–leukemia (ATLL)

This unusual T-cell malignancy is composed of neoplastic lymphoid cells of various sizes, exhibiting irregular nuclei, some containing nucleoli, often with marked convolutions of the nuclear contours. Lymph node biopsy characteristically shows a leukemic pattern of infiltration. Seen predominantly in Japan and in blacks of the West Indies, the Caribbean nations and the south-eastern United States, ATLL typically shows rapid progression, with early involvement of lymph nodes, skin, bone, blood and bone marrow. Hypercalcemia often develops. The lung, liver, G1 tract and CNS may also be involved. The disease is now known to be caused by a C-type RNA retrovirus known as human T-cell lymphoma–leukemia virus (HTLV-1).

MISCELLANEOUS LYMPHOMAS
Marginal zone lymphoma (nodal and extranodal)

This low-grade B-cell derived non-Hodgkin's lymphoma tends to involve lymph node sinuses and interfollicular zones and to surround follicles in a marginal zone pattern. Monocytoid B-cells have small nuclei with irregular outlines and fairly abundant pale cytoplasm and may involve bone marrow and extranodal sites such as salivary gland, with an indolent clinical course. The normal cellular counterpart of marginal zone lymphomas may be the marginal zone cells in the spleen. Although similar in appearance to hairy cell leukemia cells, marginal zone B-cell neoplasms are CD103 negative, while hairy cells are usually CD103 positive.

T-cell rich B-cell lymphoma

In this subtype of large cell non-Hodgkin's lymphoma of B-cell origin, the majority of cells at the site of involvement are reactive and not neoplastic T-cells. T-cell rich B-cell lymphoma may be mistaken for a T-cell lymphoma but can be demonstrated to be a B-cell derived neoplasm by immunohistochemical methods or by molecular diagnostic methods to detect immunoglobulin gene rearrangements.

EXTRANODAL LYMPHOMAS

Non-Hodgkin's lymphomas often secondarily invade visceral sites, resulting in stage IV disease. Primary involvement of extranodal sites is less common, occurring in up to 25% of cases. Extranodal lymphomas may arise in almost any site, particularly the skin, thyroid, orbit, Waldeyer's ring, central nervous system, lung, GI tract, reproductive organs, breast, stomach and kidneys. The vast majority of these cases respond to combination chemotherapy, with or without local radiotherapy.

Lymphoma of the breast

Primary lymphomas of the breast, which are rare, may present as an expanding breast mass, clinically simulating breast carcinoma. Therefore, biopsy specimens must be carefully examined, with the use of surface marker studies when possible, to avoid an unnecessary mastectomy. Most lymphomas of the breast are derived from B-cells and are DLCL or marginal zone lymphoma, although rare cases of the nodular (follicular) lymphoma and other types have been reported.

Lymphoma of the gastrointestinal tract

The gastrointestinal tract is the most common site of primary extranodal lymphoma, which accounts for approximately 2% of GI neoplasms, and most commonly involves the stomach followed by small intestine and then colon. Approximately 5% of gastric neoplasms are malignant lymphomas, the majority of which are DLCL of B-cell lineage. They most commonly occur in middle or late adulthood, typically arising in the body of the stomach; they are often large and diffuse or may appear as nodular masses. Direct spread to the liver or spleen, as well as dissemination to other areas, occasionally occurs. Gastric lymphomas carry a better prognosis than gastric carcinomas; the 5-year survival rate is approximately 50% for all stages.

Extranodal marginal zone lymphomas of mucosa-associated lymphoid tissue (MALT) accounts for a significant percentage of GI lymphomas and also occurs in a number of other extranodal sites that normally contain MALT, including breast, lung, head and neck areas, including thyroid, and the urogenital tract. It may be low grade or high grade. Low-grade MALT lymphoma is composed of small B-cells with round to irregular nuclear outlines, notable cytoplasm, associated plasma cells and a tendency to invade epithelium, resulting in characteristic lymphoepithelial lesions. Tumor cells are immunoreactive for pan-B cell markers (e.g. CD20) but not CD5, seen in other low-grade B-cell lymphomas, or CD10, seen in follicular center cell lymphomas. Low-grade MALT lymphomas tend not to disseminate widely and surgical excision results in an excellent long-term prognosis. Other relatively common types of GI non-Hodgkin's lymphoma include mantle cell lymphoma, which presents as multiple lymphomatous polyposis with a tendency to early wide dissemination, and small non-cleaved cell lymphoma, a high-grade tumor. Of note, NHL (particularly low-grade MALT type) affecting the stomach but not other sites is associated with previous *Helicobacter pylori* infection (Parsonnet *et al.*, 1994). Despite lymphoma regression with therapy for *H. pylori*, the causative role, while plausible, still remains unproven (Isaacson, 1994).

Lymphoma of the kidney

Although primary renal lymphoma is rare, about 5–10% of patients with disseminated lymphoma exhibit clinically detectable renal involvement and up to 50% of cases reveal renal lesions at autopsy. High-grade lymphomas are most commonly encountered, particularly Burkitt's lymphoma. Occasionally, patients present with renal failure owing to infiltration of the kidney by lymphoma cells, with resultant bilateral enlargement.

Intravascular lymphomatosis

Also referred to as malignant angio-endotheliomatosis, this rare B- or T-cell derived neoplastic proliferation of large pleomorphic mononuclear cells may preferentially involve the lumens of small arteries and veins, and capillaries, without significant infiltration of vessel walls or parenchymal involvement that may be seen in angiocentric T-cell lymphoma. Intravascular lymphomatosis involves multiple organs, with effects particularly notable in the central nervous system (associated dementia and neurologic impairment) and skin (plaques and nodules), and is usually rapidly fatal.

CLINICAL EVALUATION AND STAGING

The staging workup for all patients includes a detailed history and physical examination, CBC with differential, blood chemistries, serum protein electrophoresis, chest radiograph (and, if abnormal, chest CT scan), CT scan of the abdomen and pelvis and bone marrow aspiration with biopsy. Selected patients may require the following additional studies for complete evaluation: lymphangiography, MRI (to evaluate bone marrow tumor), bone scan, gallium-67 citrate scan (also useful in following response), GI series, CT scan of the head (in the presence of symptoms of lymphoma in the head and neck area) and lumbar puncture. Evaluation of the peripheral blood by a sensitive cytofluorometric technique (cell sorter) may reveal circulating monoclonal lymphocytes, especially in B-cell lymphomas. Staging laparotomy is usually not performed, because most patients have advanced disease and the choice of therapy will not be altered by the surgical findings.

The Ann Arbor staging system is employed for non-Hodgkin's lymphomas, except that the designation of stages III$_1$ and III$_2$ as applied to Hodgkin's disease is not necessary (*see* Fig. 14.13). This system, however, is not optimal, for it does not reflect important prognostic factors such as size, or 'bulk', of the tumor, the number of extranodal sites of disease, performance status or the lactate dehydrogenase (LDH) level. Separate staging classification systems have been devised for childhood lymphomas, particularly Burkitt's lymphoma and lymphoblastic lymphoma.

CLINICAL MANIFESTATIONS

In contrast to Hodgkin's disease, most patients with non-Hodgkin's lymphoma present with advanced disease (stage III or IV), which is often reflected by generalized adenopathy. In addition, the disease may occur at unusual sites, such as epitrochlear or popliteal nodes, Waldeyer's ring (nasopharynx), skin, GI tract, brain and ovaries or testes – sites rarely affected in Hodgkin's disease. Patients with low-grade lymphomas have a long history of slowly progressing disease, which may temporarily regress – so-called 'spontaneous' remission – in 5–10% of cases. High-grade and aggressive intermediate-grade lymphomas, on the other hand, usually have a more rapidly progressive course, with 40–50% of patients developing B symptoms. Although the presence of B symptoms has been considered an adverse prognostic factor, multivariate analysis after modern intensive chemotherapy programs reveals that B symptoms no longer affect survival.

Bone marrow involvement occurs in 10–40% of cases. The incidence is highest in lymphoblastic, Burkitt's and Burkitt-like lymphocytic lymphomas (20–40%) and lowest in large cell lymphoma (10–15%). Such involvement is often mainly focal, without affecting peripheral blood counts. In some patients, such as those with lymphoblastic, Burkitt's and Burkitt-like lymphoma, the marrow may be extensively infiltrated, leading to the development of pancytopenia or a leukemic phase. The leukemic phase of a lymphoma may also be a terminal event associated with disseminated disease. Immunofluorescent microscopy has revealed small numbers of monoclonal B-cells in the peripheral blood in about one-third of patients with low-grade lymphomas and in 15–20% of those with intermediate- and high-grade lymphomas.

PROGNOSTIC FACTORS

Modern combination chemotherapy programs have dramatically improved the prognosis, particularly in intermediate- and high-grade lymphomas. While formerly only 10% of patients were cured, 50–60% are now cured with intensive multidrug regimens. Owing to the clinical, histologic and immunobiologic heterogeneity of NHL, many prognostic factors have been identified that separate patients into various risk categories for relapse and decreased survival. This allows for planning of lesser or greater intensity of treatment (*see* Table 14.2).

A prognostic index has been developed by the International Non-Hodgkin's Lymphoma Prognostic Factors Project based upon patient data from 16 single institutions and co-operative groups (Shipp, 1994, Shipp *et al.*, 1993; 1994). A total of 2031 evaluable patients with aggressive NHL (NCI categories E–H; *see* Fig. 14.35) were treated with doxorubicin-containing regimens between 1982 and 1987. Multiple clinical and laboratory features were analyzed to define adverse prognostic factors that were present at the time of diagnosis and predicted for relapse and death. The International Index Model, based upon age, stage, serum LDH, performance status and number of extranodal disease sites, identified four risk groups with predicted 5-year survivals of 73%, 51%, 43% and 26% (*see* Tables 14.3 and 14.4). It was found that while older patients (>60 years) had similar complete remissions (CRs) to younger patients (<60 years), they were less likely to maintain their CR than younger patients, especially low- and low–intermediate-risk patients, with resultant shorter survival. Survival curves for the age-adjusted International Index are noted in Figure 14.36. The

Abbreviated updated (1992) NCI Working Formulation equivalent	WHO Classification	
	B-cell neoplasms	**T-cell neoplasms**
Low-grade malignant lymphoma	Precursor B-cell lymphoblastic leukemia/lymphoma	Precursor T-cell lymphoblastic leukemia/lymphoma
A Small lymphocytic (and small lymphocytic-plasmacytoid)	Mature B-cell neoplasms	Mature T-cell and natural killer cell neoplasms
B Follicular, predominantly small cleaved cell	B-cell chronic lymphocytic leukemia/small lymphocytic lymphoma	T-cell prolymphocytic leukemia
		T-cell large granular lymphocytic leukemia
C Follicular, mixed, small cleaved and large cell	B-cell prolymphocytic leukemia	Aggressive natural killer cell leukemia
II Intermediate-grade malignant lymphoma	Lymphoplasmacytic lymphoma (lymphoplasmacytoid lymphoma)	T/natural killer cell lymphoma, nasal and nasal-type (angiocentric lymphoma)
D Follicular, predominantly large cell	Mantle cell lymphoma	Mycosis fungoides
E Diffuse small cleaved cell	Follicular lymphoma (follicle center lymphoma)	Sezary syndrome
F Diffuse mixed, small and large cell	Cutaneous follicle center lymphoma	Angio immunoblastic T-cell lymphoma
G Diffuse large cell, cleaved/noncleaved	Marginal zone B-cell lymphoma of mucosa-associated lymphoid tissue type	Peripheral T-cell lymphoma (unspecified)
III Hight-grade malignant lymphoma	Nodal marginal zone lymphoma =/- monocytoid B-cell	Adult T-cell leukemia/lymphoma (HTLV1 +)
H Diffuse large cell immunoblastic		Anaplastic large-cell lymphoma (T – and null-cell types)
I Lymphoblastic (convoluted/nonconvoluted)	Splenic marginal zone B-cell lymphoma	Primary cutaneous CD 30 positive T-cell lymphoproliferative disorders (cutaneous
	Hairy cell leukemia	Anaplastic large cell lymphoma)
J Small noncleaved cell (Burkitt's/non-Burkitt's types)	Diffuse large B-cell lymphoma	Subcutaneous panniculitis-like T-cell lymphoma
	Mediastinal (thymic)	
IV Miscellaneous	Intravascular	Enteropathy-type intestinal T-cell lymphoma
Composite	Primary effusion lymphoma	Hepatosplenic g/d T-cell lymphoma
Mycosis fungoides	Burkitt's lymphoma	
True histiocytic	Plasmacytoma	
Unclassified	Plasma cell myeloma	

Fig. 14.35 Comparison of the updated (1992) National Cancer Institute's (NCI) International Working Formulation classification and the WHO classification (1999) of non-Hodgkin's lymphomas.

advantage of a prognostic index is that good-risk patients can be identified for conventional therapy while poor-risk (high-relapse) patients can be identified for new research protocols to improve the cure rate. Furthermore, treatment results among institutions and co-operative groups can be compared since standardized prognostic factors will have been utilized.

Additional poor prognostic factors include long time to achieve CR, lower dose intensity and schedule, T-cell phenotype vs B-cell phenotype (data, however, are not uniformly in agreement), elevated serum β_2-microglobulin level, increased expression of adhesion molecules (CD44), increased serum level of IL-10, bcl-2-MBR gene

rearrangement and lack of rearrangement of the bcl-6 gene (Shipp, 1994; Blay et al., 1993; Tang et al., 1994; Offit et al., 1994).

The majority of low-grade follicular lymphomas will eventually progress (transform) to an aggressive intermediate- or high-grade lymphoma. Specific genetic changes have recently been described that are associated with the latter, including p53 mutation and alterations in c-myc (Sander et al., 1993; Chang et al., 1994). An understanding of the molecular mechanisms predating or coinciding with clonal evolution of malignant lymphoma may permit early detection of this event so that effective (intensive) therapy can be employed when the tumor burden is minimal.

Table 14.1 Frequency of non-Hodgkin's lymphoma subgroups according to the NCI Working Formula classification, together with survival range by gradea compiled from data in Rosenberg 1980, and Newell et al., 1987).

NCI Working Formulation			
Category	Subgroup	Frequency (%)[b]	Survival range (yr)
Low-grade	A	14	
	B	26	] 5–10
	C	19	
Intermediate-grade	D	4	
	E	8	
	F	7	] 2–5
	G	22	
High-grade	H	9	
	I	5	] 0.5–2
	J	6	

See Figure 14.35 for definitions. Working Formulation subgroups G and H are often called diffuse large cell lymphoma (DLCL) and treated as high-grade or poor-prognosis lymphomas 'Aggressive' lymphomas refer to subgroups E–H. 'Very aggressive' lymphomas refer to subgroups I and J.

[b]Frequency in US whites.

Table 14.2 Prognostic factors in aggressive NHL. Association between host/tumor characteristics and clinical prognostic features in aggressive NHL*

Host/tumor characteristics	Clinical prognostic factors
Tumor's growth and invasive potential	Serum LDH No of nodal and extranodal sites of disease Mass size Stage according to Ann Arbor classification BM involvement
Patient's response to the tumor	Systemic B symptoms Performance status
Patient's ability to tolerate intensive therapy	Age at diagnosis Performance status BM involvement

*Aggressive lymphomas = categories E–H; see Table 14.1.

Table 14.3 Prognostic factors in aggressive NHL. Prognostic risk factors for survival in International index patients. (From Shipp, 1994)

	Relative risk	P value
Patients of all ages		
• Age (≤ 60 years v > 60 years)	1.96	< .001
• LDH (≤nl v > nl)	1.85	< .001
• Performance status (0.1 v 2–4)	1.80	< 001
• Stage (I/II v III/IV)	1.47	< .001
• Extranodal involvement		
(≤ I site v > I site)	1.48	< .001
Patients ≤ 60 yrs of age		
• Stage (I/II v III/IV)	2.17	< .001
• LDH (≤ nl v > nl)	1.95	< .001
• Performance status (0, I v 2–4)	1.81	< .001

Table 14.4 Prognostic factors in patients of all ages in aggressive NHL. The International Index. (From Shipp, 1994)

Risk group	Risk factors	Distirbution of cases (%)	CR rate (%)	RFs of CRs (%)		Survival (%)	
				2-yr rate	5-yr rate	2-yr rate	5-yr rate
Low (L)	0.1	35	87	79	70	84	73
Low-intermediate (LI)	2	27	67	66	50	66	51
High-intermediate (HI)	3	22	55	59	49	54	43
High (H)	4.5	16	44	58	40	34	26

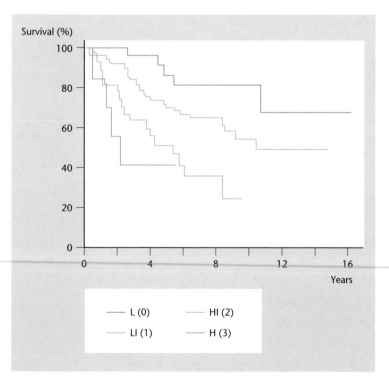

Fig. 14.36 Prognostic factors in aggressive NHL. Overall predicted survival in patients under 60 using the age-adjusted International Index. Risk groups are defined from risk factors noted in Table 14.4: low (L); low-intermediate (LI); high-intermediate (HI) and high (H). The number in parentheses refer to the number of risk factors. (Modified with permission from Shipp et al., 1993.)

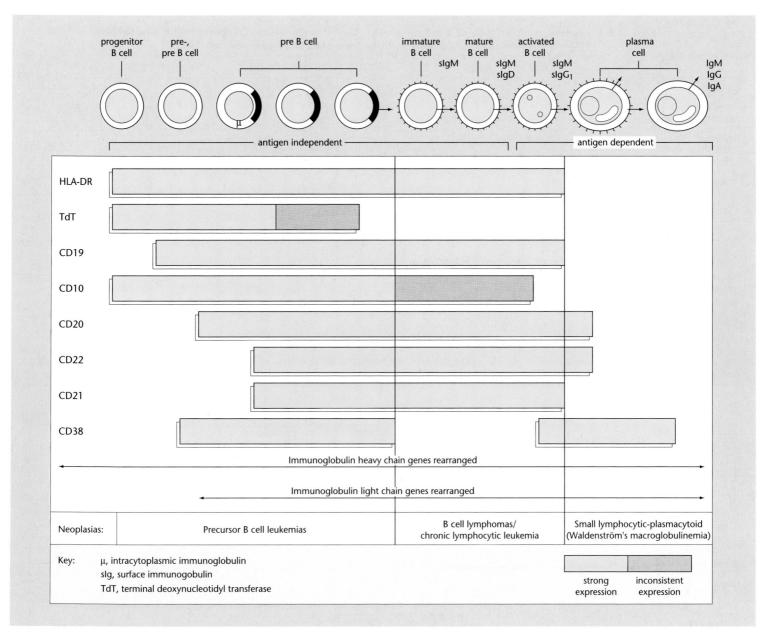

Fig. 14.37 Monoclonal antibodies to human B-cell surface antigens can be used to detect sequential stages in B-cell maturation. The malignant lymphomas and leukemias reflect these stages of normal B-cell development. (Modified with permission from Jaffe, 1990, with additional data from Uckun, 1990.)

Table 14.5 Predominant phenotypes of B-cell neoplasms. Cluster designation (CD) groupings are noted as well as the commonly used terms. (Modified from Stetter–Stevenson et al., 1995)

	CD19	CD20	CD22	CD10	CD5	CD25	CD11c	CD21	CD38	TdT
Common ALL	+	±	±	+	–	–	–	–	+/–	+
Small non-cleaved Burkitt's lymphoma	+	+	+	+	–	–	–	+/–	–	–
Large cell/large cell immunoblastic lymphoma	+	+	+	±	–	±	–	±	+	–
Nodular (follicular) lymphomas	+	+	+	+	–	–	–	+	+/–	–
Mantle cell lymphoma	+	+	+	–/+	+	–	–	+/–	–	–
Marginal zone lymphoma	+	+	+	–	–	+/–	+/–	–	+/–	–
Small lymphocytic/CLL	+	+	+	–	+	–	–	+/–	–	–
Small lymphocytic-plasmacytoid (Waldenstrom's macroglobulinemia)	+/–	+/–	+/–	–	+/–	+	–	–	+	–
Hairy cell leukemia	+	+	+	–	–	+	+	–	–/+	–
Myeloma	–	–	–	–	–	–	–	–	+	–

Key: +, nearly always positive; ±, sometimes positive; –, usually negative; ALL, acute lymphoblastic leukemia; CLL, chronic lymphocytic leukemia; TdT, terminal deoxynucleotidyl transferase.

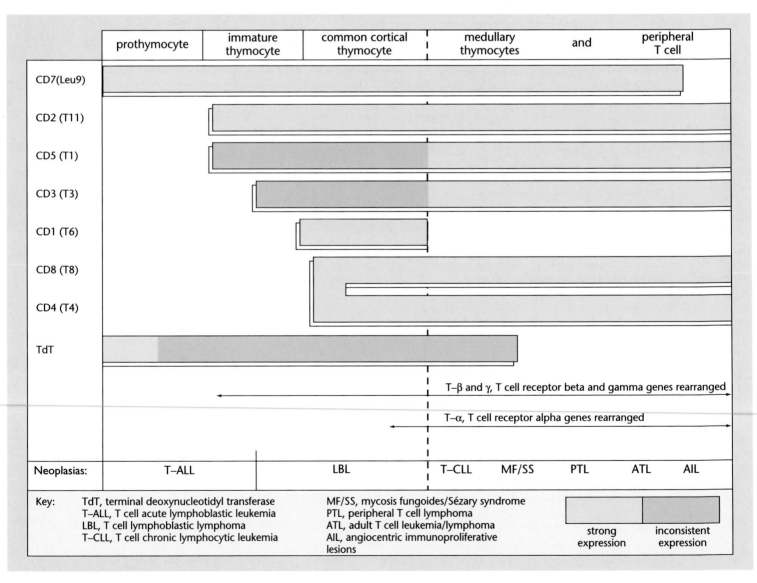

Fig. 14.38 Monoclonal antibodies to human T-cell surface antigens can be used to detect sequential stages in T-cell development. Malignancies can be phenotypically related to stages of normal T-cell maturation. CD4 (T4) (helper/inducer) cells represent 60–70% of peripheral blood cells, while CD8 (T8) (cytotoxic/suppressor) cells constitute 30–40%. (Modified with permission from Jaffe, 1990.)

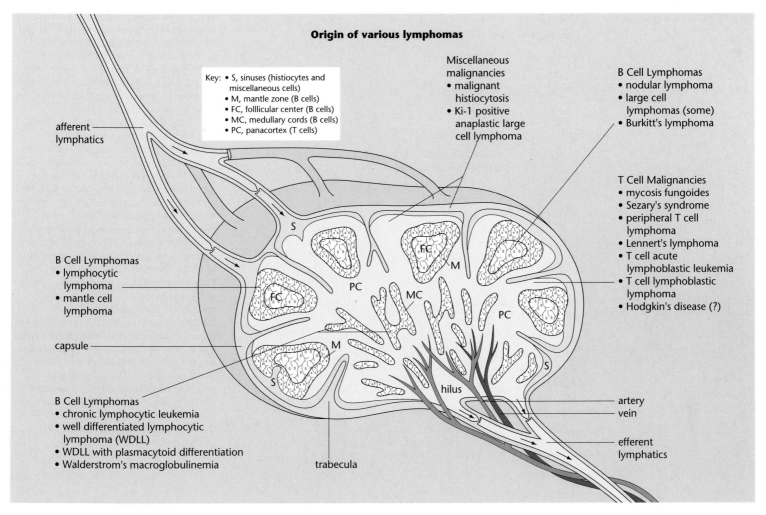

Origin of various lymphomas

Key:
• S, sinuses (histiocytes and miscellaneous cells)
• M, mantle zone (B cells)
• FC, folllicular center (B cells)
• MC, medullary cords (B cells)
• PC, panacortex (T cells)

afferent lymphatics

Miscellaneous malignancies
• malignant histiocytosis
• Ki-1 positive anaplastic large cell lymphoma

B Cell Lymphomas
• nodular lymphoma
• large cell lymphomas (some)
• Burkitt's lymphoma

T Cell Malignancies
• mycosis fungoides
• Sezary's syndrome
• peripheral T cell lymphoma
• Lennert's lymphoma
• T cell acute lymphoblastic leukemia
• T cell lymphoblastic lymphoma
• Hodgkin's disease (?)

B Cell Lymphomas
• lymphocytic lymphoma
• mantle cell lymphoma

capsule

B Cell Lymphomas
• chronic lymphocytic leukemia
• well differentiated lymphocytic lymphoma (WDLL)
• WDLL with plasmacytoid differentiation
• Walderstrom's macroglobulinemia

trabecula

hilus

artery
vein

efferent lymphatics

Fig. 14.39 Origins of various lymphomas. This diagram represents anatomic areas and functionally related compartments of a lymph node at which different lymphoid malignancies arise. For example, B-cell lymphomas arise from the follicles (mantle zone and follicular center), whereas T-cell lymphomas arise from the paracortical areas normally populated by T-lymphocytes.

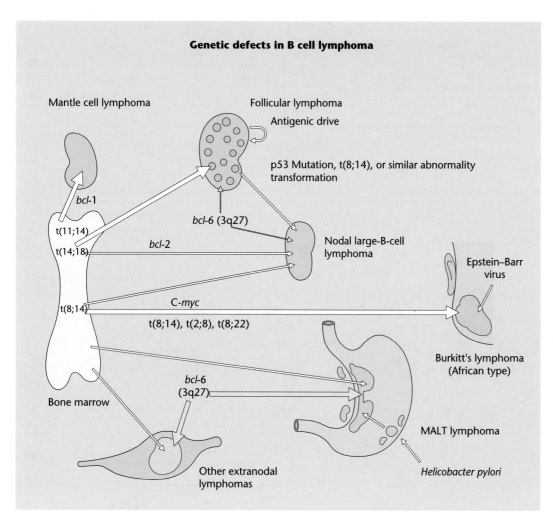

Genetic defects in B cell lymphoma

Mantle cell lymphoma

Follicular lymphoma

Antigenic drive

bcl-1

t(11;14)

t(14;18)

bcl-2

p53 Mutation, t(8;14), or similar abnormality
transformation

bcl-6 (3q27)

Nodal large-B-cell
lymphoma

Epstein–Barr
virus

t(8;14)

C-*myc*

t(8;14), t(2;8), t(8;22)

Burkitt's lymphoma
(African type)

bcl-6
(3q27)

Bone marrow

MALT lymphoma

Other extranodal
lymphomas

Helicobacter pylori

Fig. 14.40 Genetic defects in B-cell lymphoma. The translocations t(14;18) and t(11;14), and some t(8;14) translocations, probably occur in primitive B-cells in the bone marrow. Lymphomas arise after these genetically damaged B-cells mature, leave the bone marrow and acquire additional genetic lesions because of unknown secondary events (the arrows do not imply that lymphomas themselves arise in the bone marrow). These secondary events may include the antigen-driven proliferation of B-cells. Other events in B-cells carrying the t(14;18) translocation may lead directly to primary (nodal) large B-cell lymphomas. Bcl-6 rearrangements at band 3q27 occur mainly in primary extranodal lymphomas (thick blue arrows) (Offit *et al.*, 1994). Additional gene rearrangements occur in follicular lymphoma (thin blue arrows). Because nothing is known about the origin of breakpoints at 3q27 during B-cell maturation, these arrows have no identifiable starting point. Other oncogenic factors include the direct infection of B-cells by Epstein–Barr virus in Burkitt's lymphoma and the possible stimulation of MALT lymphoma cells by *Helicobacter pylori* infection. All lymphomas may subsequently spread to lymph nodes, the bone marrow or other sites, but this process is not shown in the figure. (Modified and reprinted with permission from Kluin, 1994.)

Table 14.6 Most Common Molecular Abnormalities Studied in Non-Hodgkin's Lymphoma

Gene studied	Chromosomal site	Most common disease associations
Immunoglobulin heavy chain (*IgH*) rearrangements	14q32	B-cell neoplasms*
Immunoglobulin κ light chain (*Igκ*) rearrangements	2p11	B-cell neoplasms
J_H/BCL-1	t(11;14)(q13;q32)	Mantle cell lymphoma
J_H/BCL-2	t(14;18)(q32;q21)	Follicular lymphoma, some diffuse large B-cell lymphomas
PAX5/IgH	t(9;14)(p13;q32)	Lymphoplasmacytic lymphoma
AP12/MLT	t(11;18)(q21;q21)	Extranodal marginal zone lymphoma
BCL-6 translocations	t(3;n)(q27;n)	Some diffuse large B-cell lymphomas
C-MYC translocations	t(8;n)(q24;n)	Burkitt's lymphoma
T cell receptor β chain (*TCRβ*) rearrangements	7q34	T-cell neoplasms*
T cell receptor γ chain (*TCRγ*) rearrangements	7q15	T-cell neoplasms*
NPM/ALK	t(2;5)(p23;q35)	Anaplastic large cell lymphoma

*Lineage infidelity may occur in some neoplasms, particularly lymphoblastic leukemias and lymphomas, which may result in detection of aberrant gene rearrangements (see text).
(Adapted from Arber, 2000.)

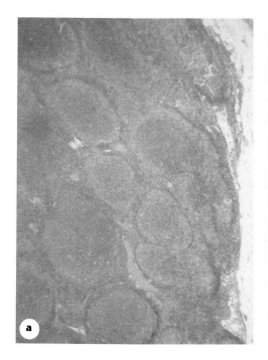
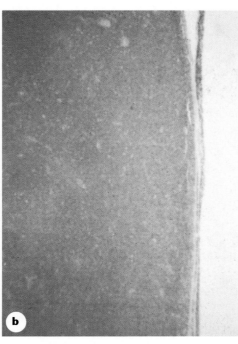

Fig. 14.41 Nodular vs diffuse lymphomas. (**a**) Low magnification of a nodular lymphoma shows many of the architectural features that are helpful in the diagnosis of follicular lymphomas. These features include complete effacement of lymph node architecture, high density of follicles with a back-to-back arrangement, infiltration of the lymph node capsule by follicles with extension into perinodal fat and loss of a distinct boundary separating the follicles from the surrounding peripheral cuff of lymphocytes. (**b**) Low magnification of a diffuse lymphoma reveals complete effacement of the normal nodal architecture by a diffuse lymphomatous process.

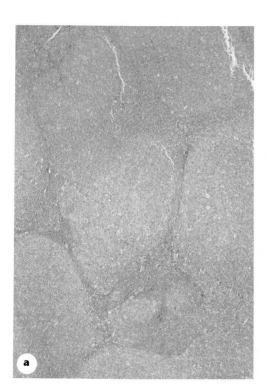
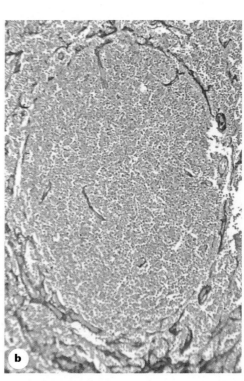

Fig. 14.42 Nodular (follicular) lymphoma. (**a**) The well-defined, uniform follicles seen in this low-power photomicrograph are due to compression of reticulin around the neoplastic follicles, shown (**b**) in this high-power view (reticulin stain).

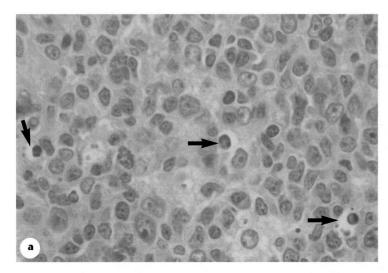
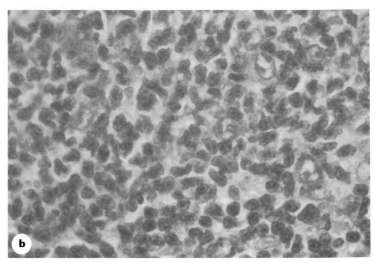

Fig. 14.43 (**a**) Apoptosis (programmed cell death) is a normal finding in germinal centers where scattered, individual necrotic cells are readily identified (arrows). In contrast, the nodular infiltrates of follicular center cell-derived nodular lymphomas (**b**) have far fewer apoptotic cells. Follicular center cell lymphomas typically exhibit a t(14;18) chromosomal translocation, which results in deregulation of expression of the *bcl*-2 proto-oncogene on chromosome 18. This gene blocks apoptosis and its overexpression results in prolongation of the lifespan of involved cells, contributing to the pathogenesis of lymphoma. Approximately 20% of diffuse non-Hodgkin's lymphomas of follicular center cell origin exhibit the t(14;18) translocation as well.

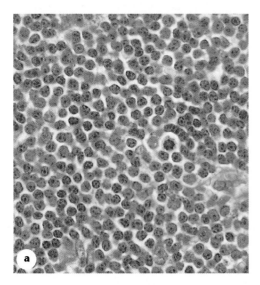
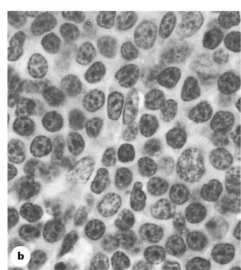
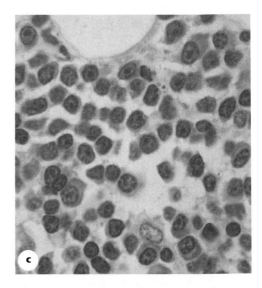

Fig. 14.44 Chronic lymphocytic leukemia (small lymphocytic lymphoma) (NCI subgroup A). (**a**) Sheets of small lymphocytes have completely destroyed the normal lymph node architecture. Virtually all cases show a diffuse pattern. (**b**) Such monotonous sheets of mature lymphocytes may also be seen in the lymph nodes in chronic lymphocytic leukemia. (**c**) This example shows plasmacytoid differentiation. All cases are of B-cell origin and usually exhibit aberrant immunoreactivity for CD5, a T-cell marker.

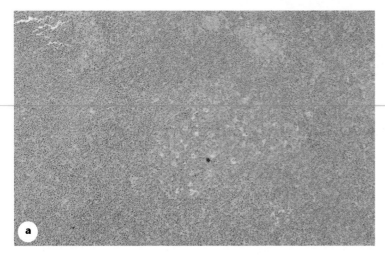
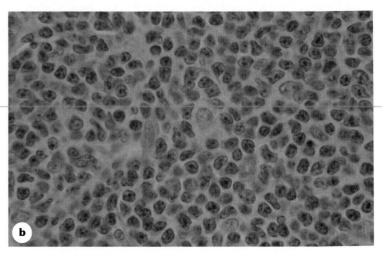

Fig. 14.45 Mantle cell lymphoma. (**a**) A vaguely nodular proliferation of small lymphocytes surrounds germinal centers in a mantle zone pattern, effacing normal lymph node architecture. Mantle cell lymphoma may also present with a diffuse pattern of lymph node involvement, usually with residual germinal centers present as well. (**b**) Higher power reveals uniform, small lymphoid cells with scant cytoplasm and small irregular to notched or cleaved nuclei with coarse chromatin. All cases are of B-cell origin and usually exhibit aberrant immunoreactivity for CD5. A significant percentage of cases exhibit a t(11;14) chromosomal translocation.

Table 14.7 Comparison of low-grade lymphomas.

Characteristic	Small lymphocytic lymphoma (SLL) chronic lymphocytic leukemia (CLL)	Mantle cell lymphoma (MCL)	Small cleaved FCC lymphoma	Marginal zone lymphoma monocytoid B cell MALT types
Nuclear appearance	Round	Irregular	Cleaved	Round to irregular
Lymph node infiltration patterns	Diffuse	Diffuse or mantle zone	Diffuse or follicular	Sinusoid interfollicular diffuse
Immunoreactivity for CDS (T1)	+	+ (–)	–	–
CD10 (CALLA)	–	– (+)	+	–
CD23	+	–	+/–	–
Surface immunoglobulin (Ig) expression	IgM weak	IgM/D intermediate	IgG bright	IgM/A
Genotypic features	(*bcl*-1)**	*bcl*-1	*bcl*-2	*bcl*-1 (–) *bcl*-2 (–)
Cytogenic features	+ 12	t(11;14)	t(14;18)	
Median survival	5–7 yrs	2–5 yrs	Diffuse 3–4 yrs Follicular 7–8 yrs	Indolent course
Salient clinical features	Autoimmune phenomena Richter's transformation	Splenomegaly GI lesions	Spontaneous remission Transformation	Tend to remain localized

*B-cell markers expressed (CD19, CD20, CD22). Low grade lymphomas of T-cell lineage are not common, but include T-cell CLL, peripheral T-cell lymphoma and Sezary's syndrome.
**t(11;14) and upregulation of *bcl*-1 is uncommon in CLL/SLL.

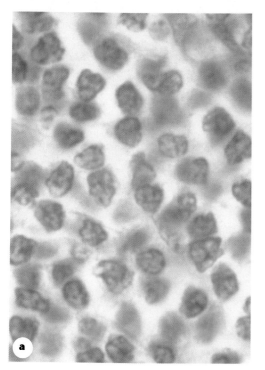
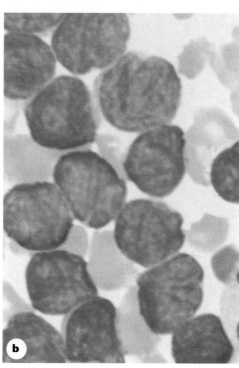

Fig. 14.46 Follicular lymphoma, grade I. (**a**) High-power microscopic section shows small cells with nuclear irregularity including cleaves (notches) and indentations. (**b**) Touch prep of a lymph node demonstrates classic cleaved cells, some with split nuclei. Lymph node architecture may be either nodular or diffuse. All cases are of B-cell origin.

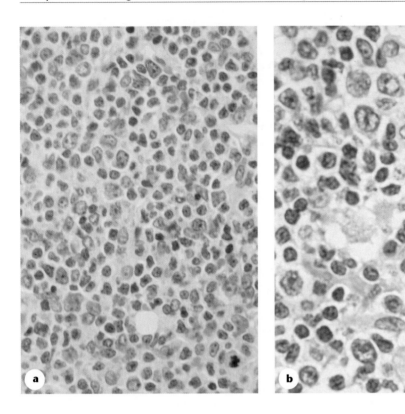

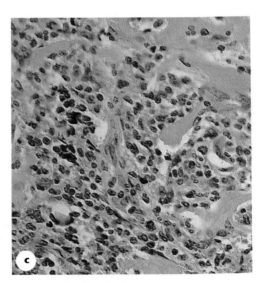

Fig. 14.47 Follicular lymphoma, grade II. (a) Low- and (b) high-power photomicrographs demonstrate a lymphoma composed of both small lymphocytes and large lymphoid cells. Lymph node architecture may be either nodular (NM, NCI subgroup C) or diffuse (DM, NCI subgroup F).

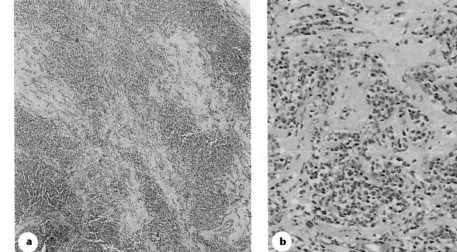

Fig. 14.48 Follicular lymphoma, grade II, diffuse. (a) Low-power photomicrograph of a retroperitoneal lesion shows a sclerosing mixed lymphoma exhibiting broad birefringent bands of collagen. (b) In other areas, the compartmentalizing bands are hyalinized. This pattern of sclerosis is also seen with diffuse large cell lymphomas, particularly in the mediastinum. (c) High-power view of areas compartmentalized by hyalinized collagenous bands shows that the tumor is composed of small and large cleaved follicular center cells.

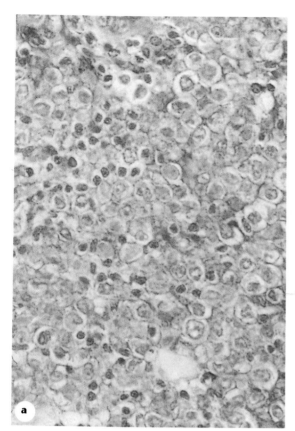

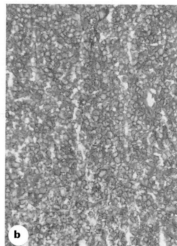

Fig. 14.49 Non-Hodgkin's lymphomas. Unlike poorly differentiated carcinomas and sarcomas, lymphomas show (**a**) strong reactivity with immunoperoxidase staining for LCA (CD45), as can be seen in this case of a diffuse large cell lymphoma. Monoclonality in B-cell lymphoma is documented by positive immunoperoxidase staining for one light chain type; (**b**) in this case, the light chain is positive, as compared (**c**) with the light chain. Immunophenotyping is carried out with a panel of monoclonal antibodies (*see* Fig. 14.37).

Table 14.8 Histologic subtypes of diffuse large cell lymphoma (DLCL). Various morphologic or descriptive types are listed with the cell of origin. Considerable heterogeneity is noted.

Subtype	NCI subgroup	Cell of origin
Large cleaved follicular center cell	G	B
Large noncleaved follicular center cell	G	B
Mixed cleaved/noncleaved follicular center cell	G	B
Large clear cell	G	B
Immunoblastic	H	B (80%), T (20%)
Multilobulated cell	–	T (90%), B (10%)
KI-1 lymphoma	–	T (80%), B (10%) undefined (10%)
True diffuse histiocytic lymphoma	IV	Monocyte (histiocytes)
Unclassified	IV	Undefined

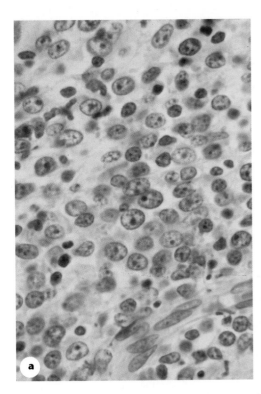

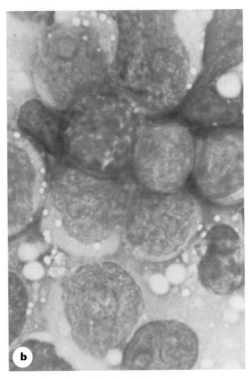

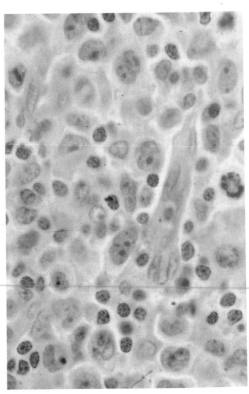

Fig. 14.50 Large cell lymphoma (large, non-cleaved cell type) (NCI subgroup G). **(a)** High magnification reveals large cells with predominantly round nuclei, distinct nucleoli and a moderate amount of cytoplasm. Small lymphocytes in the background allow size comparison. Note the lack of well-defined cell borders and an absence of an organoid pattern, features more commonly associated with carcinomas. **(b)** Touch prep of a lymph node shows large cells with large, prominent nucleoli and basophilic cytoplasm.

Fig. 14.51 Large cell lymphoma (large, cleaved cell type) (NCI subgroup G). Large cells are part of a heterogeneous population composed predominantly of irregular and cleaved cells, as well as occasional round forms.

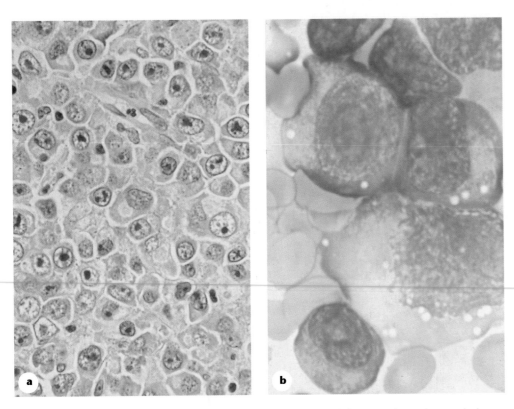

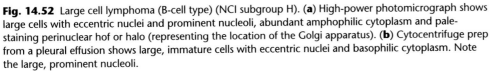

Fig. 14.52 Large cell lymphoma (B-cell type) (NCI subgroup H). **(a)** High-power photomicrograph shows large cells with eccentric nuclei and prominent nucleoli, abundant amphophilic cytoplasm and pale-staining perinuclear hof or halo (representing the location of the Golgi apparatus). **(b)** Cytocentrifuge prep from a pleural effusion shows large, immature cells with eccentric nuclei and basophilic cytoplasm. Note the large, prominent nucleoli.

Fig. 14.53 Large cell lymphoma (T-cell type) (NCI subgroup H). The predominant cell population is composed of large cells with round to lobated nuclei, prominent magenta nucleoli and abundant pale cytoplasm. Note the range of cell sizes and scattered eosinophils.

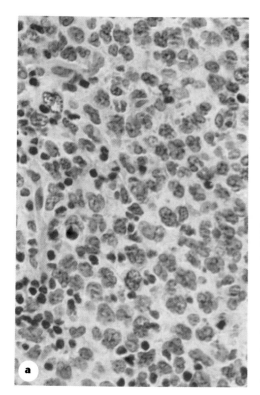

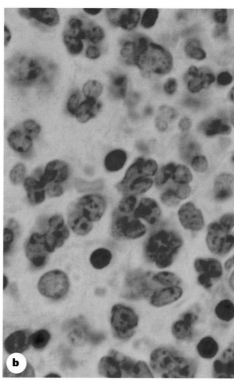

Fig. 14.54 Large cell lymphoma (multilobulated cell type). (**a, b**) This high-grade lymphoma, most often arising from peripheral (post-thymic) T-lymphocytes, is marked by large, multilobulated or multisegmented nuclei, with relatively fine chromatin and small to inconspicuous nucleoli. Under high magnification, the nucleus of a typical cell has a 'popcorn' shape. (Courtesy of Dr G Pinkus, Pathology Department, Brigham and Women's Hospital, Boston, MA.)

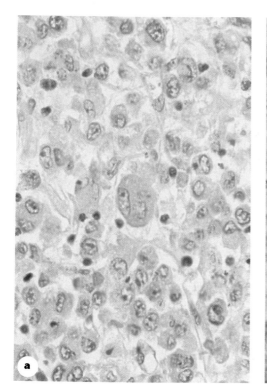

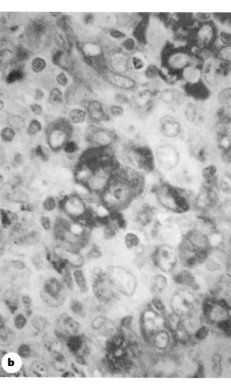

Fig. 14.55 Large cell lymphoma (true histiocytic type). (**a**) Large cells with membranes are present together with occasional focal erythrophagocytosis, a helpful but non-specific indicator of this type of lymphoma. Nuclei typically exhibit conspicuous lobulation, often appearing multinucleate. Confirmatory histochemical staining shows positivity for (**b**) α1-antichymotrypsin and (not shown) α1-naphthylacetate esterase (non-specific esterase), lysozyme and acid phosphatase in some cases. In this patient, monoclonal antibodies to MO-1 (a monocyte marker), LCA (CD45), lysozyme and epithelial membrane antigen (EMA) were positive; B- and T-cell markers were all negative. Ultrastructural studies showed pseudopod-like projections of the plasma membrane, microfilaments, phagolysosomes and phagocytized material.

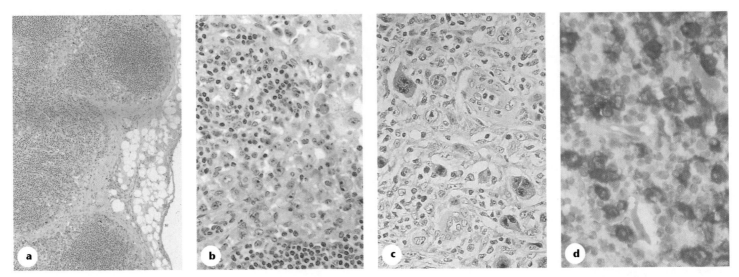

Fig. 14.56 Anaplastic large cell lymphoma (ALCL). (**a**) Low-power photomicrograph demonstrates sinusoidal and paratrabecular infiltration by lymphoma cells surrounding intact, uninvolved germinal centers. (**b**) With higher magnification, the bizarre cells of the sinusoidal infiltrate can be better appreciated. The cells have irregular nuclei and prominent nucleoli. An uninvolved germinal center is seen in the lower part of the field.

(**c**) Under high magnification, some of the typically large, bizarre lymphoma cells are suggestive of Reed–Sternberg cells. (**d**) Immunoperoxidase staining shows immunoreactivity for Ki-1 (CD30) antigen; there was no reactivity for CD15 (Leu-M1) antigen (not shown). This lymphoma may be misdiagnosed as Hodgkin's disease or metastatic carcinoma unless appropriate studies are carried out (*see* Table 14.9).

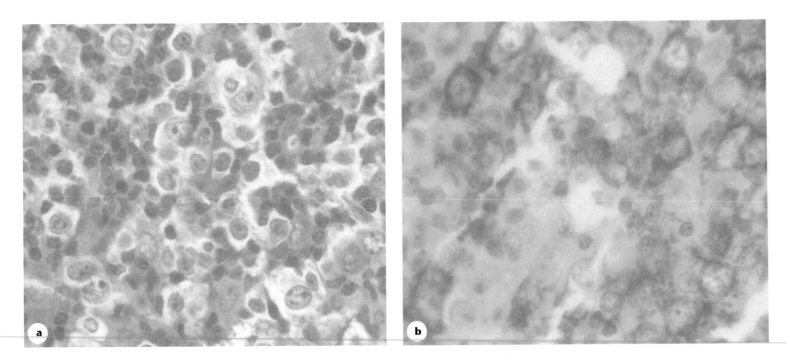

Fig. 14.57 Large cell lymphoma (T-cell rich B-cell type). (**a**) Nodal architecture is effaced by a diffuse infiltrate composed mainly of small lymphoid cells with interspersed large mononuclear cells. (**b**) Immunoperoxidase studies reveal that the small cells are reactive T-cells (not shown), while the large cells are a clonal population of B-cells, here shown to be reactive for B-cell marker CD20. Clinical features parallel those of other B-cell large cell lymphoma patients, although about 30% of patients have splenomegaly (Rodriguez *et al.*, 1993). It is important not to confuse T-cell rich B-cell lymphoma with Hodgkin's disease or cases of peripheral T-cell lymphoma which require different therapy.

Table 14.9 Monoclonal antibodies useful in the diagnosis of large cell lymphomas, Hodgkin's disease, and undifferentiated metastatic carcinomas.

Monoclonal antibody	Hodgkin's disease[a]	Diffuse large cell lymphoma (DLCL)				Undifferentiated metastatic carcinoma
		T cell	B cell	ALCL type[b]	True DHL	
Ki-1 (CD30)	+	–	–	+		–
CD15 (Leu-MI)	+	–	–	–	–	±
T cell markers	–	+	–	±	–	–
B cell markers	–	–	+	±	–	–
LCA (CD45)	–	+	+	+	+	–
EMA	–	–	–	+	+	+

[a]Reed–Sternberg cells (excluding the lymphocyte predominance type)

[b]A small percentage of T and B cell lymphomas are positive for Ki-1 (CD30) antigen.

Key: DHL, diffuse histlocytic lymphoma; LCA, leukocyte common antigen; EMA, epithelial membrane antigen; +, positive; –, negative; ±, may be positive or negative.

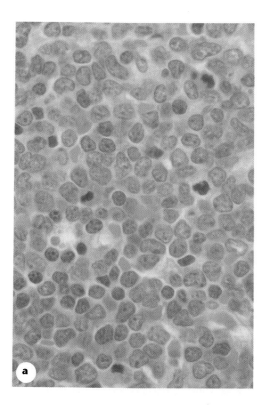

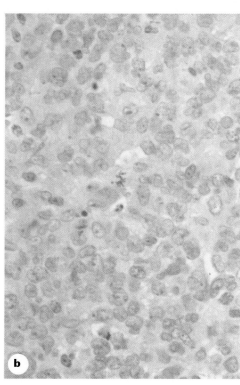

Fig. 14.58 Lymphoblastic (precursor T-cell) lymphoma (NCI subgroup I). (**a**) Malignant cells are small and light staining and have round to convoluted nuclei with delicate, evenly dispersed chromatin and indistinct nucleoli. (**b**) Most lymphoblasts show characteristic prominent nuclear convolutions or cerebriform shapes, although rare, non-convoluted types exist. Mitoses are often seen, as well as a 'starry sky' appearance. In most instances, the cells are derived from immature T-lymphocytes, although a B-cell phenotype can be seen in rare cases.

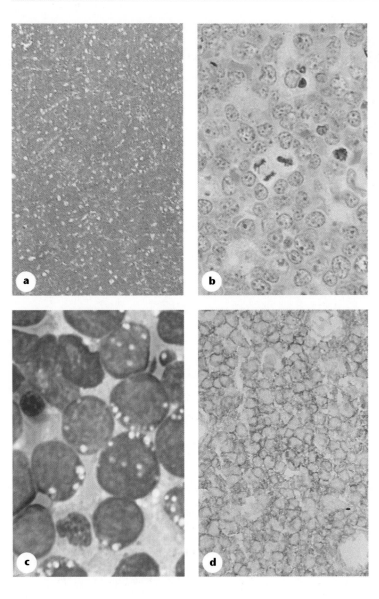

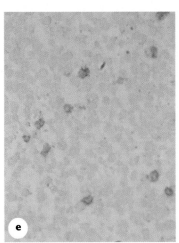

Fig. 14.59 Burkitt's lymphoma (NCI subgroup J). (**a**) Low-power photomicrograph reveals a 'starry sky' appearance resulting from the presence of benign macrophages, which are active in the phagocytosis of necrotic cells and debris. This pattern is non-specific and can be seen with any rapidly proliferating lymphoma. (**b**) With higher magnification, monotonous small-to intermediate-sized cells can be seen; these cells have round nuclear outlines, multiple basophilic nucleoli and abundant mitoses. (**c**) Bone marrow aspirate shows small, immature cells with deep basophilic cytoplasm containing many vacuoles. Distinct nucleoli are seen in several of the cells. (**d**) Immunoperoxidase staining demonstrates immunoreactivity for CD20 (B1) antigen; (**e**) only background, scattered benign T-cells are present, which show reactivity for CD2 (T11) antigen.

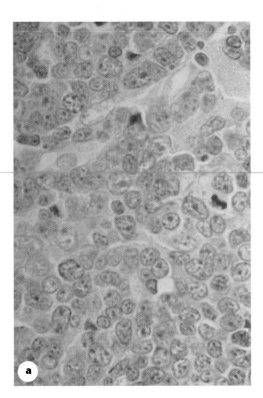

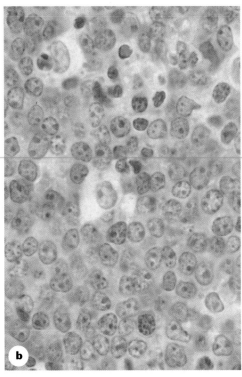

Fig. 14.60 Burkitt-like lymphoma (NCI subgroup J). (**a**) Lymph node biopsy specimen shows diffuse replacement by small-to intermediate-sized lymphoid cells having sparse cytoplasm, round to irregular nuclei and distinct nucleoli. Many mitoses are evident. (**b**) Benign histiocytes are scattered in the background. Immunoperoxidase studies (not shown) demonstrated positivity for LCA (CD45), CD20 (B1) and CD 22, with monotypic expression of light chains. Morphologically, non-Burkitt's lymphoma differs from Burkitt's lymphoma by a greater variation in cell size and shape, as well as a larger, more distinct, single central nucleolus, as shown here. Unlike Burkitt's lymphoma, this subtype usually does not have c-*myc* gene rearrangement (Yano *et al.*, 1992).

Table 14.10 Monoclonal antibodies useful in the diagnosis of T cell lymphomas.

	Pan T-cell markers			Other T-cell markers		Other markers			
	CD2	CD3	CD5	CD4	CD8	CD10	CD30	ALK	TdT
T PLL	+	+	+	+/–	–/+	–	–	–	–
Cerebriform (mycosis fungoides)	+	+	+	+	–	–	–	–	–
Pleomorphic (small cell; mixed small and large cell; large cell)	+	+	+	+/–	–/+	–	–/+	–	–
Anaplastic large cell*	+/–	+/–	+/–	+/–	–/+	–	+	+	–
Precursor T-cell (lymphoblastic)*	+/–	+/–	+/–	+/–	–/+	+/–	–	–	+

*Some cases may express B-cell markers.

Keys: ALK, ALK protein; TdT, terminal deoxynucleotidyl transferase; PLL, prolymphocytic leukemia; +, positive; –, negative; +/–, more often positive than negative; –/+, more often negative than positive.

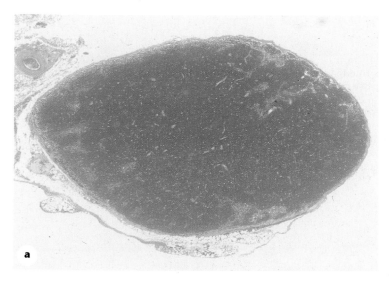

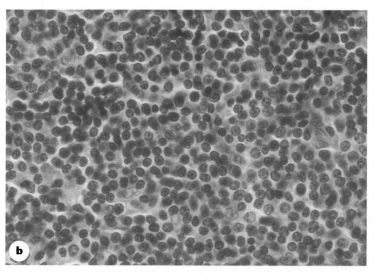

Fig. 14.61 Peripheral T-cell non-Hodgkin's lymphoma, small lymphocytic type. (**a, b**) Nodal architecture is effaced by a uniform population of small lymphoid cells with scant cytoplasm and small nuclei with coarse chromatin and round, slightly irregular nuclear outlines. The lymphoid cells are immunoreactive for pan-T cell markers (not shown). T-cell lymphoma of small lymphocytic type often has associated inv(14) and +8q chromosomal abnormalities.

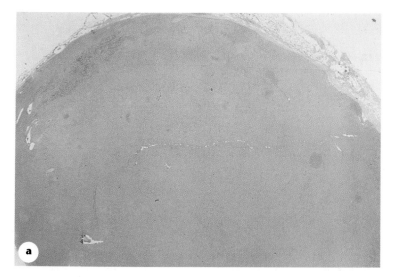

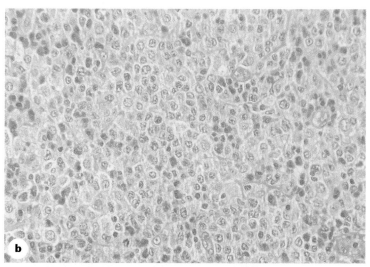

Fig. 14.62 Peripheral T-cell non-Hodgkin's lymphoma, unspecified. (**a, b**) A cervical lymph node biopsy from a 50-year-old man reveals architectural effacement by a diffuse infiltrate composed of small- to large-sized cells, most with prominent nuclear irregularity, and with moderate amounts of pale cytoplasm in the larger cells. Note the presence of numerous admixed eosinophils, a finding frequently seen in T-cell lymphomas.

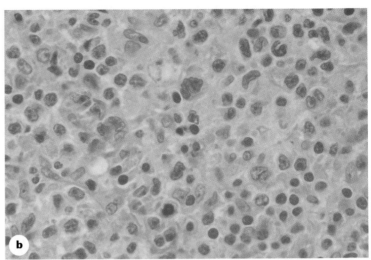

Fig. 14.63 Peripheral T-cell non-Hodgkin's lymphoma, unspecified. (**a, b**) A 71-year-old man presented with left axillary lymphadenopathy. Biopsy revealed a diffuse infiltrate of large lymphoid cells with pale cytoplasm and large irregular to cleaved nuclei, including occasional Reed–Sternberg-like cells with pale prominent nucleoli. Tumor cells were immunoreactive for pan-T cell markers, including CD2 and CD5, and were non-reactive for pan-T cell marker CD7, consistent with the phenomenon of antigen deletion frequently observed in T-cell non-Hodgkin's lymphomas. No immunoreactivity was evident for Leu M1 (CD15), a marker of Reed–Sternberg cells seen in Hodgkin's disease.

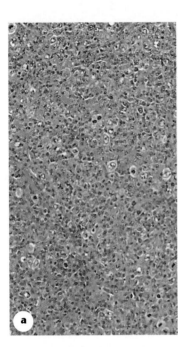

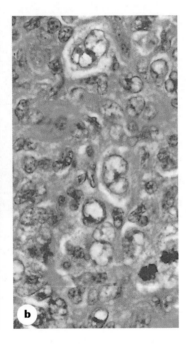

Fig. 14.64 Adult T-cell lymphoma-leukemia (ATLL). (**a**) Low-power microscopic section of lymph node shows replacement of the normal architecture by pleomorphic lymphoid cells. (**b**) Under high magnification, occasional bizarre, polylobulated giant cells and prominent mitotic figures can be seen.

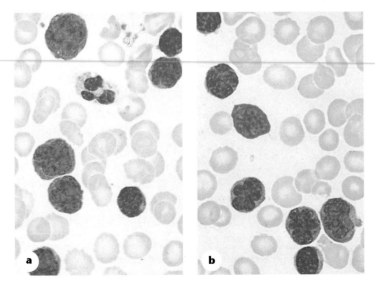

Fig. 14.65 Adult T-cell lymphoma-leukemia (ATLL). (**a, b**) Peripheral blood films reveal characteristic abnormal lymphocytes with convoluted nuclei. (Courtesy of Dr D Catovsky.)

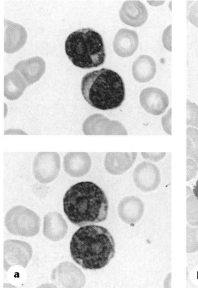

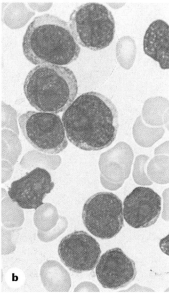

Fig. 14.66 Leukemic transition of lymphoma. Peripheral blood films show (**a**) lymphoid cells, two of which exhibit prominent nuclear clefts, in a patient with nodular, poorly differentiated lymphocytic (NPDL) lymphoma. (**b**) In a patient with widely disseminated, terminal large cell lymphoma, abnormal large- and medium-sized immature lymphoid cells are present in peripheral blood, exhibiting abundant cytoplasm and prominent nucleoli.

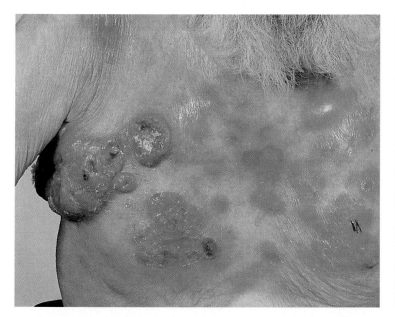

Fig. 14.67 Cutaneous involvement in diffuse large cell lymphoma. Large nodules and fungating tumors, often of a deep red or plum color, may occur. Skin biopsy is essential for diagnosis and distinction from mycosis fungoides. Although T-cell lymphomas often involve the skin, B-cell lymphomas may also occasionally spread to the skin and subcutaneous tissues. Dissemination to other organs eventually occurs in most cases.

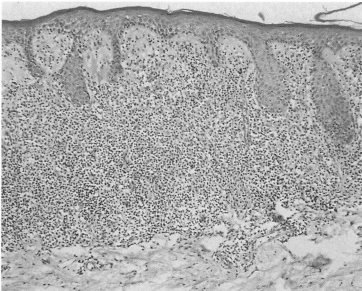

Fig. 14.68 Cutaneous involvement in systemic lymphoma. The epidermis is not affected and a grenz zone (a band like area of uninvolvement between epidermis and tumor) is present. The latter and the absence of Pautrier's microabscesses are features that help distinguish B-cell lymphomas from mycosis fungoides and other cutaneous T-cell lymphomas. A dense band-like infiltrate of poorly differentiated lymphocytic cells occupies the upper and mid-dermis. Infiltration of hair follicles or sebaceous glands (not shown) is a common feature of most lymphomas that secondarily involve the skin.

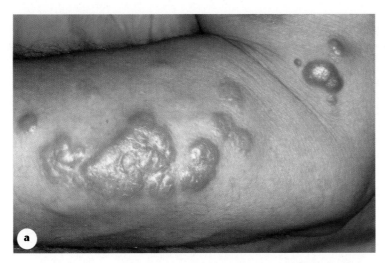

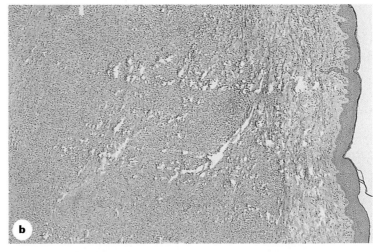

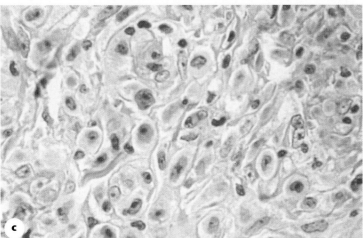

Fig. 14.69 Cutaneous anaplastic large cell lymphoma. This 68-year-old man presented with slowly progressive cutaneous lesions, together with retroperitoneal and groin adenopathy. (**a**) Close-up view of the arm shows multiple raised, firm, irregular lesions. (**b**) Low-power microscopic section of a skin biopsy reveals diffuse involvement of the reticular dermis by a blue cell infiltrate. (**c**) Higher magnification shows large cells with bizarre, hyperlobated nuclei, prominent nucleoli and abundant cytoplasm.

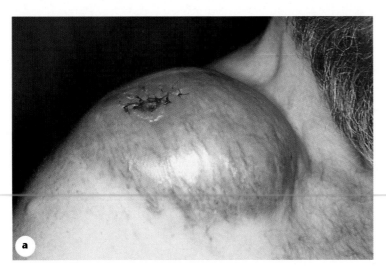

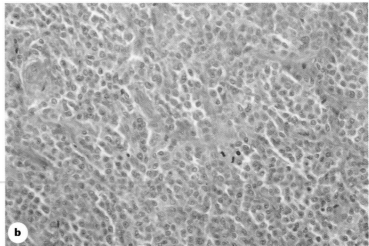

Fig. 14.70 Cutaneous involvement in peripheral T-cell lymphoma, unspecified. (**a**) This 57-year-old man developed a large mass in the right shoulder, with no other lesions or adenopathy found on extensive evaluation. (**b**) Biopsy of the lesion shows intermediate- to large-sized lymphoid cells with round to irregular nuclear outlines, indistinct nucleoli and pale eosinophilic cytoplasm. The lesion diffusely infiltrates from the dermis into the subcutaneous tissue but shows no epidermotrophism. The malignant cells stained positive for LCA (CD45) and CD4 but were negative for CD5, CD3, CD1, CD8, CD2 and B-cell antigens (not shown). Primary cutaneous T-cell lymphoma is not common. The patient responded to chemotherapy followed by local radiotherapy. (Courtesy of Dr D Roberts, Department of Pathology, Brigham and Women's Hospital, Boston, MA.)

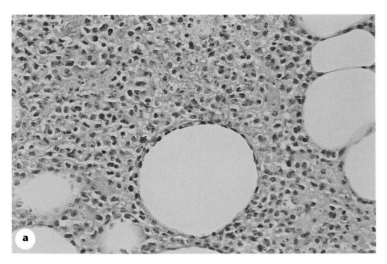

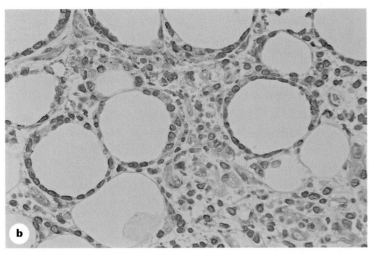

Fig. 14.71 Subcutaneous panniculitis-like T-cell lymphoma, which occurs in young patients, typically involves the subcutaneous tissues of the extremities and may be associated with a hemophagocytic syndrome. (**a**) Intermediate size

T-cells infiltrate subcutaneous and adipose tissues and are typically immunoreactive for (**b**) CD3, CD8 and cytotoxic markers TIA-1 and perforin.

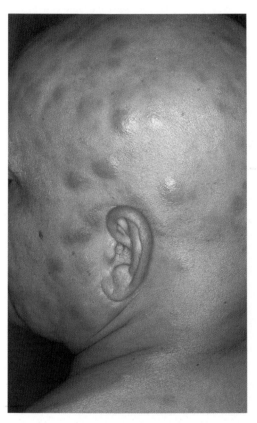

Fig. 14.72 NK cell lymphoma in a 46-year-old man. Numerous scalp and other cutaneous lesions are noted. The malignant cells were positive for both CD3 and CD56. He eventually developed generalized lymphadenopathy, a leukemic phase and CNS involvement, including spread to the spinal fluid. While initial response to chemotherapy was dramatic, progressive recurrent disease was fatal. A more indolent NK cell lymphoma (also called large granular lymphocyte lymphoma or leukemia) is positive for CD3 but negative for CD56 antigens and a third type is negative for CD3 and positive for CD56.

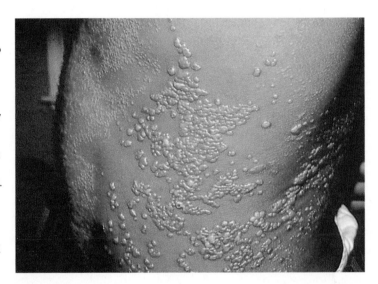

Fig. 14.73 Cutaneous involvement in adult T-cell lymphoma–leukemia. This unusual lymphoproliferative malignancy typically involves the skin, as well as lymph nodes, early in its course. Skin involvement in this case is extensive. (Courtesy of Dr JW Clark.)

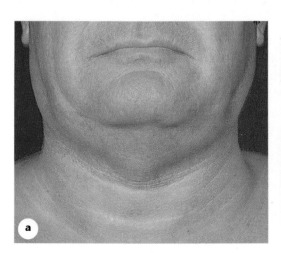

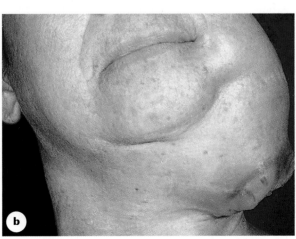

Fig. 14.74 Cervical adenopathy in non-Hodgkin's lymphoma. (**a**) Bilateral cervical lymphadenopathy is present in this patient with follicular lymphoma. (**b**) In another patient with diffuse large cell lymphoma, massive enlargement of lymph nodes in the left submandibular area has occurred together with extensive ulceration of the overlying skin.

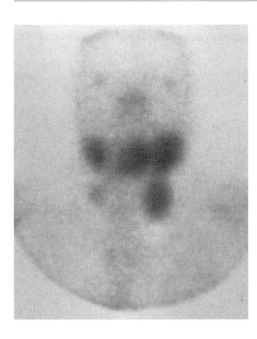

Fig. 14.75 Cervical adenopathy in diffuse large cell lymphoma (stage IIA). Gallium-67 citrate scan in a 55-year-old man who presented with bulky lymphadenopathy involving only the neck nodes shows intense uptake in the submandibular and submental nodes and lower neck bilaterally. Gallium scan is useful in detecting sites of disease that are not palpable, as well as in following the response to therapy.

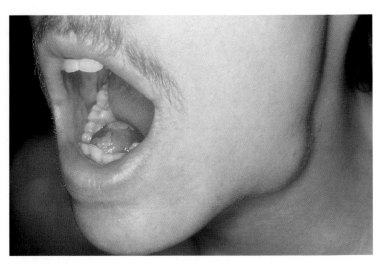

Fig. 14.76 Mandibular and intraoral involvement in Burkitt-like lymphoma. This 22-year-old man presented with a prominent tumor mass in the mandible and was found to have widespread disease. Note also the lymphomatous mass protruding through the floor of the mouth; superficial ulceration is present. Jaw lesions are particularly common in both Burkitt's and Burkitt-like types of high-grade lymphomas. Intensive chemotherapy resulted in a rapid and complete remission.

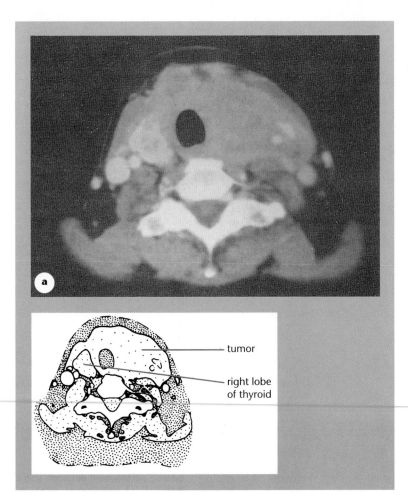

tumor

right lobe of thyroid

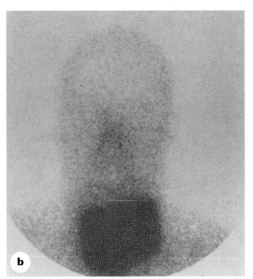

Fig. 14.77 Thyroid involvement in diffuse large cell lymphoma (stage I_E). (**a**) CT scan of a 68-year-old woman who presented with a large neck mass shows extensive involvement of the anterior neck and left portion of the thyroid. The normal thyroid has a high attenuation number because of its normal iodine content. (**b**) A gallium-67 citrate scan shows uptake in the primary mass.

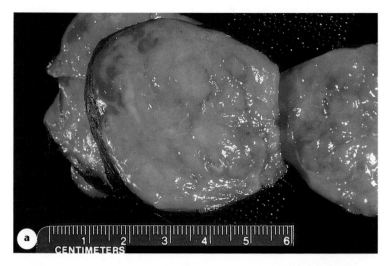

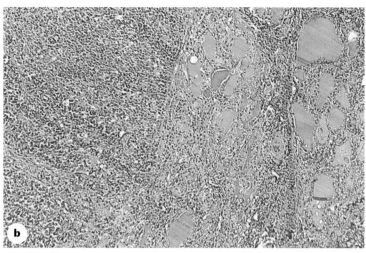

Fig. 14.78 Thyroid involvement in diffuse large cell lymphoma (DLCL). (**a**) Diffusely enlarged, focally hemorrhagic and necrotic thyroid involved by DLCL. (**b**) Histologic section of thyroid shows sheets of neoplastic cells on the left adjacent to residual colloid-filled acini on the right. Immunoperoxidase staining for light chains confirmed the monoclonality of the tumor cells. Although thyroid involvement is most common with large cell lymphomas, particularly B-cell immunoblastic lymphoma, occasional lymphocytic and nodular lymphomas have been reported. Most patients have evidence of coexisting Hashimoto's thyroiditis.

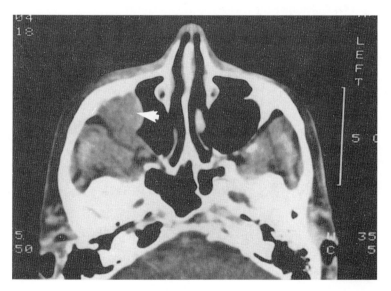

Fig. 14.79 Nasopharyngeal involvement in diffuse large cell lymphoma (stage I$_E$). CT scan of a 34-year-old man who presented with frontal headaches and swelling around the eye reveals a tumor mass (arrow) primarily arising from the right maxillary sinus. He was treated successfully with surgery and radiotherapy; subsequently he developed a testicular mass and was placed on intensive combination chemotherapy.

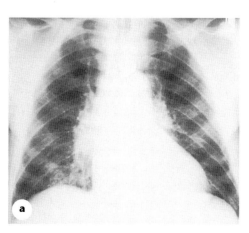

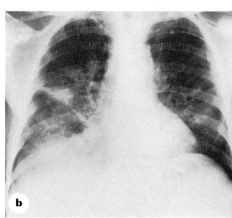

Fig. 14.80 Mediastinal and pulmonary involvement in follicular lymphoma. Chest radiographs show (**a**) bilateral hilar lymph node enlargement and (**b**) interstitial and confluent shadowing, particularly in the lower and mid-zones, which biopsy showed to be due to lymphomatous infiltration.

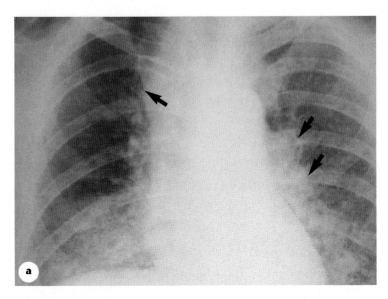

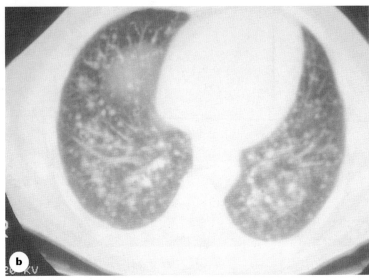

Fig. 14.81 Mediastinal and pulmonary involvement in diffuse large cell lymphoma. (**a**) Frontal chest radiograph shows innumerable tiny bilateral lung nodules. The mediastinum is also widened because of adenopathy, particularly in the right paratracheal region (black arrow), and the left hilum is enlarged and lobular in contour (arrowheads). (**b**) CT image at the level of the lung bases displayed with lung windows also demonstrates the many tiny, well-defined nodules in both lungs. The patient, a 66-year-old man, had presented with a follicular lymphoma several years earlier. Transition to a large cell lymphoma occurs in over 30% of patients with low- or intermediate-grade lymphomas, particularly with long-standing disease (*see* Fig. 14.88).

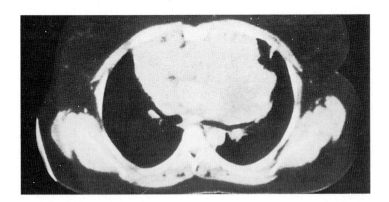

Fig. 14.82 Mediastinal involvement in precursor T-cell lymphoblastic lymphoma. CT scan through the mid-thorax shows gross enlargement of anterior mediastinal lymph nodes. This high-grade NHL of early T-cell lineage may arise in the mediastinum and occurs mainly in boys and adolescent males, which contrasts with mediastinal diffuse large cell lymphoma of B-cell lineage. With the latter, women outnumber men 2 : 1 and the median age at presentation is less than 30 years (*see* Fig. 14.83) (Aisenberg, 1993).

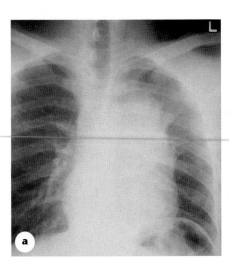

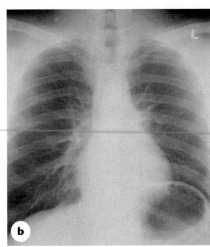

Fig. 14.83 Mediastinal involvement in diffuse large cell lymphoma. Chest film shows bulky mediastinal adenopathy in an 18-year-old man with stage I before (**a**) and after (**b**) complete remission, which was achieved in only 6 weeks after the initiation of combination chemotherapy. The patient was disease free more than 17 years later. Microscopically, primary large cell lymphoma is associated with dense sclerosis in about half of the cases. Clinically, adverse prognostic features include bulky (>7 cm) masses, extranodal disease, pleural effusion, elevated LDH or persistent gallium-67 avidity after treatment (Kirn *et al.*, 1993).

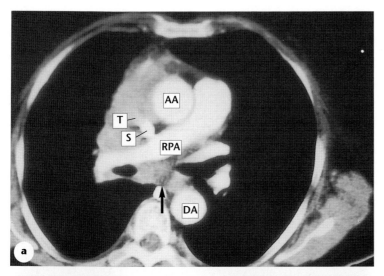

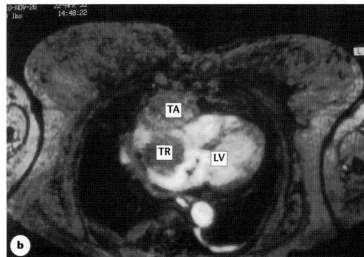

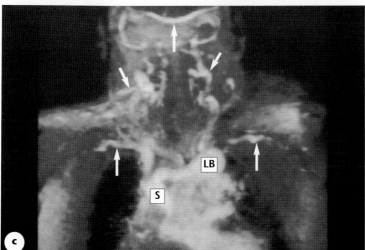

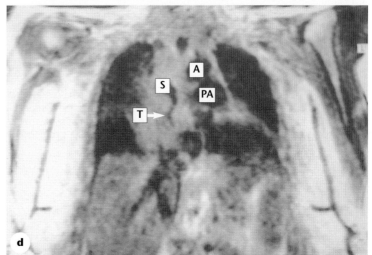

Fig. 14.84 Superior vena cava (SVC) syndrome in diffuse large cell lymphoma. (**a**) CT image with intravenous contrast at the level of the right pulmonary artery (RPA) showing tumor (T) infiltrating into the area of the SVC (S) which is narrowed. Tumor is also present in the subcarinal space (arrow). AA, ascending aorta; DA, descending aorta. (**b**) MR image in the axial plane at the level of the left ventricle (LV) using a sequence which produces a high signal from flowing blood. Tumor is seen both anterior to the heart (TA) and protruding into the lumen of the right atrium (TR). A small left pleural effusion is also present

(arrow). (**c**) MR image in the coronal plane at the level of the anterior neck using a sequence which produces a high signal from flowing blood. Numerous tortuous and dilated neck collateral vessels are present (arrows), indicating obstruction of venous return. LB=left brachiocephalic vein; S=superior vena cava. (**d**) T1-weighted MR image in the coronal plane through the main pulmonary artery (PA). Tumor is seen filling the right atrium (T). A markedly narrowed superior vena cava (S) passes through the tumor, tapering to a slit inferiorly (arrow). A, aortic arch.

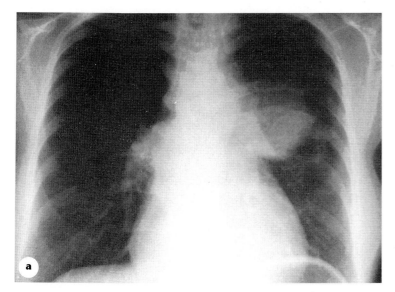

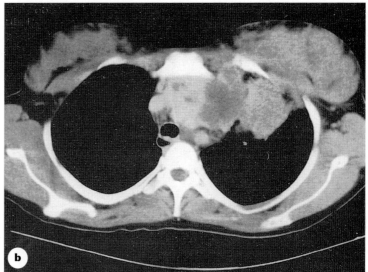

Fig. 14.85 Mediastinal involvement in diffuse large cell lymphoma (stage IVB). (**a**) Chest film of a 30-year-old woman who presented with cough, fever and weight loss shows a large upper mediastinal mass. (**b**) On CT scan, the mass appears heterogeneous, a result of necrosis within the tumor. There is also a second mass extending from the mediastinum and involving the lung

parenchyma. Spread of the lymphoma through the chest wall and into the pectoralis muscles and breast is evident. Biopsy showed a B-immunoblastic sarcoma (BIBS) subtype of large cell lymphoma. A complete remission was obtained with combination chemotherapy.

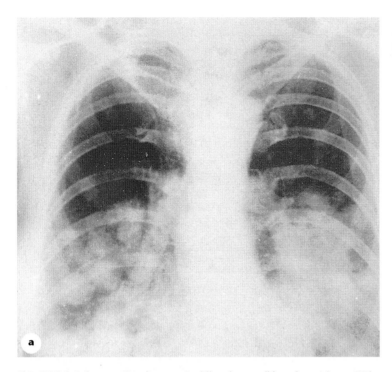

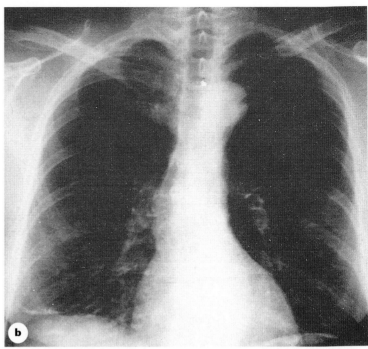

Fig. 14.86 Pulmonary involvement in diffuse large cell lymphoma (stage IVB). (**a**) A 64-year-old woman who presented with fever, weight loss and dyspnea was found to have multiple pulmonary nodules on chest radiography. Biopsy yielded the diagnosis. (**b**) Two months after chemotherapy, there is complete remission. Non-Hodgkin's lymphomas in the lung exhibit a broad spectrum of radiographic findings, ranging from purely linear or 'reticular' (reticulonodular) infiltrates to the extensive large nodules seen in this case. Less commonly, a single nodule or a focal infiltrate resembling pneumonia may be seen.

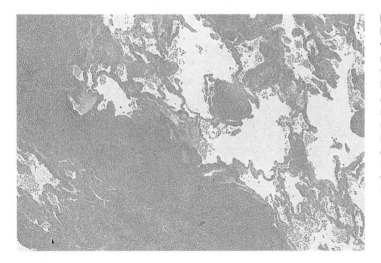

Fig. 14.87 Primary pulmonary lymphocytic lymphoma. Low-power view of a lung biopsy shows sheets of neoplastic lymphocytes at the edge of the tumor infiltrating the surrounding lung along bronchovascular bundles and alveolar septa. Primary pulmonary non-Hodgkin's lymphomas are uncommon, although lung involvement is frequent as part of disseminated disease, most often with DLCL. In some patients morphologic features are diagnostic of a low-grade MALT lymphoma.

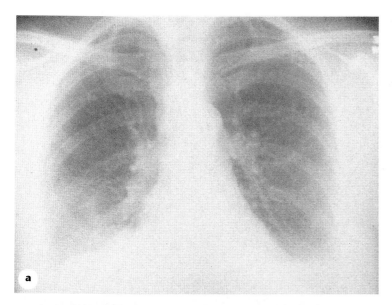

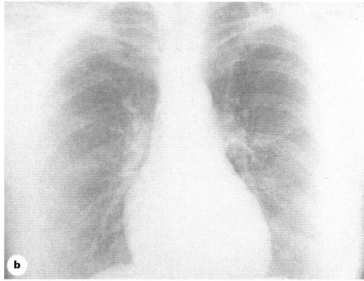

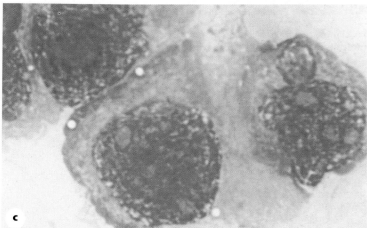

Fig. 14.88 Malignant pleural effusion in follicular lymphoma (stage IVA). (**a**) Chest film of a 57-year-old woman who presented with increasing dyspnea and cough shows small bilateral pleural effusions. Further workup revealed retroperitoneal adenopathy with ascites. A dramatic response occurred within 3 weeks of initiation of combination chemotherapy. (**b**) Followup film shows complete resolution of the pleural effusions. Four years later, fever and weight loss occurred, in association with pleural effusions, adenopathy and subcutaneous nodules. (**c**) Cytocentrifuge preparation of pleural fluid shows large malignant cells with irregular nuclei containing prominent nucleoli, findings diagnostic of a large cell lymphoma. Lymph node biopsy (not shown) confirmed histologic progression to a diffuse large cell lymphoma (*see* Fig. 14.81).

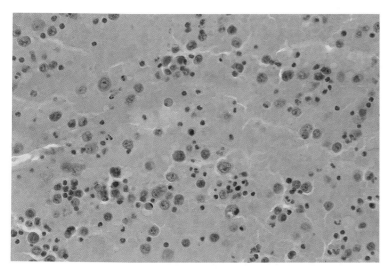

Fig. 14.89 Primary effusion lymphoma, typically found in HIV-positive patients, presents in pleural, pericardial or ascitic fluid without a tumor mass. It is a high-grade B-cell lymphoma with a poor prognosis (median survival <1 year). Neoplastic cells are CD45, CD30, HLA-DR positive as well as being positive for Kaposi's sarcoma-associated herpesvirus, HHV8 and Epstein–Barr virus.

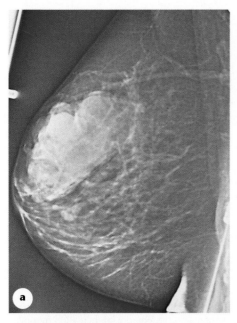

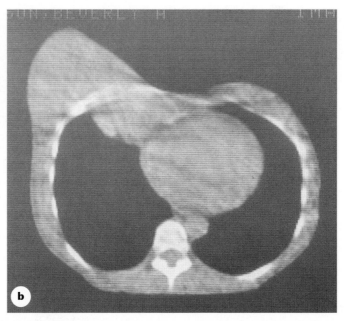

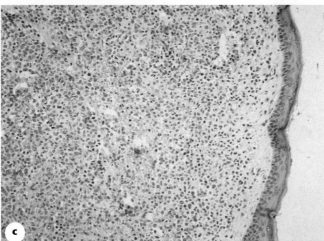

Fig. 14.90 Lymphoma of the breast (stage I$_E$). (a) Mammogram of a 35-year-old woman who presented with a large upper left breast mass shows a soft tissue mass with no suspicious calcifications. The differential diagnosis included adenocarcinoma of the breast, cystosarcoma phylloides, lymphoma and, less likely, metastases or a benign process. Biopsy was positive for a diffuse large cell lymphoma (DLCL). (b) Staging CT scan in another patient, who developed rapid enlargement of the right breast and axillary adenopathy, dramatically reveals how extensively the tumor has infiltrated the breast; there is also extension of the lymphoma into the internal mammary nodes. Biopsy also showed a DLCL. (c) Microscopic section of a breast biopsy from a woman who presented with an inflammatory breast lesion demonstrates involvement by a DLCL. Primary lymphomas of the breast represent a B-cell spectrum, varying from high-grade to low-grade follicular and MALT types (Mattia *et al.*, 1993).

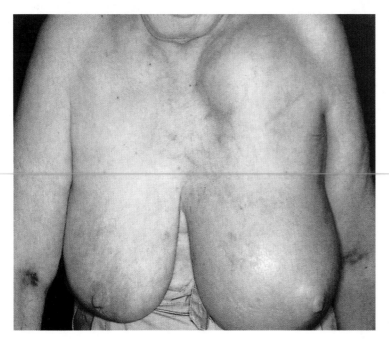

Fig. 14.91 Involvement of the breast in lymphoma (stage IV). This 75-year-old woman presented with advanced diffuse large cell lymphoma including involvement of lung and heart. Note the enlarged left breast with inflammatory skin changes due to lymphatic obstruction, simulating primary inflammatory breast carcinoma. A greatly enlarged left upper chest wall mass is also evident, arising from underlying adenopathy.

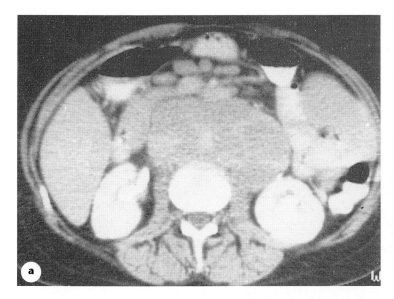

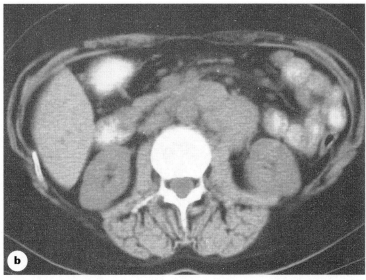

Fig. 14.92 Retroperitoneal involvement in follicular lymphoma (stage IIIA). (**a**) Staging CT scan in a 42-year-old woman who presented with generalized adenopathy shows enlarged retroperitoneal nodes which demonstrated marked uptake on gallium-67 citrate scan (not shown). (**b**) Following combination chemotherapy, there is dramatic regression in the retroperitoneal nodes.

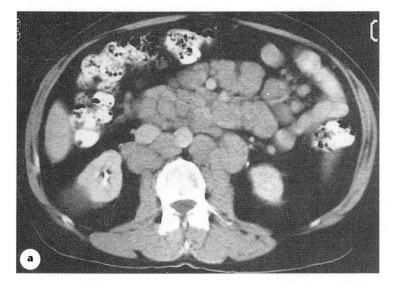

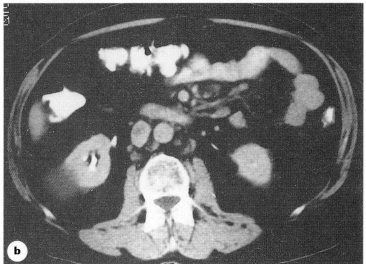

Fig. 14.93 Mesenteric and retroperitoneal involvement in small lymphocytic lymphoma (stage IVA). A 58-year-old man presented with generalized adenopathy, mild anemia and thrombocytopenia. Bone marrow biopsy revealed infiltration by small, well-differentiated lymphocytes. Surface marker studies were consistent with a monocolonal population of B-lymphocytes. (**a**) Abdominal CT scan demonstrates many enlarged mesenteric and retroperitoneal lymph nodes. (**b**) Followup CT scan 16 months later after intermittent chemotherapy shows regression in all nodes, confirming a complete clinical remission. As an incidental finding, note the benign renal cyst in the right kidney.

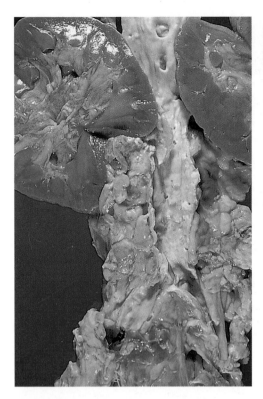

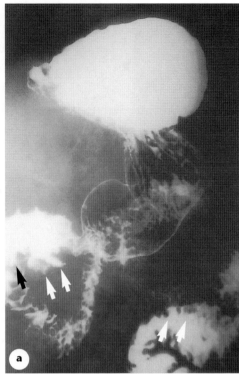

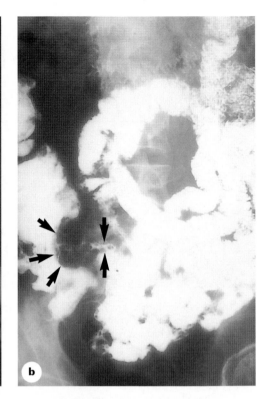

Fig. 14.94 Retroperitoneal involvement in diffuse large cell lymphoma. Confluent adenopathy of retroperitoneal lymph nodes has led to bilateral encasement and compression of the ureters by pink-tan, fleshy tumor.

Fig. 14.95 Mucosa-associated lymphoid tissue (MALT) marginal zone lymphoma of the gastrointestinal tract. (**a**) Abdominal film from upper gastrointestinal series showing thickened nodular folds in the duodenum (arrows) and less prominent nodularity of the mucosa in the jejunum (arrowheads) consistent with infiltrative process in the small bowel mucosa. (**b**) Abdominal film from a small bowel follow-through series showing the relatively normal appearance of the distal jejunum and proximal ileum, but marked narrowing and irregularity of the terminal ileum (arrowheads), with a large filling defect in the region of the ileocecal valve (arrows), consistent with markedly thickened, infiltrated mucosa (*see also* Fig. 14.96).

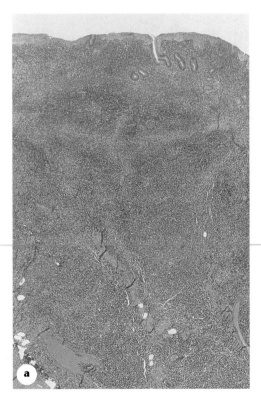

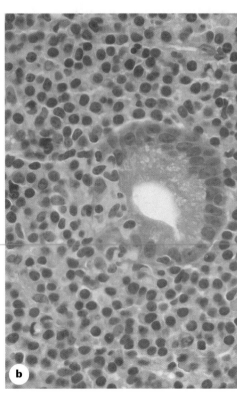

Fig. 14.96 Marginal zone lymphoma of MALT of the stomach. (**a, b**) The stomach wall is extensively infiltrated by small lymphoid cells with a moderate amount of cytoplasm and round to irregular nuclei, with occasional plasma cells and scattered germinal centers. (**b**) Higher power reveals scattered lymphoepithelial lesions. The lymphoid cells are positive for pan-B cell markers and negative for CD5 and CD10. Some patients appear to respond to therapy for *Helicobacter pylori* infection which has been implicated as an etiologic agent (Isaacson, 1994).

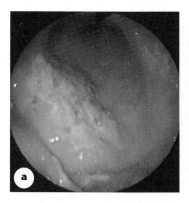 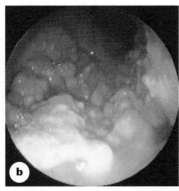

Fig. 14.97 Lymphoma of the stomach. (**a, b**) These endoscopic views show diffuse nodular involvement of the gastric wall by a diffuse large cell lymphoma. This lesion was associated with a protein-losing enteropathy.

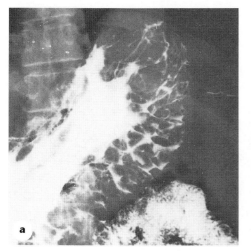 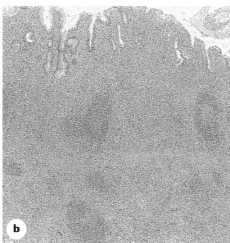

Fig. 14.98 Lymphoma of the stomach. (**a**) Barium study shows mucosal and mural involvement of the fundus and body of the stomach. (**b**) Histologic section reveals invasion of the gastric glands, lamina propria, and deeper areas by sheets of tumor cells of a diffuse large cell lymphama. (**a**: Courtesy of Dr. D. Nag)

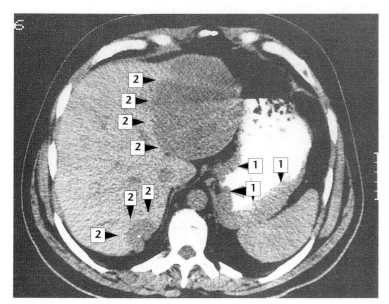

Fig. 14.99 Lymphoma of the stomach. CT scan of a 45-year-old man who presented with weight loss and epigastric distress shows thickening of the wall of the body of the stomach (arrows 1), as well as two low-attenuation masses in the liver (arrows 2). Although these abnormalities are compatible with the diagnosis of lymphoma, there is no way to distinguish them from gastric adenocarcinoma with metastases to the liver. Endoscopic gastric biopsy showed a diffuse large cell lymphoma.

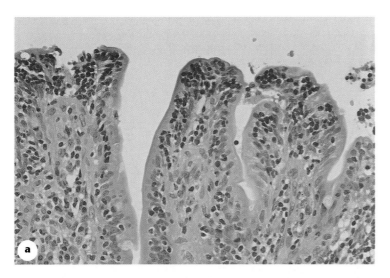

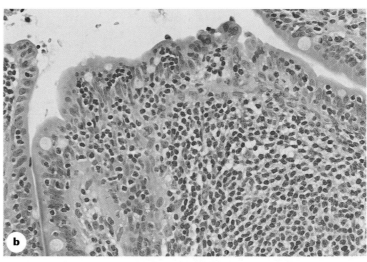

Fig. 14.100 Enteropathy-type T-cell lymphoma occurs in older patients, many of whom have a history of celiac disease. Neoplastic T-cells infiltrate segments of small bowel (**a**) leading to villous blunting, atrophy and malabsorption (**b**). The neoplastic cells are immunoreactive for pan-T cell markers such as CD3 as well as CD103.

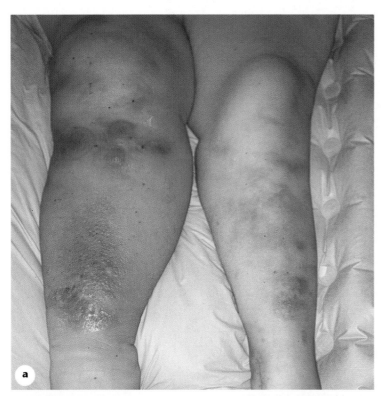

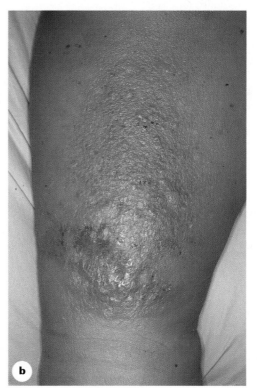

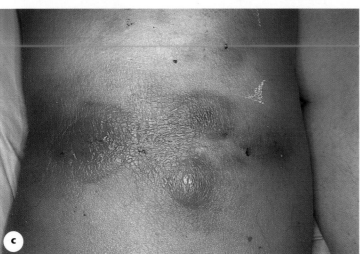

Fig. 14.101 Mantle cell lymphoma of soft tissue in a 66-year-old woman. (**a**) This aggressive lymphoma arose in an unusual location with subsequent destruction of the tibia and fibula. (**b,c**) Close-up views show involvement of skin with diffuse thickening and nodular lesions.

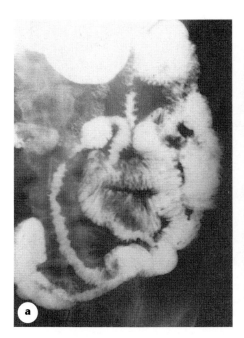
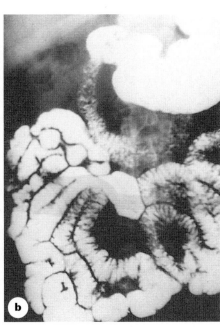

Fig. 14.102 Gastrointestinal involvement in B-cell large cell lymphoma. A 55-year-old man presented with abdominal complaints. On workup, he was found to have mediastinal, hilar and peripheral adenopathy, as well as (**a**) diffuse narrowing and irregularity of several loops of small bowel, consistent with involvement by lymphoma. A mass effect in the right lower quadrant can also be seen. (**b**) Combination chemotherapy resulted in complete remission, as can be seen in this followup barium film.

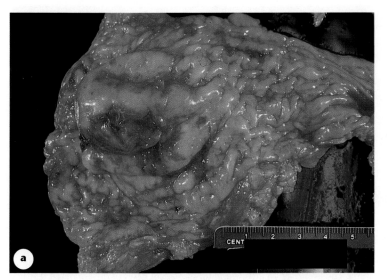

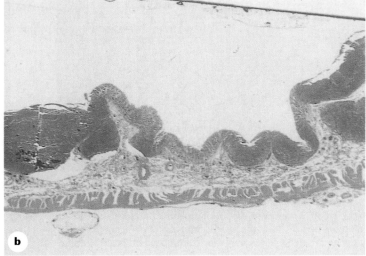

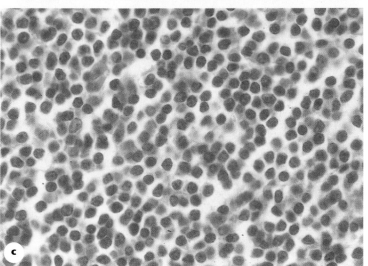

Fig. 14.103 Mantle cell lymphoma of the colon, presenting as multiple lymphomatous polyposis. A 67-year-old woman presented with GI bleeding. Biopsies and subsequent resection reveal multiple submucosal tumor masses in the right colon and ileum which focally erode the mucosa and infiltrate to lamina propria (**a, b**). The infiltrate is composed of small lymphoid cells with irregular to cleaved nuclei (**c**). Tumor was present in numerous pericolic lymph nodes and, at autopsy, was found to have spread extensively with the retroperitoneum and to involve lung, liver, spleen and bone marrow. Early, wide dissemination is a characteristic feature in multiple lymphomatous polyposis. Tumor cells are positive for pan-B cell markers and CD5.

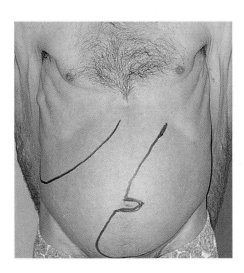

Fig. 14.104 Splenic and liver involvement in follicular lymphoma. Massive enlargement of the spleen and hepatomegaly are apparent in this patient.

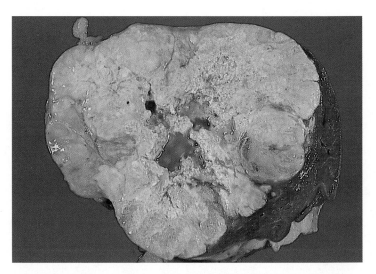

Fig. 14.105 Splenic involvement in B-cell diffuse large cell lymphoma. This spleen, removed at laparotomy, has been sectioned to show widespread replacement of tissue by pale tumor with extensive areas of necrosis.

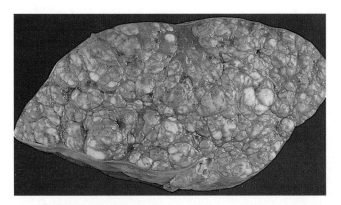

Fig. 14.106 Splenic involvement in follicular lymphoma. Coarse, nodular deposits of pale tumor have diffusely replaced normal tissue in this greatly enlarged spleen. Involvement of the spleen is very common, particularly in the nodular subtypes of non-Hodgkin's lymphoma. Splenomegaly may cause destruction of red cells, white cells, or platelets (hypersplenism).

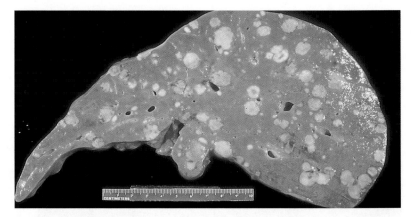

Fig. 14.107 Hepatic involvement in B-cell diffuse large cell lymphoma. A 64-year-old woman with a stage IV DPDL lymphoma responded to treatment at first, but then relapsed with a downhill course despite further therapy. Autopsy showed widespread disease and histologic examination revealed transition to a high-grade lymphoma. The liver may be involved in up to 50% of cases of disseminated disease. Histologic progression from a low-grade to an intermediate- or high-grade lymphoma occurs clinically in about 30% of cases, but at autopsy as many as 60–70% of cases show a change in histology to a higher-grade (aggressive) lymphoma.

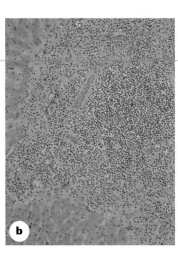

Fig. 14.108 Hepatic involvement in follicular lymphoma. (**a**) Dark patches of lymphocytic tumor cells infiltrate the liver, causing (**b**) expansion of a portal tract. This type of periportal involvement is often seen in lymphocytic lymphomas and may not be associated with very abnormal liver chemistry tests.

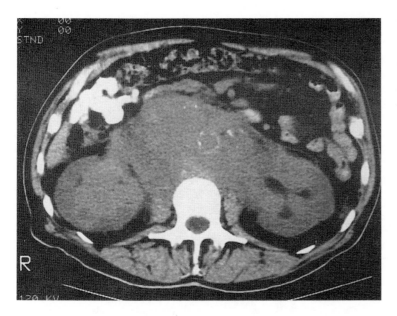

Fig. 14.109 Renal involvement in diffuse large cell lymphoma. A 54-year-old man who had a stage III NPDL lymphoma for 7 years suddenly developed increasing abdominal distension. This CT scan shows diffuse retroperitoneal adenopathy encasing the aorta and extending directly into the renal parenchyma bilaterally. A cauda equina syndrome developed and CSF examination showed large lymphoma cells, indicating histologic conversion to an aggressive malignancy.

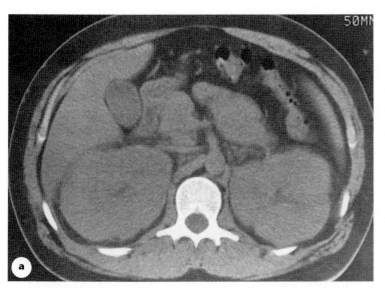

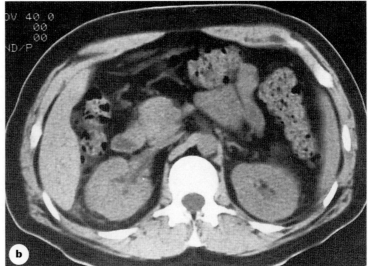

Fig. 14.110 Renal involvement in precursor T-cell lymphoblastic lymphoma. A 31-year-old man presented with weight loss, fatigue and low back pain. Evaluation revealed acute renal failure. (**a**) Abdominal CT scan shows greatly enlarged kidneys, which on biopsy yielded the diagnosis. Bone marrow was also involved by lymphoma. Immunophenotyping of bone marrow cells showed positivity for CD2 71%, CD5 53%, CD3 (22%), CD8 (30%) and CD4 (8%). The patient's condition improved dramatically with intensive chemotherapy. (**b**) Followup CT scan 1 month later shows essentially normal kidneys.

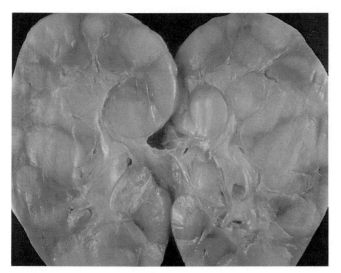

Fig. 14.111 Renal involvement in diffuse large cell lymphoma. There is little remaining parenchyma in this specimen, which exhibits many large, gray-white nodules of tumor.

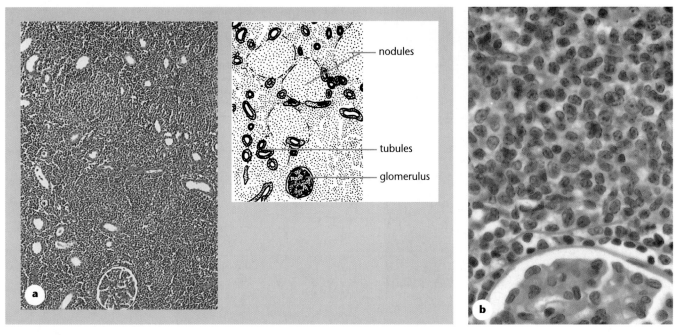

Fig. 14.112 Renal involvement in follicular lymphoma. (**a**) The presence of nodular infiltrates in the renal cortex is consistent with involvement by a B-cell lymphoma. (**b**) Higher magnification demonstrates that the infiltrate is composed of a mixture of large and small lymphocytes, as well as scattered small, cleaved cells typical of a follicular center cell lymphoma. (Reproduced from Schumann and Weiss, 1981.)

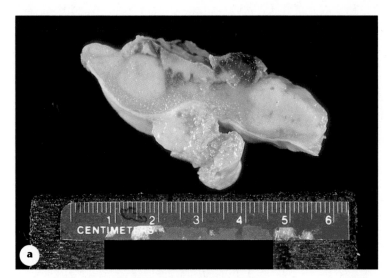

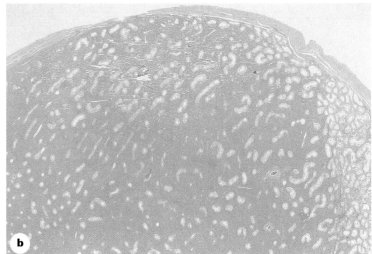

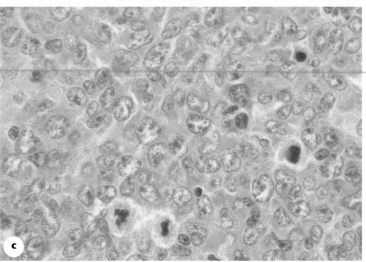

Fig. 14.113 Testicular involvement by diffuse large cell lymphoma (DLCL). (**a**) A tan-pink tumor mass accounts for the testicular enlargement in a 51-year-old man. (**b**) Low-power view of the interstitial DLCL infiltrate which characteristically surrounds seminiferous tubules. (**c**) High-power view reveals a population of large lymphoid cells, many with irregular and cleaved nuclei. Non-Hodgkin's lymphoma is the most common testicular tumor in men over 60 years of age and is most commonly large cell type and of B-cell origin, as was true in this case.

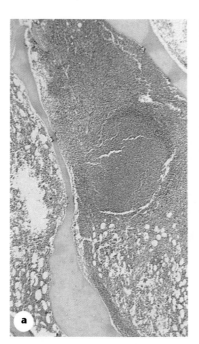
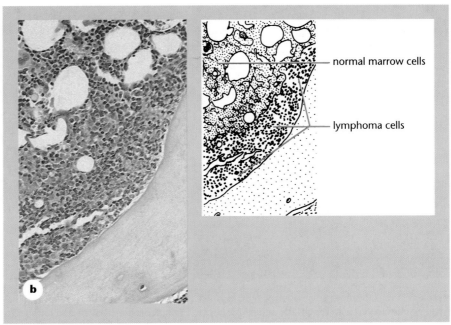

Fig. 14.114 Bone marrow involvement in follicular lymphoma. (**a**) Low-power microscopic section of a needle biopsy specimen reveals almost complete replacement of normal hematopoietic tissue in the upper portion of the field and a paratrabecular collection of neoplastic lymphoid cells below. (**b**) Higher magnification shows the demarcation between the paratrabecular lymphoid cells and the normal hematopoietic cells and fat.

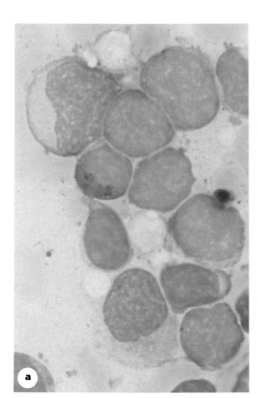
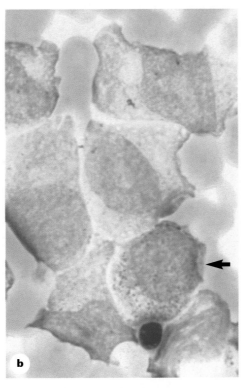
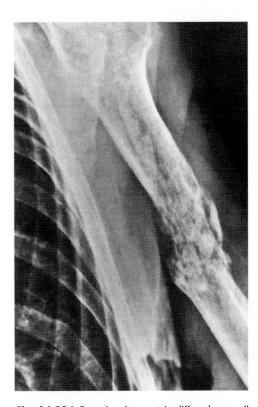

Fig. 14.115 Bone marrow involvement in non-Hodgkin's lymphoma. (**a**) Smear from a bone marrow aspiration in a patient with follicular lymphoma shows small, poorly differentiated cells with scanty cytoplasm; irregular nuclear contours are apparent, with slight indentations in some of the cells. Nuclear chromatin is fine and light staining. Nucleoli are not evident. (**b**) In this patient with a diffuse large cell lymphoma, immature cells have large, prominent nucleoli. A promyelocyte (granulated cell) is seen in the lower right field (arrow).

Fig. 14.116 Bone involvement in diffuse large cell lymphoma (stage 1_E). Radiograph of the left upper arm of a 45-year-old man who complained of sudden onset of pain shows a pathologic fracture through an area of permeative destruction of cortical and medullary bone. The fracture is quite recent, as there is little or no periosteal reaction either to the tumor itself or to the complicating fracture. Biopsy yielded the diagnosis.

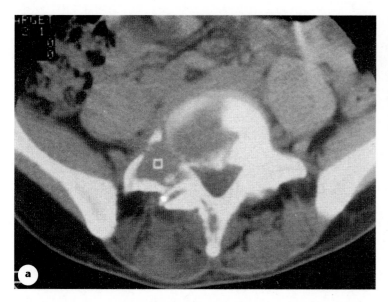

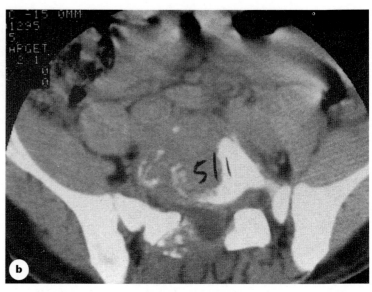

Fig. 14.117 Bone involvement in Burkitt-like lymphoma (stage IVB). (**a,b**) CT scans in an 18-year-old man who presented with weight loss and severe low back pain reveal destruction at the L5–S1 vertebrae. Further workup disclosed multiple bone lesions and retroperitoneal adenopathy.

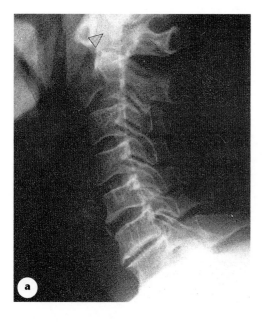

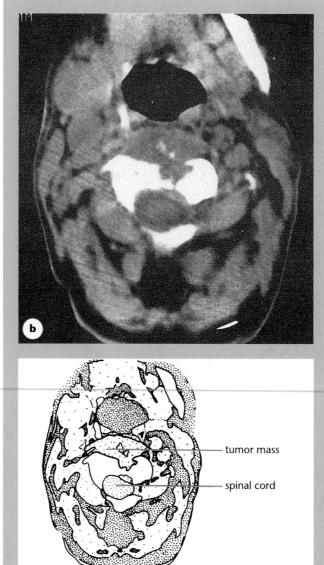

Fig. 14.118 Bone involvement in follicular lymphoma (stage IV). A 62-year-old man with a 3-year history of lymphoma, involving mainly the bone marrow and lymph nodes, showed a partial response with chemotherapy but suddenly developed severe neck pain. (**a**) Plain radiograph of the cervical spine shows lytic destruction of the body of C1 (arrowhead). (**b**) CT scan reveals tumor invasion of C1–C2 with extension into the spinal canal. Stabilization of the neck was achieved by a bone graft. Further workup disclosed other bone lesions and retroperitoneal adenopathy.

tumor mass

spinal cord

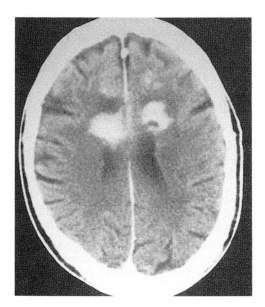

Fig. 14.119 CNS involvement in diffuse large cell lymphoma. A 62-year-old man who was diagnosed 3 years earlier with a stage IIA lymphoma involving the mediastinum achieved complete remission with chemotherapy. Subsequently, a testicular mass developed, followed by headaches. This CT scan shows several enhancing periventricular lesions consistent with CNS involvement by lymphoma.

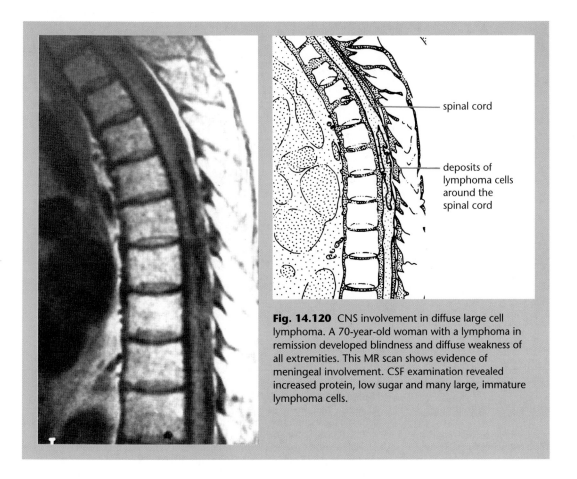

spinal cord

deposits of lymphoma cells around the spinal cord

Fig. 14.120 CNS involvement in diffuse large cell lymphoma. A 70-year-old woman with a lymphoma in remission developed blindness and diffuse weakness of all extremities. This MR scan shows evidence of meningeal involvement. CSF examination revealed increased protein, low sugar and many large, immature lymphoma cells.

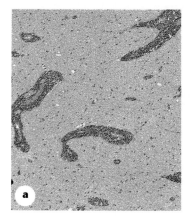
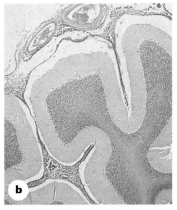

Fig. 14.121 CNS involvement in precursor T-cell lymphoblastic lymphoma. (**a**) Invasion has occurred along perivascular spaces and (**b**) the meninges are extensively involved. A similar pattern occurs in primary lymphoma of the brain, which in most cases is an undifferentiated or large cell lymphoma. Primary lymphoma of the brain is an AIDS-defining illness and the second most frequent extranodal disease site after the GI tract. Almost all cases are of B-cell type. Epstein–Barr virus is thought to have a role in the pathogenesis of CNS lymphomas in immunocomprised patients, including AIDS patients (*see* Chapter 17).

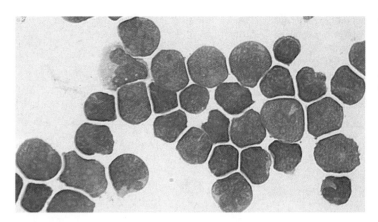

Fig. 14.122 CNS involvement in precursor T-cell lymphoblastic lymphoma. High-power view of a cytospin preparation of CSF shows typical T-lymphoblasts. The nucleus in many of the cells has a convoluted or cloverleaf appearance. Another high-grade lymphoma, small non-cleaved cell lymphoma, Burkitt's-type, also has a predilection for involvement of the meninges.

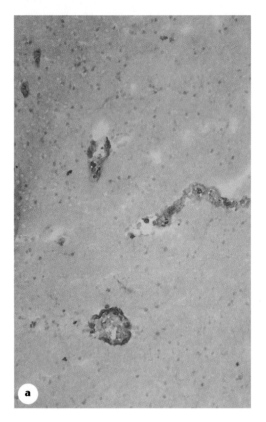
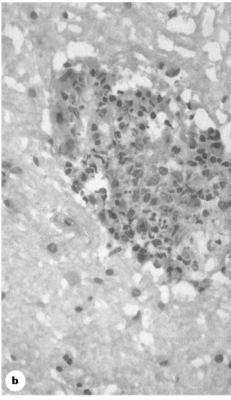

Fig. 14.123 CNS involvement in intravascular lymphomatosis (IVL). (**a**) Low-power view of the brain shows several intravascular foci of lymphoma cells in a 43-year-old man who presented with confusion and other neurologic features (immunoperoxidase stain for leukocyte common antigen). (**b**) Higher-power view shows cluster of large lymphoid cells within a vessel. Immunophenotyping revealed monoclonal B-lymphocytes (not shown). The patient had widespread involvement of the CNS as well as blood vessels of the lungs. IVL is an unusual aggressive lymphoma with a variety of CNS, cutaneous and pulmonary manifestations (Demirer *et al.*, 1994). Few cases are diagnosed *ante mortem*. The mechanisms for trapping of neoplastic lymphocytes within small vessels of diffuse organs remain unexplained. (Courtesy of Dr M. Kilo.)

REFERENCES

Abbondanzo S, Wenig G: Non-Hodgkin's lymphoma of the sinonasal tract. Cancer 1995; 75 : 1281–1291.

Arber DA: Molecular diagnostic approach to non-Hodgkin's lymphoma. J Mol Diagnos 2000; 2 : 178–190.

Arnold A, Cossman J, Bakhshi A, *et al.*: Immunoglobulin–gene rearrangements as unique clonal markers in human lymphoid neoplasms. N Engl J Med 1983; 309 : 1593–1599.

Baddoura F, Chan W, Masih A, *et al.*: T-cell-rich B-cell lymphoma. Am J Clin Pathol 1995; 103 : 65–75.

Berger F, Felman P, Thiebelemont C, *et al.*: Non-MALT marginal zone B-cell lymphomas: a description of clinical presentation and outcome in 124 patients. Blood 2000; 95 : 1950–1956.

Blay JY, Bardin N, Rousset F, *et al.*: Serum interleukin-10 in non-Hodgkin's lymphoma: a prognostic factor. Blood 1993; 82(7):2169–2174.

Braziel RM, Arber DA, Slovak ML, *et al.*: The Burkitt-like lymphomas: a Southwest Oncology Group study delineating phenotypic, genotypic, and clinical features. Blood 2001; 97 : 3713–3720.

Carey JL, Hanson CA: Flow cytometric analysis of leukemia and lymphoma. In: Keren DF, Hanson CA, Hurtubise PE, eds: Flow Cytometry and Clinical Diagnosis. American Society of Clinical Pathologists, Chicago, 1994; pp. 197–308.

Chan JKC, Banks PM, Clearly ML, *et al.*: A revised European–American classification of lymphoid neoplasms proposed by the International Lymphoma Study Group. Am J Clin Pathol 1995; 103 : 543–560.

Chang H, Benchimol S, Minden MD, *et al.*: Alterations of p53 and c-myc in the clonal evolution of malignant lymphoma. Blood 1994; 83(2):452–459.

Clarke C, Glaser SL. Changing incidence of non-Hodgkin Lymphomas in the United States. Cancer 2002; 94:2015–23

Cordier JF, Chailleux E, Lauque D, *et al.*: Primary pumonary lymphomas: a clinical study of 70 cases in nonimmunocompromised patients. Chest 1993; 103 : 201–208.

Dabbs DJ, Moul-Manager L, Mignon F, *et al.*: Glomerular lesions in lymphomas and leukemias. Am J Med 1986; 80 : 63–70.

Demirer T, Dail DH, Aboulatia DM: Four varied cases of intravascular lymphomatosis and a literature review. Cancer 1994; 73 : 1738–1745.

Fisher R, Dahlberg S, Hathwani B, *et al.*: A clinical analysis of two indolent lymphoma entities: mantle cell lymphoma and marginal zone lymphoma (including the mucosa-associated lymphoid tissue and monocytoid B-cell subcategories): a Southwest Oncology Group study. Blood 1995; 85 : 1075–1082.

Freedman AS, Nadler LM: Cell surface markers in hematologic malignancies. Semin Oncol 1987; 14 : 193–212.

Harris NL, Jaffe ES, Stein H, *et al.*: A revised European–American classification of lymphoid neoplasms: a proposal from the International Lymphoma Study Group. Blood 1994; 84 : 1361–1392.

Harris NL, Jaffe ES, Diebold J, *et al.*: World Health Organization classification of neoplastic diseases of the hematopoietic and lymphoid tissues: report of the clinical advisory committee meeting, Airlie House, Virginia, November 1997. J Clin Oncol 1999; 17 : 3835–3849.

Hecht JL, Aster JC: Molecular biology of Burkitt's lymphoma. J Clin Oncol 2000; 18 : 3707–3721.

Hicks D, Gokan T, O'Keepe R, *et al*.: Primary lymphoma of bone: correlation of magnetic resonancy imaging features with cytokine production by tumor cells. Cancer 1995; 75 : 973–980.

Hsu S-M, Waldron JW, Hsu P-L, *et al*.: Cytokines in malignant lymphomas: review and prospective evaluation. Hum Pathol 1993; 24 : 1040–1057.

Isaacson PG: Gastric lymphoma and *Helicobacter pylori*. N Engl J Med 1994; 350(18):1310–1311.

Isaacson PG, Norton AJ: Extranodal Lymphomas. Churchill Livingstone, New York, 1999.

Jaffe ES: The role of immunophenotypic markers in the classification of non-Hodgkin's lymphomas. Semin Oncol 1990; 17 : 11–19.

Kadin ME: Ki-1/CD30+ (anaplastic) large-cell lymphoma: maturation of a clinicopathologic entity with prospects of effective therapy. J Clin Oncol 1994; 12(5):884–887.

Kaleem Z, White G, Vollmer RT: Critical analysis and diagnostic usefulness of limited immunophenotyping of B-cell non-Hodgkin lymphomas by flow cytometry. Am J Clin Pathol 2000; 115 : 136–142.

Kirn D, Mauch P, Shaffer K, *et al*.: Large cell and immunoblastic lymphoma of the mediastinum: prognostic features and treatment outcome in 57 patients. J Clin Oncol 1993; 11 : 1336.

Kluin P: bcl-6 in lymphoma – sorting out a wastebasket? N Engl J Med 1994; 331 : 116–118.

Lamy T, Loughran TP Jr: Large granular lymphocyte leukemia. Cancer Control 1998; 5 : 25.

Mattia AR, Ferry JA, Harris NL: Breast lymphoma: a B-cell spectrum including the low grade B-cell lymphoma of mucosa associated lymphoid tissue. Am J Surg Pathol 1993; 17 : 574–587.

Nathwani BN, Mohrmann RL, Brynes RK, *et al*.: Monocytoid B-cell lymphomas: an assessment of diagnostic criteria and a perspective on histogenesis. Hum Pathol 1992; 23 : 1061–1071.

Newell GR, Cabanillas FG, Hagemeister FJ, *et al*.: Incidence of lymphoma in the US classified by the working formulation. Cancer 1987; 59 : 857–861.

Non-Hodgkin's Lymphoma Classification Project: A clinical evaluation of the international study group classification of non-Hodgkin's lymphoma. Blood 1997; 89 : 3909–3918.

Offit K, Lo Coco F, Louie DC, *et al*.: Rearrangement of the bcl-6 gene as a prognostic marker in diffuse large-cell lymphoma. N Engl J Med 1994; 331 : 74–80.

Parsonnet J, Hansen S, Kodriguez L, *et al*.: Helicobacter pylori infection and gastric lymphoma. N Engl J Med 1994; 330 : 1267–1271.

Penny RJ, Blaustein JC, Longtime JA, Pinkus GS: Ki-1-positive large cell lymphomas, a heterogenous group of neoplasms: morphologic, immunophenotypic, genotypic, and clinical features of 24 cases. Cancer 1991; 68 : 362–373.

Pinkus GS, O'Hara CJ, Said JW: Peripheral/post-thymic T-cell lymphomas: a spectrum of disease. Cancer 1990; 65 : 971–998.

Pinkus GS, Lones M, Shintaku IP, Said JW: Immunohistochemical detection of Epstein–Barr virus-encoded latent membrane protein in Reed–Sternberg cells and variants of Hodgkin's disease. Modern Pathol 1994; 7 : 454–461.

Rosenberg SA: National Cancer Institute sponsored study of classifications of non-Hodgkin's lymphomas: summary and description of a working formulation for clinical usage. Cancer 1980; 45 : 2188–2193.

Sander CA, Yano T, Clark HM, *et al*.: p53 mutation is associated with progression in follicular lymphomas. Blood 1993; 82(7):1994–2004.

Shipp MA: Prognostic factors in aggressive non-Hodgkin's lymphoma: who has 'high-risk' disease? Blood 1994; 83 : 1165–1173.

Shipp MA, Harrington DP, Anderson JR, *et al*.: Development of a predictive model for aggressive lymphoma: the International Non-Hodgkin's Lymphoma Prognostic Factors Project. N Engl J Med 1993; 329 : 987–994.

Shivdasani RA, Hess JL, Skarin AT, *et al*.: Intermediate lymphocytic lymphoma: clinical and pathologic features of a recently characterized subtype of non-Hodgkin's lymphoma. J Clin Oncol 1993; 11(4):802–811.

Siebert JD, Mulvaney DA, Potter KL, *et al*.: Relative frequencies and sites of presentation of lymphoid neoplasms in a community hospital according to the revised European–American classification. Am J Clin Pathol 1999; 111 : 379–386.

Siebert JD, Harvey LAC, Fishkin PAS, *et al*.: Comparison of lymphoid neoplasm classification. Am J Clin Pathol 2001; 115 : 650–655.

Siegal RS, Pandolfino T, Guitart J, *et al*.: Primary cutaneous T-cell lymphoma: review of current topics. J Clin Oncol 2000; 18 : 2908–2925.

Skarin AT: Non-Hodgkin's lymphoma. In: Stollerman GH, Harrington WJ, La Mont JT, *et al*., eds: Annals of Internal Medicine. Year Book Medical Publishers, Chicago, 1989; pp. 34 : 209–242.

Staudt LM: The molecular and cellular origins of Hodgkin's disease. J Exp Med 2000; 191 : 207–212.

Stetter-Stevenson M, Medeiros L, Jaffe E: Immunophenotypic methods and findings in the diagnosis of lymphoproliferative disorders. In: Jaffe E, ed: Surgical Pathology of the Lymph Nodes and Related Organs. Sanders, Philadelphia, 1995; pp. 22–57.

Tang SC, Visser L, Hepperle B, *et al*.: Clinical significance of bcl-2-MBR gene rearrangement and protein expression in diffuse large-cell non-Hodgkin's lymphoma: an analysis of 83 cases. J Clin Oncol 1994; 12(1):149–154.

Taylor MA, Kaplan HS, Nelsen TS: Staging laparotomy with splenectomy for Hodgkin's disease: the Stanford experience. World J Surg 1985; 9 : 449.

Uckun FM: Regulation of human B-cell ontogeny. Blood 1990; 76 : 1908–1923.

Van Besien K, Kelta M, Bahaguna P. Primary mediastinal B-cell lymphoma: A review of pathology and management. J Clin Oncol 19: 1855–1864, 2001.

Waldmann TA, Davis MM, Bongiovanni KF, *et al*.: Rearrangements of genes for the antigen receptor on T cells as markers of lineage and clonality in human lymphoid neoplasms. N Engl J Med 1985; 313 : 776–783.

Weisenberger DD, Armitage JO: Mantle cell lymphoma – an entity comes of age. Blood 1996; 87 : 4483–4494.

Whang-Peng J, Knutsen T, Jaffe ES, *et al*.: Sequential analysis of 43 patients with non-Hodgkin's lymphoma: clinical correlations with cytogenetic, histologic, immunophenotyping, and molecular studies. Blood 1995; 85 : 203–216.

Yunis JJ, Frizzera G, Oken MM, *et al*.: Multiple recurrent genomic defects in follicular lymphoma. N Engl J Med 1987; 316 : 79–84.

FIGURE CREDITS

The following books published by Gower Medical Publishing are sources of figures in the present chapter. The figure numbers given in the listing are those of the figures in the present chapter. The page numbers given in parentheses are those of the original publication.

Bullough PG, Boachie-Adjei O: Atlas of Spinal Diseases. Lippincott/Gower Medical Publishing, Philadelphia/New York, 1988; Fig. 14.30 (p. 203).

Bullough PG, Vigorita VJ: Atlas of Orthopedic Pathology. University Park Press/Gower Medical Publishing, Baltimore/New York, 1984: Figs 14.7 (p. 13.8), 14.31 (p. 13.8), 14.116 (p. 13.6).

Cawson RA, Eveson JW: Oral Pathology and Diagnosis. Heinemann Medical Books/Gower Medical Publishing, London, 1987: Figs 14.5 (p. 18.15), 14.11 (p. 18.15), 14.42 (p. 18.10), 14.44a (p. 18.10), 14.44b,c (p. 18.12).

du Bois RM, Clarke SW: Fibreoptic Bronchoscopy in Diagnosis and Management. Lippincott/Gower Medical Publishing, Philadelphia/London, 1987: Fig. 14.16 (p. 3.17).

du Vivier A: Atlas of Clinical Dermatology. Churchill Livingstone/Gower Medical Publishing, Edinburgh/London, 1986: Figs 14.67 (p. 8.14), 14.68 (p. 8.15).

Fletcher CDM, McKee PH: An Atlas of Gross Pathology. Edward Arnold/Gower Medical Publishing, London, 1987: Figs 14.25b (p. 52), 14.106 (p. 52).

Hewitt PE: Blood Diseases (Pocket Picture Guides). Gower Medical Publishing, London, 1985: Fig. 14.18 (p. 43).

Hoffbrand AV, Pettit JE: Clinical Haematology Illustrated. Churchill Livingstone/Gower Medical Publishing, Edinburgh/London, 1987: Figs 14.1 (p. 10.4), 14.3a (p. 10.4), 14.09 (p. 10.5), 14.10 (p. 10.5), 14.12 (p. 10.6), 14.13 (p. 10.6), 14.21 (p. 10.2), 14.25a (p. 10.3), 14.27 (p. 10.2), 14.28 (p. 10.2), 14.34 (p. 10.3), 14.64 (p. 10.18), 14.65 (p. 10.18), 14.66 (p. 10.13), 14.73 (p. 10.18), 14.74 (p. 10.8), 14.78 (p. 10.15), 14.80 (p. 10.14), 14.81 (p. 10.14), 14.87 (p. 10.15), 14.98 (p. 10.15), 14.104 (p. 10.9), 14.105 (p. 10.9), 14.114 (p. 10.13), 14.121 (p10.15), 14.122 (p. 10.16).

Kassner EG, ed.: Atlas of Radiopathic Imaging. Lippincott/Gower Medical Publishing, Philadelphia/New York, 1989: Fig. 14.22 (p. 8.39).

Misiewicz JJ, Bartram CI, Cotton PB, *et al*.: Atlas of Clinical Gastroenterology. Gower Medical Publishing, London, 1985: Fig. 14.108 (p. 19.6).

Schumann GB, Weiss MA: Atlas of Renal and Urinary Tract Cytology and Its Histopathologic Bases. Lippincott, Philadelphia, 1981: Fig. 14.112.

Silverstein FE, Tytgat GNJ: Atlas of Gastrointestinal Endoscopy. Saunders/Gower Medical Publishing, Philadelphia/New York, 1987: Fig. 14.97 (p. 6.11).

Weiss MA, Mills SE: Atlas of Genitourinary Tract Disorders. Lippincott/Gower Medical Publishing, Philadelphia/New York, 1988: Figs 14.47a,b (p. 8.25), 14.47c (p. 8.26), 14.94 (p. 8.24), 14.111 (p. 11.58).

15 Multiple myeloma and plasma cell dyscrasias

Faith E. Davies, Kenneth C. Anderson, David M. Dorfman,
Arthur T. Skarin

Multiple myeloma and related disorders comprise a spectrum of diseases that are characterized by the autonomous proliferation of differentiated lymphoid cells and plasma cells whose physiologic function is to secrete immunoglobulins. Plasma cell dyscrasias account for 1% of all cancers in the United States and approximately 10% of hematological malignancies. Multiple myeloma is the most common of the dyscrasias, representing about 75% of cases and affecting approximately 12 000 individuals each year. Waldenstrom's macroglobulinemia accounts for about 20% of cases, with the remainder consisting of other types of heavy chain disease.

MULTIPLE MYELOMA

Multiple myeloma (MM) is a malignancy of clonal plasma cells involving primarily the bone and bone marrow. The median age at diagnosis is approximately 65 years and fewer than 3% of patients are younger than 40 years. The outlook for patients is poor with a median survival of approximately 3.5 years. In 2001, 14 400 patients will be diagnosed and 11 200 patients will die from the disease (Greenlee *et al.*, 2001).

Disease biology

The available evidence suggests that the clonal precursor cell in MM is a B-cell that has undergone somatic hypermutation and passed through the germinal center. Within the lymph node illegitimate immunoglobulin class switching occurs, resulting in chromosome 14q32 translocations and the dysregulation of a number of oncogenes (FGFR3/MMSET, cyclin D1, c-*maf*). Adhesion molecules then mediate homing of the immortalized MM cells from the lymph node to the bone marrow (BM), where binding of MM cells to bone marrow stromal cells (BMSC) occurs, localizing the MM cells within the BM microenvironment. Adhesion of MM cells results in an increase in the transcription and secretion of a number of cytokines involved in MM cell growth and survival, including interleukin-6 (IL-6), tumor necrosis factor-α (TNF-α) and transforming growth factor-β (TGF-β). Other cytokines are produced that promote bone resorption, tumor migration and invasion, including matrix metalloproteinase-1, interleukin-1β and vascular endothelial growth factor (VEGF). As disease progresses, the development of plasma cell leukaemia (PCL) is characterized by increasing genetic instability of the MM cell associated with a high frequency of chromosomal abnormalities including RAS, p53 and c-*myc* mutations. This is accompanied by a decreased expression of certain adhesion molecules, which facilitates tumor cell mobilization into the peripheral blood. The acquisition of other adhesion molecules on the MM cell surface leads to the metastasis of MM cells to sites outside the bone marrow and the development of extramedullary plasmacytoma.

Diagnosis and morphology

Major and minor diagnostic criteria have been identified. These include the presence of excess monotypic marrow plasma cells, monoclonal immunoglobulin in either the serum or urine, decreased normal immunoglobulin levels and lytic bone lesions. It must be distinguished from other disorders characterized by monoclonal gammopathies, both malignant and otherwise. These include monoclonal gammopathy of undetermined significance (MGUS), Waldenstrom's macroglobulinemia, non-Hodgkin's lymphoma, light chain amyloid, idiopathic cold agglutinin disease, essential cryoglobulinemia and heavy chain disease.

The morphology of plasma cells in MM varies from typical small, mature cells that appear normal to larger cells with immature nuclei containing prominent clear nucleoli, little or no perinuclear clear area (hof) and a rim of basophilic cytoplasm. In between these extremes are medium-sized cells, often characterized by an eccentric nucleus with one or several small nucleoli, a diffuse chromatin pattern, perinuclear hof and a variable amount of blue cytoplasm. On biopsy normal bone marrow architecture is lost and the plasma cells are found as single cells or small clusters between adipocytes. As the disease progresses, diffuse marrow replacement occurs, resulting in a packed marrow.

The diagnosis of MM can be confirmed by immunoperoxidase staining that demonstrates the presence of monoclonal cytoplasmic staining light chains (κ or λ) or monoclonal heavy chains (IgG, IgA or IgD). As plasma cells are terminally differentiated B-cells, they express a number of B-cell antigens as well as myeloma-associated antigens including CD38, CD138 (syndecan-1), Muc-1 and PCA-1. They lack CD10, CD20, CD23, CD34 and CD45RO.

Staging of multiple myeloma

The Durie–Salmon staging system reliably separates patients into prognostic groups using simple laboratory measurements. In addition to a full physical examination, a complete blood count with blood smear and blood chemistries, including renal studies, is required. Serum electrophoresis with quantification of protein, as well as a 24-hour urine electrophoresis and quantification of Bence-Jones protein (light chains), should also be performed. Bone marrow aspirate and biopsy are indicated. An estimation of the extent of bone disease using a skeletal bone survey is advisable, although in many centers this has now been superceded by magnetic resonance imaging.

Clinical manifestations

The clinical picture of MM involves a combination of bone destruction leading to pain or fracture with hypercalcemia; infection due to immune deficiency; bone marrow failure leading to anemia and, less commonly, thrombocytopenia; and renal failure due to hypercalcemia, direct damage from paraprotein or precipitation of light chain in renal tubules. A hyperviscosity syndrome may occur in some patients and neurological complications such as spinal cord compression and peripheral neuropathy may be seen.

A number of studies have evaluated various parameters for prognostic significance. β2-microglobulin (β2 m), a polypeptide that forms the extracellular portion of the light chain of the class I histocompatibility complex, is the single most important variable. Levels correlate with a high tumor burden and decreasing renal function. The extent and type of bone marrow infiltration are also important: patients with a plasmablastic morphology have a much shorter median survival compared to patients with other morphological subtypes. Measures of tumor cell proliferation, such as the plasma cell labeling index (PCLI), are also useful; a high PCLI correlates with a shorter survival time independent of tumor cell mass. The presence of certain cytogenetic abnormalities also has prognostic significance: patients with partial or complete deletions of chromosome 13 or abnormalities of 11 q have an adverse outcome.

Therapy

Current therapy includes the use of conventional low-dose chemotherapy or high-dose chemotherapy with autologous or allogeneic stem cell transplantation. Although these regimens are able to reduce tumor burden, complete molecular remission of disease is rare and all patients eventually relapse. Novel pharmacological (e.g. thalidomide and proteasome inhibitors) and immunological-based treatment approaches (e.g. vaccination, antibody therapy) are currently being evaluated which will be used, either alone or in combination with conventional and high-dose chemotherapy, to improve response and outcome.

PLASMA CELL LEUKEMIA

Plasma cell leukemia (PCL) is characterized by the presence of more than 2×10^9/l plasma cells within the peripheral blood, which constitutes 20% of all circulating cells. The majority (60%) of cases are *de novo* or primary, in which a leukemic picture develops in the absence of documented preceding myeloma, whereas 40% of cases are secondary and occur in 1% of myeloma patients with advanced myeloma that is refractory to treatment. The symptoms of primary disease are similar to myeloma, although the disease course is often more aggressive with symptoms relating to extramedullary disease (plasmacytomas and hepatosplenomegaly) and bone marrow failure (anemia, infections and bleeding).

MONOCLONAL GAMMOPATHY OF UNDETERMINED SIGNIFICANCE

Monoclonal gammopathy of undetermined significance (MGUS) describes a condition characterized by the presence of a low level of paraprotein in the absence of other clinical features of multiple myeloma, Waldenstrom's macroglobulinemia or other B-cell lymphoproliferative disorders. The incidence of MGUS increases with age, with 1% of the population under the age of 60 years and between 4–5% of the population over the age of 80 years being affected. The previous term 'benign monoclonal gammopathy' is a misleading description of the disease, since approximately 25% of patients will go on to develop an overt plasma cell disorder.

WALDENSTROM'S MACROGLOBULINEMIA

Waldenstrom's macroglobulinemia (WM) is a chronic B-cell lymphoproliferative disorder in which most of the clinical manifestations are due to the presence of a high level of serum IgM paraprotein. It is predominantly a disease of the elderly, with a median age at presentation of 65 years and remains incurable with a median survival of 5 years. The disorder is characterized by bone marrow infiltration with small lymphocytes, plasma cells and characteristic lymphoplasmacytoid cells, which have the nucleus of a lymphocyte and cytoplasm of a plasma cell. The immunophenotype of WM cells is between that of well-differentiated small lymphocytes and plasma cells, as cells express monoclonal surface and cytoplasmic IgM pan-B cell markers CD19, 20 and 22 and late B-cell differentiation markers such as CD38 and FMC7 but lack CD5, 10 and 23. Most patients develop symptoms due to tumor cell infiltration of bone marrow resulting in anemia, increased infections and bleeding. Splenomegaly, hepatomegaly and lymphadenopathy are common. Many patients present with hyperviscosity syndrome accompanied by headache, confusion and blurred vision. Cryoglobulinemia, cold agglutinin disease and neurological manifestations may also occur. In contrast to other plasma cell disorders, there is an absence of bony changes and lytic lesions.

LIGHT CHAIN-ASSOCIATED AMYLOIDOSIS

Light chain amyloid, previously called primary amyloid, is characterized by the extracellular deposition of fibrillar protein derived from monoclonal light chains. The fragments form β-pleated sheets which become insoluble and resistant to degradation following the deposition of glycosaminoglycans and the normal protein serum amyloid P component (SAP). The clinical features depend on the spectrum of organ involvement, with the most commonly affected organs being the heart, kidneys and peripheral nerves. Other features include macroglossia (infrequent but pathognomonic), GI malabsorption, hepatosplenomegaly and skin involvement including papular and nodular lesions and characteristic purpura around the eyes. A monoclonal component is usually present in the serum or urine, although immunofixation is often required to demonstrate its presence as the peak may be small. Amyloid may occur as a long-term complication of most clonal B-cell disorders, especially myeloma and, less commonly, Waldenstrom's macroglobulinemia.

HEAVY CHAIN DISORDERS

This group of rare plasma cell disorders is characterized by the production of a monoclonal immunoglobulin that is formed from truncated heavy chains with no associated light chains. α-Heavy chain disease, a subtype of immunoproliferative small intestine disease (IPSID), is diagnosed by the identification of monoclonal immunoglobulin α-heavy chain fragments in the plasma or urine. The pathologic process consists of a lymphoma-like proliferation of lymphoid cells and plasma cells in the lamina propria of the small intestine and in mesenteric nodes accompanied by diarrhea and malabsorption. Occasionally the disease may present with respiratory symptoms due to infiltrations in the respiratory tract. It was previously referred to as Mediterranean abdominal lymphoma but it may also be identified in patients of non-Mediterranean ancestry.

Table 15.1 Diseases associated with the production of paraprotein

Stable production	Uncontrolled production
MGUS	MGUS
Idiopathic cold agglutinin disease	Smoldering myeloma
Essential cryoglobulinemia	Multiple myeloma
Transient M-proteins	Light chain amyloidosis
Occasionally metastatic carcinoma, connective tissue disorders and skin disorders	Waldenstrom's macroglobulinemia
	Heavy chain disease
	Non-Hodgkin's lymphoma

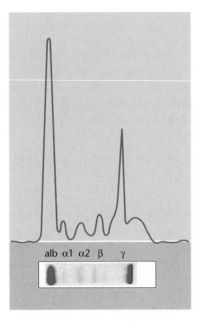

alb α1 α2 β γ

Fig. 15.1 Benign monoclonal gammopathy. Serum protein electrophoresis shows M-protein in the γ region. Unlike the pattern in multiple myeloma, there is no reduction in the background normal β and γ globulins. In about 25% of cases, multiple myeloma or a lymphoproliferative disorder will develop within 10 years. For the remaining 75%, no significant illness may become apparent within that time interval.

Fig. 15.2 Diagnostic criteria for multiple myeloma.

Criteria for the diagnosis of multiple myeloma

Major criteria

1. Plasmaytoma on tissue biopsy
2. Bone marrow plasmacytosis (>30% plasma cells)
3. Monoclonal immunoglobulin spike on serum electrophoresis
IgG>3.5g/dl or Iga>2.0g/dl; K or l light chaine excretion >1.0g/day on 24-hour urine electrophoresis

Minor criteria

a. Bone marrow plasmacytosis (10-30% plasma cells)
b. Monoclonal immunoglobulin spike present but of lesser magnitude than above
c. Lytic bone lesions
d. Normal IgM<50mg/dl, IgA<100mg/dl or IgG<600mg/dl

Any of the following criteria will confirm the diagnosis:
Any two major criteria
Major criteria 1 plus minor criteria b, c or d
Major criteria 3 plus minor criteria a or c
Minor criteria a, b and c or a, b and d

Fig. 15.3 Staging system for multiple myeloma. (Modified from Durie and Salmon, 1985.)

537

	Criteria	Measured myeloma cell mass (cells × 10^{12}/m²)

Stage I	All of the following:
	
	1. Hemoglobin value > 10 g/100 mL
	2. Serum calcium value normal (< 12 mg/100 mL)
	3. On radiograph, normal bone structure (scale 0) or solitary bone plasmacytoma only
	4. Low M-component production rates
	   A. IgG value < 5 g/100 mL
	   B. IgA value < 3 g/100 mL
	   C. Urine light chain M-component on electrophoresis < 4 g/24 h
		<0.6 (low)

Stage II	Fitting neither stage I nor stage III	0.6–1.20 (intermediate)

Stage III	One or more of the following:
	
	1. Hemoglobin value < 8.5 g/100 mL
	2. Serum calcium value > 12 mg/100 mL
	3. Advanced lytic bone lesions (scale 3)
	4. High M-component production rates
	   A. IgG value > 7 g/mL
	   B. IgA value > 5g/mL
	   C. Urine light chain M-component on electrophoresis > 12 g/24
		> 1.20 (high)

Subclassifications
A = relatively normal renal function (serum creatinine value < 2.0 mg/100 mL)
B = abnormal renal function (serum creatinine value ≥ 2.0 mg/100 mL)

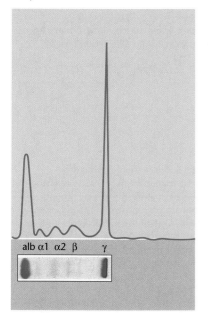

Fig. 15.4 Multiple myeloma. Serum protein electrophoresis demonstrates an M-protein in the γ globulin region and a reduced level of background γ globulin. This 'spike' and deficiency pattern is typical of patients with myeloma.

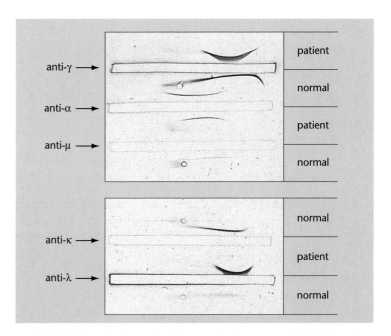

Fig. 15.5 Multiple myeloma (IgG-λ type). Normal protein is recognized by characteristic arc patterns on immunoelectrophoresis. In the reactions against anti-γ and anti-λ, the IgG-λ M-protein maintains its electrophoretic position but appears as a 'bow' or thickened arc with a smaller than usual radius. Reduced levels of IgA and IgM are reflected in small or absent arcs in the reactions with anti-α and anti-μ.

Table 15.2 Frequency of M-protein types in multiple myeloma.

Types	Frequency (%)
IgG	52
IgA	22
κ only	9
λ only	7
IgD	2
Biclonal	1
IgM	0.5
Negative	6.5

IgM rarely occurs since it usually indicates Waldenstrom's monoglobulinemia. Light chain disease is defined by circulating light chains only with Bence-Jones proteinuria and hypogammaglobulinemia. As the result of imbalanced immunoglobulin production, most patients with an 'M' component also have monoclonal light chains that vary from barely detectable levels to grams per day. (Data from 984 patients with multiple myeloma at the Mayo Clinic, 1982–1994.)

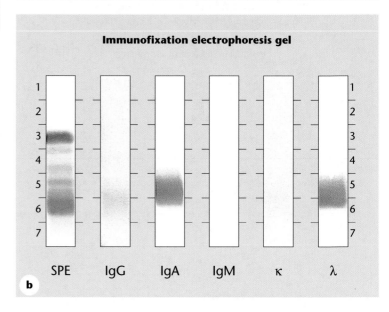

Serum protein electrophoresis

	Percentage	Normal range
Albumin	32.3	56.4–71.6
α_1	3.6	1.9–4.5
α_2	5.3	7.3–15.0
β	6.8	6.2–11.5
γ	52.0	7.8–18.2

Quantitative immunoglobulin

	mg/dL	Normal range
IgG	275	600–1450
IgA	2964	60–340
IgM	10.4	25–200

a

Immunofixation electrophoresis gel

SPE   IgG   IgA   IgM   κ   λ

b

Fig. 15.6 Multiple myeloma (IgA-λ type). Immunoelectropherogram shows an excess of γ globulin, which is overwhelmingly IgA-λ. SPE, serum protein electrophoresis.

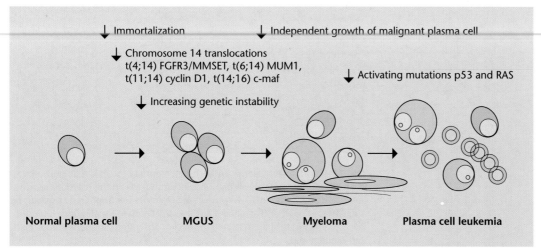

↓ Immortalization   ↓ Independent growth of malignant plasma cell

↓ Chromosome 14 translocations
t(4;14) FGFR3/MMSET, t(6;14) MUM1,
t(11;14) cyclin D1, t(14;16) c-maf   ↓ Activating mutations p53 and RAS

↓ Increasing genetic instability

Normal plasma cell   MGUS   Myeloma   Plasma cell leukemia

Fig. 15.7 It is thought that the transformation from MGUS to MM and PCL occurs in an orderly fashion, although not all stages are present within the individual patient. One of the initial events involves the translocation of chromosome 14q32 with oncogene dysregulation during immunoglobulin class switching. This results in genetic instability and later independent cell growth. A high frequency of chromosomal abnormalities including RAS, p53 and c-*myc* mutations characterizes plasma cell leukaemia.

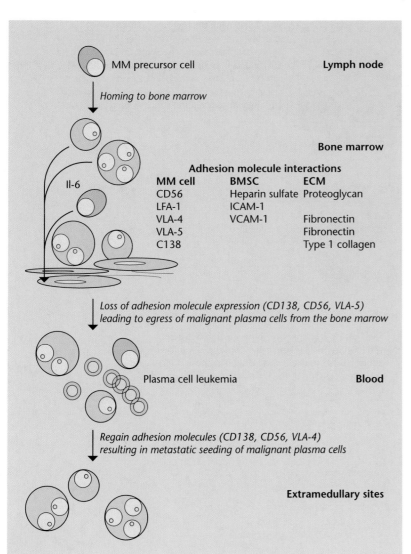

MM precursor cell   **Lymph node**

Homing to bone marrow

                                                                Bone marrow

Il-6

Adhesion molecule interactions

MM cell	BMSC	ECM
CD56	Heparin sulfate	Proteoglycan
LFA-1	ICAM-1	
VLA-4	VCAM-1	Fibronectin
VLA-5		Fibronectin
C138		Type 1 collagen

Loss of adhesion molecule expression (CD138, CD56, VLA-5) leading to egress of malignant plasma cells from the bone marrow

Plasma cell leukemia   **Blood**

Regain adhesion molecules (CD138, CD56, VLA-4) resulting in metastatic seeding of malignant plasma cells

                                                                Extramedullary sites

Fig. 15.8 Adhesion molecules mediate the homing of MM cells from the lymph node to the bone marrow (BM), where binding of MM cells to bone marrow stromal cells (BMSC) occurs. As disease progresses, there is a decreased expression of some adhesion molecules, which facilitates tumor cells mobilization into the peripheral blood. The acquisition of other adhesion molecules on the MM cell surface leads to the metastasis of MM cells to sites outside the bone marrow.

Table 15.3 Criteria for the diagnosis of MGUS, smoldering myeloma and multiple myeloma

	MGUS	Smoldering myeloma	Multiple myeloma
M component	<30g/l	>30g/l	>30g/l
% BM plasma cells	<10%	>10% <30%	>30%
Symptoms	Nil	Nil	Yes
Bone lesions	Nil	Nil	Present
Anemia, hypercalcemia or renal impairment	Nil	Nil	Present
Followup	Stable	Stable initially, once progressed similar to MM	Median survival 3.5 years

Table 15.4 Cytokines involved in multiple myeloma disease biology

Cytokine	Role
Interleukin-6	Proliferation and survival of MM cells
Vascular endothelial growth factor	Proliferation and migration of MM cells; angiogenesis
Tumor necrosis factor-α	Upregulation of adhesion molecules on MM cell surface; osteoclast activation
Transforming growth factor-β	Increased IL-6 secretion by bone marrow stromal cells; inhibition of T-cell proliferation
Insulin-like growth factor	Proliferation and survival of MM cells
Interleukin-1β	Osteoclast activation; induction of IL-6 secretion by osteoblasts; increased expression of adhesion molecules on MM cell surface
Lymphotoxin	Osteoclast activation
TRANCE/RANKL	Differentiation and maturation of osteoclast progenitors
Interleukin-11	Stimulation of osteoclastogenesis and inhibition bone formation.
Hepatocyte growth factor	Induction of IL-11 secretion by osteoblasts

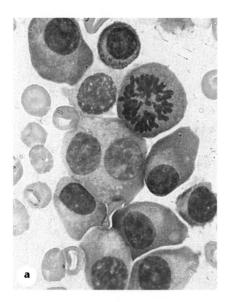
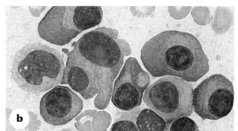
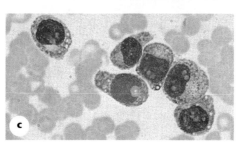
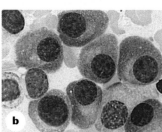

Fig. 15.9 Multiple myeloma. These bone marrow aspirates demonstrate the morphology of abnormal plasma cells (**a**) Some myeloma cells are binuclear, with nucleoli; one mitotic figure can be seen. (**b**) The nuclei of a single binucleate cell vary greatly in size. (**c**) Abnormal cytoplasmic and nuclear vacuolation can also be encountered.

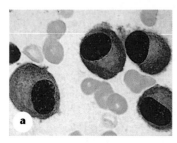
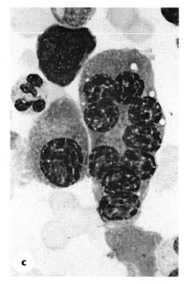

Fig. 15.10 Multiple myeloma. (**a,b**) Considerable variation in nuclear size and cytoplasmic volume of abnormal plasma cells can be seen in these bone marrow aspirates. (**c**) One of the myeloma cells is multinucleate.

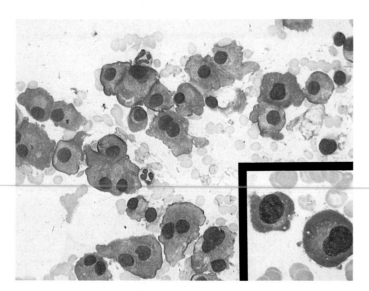
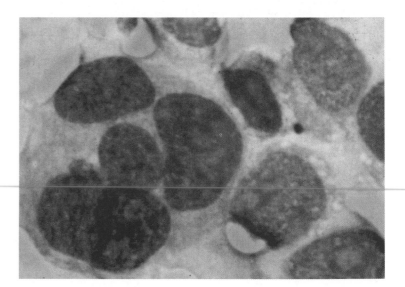

Fig. 15.11 Multiple myeloma. Numerous thesaurocytes – large plasma cells with small, sometimes pyknotic, nuclei and expanded fibrillary cytoplasm that also shows 'flaming' of the cell rim (inset) – are evident in this bone marrow aspirate. Although 'flaming cells' occur most frequently with IgA production, they may also be seen with M-protein of other classes. The red color results from the high carbohydrate content of IgA protein.

Fig. 15.12 Bone marrow aspirate from a patient with rapidly progressive disease shows large bizarre multinucleate plasmablasts. Plasmablasts have a fine reticular chromatin pattern, large nucleoli and less abundant cytoplasm (less than half of the nuclear area). This morphological subset is associated with a high PCLI, more advanced and aggressive disease and a worse prognosis. Histologically it may be mistaken for metastatic carcinoma or large cell lymphoma; however, immunophenotyping is diagnostic for a monoclonal population of malignant plasma cells. It was formerly called 'anaplastic' myeloma.

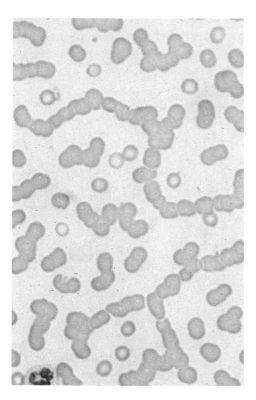

Fig. 15.13 Multiple myeloma. Peripheral blood film demonstrates marked rouleaux formation of red cells and increased background staining due to the high protein level.

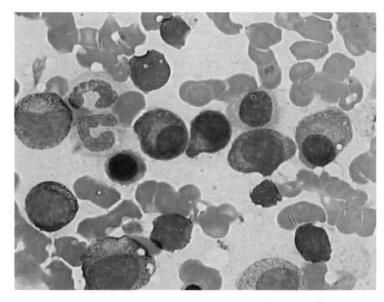

Fig. 15.14 The peripheral blood is characterized by the presence of a large number of circulating plasma cells, which may be morphologically normal or have blastic features. Anemia is invariably present and both neutropenia and thrombocytopenia are common. Rouleaux formation is usually also present with a high non-specific background staining, especially in secondary PCL cases where the level of paraprotein is often high. (From Wickramasinghe & McCullough, Blood and Bone Marrow Pathology. © 2003 Churchill Livingstone.)

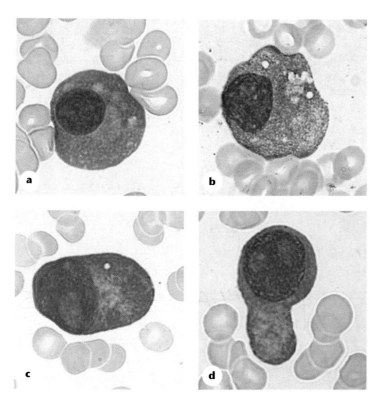

Fig. 15.15 Multiple myeloma. (**a–d**) Isolated myeloma cells are visible in peripheral blood smears from two patients. Plasma cell leukemia is rare, occurring in 2–5% of patients. It may be the presenting feature or may occur as a terminal event. Most cases exhibit rapidly progressive disease, with prominent bone symptoms, marked anemia, azotemia and infiltration of organs and tissues.

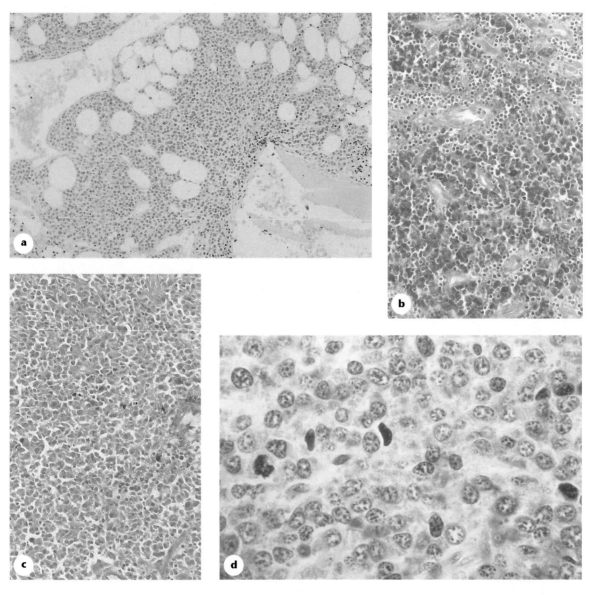

Fig. 15.16 Multiple myeloma. (a) Low-power view of a bone marrow core biopsy specimen shows diffuse replacement of marrow by a monoclonal population of plasma cells. Plasma cells stain positive for anti-κ light chain (b) but not anti-λ light chain (c) with the immunoperoxidase technique. (d) At high power, plasma cells are characterized by clumped 'clock-face' chromatin, eccentric nuclei and perinuclear hof (halo).

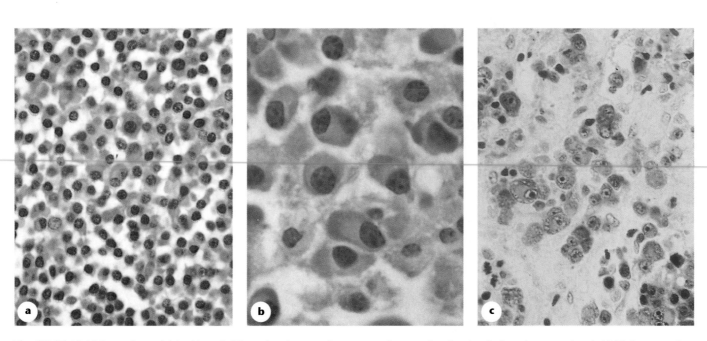

Fig. 15.17 Multiple myeloma. (a) In this well-differentiated tumor, the deposits consist of plasma cells. (b) At higher power, the typically eccentric nuclei, relatively large areas of basophilic or amphophilic cytoplasm, and perinuclear hof can be appreciated. (c) High-power view of a poorly differentiated myeloma tumor containing plasma cells with prominent nucleoli and multinucleate cells.

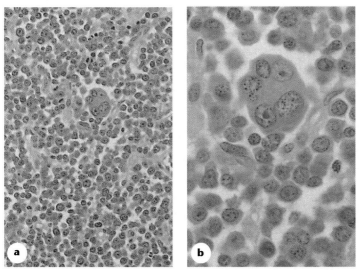
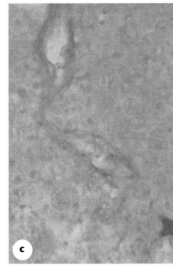
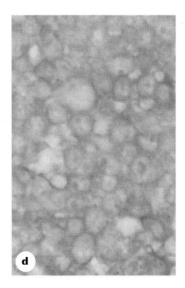

Fig. 15.18 Extramedullary plasmacytoma. (**a**) This anterior chest wall lesion exhibits scant, delicate connective tissue stroma and a relatively monomorphous population of cells, unlike the findings in plasma cell granuloma. (**b**) Plasma cells have eccentric nuclei with a 'clock-face' chromatin pattern and amphophilic cytoplasm. This tumor contains many immature forms and occasional multinucleate cells. (**c,d**) Demonstration of a single light chain class by immunoperoxidase staining confirms the presence of a monoclonal (neoplastic) population of plasma cells (**c**: κ negative; **d**: λ positive). (Courtesy of S. Swerdlow MD, Cincinnati, OH.)

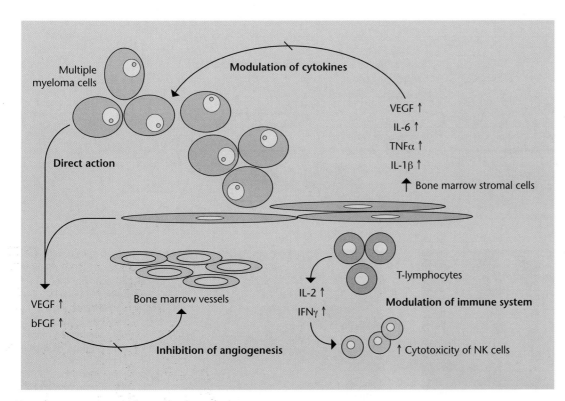

Fig. 15.19 Although the exact mechanism of action of thalidomide in myeloma is unclear, it can be postulated that its pharmacological effects may be mediated via a number of pathways involving both the tumor cell and the bone marrow microenvironment: (**a**) a direct effect on tumor or bone marrow stromal cells, (**b**) an alteration in the adhesion profile between myeloma and bone marrow stromal cells, (**c**) an inhibition of cytokine release from bone marrow stromal cells, (**d**) an antiangiogenic effect, or (**e**) an immunomodulatory effect.

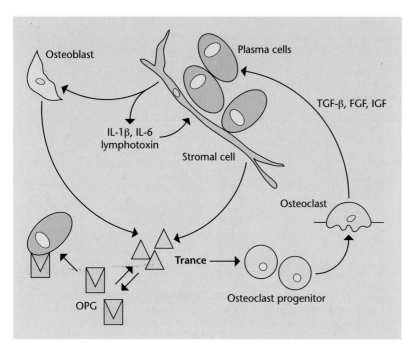

Fig. 15.20 There is an uncoupling of normal bone remodeling with increased bone resorption and decreased bone formation. When MM cells bind to bone marrow stroma cytokines are produced which stimulate bone marrow stromal cells and osteoblasts to produce TRANCE, which leads to the differentiation and maturation of osteoclast progenitors. Osteoprotegerin (OPG) directly regulates osteoclast activity by acting as an alternative receptor for TRANCE. However, syndecan produced by MM cells traps OPG, leading to an excess of TRANCE. The increased osteoclast activity results in bone resorption and secretion of cytokines, further stimulating MM cell growth.

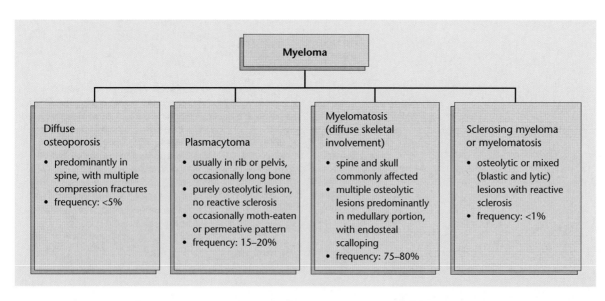

Fig. 15.21 Variants in the radiographic presentation of myeloma.

Diffuse osteoporosis
- predominantly in spine, with multiple compression fractures
- frequency: <5%

Plasmacytoma
- usually in rib or pelvis, occasionally long bone
- purely osteolytic lesion, no reactive sclerosis
- occasionally moth-eaten or permeative pattern
- frequency: 15–20%

Myelomatosis (diffuse skeletal involvement)
- spine and skull commonly affected
- multiple osteolytic lesions predominantly in medullary portion, with endosteal scalloping
- frequency: 75–80%

Sclerosing myeloma or myelomatosis
- osteolytic or mixed (blastic and lytic) lesions with reactive sclerosis
- frequency: <1%

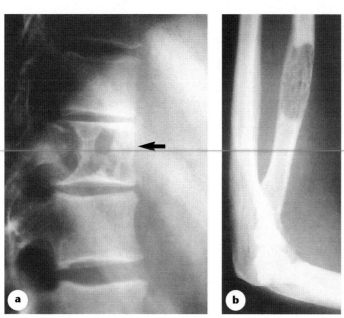

Fig. 15.22 Multiple myeloma. (**a**) Plain film of the thoracic spine shows multiple radiolucencies in the body of T12 (arrow). (**b**) In another patient, a deposit of myeloma is apparent in the midshaft of the radius.

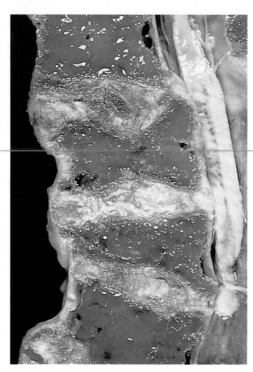

Fig. 15.23 Multiple myeloma. This segment of the lower thoracic spine has been sectioned to show extensive replacement of the bone and marrow by gelatinous red tissue. The resultant osteoporosis has caused multiple compression fractures. (Courtesy of Howard Dorfman MD.)

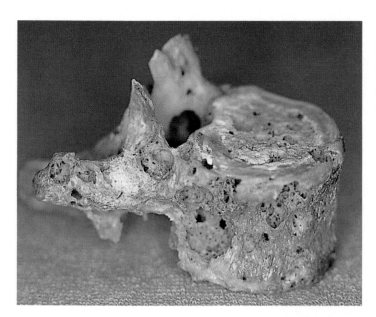

Fig. 15.24 Multiple myeloma. A macerated vertebral body exhibits many destructive round defects throughout the bone. (Specimen from the collection of the Smithsonian Institute; courtesy of Dr Donald J. Ortner.)

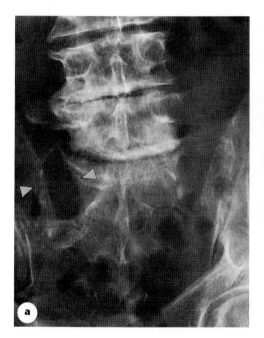

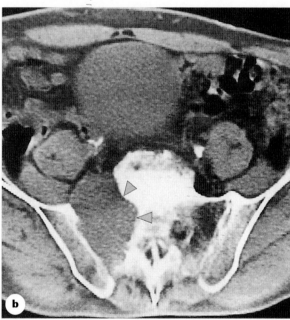

Fig. 15.25 Plasmacytoma. (**a**) Anteroposterior view of the lumbosacral spine in a 68-year-old man who presented with lower back pain shows a large lytic lesion (arrows) in the right side of the sacrum adjacent to the sacroiliac joint. (**b**) CT scan demonstrates an adjacent soft tissue mass (arrows). On the basis of these findings, a solitary plasmacytoma, a metastatic lesion, malignant fibrous histiocytoma and fibrosarcoma were considered in the differential diagnosis. A fluoroscopy-guided biopsy yielded the diagnosis.

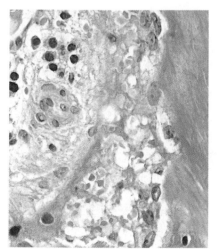

Fig. 15.26 Multiple myeloma. Although plasma cells are seen in the upper left of this bone biopsy specimen, osteoclasts (the multinucleate cells at the bone–intertrabecular tissue interface) are the cells responsible for the bone absorption around the osteolytic lesion.

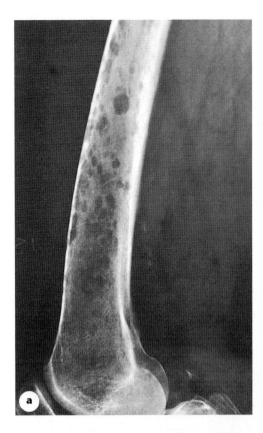
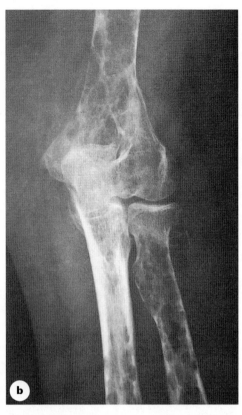

Fig. 15.27 Multiple myeloma. (**a**) Lateral radiograph of the distal femur shows numerous classic punched-out lytic lesions. (**b**) Plain film of the elbow in a 65-year-old woman demonstrates endosteal scalloping of the cortex, typical of diffuse myelomatosis.

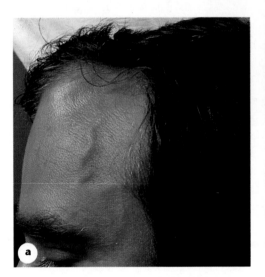
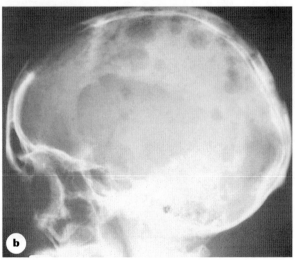

Fig. 15.28 Multiple myeloma. (**a**) A 35-year-old man developed multiple osseous lesions; in this instance, a plasmacytoma involves the forehead. (**b**) Skull radiograph reveals other osteolytic areas in addition to the large frontal lesion. Bone marrow aspirations were normal. A small amount of Bence-Jones protein was detected in concentrated urine by immunoelectrophoresis.

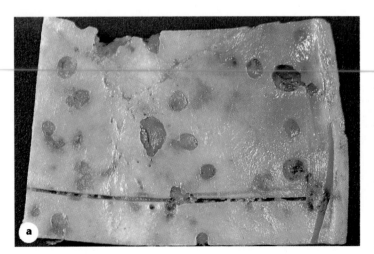
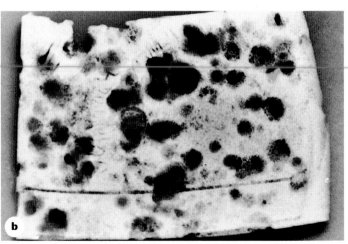

Fig. 15.29 Multiple myeloma. (**a**) A portion of the skull removed from a patient with multiple myeloma shows many round defects filled with pinkish-gray tissue. (**b**) Specimen radiograph of the portion of skull demonstrates the clearly demarcated lytic lesions.

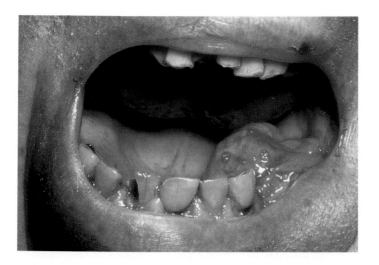

Fig. 15.30 Plasmacytoma. This 60-year-old man with IgD multiple myeloma presented with a lesion of the lower mandible, with soft tissue extension into the floor of the mouth. He also had severe anemia and uremia.

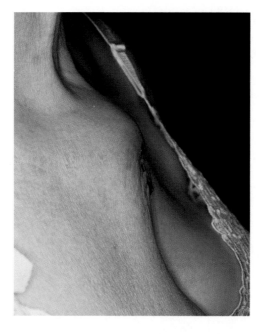

Fig. 15.31 Plasmacytoma. This 78-year-old woman presented with a painful slowly enlarging mass protruding from her upper sternum.

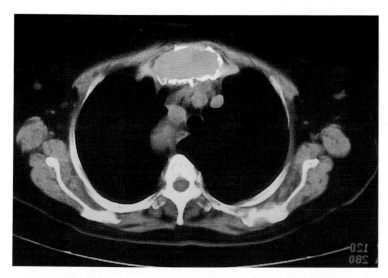

Fig. 15.32 CT scan shows a destructive, expansile mass of the manubrium. Biopsy was diagnostic of a plasmacytoma composed of monoclonal IgG$_K$ plasma cells. Of note, iliac crest bone marrow biopsy showed 5% involvement by IgG$_L$ plasma cells.

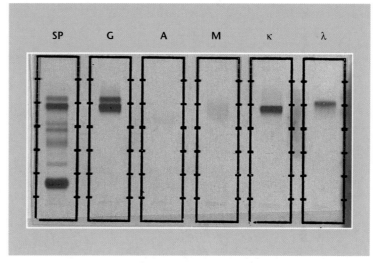

Fig. 15.33 Serum protein electrophoresis demonstrates a 'biclonal gammopathy' with two IgG 'M' components in the γ globulin region. Biclonal gammopathies are unusual, seen in only about 1% of cases of multiple myeloma. Of note, 6 months later, the patient's 42-year-old son presented with a pathologic lumbar spine fracture and was found to have stage IIIB myeloma. Familial multiple myeloma is not common, but is occasionally reported.

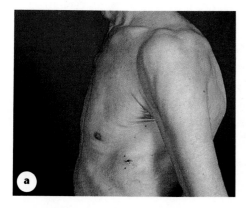
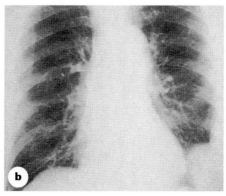
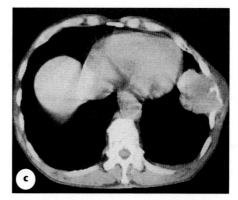

Fig. 15.34 Solitary osseous plasmacytoma. (**a**) A firm, ovoid mass, measuring 9 cm in diameter, is visible over the lower lateral aspect of the left chest wall. Protein studies, CBC and bone marrow were normal. No other skeletal lesions were detected. (**b**) Chest film shows a well-defined mass, approximately 5 cm in diameter, in the lower left chest; the mass is pleural in position and arises from the ninth rib. (**c**) On CT scan, erosion of the rib is apparent, together with a soft tissue mass extending both into the pleural space and outward.

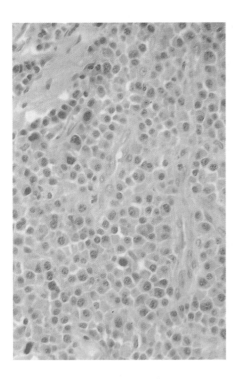

Fig. 15.35 Solitary osseous plasmacytoma. Bone biopsy specimen reveals dense collections of plasma cells supported by a vascular stroma.

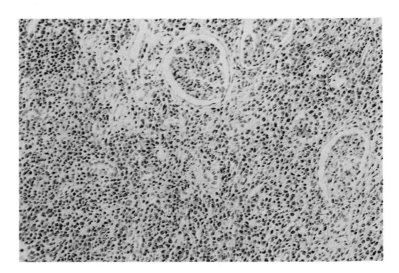

Fig. 15.36 Multiple myeloma (renal involvement). Photomicrograph of renal tissue from a patient who died from advanced multiple myeloma shows replacement of the majority of the stroma by tumor cells; several glomeruli and tubules are spared. Both kidneys were diffusely infiltrated by plasma cells, which led to renal failure.

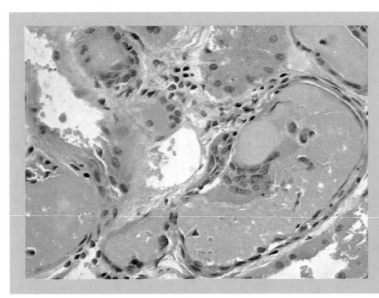

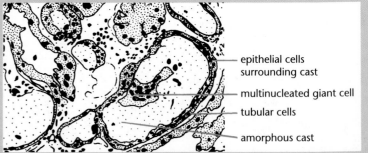

- epithelial cells surrounding cast
- multinucleated giant cell
- tubular cells
- amorphous cast

Fig. 15.37 Multiple myeloma (renal involvement). Histologic section of kidney shows a cast lined by epithelial cells within a dilated renal tubule. There is also a giant cell reaction to the proteinaceous material within the cast. 'Myeloma kidney' refers to a variety of findings, like those shown here, including tubular atrophy and the presence of chronic inflammatory cells. The tubular, often laminated proteinaceous material consists of Bence-Jones protein, albumin and often fibrinogen.

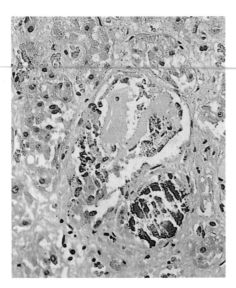

Fig. 15.38 Multiple myeloma (nephrocalcinosis). Irregular fractured hematoxylinophilic deposits of calcium are seen in this fibrotic renal tissue.

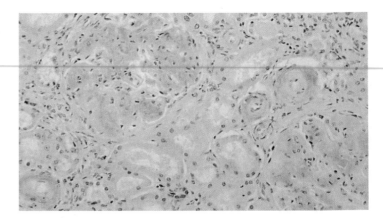

Fig. 15.39 Multiple myeloma (renal amyloid disease). Microscopic section of renal tissue reveals extensive amyloid deposition in the glomeruli and associated arterioles.

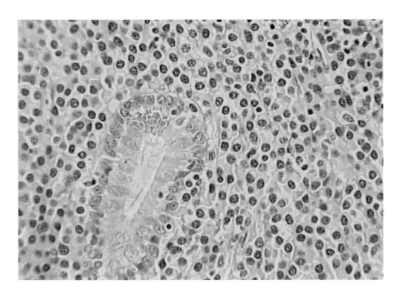

Fig. 15.40 Plasma cells are deposited throughout the gut in this unusual presentation of IgA extrameduallary disease. (From Wickramasinghe & McCullough, Blood and Bone Marrow Pathology. © 2003 ChurchillLivingstone.)

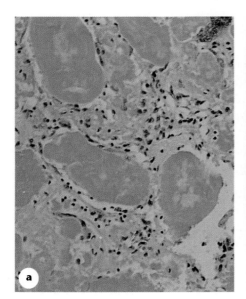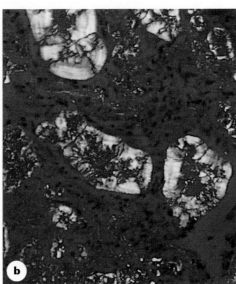

Fig. 15.41 Amyloid. (**a**) Exceptionally large amounts of amyloid are evident in this microscopic section as homogeneous masses staining positive with Congo red. (**b**) Under polarized light, these areas show brilliant apple-green birefringence. Amyloidosis is a well-recognized complication in about 20% of cases of multiple myeloma, in which circumstance the characteristic β-pleated sheets of fibrillary protein are composed of abnormal immunoglobulin light chains. Most often there is diffuse deposition in the kidneys, heart, vessels, skin and gastrointestinal tract. Nodular, tumor-like deposition, as seen here, is extremely unusual.

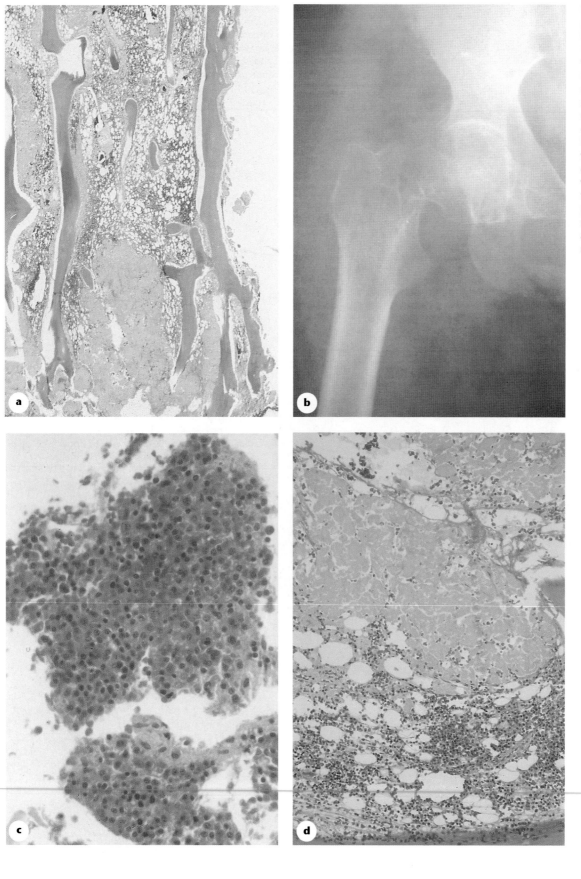

Fig. 15.42 Amyloid. (**a**) Low-power photomicrograph of a bone marrow biopsy from a patient with multiple myeloma involving bone marrow as well as extensive deposits of myeloma-associated amyloid within marrow, and also involving the joint space and surrounding soft tissue. (**b**) Hip film revealing the presence of a pathologic fracture of the right hip and lytic lesions within the femur, as well as radiolucent deposits consistent with amyloid within the joint and surrounding soft tissue. (**c**) Homogeneous nodule of plasma cells within the bone marrow. (**d**) Amorphous eosinophilic amyloid deposit within bone marrow.

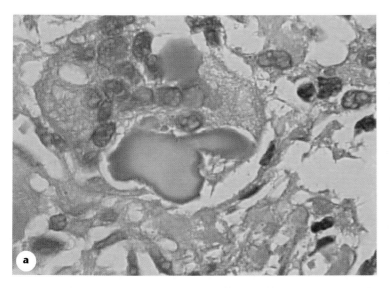

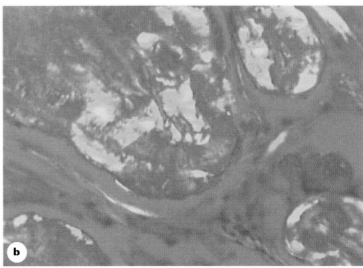

Fig. 15.43 An unusual presentation of light chain amyloid within the postnasal space. (**a**) On H&E staining there are scattered plasma cells.

(**b**) Fibrils stain apple green under polarized light. (From Wickramasinghe & McCullough, Blood and Bone Marrow Pathology. © 2003 Churchill Livingstone.)

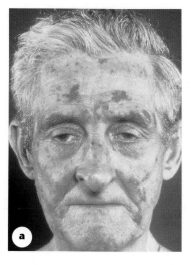

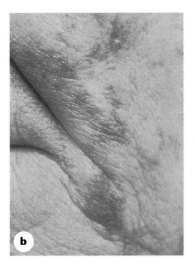

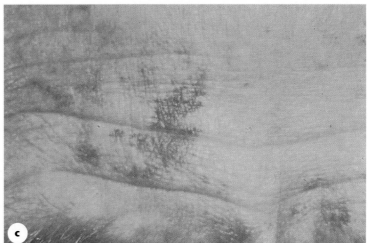

Fig. 15.44 Amyloid skin deposits. (**a–c**) The purpuric skin lesions visible on the face of this man can be ascribed to the deposition of amyloid in cutaneous blood vessels.

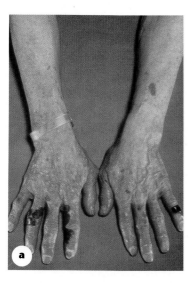

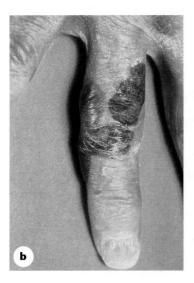

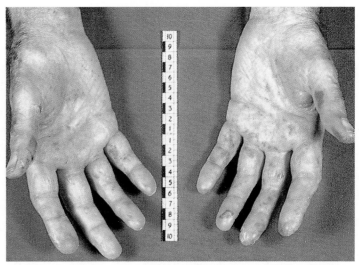

Fig. 15.45 Amyloid skin deposits. Large purpuric lesions have developed on the hands and fingers, exacerbated by minimal friction and pressure.

Fig. 15.46 Amyloid skin deposits. Purpuric skin lesions with characteristic smooth, yellowish deposits can be seen in this patient with multiple myeloma. The skin is hard, dense and waxy.

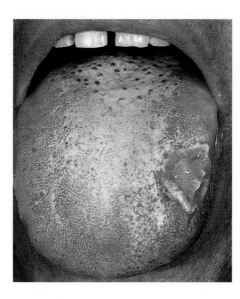

Fig. 15.47 Amyloid. The tongue exhibits macroglossia and a deep ulcer on the upper and anterolateral surfaces. The floor of the ulcer has the waxy appearance typical of amyloid deposition.

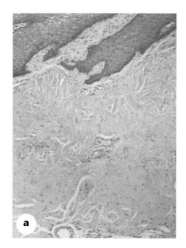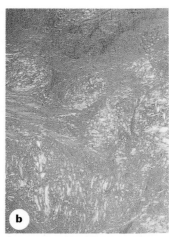

Fig. 15.48 Amyloid. (**a**) Photomicroscopic section of the ulcer seen in Figure 15.47 shows extensive deposition of pale-staining acidophilic material. (**b**) Stained with Congo red, this material shows the characteristic green birefringence of amyloid.

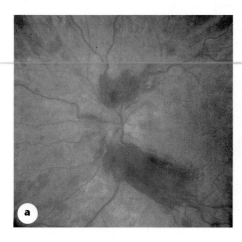

Fig. 15.49 Amyloid disease. These nodular deposits of amyloid contrast with the diffuse enlargement shown in Figure 15.47. Similar nodules are also evident on the lips. Changes in taste sensation may occur.

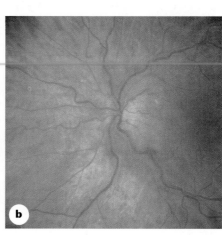

Fig. 15.50 Multiple myeloma (ecchymoses). Abnormal bleeding is noted in 10–20% of patients at presentation. Cutaneous hemorrhages and epistaxis are the most common bleeding manifestations. This patient had recurrent 'blood blisters' in the mouth, combined with periorbital hematomas and subconjunctival hemorrhages. The pathogenesis is complex but probably involves interference with platelet–capillary interaction and/or with clotting factors by the paraprotein. Uremia and thrombocytopenia may contribute.

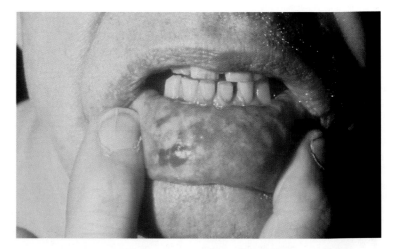

Fig. 15.51 Multiple myeloma (hyperviscosity syndrome). (**a**) Distension of retinal veins and widespread hemorrhage accompany the hyperviscosity syndrome. The patient presented with some loss of vision and headache. (**b**) Two months after plasmapheresis and chemotherapy, the vessels are normal and almost all hemorrhage has cleared. (Courtesy of Prof. J.C. Parr.)

Table 15.5 Causes of hyperviscosity syndrome

Causes	Diseases
M-proteins	Waldenström's macroglobulinemia
	Multiple myeloma
Polycythemia	Polycythemia vera
	Severe secondary polycythemia
Leukostasis	Chronic myelogenous leukemia
	Acute nonlymphocytic leukemias with white cell counts > 100 000/mm³
Hyperfibrinogenemia	Following factor VIII replacement therapy with large amounts of cryoprecipitate

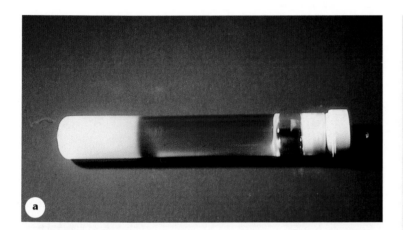

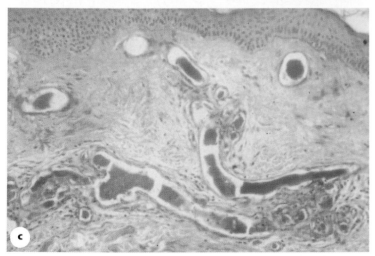

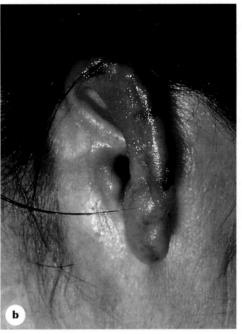

Fig. 15.52 Multiple myeloma (IgG cryoglobulinemia). This patient experienced severe pain in the extremities, face and ears on exposure to cold. (**a**) The concentration of cryoglobulin (6g/100ml) was vividly demonstrated by keeping the plasma in a refrigerator overnight, resulting in precipitation. (**b**) Crusted hemorrhagic lesions are present on the ears. (**c**) Skin biopsy reveals precipitation of cryoglobulin in small cutaneous vessels.

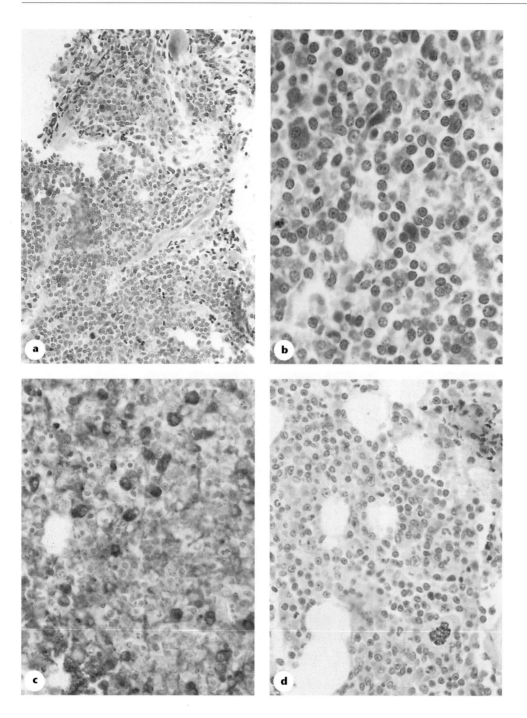

Fig. 15.53 Waldenström's macroglobulinemia. (**a**) Low-power photomicrograph of a bone marrow core biopsy specimen shows marked hypercellularity with loss of the normal 50 : 50 fat-to-cell ratio due to infiltration by tumor cells. (**b**) High magnification reveals lymphocytes, plasma, cells and lymphoplasmacytoid cells typical of Waldenström's macroglobulinemia. The presence of mast cells, with their distinctive granules that stain purple with Giemsa, is sometimes a helpful diagnostic feature because of their association with this disease. Immunoperoxidase studies reveal that the plasmacytoid cells are (**c**) strongly immunoreactive for IgM heavy chains but (**d**) negative for IgG. The cells were also positive for κ light chains but negative for λ light chains (not shown).

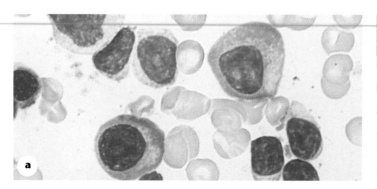
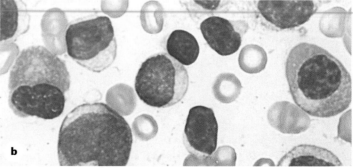

Fig. 15.54 Waldenstrom's macroglobulinemia. (**a,b**) Characteristically, the cells have features combining those of classic lymphocytes with those of plasma cells. For example, some cells have the nuclear appearance of a lymphocyte and the cytoplasmic features of a plasma cell. The chromatin patterns in the larger nuclei are more open and primitive.

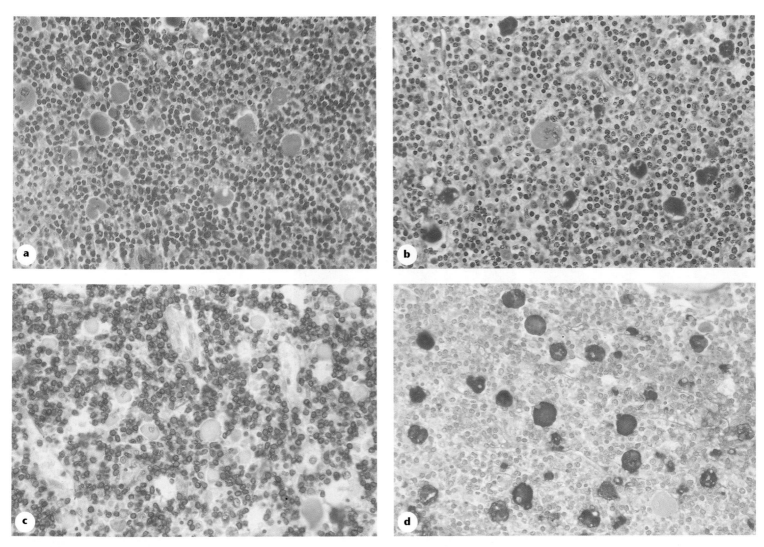

Fig. 15.55 Waldenstrom's macroglobulinemia. (**a**) Low-power photomicrograph of a bone marrow biopsy reveals a diffuse cellular infiltrate composed of small lymphocytes as well as lymphoplasmacytoid cells and plasma cells, many of which contain prominent intracytoplasmic immunoglobulin inclusions, which are PAS positive (**b**). The small lymphocytes are immunoreactive for B-cell marker CD74 (**c**) and immunoglobulin inclusions exhibit positive staining for IgM (**d**).

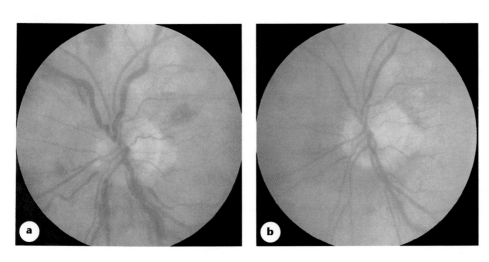

Fig. 15.56 Waldenstrom's macroglobulinemia (hyperviscosity syndrome). (**a**) The retina of a patient who presented with blurred vision, headache and dizziness exhibits gross distension of vessels, particularly the veins, which show bulging and constriction (the 'linked sausage' effect), as well as areas of hemorrhage. (**b**) After plasmapheresis, the vascular diameters are normal and the hemorrhagic areas have cleared.

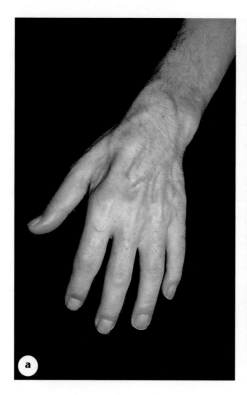

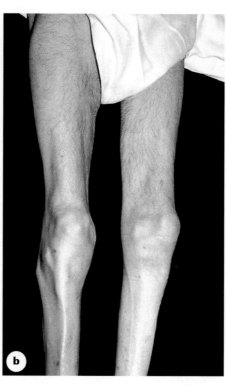

Fig. 15.57 Waldenstrom's macroglobulinemia (neuropathy). This 75-year-old man developed severe hand and leg weakness due to peripheral neuropathy. (**a**) Evaluation of the hand shows marked atrophy of the interosseous muscles. (**b**) The legs show marked muscle atrophy. These features are mainly the result of amyloid deposition in small vessels supplying nerves.

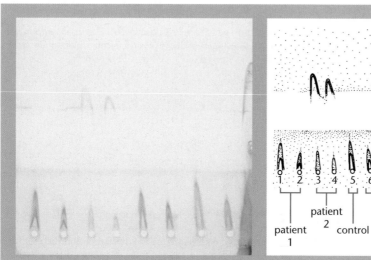

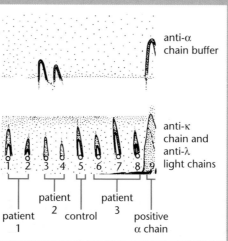

Fig. 15.58 α-Heavy chain disease. Gel electrophoresis results are shown for a case of α-chain disease (patient 2) with accompanying positive control (9). Patients 1 and 3 are negative. The numbered wells contain the sera to be tested. When they migrate across the plate under the influence of an electrophoretic current, the light chains are precipitated in the proximal one-third of their course by the anti-κ and anti-λ in the gel. Any serum containing heavy chains is precipitated in the distal third of the gel by anti-α chain. (Courtesy of Dr A. Howard.)

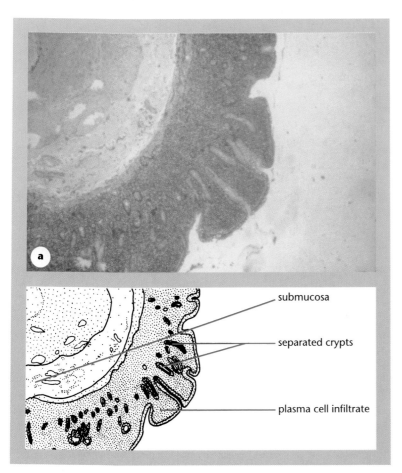

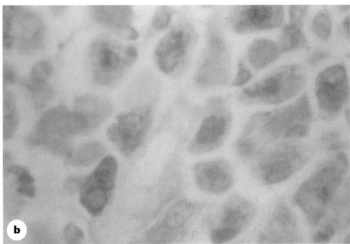

Fig. 15.59 α-heavy chain disease. (**a**) At the stage prior to a frank tumor, the mucosa of the small intestine is diffusely infiltrated by mature plasma cells that push the crypts apart. (**b**) The immunoperoxidase technique demonstrates only IgA (staining brown) in the plasma cells and no light chain.

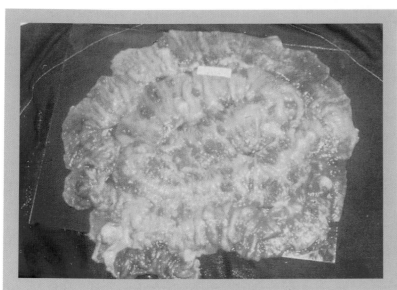

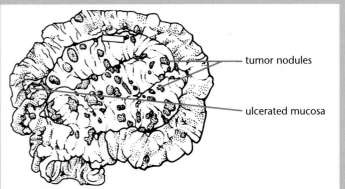

Fig. 15.60 α-heavy chain disease. This surgical specimen of ileum shows frank tumor nodules clearly visible in the mesentery, ulcerating the ileal mucosa. (Courtesy of Dr F. Asselah.)

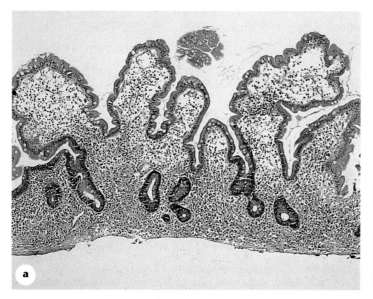

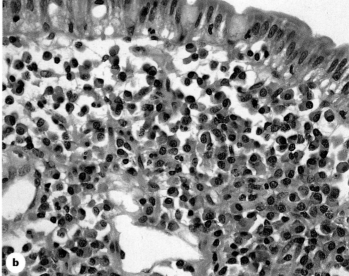

Fig. 15.61 α-heavy chain disease. A 25-year-old Algerian man presented with malabsorption syndrome consisting of weight loss, chronic diarrhea, steatorrhea and hypocalcemia, which responded to broad-spectrum antibiotics. (**a**) Biopsy specimen of small intestine shows diffuse infiltration of the lamina propria by (**b**) a mixture of lymphocytes, plasma cells and plasmacytoid cells. Immunocytochemical staining showed that the vast majority of these cells contained α-heavy chains without κ or λ light chains. Serum and urine samples revealed a broad band in the α2 region, which precipitated with an anti-IgA antiserum but showed no reactivity to anti-κ or anti-α. (Courtesy of Dr J.E. McLaughlin.)

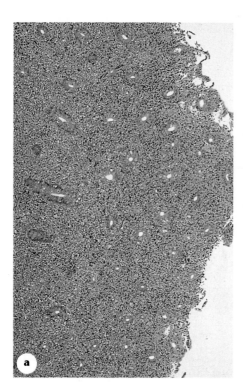

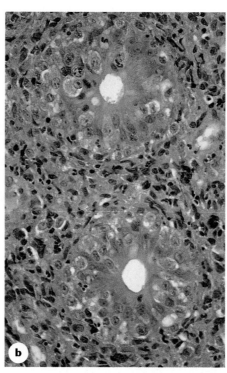

Fig. 15.62 α-heavy chain disease. Two years after presentation, the same patient as presented in Figure 15.61 developed small intestinal obstruction. After resection, the small bowel was found to be heavily infiltrated by a large cell immunoblastic lymphoma, with an additional mixed infiltrate of neutrophils, plasma cells and macrophages. Despite intensive chemotherapy, the tumor relapsed, involving the large and small bowel and intra-abdominal lymph nodes, which showed similar histologic findings. The rectal mucosa seen at (**a**) low and (**b**) high power shows complete loss of normal architecture; remaining crypt cells are surrounded by a diffuse infiltrate composed of large malignant cells and mixed inflammatory cells. The α-heavy chain could still be detected in serum but not in urine at this relapse. (Courtesy of Dr J.E. McLaughlin.)

Acknowledgements

We are extremely grateful to Dr Andrew Jack and Professor Gareth Morgan (Haematological Malignancy Diagnostic Service, Leeds General Infirmary, Leeds, UK) for allowing us to use some of their figures.

REFERENCES

Avet-Loiseau H, Brigaudeau C, Morineau N, *et al.*: High incidence of cryptic translocations involving the Ig heavy chain gene in multiple myeloma as shown by fluorescence in situ hybridization. Genes Chromosomes Cancer 1999; 24 : 9–15.

Bartl R, Frisch B, Fateh-Moghadam A, *et al.*: Histological classification and staging of multiple myeloma. A retrospective and prospective study of 674 cases. Am J Clin Hematol 1987; 87 : 342–355.

Corradini P, Ladetto M, Voena C, *et al.*: Mutational activation of N- and K-ras oncogenes in plasma cell dyscrasias. Blood 1993; 81 : 2708–2713.

Dankbar B, Padro T, Leo R, *et al.*: Vascular endothelial growth factor and interleukin 6 in paracrine tumour-stromal cell interaction in multiple myeloma. Blood 2000; 95 : 2630–2636.

Davies FE, Anderson KC: Novel therapeutic targets in multiple myeloma. Eur J Haematol 2000; 64 : 359–367.

Dimopoulos MA, Panayiotidis P, Moulopoulos LA, *et al.*: Waldenstrom's macroglobulinemia: clinical features, complications and management. J Clin Oncol 2000; 18 : 214–226.

Dimopoulos M, Moulopoulos I, Maniatis A, Alexanian R: Solitary plasmacytoma of bone and asymptomatic multiple myeloma. Blood 2000: 96 : 2037–2044.

Durie BGM, Salmon SE: A clinical staging system for multiple myeloma. Correlation of measured cell mass with presenting clinical features, response to treatment and survival. Cancer 1975; 36 : 842–854.

Falk RH, Comenzo RL, Skinner M: The systemic amyloidoses. N Engl J Med 1997; 337(13):898–909.

Fermand JP, Brouet JC: Heavy chain diseases. Hematol Oncol Clin North Am 1999; 13 : 1281–1294.

Garcia-Sanz R, Orfao A, Gonzalez M, *et al.*: Primary plasma cell leukemia: clinical, immunophenotypic, DNA ploidy and cytogenetic characteristics. Blood 1999; 93 : 1032–1037.

Gilmore JD, Hawkins PN, Pepys MB: Amyloidosis: a review of recent diagnostic and therapeutic developments. Br J Haematol 1997; 99 : 245–256.

Greenlee R, Hill-Harmon M, Murray T, Thun M: Cancer statistics 2001. CA Cancer J Clin 2001; 51(1):15–36.

Greipp PR, Leong T, Bennett JM, *et al.*: Plasmablastic morphology – an independent prognostic factor with clinical and laboratory correlates. Blood 1998; 91 : 2501–2507.

Greipp PR, Katzman JA, O'Fallon WM, *et al.*: Value of β2 microglobulin level and plasma cell labeling indices as prognostic factors in patients with newly diagnosed myeloma. Blood 1988; 72 : 219–223.

Herrington LJ, Weiss NS, Olsham AF: Epidemiology of myeloma. In: Malpass JS, Bergsagel DE, Kyle R, Anderson K, eds: Myeloma: Biology and Management. Oxford Medical Publications, Oxford, 1998: pp. 150–186.

Kyle RA: Benign monoclonal gammopathy – after 20–35 years of follow up. Mayo Clin Proc 1993; 68 : 26–36.

Kyle RA, Garton JP: The spectrum of IgM monoclonal gammopathy in 430 cases. Mayo Clin Proc 1987; 62 : 719–731.

Lust JA, Donovan KA: The role of IL-1β in the pathogenesis of multiple myeloma. Hematol Oncol Clin North Am 1999; 13 : 1117–11125.

Manolagas SC, Jilka RL: Bone marrow, cytokines and bone remodelling. N Engl J Med 1995; 332 : 305–311.

Menke D, Horny HP, Griesser H, *et al.*: Primary lymph node plasmacytomas (plasmacytic lymphomas). Am J Clin Pathol 2001; 115 : 119–126.

Milla F, Oriol A, Aguilar JL, *et al.*: Usefulness and reproducibility of cytomorphologic evaluations to differentiate myeloma from monoclonal gammopathies of unknown significance. Am J Clin Pathol 2001; 115 : 127–135

Norfolk DN, Child JA, Cooper EH, *et al.*: Serum β2 microglobulin in myelomatosis: potential value in stratification and monitoring. Br J Cancer 1980; 42 : 510–515.

Portier M, Moles JP, Makars GR, *et al.*: P53 and RAS gene mutations in multiple myeloma. Oncogene 1992; 7 : 2539–2543.

Raje N, Anderson KC: Thalidomide: a revival story. N Engl J Med 1999; 341 : 1606–1609.

Sahota SS, Leo R, Hamblin TJ, *et al.*: Ig V_H gene mutational patterns indicate different tumour cell status in human myeloma and monoclonal gammopathy of undetermined significance. Blood 1996; 87 : 746–755.

Teoh G, Anderson KC: Interaction of tumour and host cells with adhesion and extracellular matrix molecules in the development of multiple myeloma. Hematol Oncol Clin North Am 1997; 11 : 27–42.

Treon SP, Anderson KC: Interleukin-6 in multiple myeloma and related plasma cell dyscrasias. Curr Opin Hematol 1998; 5 : 42–48.

Tricot G, Barlogie B, Jaganath S, *et al.*: Poor prognosis in multiple myeloma is associated only with partial or complete deletions of chromosome 13 or abnormalities involving 11 q and not with other karyotype abnormalities. Blood 1995; 86 : 4250–4256.

Tricot G: New insights into the role of microenvironment in multiple myeloma. Lancet 2000; 335 : 248–249.

Vacca A, Ribatti D, Presta M, *et al.*: Bone marrow neovascularisation, plasma cell angiogenic potential and matrix metalloproteinase-2 secretion parallel progression of human multiple myeloma. Blood 1999; 93 : 3064–3073.

FIGURE CREDITS

16 Solid tumors in childhood

Holcombe E. Grier, Antonio Perez-Atayde, Fredric A. Hoffer

Cancer in childhood is quite rare compared with the incidence of cancer in adults; approximately 6500 new cases are diagnosed in the United States each year. Nevertheless, cancer remains the second most common cause of death during childhood. The common childhood cancers and their frequency are shown in Table 16.1. It is important to note that the relative incidence of tumors is not constant through childhood. The median age for neuroblastoma, for instance, is 1–2 years and the tumor is unusual after 5 years of age. In contrast, the incidence of Hodgkin's disease peaks in adolescence and is rare in children less than 5 years of age.

Childhood cancers have provided insights into the biology and treatment of neoplasia in general. The identification of recessive oncogenes, for example, as well as the advantage of multimodal therapy on cure rates were first described in the context of childhood malignancies such as Wilms' tumor, retinoblastoma and other solid tumors of childhood.

Several malignancies seen in adults and children are covered in other chapters and will not be reviewed here. Brain tumors and germ cell tumors are handled in Chapters 6 and 12, acute leukemias in Chapter 13 and lymphomas in Chapter 14.

RETINOBLASTOMA

Retinoblastoma is a malignancy of early childhood that arises in the retina. It is often present at birth and is rarely diagnosed later than 6 years of age. The disease is hereditary in 60% of cases and non-hereditary in the remainder. The hereditary type may be transmitted as an autosoma dominant trait from an affected parent or may occur as a spontaneous mutation. This type of retinoblastoma, which is passed on to 50% of subsequent offspring, is diagnosed earlier than the non-hereditary form and is usually multifocal at presentation. It is associated with the somatic loss of a recessive oncogene, the retinoblastoma (Rb) gene, from chromosome 13. Loss of both Rb genes leads to the tumor, thus explaining why multiple tumors occur in patients lacking one of the Rb genes (the first 'hit' of the two-hit process has occurred in all the cells). Patients are at high risk for secondary sarcomas, both at previous radiation sites and elsewhere. A staging system developed by Reese and Ellsworth predicts the likelihood of tumor control and preservation of vision, based on the location of the tumor or tumors within the orbit.

In contrast to the hereditary form, non-hereditary retinoblastoma is always unilateral and does not have a high risk of second tumors except in the radiated field. Up to 10% of unilateral tumors may be hereditary and genetic counseling along with molecular analysis of the germline Rb genes is necessary for all patients even with unilateral presentation.

Patients with retinoblastoma most commonly present with leukokoria, a whitish reflex from a mass behind the lens. In the US, the disease is usually confined to the globe at diagnosis, although it may grow along the optic tract or extend through the globe and invade bone. Microscopically, retinoblastoma cells have hyperchromatic nuclei with scanty cytoplasm. The vast majority of patients with retinoblastoma are cured with a combination of surgery and/or radiotherapy. Chemotherapy is used only for the very rare patient with extraocular disease or distant metastases.

The size and extent of retinoblastoma can be measured by many means including direct ophthalmoscopy, computed tomography, magnetic resonance imaging and sonography. Fluorescein angiography (not illustrated) will detect small vascular lesions. It is performed by intravenous injection of a fluorane dye and direct photography of the retina illuminated by an ultraviolet light.

WILMS' TUMOR

Wilms' tumor is the most common tumor of the kidney in childhood; other, rarer, malignant renal tumors of childhood include clear cell sarcoma and rhabdoid tumor. The median age at diagnosis of Wilms' tumor is between 2 and 3 years and it is uncommon after 8 years of age. The classic histologic appearance of Wilms' tumor is triphasic, comprising blastemal, epithelial (tubules and glomeruloid structures) and mesenchymal elements, although many tumors exhibit only one or two of these elements. The presence of anaplasia is associated with a poorer prognosis.

Most patients with Wilms' tumor present with an abdominal mass, usually first palpated by the parents. Less common presentations include hematuria and hypertension; systemic symptoms are rare. Bilateral tumors are found at presentation in 4–7% of cases. In 5% of cases, Wilms' tumor is associated with other abnormalities of the GU system and, more rarely with hemihypertrophy, the Beckwith–Wiedemann syndrome (macroglossia, somatic gigantism, abdominal wall defects and hypoglycemia), Drash syndrome (pseudohermaphroditism and nephropathy) and aniridia. The latter syndrome led to the discovery of an association in some patients between Wilms' tumor and loss of the WT-1 gene on the long arm of chromosome 11. This gene is a zinc-finger DNA binding protein that is expressed in the developing kidney.

The grouping system developed by the National Wilms' Tumor Study is shown in Figure 16.7. The workup for Wilms' tumor includes urinalysis, chest radiography, and abdominal and chest CT scan. The lung is the most common site of metastases. MRI of the abdomen may also be useful and may substitute for abdominal CT. MRI may help differentiate nephrogenic rests from bilateral Wilms' tumor. Either MRI or ultrasonography of the abdomen should be done preoperatively to visualize tumor within the inferior vena cava.

NEUROBLASTOMA

Neuroblastoma is the most common extracranial solid tumor in childhood and the most common cancer in infants. The median age at diagnosis is 2 years, although neuroblastoma occasionally occurs in adults. The tumor, originating in neural crest cells, can occur anywhere along the sympathetic nerve chain. By far the most common location for a primary tumor is the adrenal gland. In its most primitive form, the histology of neuroblastoma is marked by poorly differentiated small, round blue cells. At an intermediate stage of maturation, there is differentiation toward ganglion cells. Tumors composed of a mixture of neuroblasts and mature ganglion cells are classified as ganglioneuroblastomas. At the most differentiated end of the spectrum is ganglioneuroma, a benign tumor composed entirely of mature ganglion cells, neurites and Schwann cells.

The International Neuroblastoma Staging System is shown in Table 16.2.

Stage 4-S neuroblastoma is an unusual malignancy that has a high likelihood of spontaneous resolution despite the existence of extensive, generalized metastases at the time of presentation. The most common fatal complication in stage 4-S disease is respiratory compromise secondary to massive enlargement of the liver. For other patients with neuroblastoma, prognosis overall is stage and age related, with a markedly improved survival rate for patients who present before the age of 1 year.

The presenting signs and symptoms of neuroblastoma depend on the location of the primary tumor. An abdominal mass associated with an adrenal tumor is the most common presentation. Paraspinal tumors may present with cord compression and thoracic tumors are occasionally associated with Horner's syndrome. Patients with metastatic disease frequently present with proptosis and periorbital ecchymosis. Metastases occur to lymph nodes, bone, bone marrow, liver and skin. Patients frequently show systemic symptoms of irritability and poor food intake, probably occasioned by pain from extensive bone involvement. Urinary excretion of catecholamines is increased in 85–90% of patients with neuroblastoma; in fact, the diagnosis can be made on the basis of increased urinary catecholamines associated with typical neuroblastoma cells in the bone marrow. Workup should also include a bone scan and MR or CT imaging of the primary; many centers are doing MIBG scanning, utilizing the tumor uptake of the radiolabeled catecholamine precursor meta-iodobenzylguanidine. Rarely, patients present with diarrhea from secretion of vasoactive intestinal polypeptide (VIP) or with the syndrome of opsoclonus–myoclonus; the latter syndrome may be an autoimmune phenomenon and may not regress even with successful treatment of the tumor.

Neuroblastoma is one of the first tumors noted in some cases to involve amplification of a dominant oncogene. Cytogenetic studies of cell lines and fresh tumor specimens may show double minutes or homogeneous staining regions representing multiple copies of the N-*myc* oncogene. Amplification of this gene conveys a less favorable prognosis. Several other biologic variables predict outcome in neuroblastoma. The International Neuroblastoma Risk Groups committee is attempting to define patient subsets based on these variables.

HEPATIC TUMORS

The most common primary malignant tumors of the liver in childhood are hepatoblastoma and hepatoma (hepatocellular carcinoma). (*See also* text and illustrations on 'Hepatoma' in Chapter 5.) The distinguishing clinical characteristics of hepatoblastoma and hepatoma are shown in Table 16.3

Hepatoblastoma is a rare, embryonal malignant neoplasm that typically presents in infancy, showing a predilection for males. It may be associated with a variety of congenital anomalies and with the syndrome of familial polyposis coli (FPC). Children with hepatoblastoma and FPC may exhibit congenital hypertrophy of the

retinal pigment epithelium (CHRPE), which is sometimes seen with FPC. There is an increased incidence of hepatoblastoma in low birthweight infants; the cause for this association is not known. Most children with hepatoblastoma present with an asymptomatic abdominal mass, which grossly appears tan and lobulated. Workup includes measurement of α-fetoprotein (AFP), which is elevated in nearly all patients, and human chorionic gonadotrophin (HCG), of which only a small number of patients show elevation. CT scan of the lung, the most common site of metastasis, is part of patient workup, as well as abdominal MRI, ultrasonography and, finally, angiography of the liver if the potential for resection is unclear. Complete resection of the primary tumor is the most important element in curing hepatoblastoma. Adjuvant chemotherapy appears to offer some advantage in completely resected cases and neo-adjuvant chemotherapy may convert some patients' tumors from being unresectable to resectable; this approach has considerably increased the cure rate in hepatoblastoma.

RHABDOMYOSARCOMA

Rhabdomyosarcoma, a malignancy that differentiates toward striated muscle cells, is the most common soft tissue sarcoma of childhood. (*See also* text and illustrations on 'Rhabdomyosarcoma' in Chapter 10.) Pathologic sections occasionally show cross-striations, but their presence is not necessary to establish the diagnosis. Antibodies against muscle-specific proteins and electron microscopy showing bundles of actin and myosin filaments can be extremely helpful in distinguishing rhabdomyosarcoma from other tumors. Two histologic patterns have been identified: embryonal and alveolar. Cytogenetics is an important tool in the diagnosis of rhabdomyosarcoma. A vast majority of tumors with alveolar characteristics have a translocation between the FKHR gene (one of the forkhead transcription factor genes) on chromosome 13 and the PAX3 gene on chromosome 2 (or, less commonly, the PAX7 gene on chromosome 1).

The median age at presentation for childhood rhabdomyosarcoma is 2–3 years for GU tumors and 6 years for tumors of the head and neck (*see* Table 16.5). Stage is determined using the surgically based grouping system devised by the Intergroup Rhabdomyosarcoma Study (*see* Table 16.4 and Fig. 16.25), although in recent years there has been greater use of a TNM system. Proper staging requires MRI of the primary, CT of the lungs and bone marrow aspirates and biopsies.

Surgery, radiotherapy and chemotherapy are all important for long-term survival. Prognosis depends on the site of origin of the tumor and its histology: orbital, paratesticular and most GU primary tumors have a more favorable prognosis than those of the extremities, trunk and head and neck with extensive bone destruction; the alveolar histologic variant carries a less favorable prognosis than the embryonal.

THE EWING'S FAMILY OF TUMORS

Ewing's sarcoma and peripheral primitive neuroectodermal tumor (PNET) of bone and soft tissue

Ewing's sarcoma is the second most common malignant bone tumor in children and adolescents. (*See also* text and illustrations on 'Ewing's Sarcoma' in Chapter 10.) Although its cell of origin is unclear, its histology is marked by small, round blue cells, classically often containing PAS-positive material. Recently it has become clear that Ewing's sarcoma of bone and soft tissue has a continuum of differentiation, with the most differentiated form frequently termed primitive neuroectodermal tumor (PNET). The pathogenesis and cytogenetics of PNET are clearly different from the group of CNS tumors (central PNET) that unfortunately carry the same name. PNETs exhibit neuroectodermal differentiation as demonstrated on electron microscopy or by positivity with neuronal markers such as neuron-specific enolase. The clinical importance of this variation in differentiation is unclear. PNET and Ewing's sarcoma cells both stain positively to antibodies to the protein product of the MIC2 gene. Ewing's sarcoma and PNET have a high incidence of a clonal abnormality, a translocation between chromosomes 11 and 22. This translocation creates a novel chimeric protein consisting of parts of two genes: *FLI1* (an Ets-like oncogene) and *EWS*, a novel gene. Much of this information can often be obtained by needle aspiration, especially since polymerase chain reaction assays exist for the translocation. These tumors have a peak occurrence in the early second decade, but can occur in patients as young as infants or as old as 30 years of age. The disease is extremely rare in blacks and Asians.

For patients with bone primaries, the most common symptom is a painful mass. For both soft tissue and bone primaries, fever may be a symptom at presentation in about one-third of patients and occurs more commonly with large tumors or tumors with metastases. The most common bone site is the pelvis, followed closely by the femur, although the tumor can occur in virtually any bone. When a long bone is the site of a primary tumor, the midshaft of the femur is the most commonly involved area. Soft tissues in nearly every region of the body can develop PNETs, including the extremities, pelvis, retroperitoneum, etc. Most common sites include the paraspinal and thoracopulmonary regions. The paraspinal masses often impinge on the spinal cord. The thoracopulmonary tumor is commonly referred to as the Askin tumor of the chest wall and more frequently has pathologic findings of neuroectodermal differentiation than tumors in other sites.

The workup of a patient with Ewing's sarcoma/PNET should include plain films and MR scanning of the primary tumor. In addition, CT scan of the lungs, bone scan, bone marrow aspiration and biopsy and determination of lactate dehydrogenase (LDH) level are part of patient workup. The most common site of metastases is the lung, followed by bone. Poor prognosis factors for patients with bone primaries, in order of importance, are the presence of metastases, large size of the primary tumor and location of the primary. Pelvic involvement carries a worse prognosis than involvement of the femur or humerus, which in turn has a worse prognosis than involvement distal to the knee and elbow. Treatment includes systemic chemotherapy for control of micrometastatic disease, which is present in more than 90% of patients, as indicated by the cure rate achieved with amputation alone. Radiotherapy can control the primary lesion in the majority of patients and it is unclear whether or not surgical excision of the primary tumor improves local control or overall disease-free survival.

OSTEOSARCOMA

Osteosarcoma (osteogenic sarcoma) is the most common malignant tumor of bone in children and adolescents. (*See also* text and illustrations on 'osteosarcoma' in Chapter 10.) Derived from primitive mesenchymal bone-forming cells, osteosarcoma is defined histologically by malignant sarcomatous cells that form osteoid. The tumor most commonly arises in the second decade of life, with peak occurrence during the adolescent growth spurt. Most adolescents present with pain, often in conjunction with a soft tissue mass. Osteosarcoma is primarily a disease that affects the metaphysis of long bones. The distal femur is the most common primary site, followed by the proximal tibia and the proximal humerus.

Workup of a patient with presumed osteosarcoma should include plain films and MR scan of the primary lesion, as well as CT scan of the lung, bone scan and determination of LDH level. Metastases at the time of presentation are associated with a poor prognosis. Successful treatment of patients with non-metastatic osteosarcoma requires complete surgical excision of the primary tumor and adjuvant chemotherapy. It is not clear at present whether preoperative chemotherapy improves the overall survival rate.

Table 16.1 Common malignant tumors in childhood and their relative frequency.*

Malignant Tumor	Frequency (%)
Leukemia (mostly ALL, some AML)	30
Brain tumors	19
Lymphomas (Hodgkin's and non-Hodgkin's)	13
Neuroblastoma	8
Kidney (mostly Wilms' tumor)	6
Soft tissue sarcoma (rhabdomyosarcoma most common)	7
Retinoblastoma	3
Bone	5
Liver	1
Other	8

*<15 years of age.
Compiled from SEER data, National Cancer Institute.

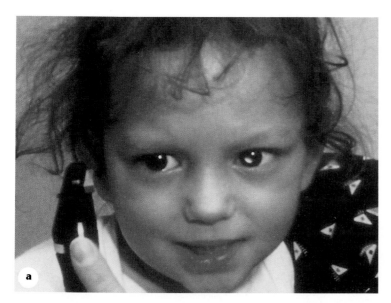

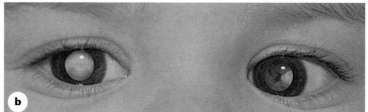

Fig. 16.1 Retinoblastoma. (**a**) Frequently, families first note leukokoria by a white reflex in the retina seen in photographs of their child. The normal red reflex is lost due to a retinal tumor. (**b**) This 1-year-old child shows gross ocular involvement. A convergent squint is also present. (**a**: Courtesy of Nancy Tarbell MD, Children's Hospital, Boston, MA.)

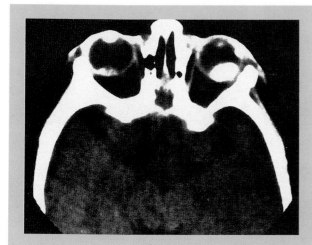

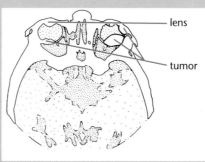

lens

tumor

Fig. 16.2 Retinoblastoma. CT scan in a child with hereditary disease shows several tumor foci involving the orbits bilaterally. (Courtesy of Roy Strand MD, Children's Hospital, Boston, MA.)

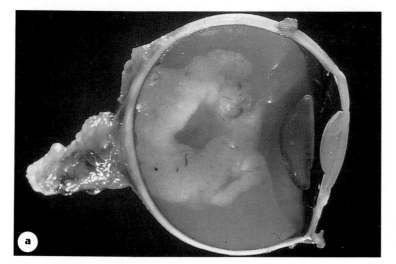

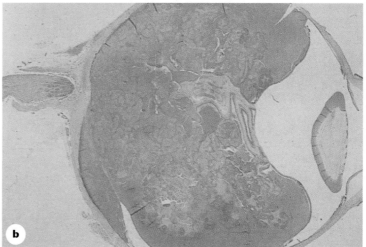

Fig. 16.3 Retinoblastoma. (**a**) Cross-section of an eye shows a tumor growing into the vitreous humor from its origin along the posterior wall of the retina.

(**b**) Whole-mount section of an eye demonstrates a similar retinoblastoma invading the vitreous and extending into the optic nerve.

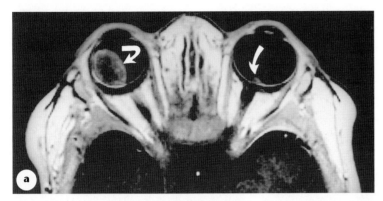

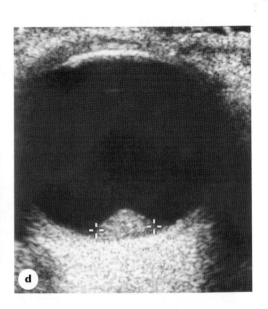

Fig. 16.4 This 3-month-old girl has bilateral retinoblastoma. (**a**) Post-contrast T1-weighted axial MR imaging demonstrates the larger right and smaller left retinal masses (curved arrows). (**b**) Longitudinal transorbital high-resolution (13 MHz) ultrasound shows the 1.4 cm diameter right globe mass (cross-hatches) nearly filling the globe. (**c**) A more medial ultrasound section demonstrates the retinal detachment (curved arrow) not seen by MR or CT. (**d**) The left retinal mass (cross-hatches) measured 5 mm on this ultrasound.

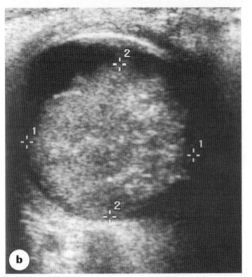
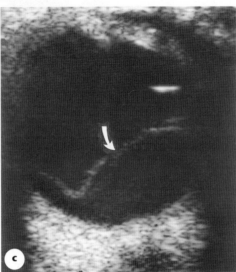

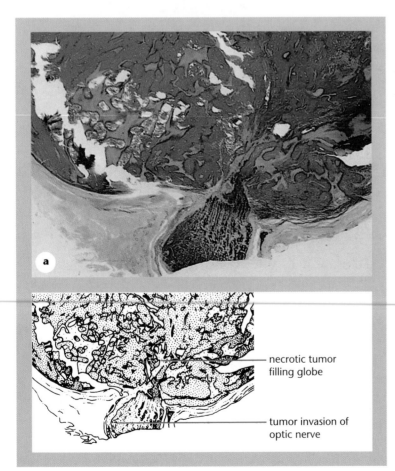

necrotic tumor filling globe

tumor invasion of optic nerve

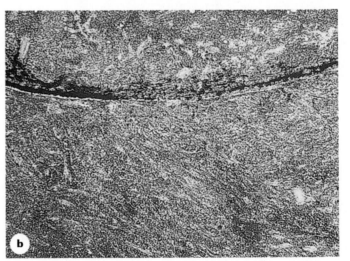

Fig. 16.5 Retinoblastoma. (**a**) Tumor completely fills the vitreal cavity and extends into the optic nerve in this microscopic section. (**b**) Photomicroscopy in another case reveals direct extension into the underlying choroid.

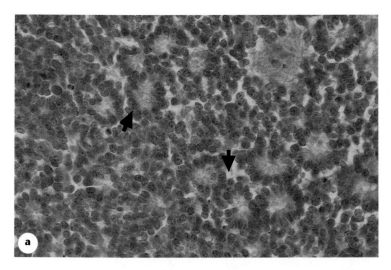

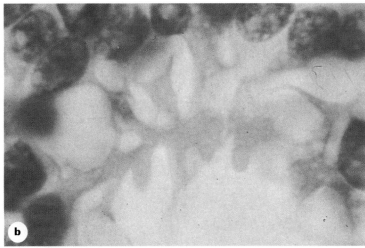

Fig. 16.6 Retinoblastoma. (**a**) Small cells with round, hyperchromatic nuclei are arranged in well-developed Flexner–Wintersteiner rosettes (arrows), which are interpreted as a primitive attempt at photoreceptor differentiation. (**b**) With high magnification, careful inspection reveals apical intraluminal protrusions indicating photoreceptor differentiation.

Fig. 16.7 National Wilms' Tumor Study grouping system.

Group 1
- Tumor limited to kidney and completely excised
- Surface of renal capsule intact
- No tumor rupture before or during removal
- No residual tumor apparent beyond margins of excision

Group II
- Tumor extending beyond kidney but completely excised
- Regional extension of tumor (i.e., penetration through outer surface of renal capsule into perirenal soft tissues)
- Vessels outside kidney substance infiltrated or contain tumor thrombus
- Tumor may have been biopsied, or local spillage of tumor confined to flank
- No residual tumor apparent at or beyond margins of excision

Group III
- Residual nonhematogenous tumor confined to abdomen, with any of the following:
- Lymph nodes (hilar, periaortic, or beyond) found on biopsy to be involved
- Diffuse peritoneal contamination by tumor (e.g., by spillage of tumor beyond flank before or during surgery or by tumor growth through peritoneal surface)
- Implants found on peritoneal surface
- Tumor extending beyond surgical margins (microscopically or grossly)
- Tumor not completely resectable due to local infiltration into vital structures

Group IV
- Hematogenous metastases
- Deposits beyond stage III (i.e., lung, liver, bone, brain)

Group V
- Bilateral renal involvement at diagnosis

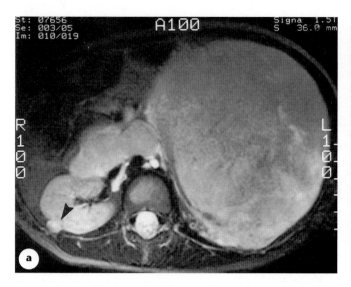

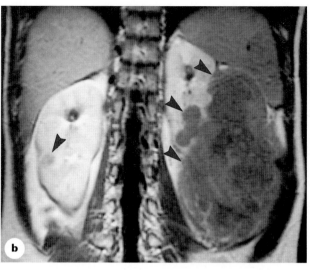

Fig. 16.8 Wilms' tumor. Physical examination easily revealed the left renal mass in this 4-year-old. (**a**) The axial T2-weighted, fat-suppressed fast spin-echo MR shows the large left Wilms' tumor extending across the midline and a second, small, round Wilms' tumor in the right kidney (arrow). (**b**) The coronal gadolinium-enhanced T1-weighted MR scan shows the bilateral Wilms' tumor, with a nodular appearance suggesting nephroblastomatosis (arrows). MR scan not only provides a good look at both kidneys, but also provides the mandatory imaging of the inferior vena cava which, if involved, has to be tied off early in surgery to prevent tumor emboli. At surgery the left kidney as well as the nodule of Wilms' tumor on the right were removed. Surgery in Wilms' tumor should always use an anterior approach so that appropriate nodes can be biopsied.

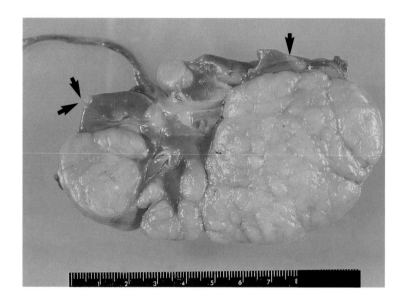

Fig. 16.9 Wilms' tumor with nephroblastomatosis. Bisected nephrectomy specimen shows multicentric Wilms' tumors. Multicentric tumors are usually associated with nephroblastomatosis, sometimes bilateral. Nephroblastomatosis is seen as small cortical nodules (arrows).

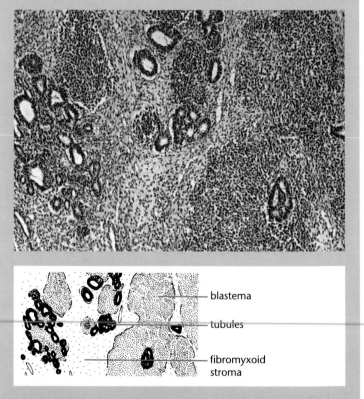

Fig. 16.10 Wilms' tumor. Its classic triphasic pattern is marked by circumscribed nodules of blastema showing variable epithelial differentiation and tubule formation, surrounded by a fibromyxoid stroma. (Reproduced with permission from Schumann and Weiss, 1981.)

	Table 16.2 INSS criteria
Stage	**Definition**
1	Localized tumor with complete gross excision, with or without microscopic residual disease; representative ipsilateral non-adherent[†] lymph nodes negative for tumor microscopically
2A	Localized tumor with incomplete gross excision; representative ipsilateral non-adherent lymph nodes negative for tumor microscopically
2B	Localized tumor with or without complete gross excision, with ipsilateral, non-adherent lymph nodes positive for tumor. Enlarged contralateral lymph nodes must be negative microscopically
3	Unresectable unilateral tumor infiltrating across the midline,[‡] with or without regional lymph node involvement or localized unilateral tumor with contralateral regional lymph node involvement or midline tumor with bilateral extension by infiltration (unresectable) or by lymph node involvement
4	Any primary tumor with dissemination to distant lymph nodes, bone marrow, liver, skin and/or other organs (except as defined for stage 4S)
4S	Localized primary tumor (as defined for stages 1, 2A or 2B), with dissemination limited to skin, liver, and/or bone marrow* (limited to infants <1 year of age)

*Marrow involvement in stage 4S should be minimal, i.e. <10% of total nucleated cells identified as malignant on bone marrow biopsy or on marrow aspirate. More extensive marrow involvement would be considered to be stage 4. The MIBG scan, if performed, should be negative in the marrow. [†]Lymph nodes attached to and removed with the primary tumor. [‡]The midline is defined as the vertebral column. Tumors originating on one side and crossing the midline must infiltrate to or beyond the opposite side of the vertebral column.

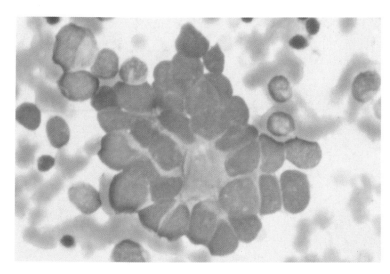

Fig. 16.11 Neuroblastoma. This bone marrow aspirate shows a clump of tumor cells in a rosette formation with central fibrillar material. The individual cells, resembling lymphoblasts, are small and have scanty cytoplasm.

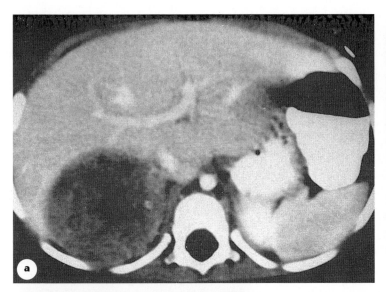

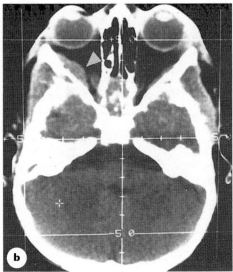

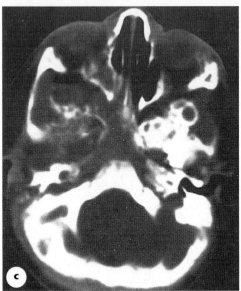

Fig. 16.12 Neuroblastoma. (**a**) Abdominal CT scan in a 2-year-old child who presented with proptosis and periorbital ecchymosis shows a right upper quadrant soft tissue mass, which was palpable on examination. (**b**) CT section at the level of the orbits reveals a mass (arrow) extending into the right orbit; (**c**) the bone destruction is extensive.

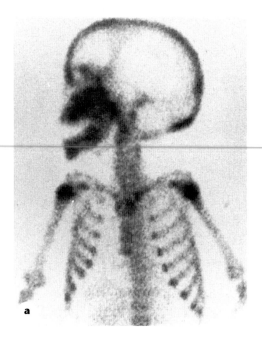

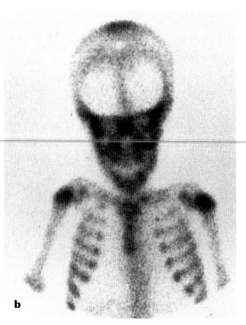

Fig. 16.13 Neuroblastoma. (**a,b**) Bone scans of the patient shown in Fig. 16.12 reveal extensive involvement of the facial bones and multiple 'hot' spots in the skull, reflecting metastatic deposits. Symmetric involvement of the long bones, in this case both proximal humeri, is common in neuroblastoma.

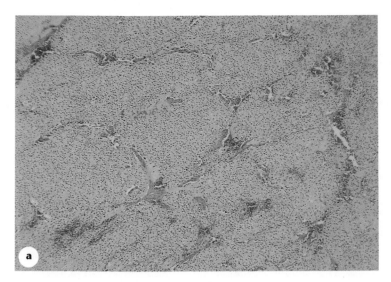

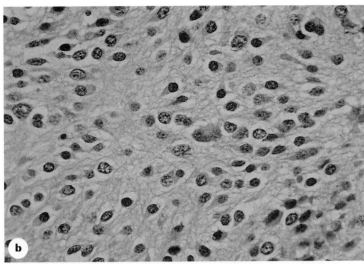

Fig. 16.14 Neuroblastoma. (**a**) This low-power view shows the characteristic lobular pattern of neuroblastoma with discrete, large nests of tumor cells surrounded by a delicate fibrovascular stroma. (**b**) A higher-power view of the same tumor reveals that small, round tumor cells are separated by an abundant, pink, fibrillary network (neuropile). The neuropile represents cytoplasmic processes (neurites). The tumor cells at the center of this photograph show signs of maturation as evidenced by the abundant cytoplasm, resembling immature ganglion cells.

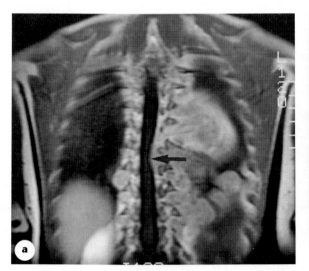

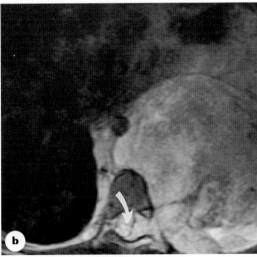

Fig. 16.15 Posterior mediastinal neuroblastoma. (**a**) This 4-year-old presented to his pediatrician with new onset of difficulty in walking. The coronal MR T1-weighted image with gadolinium demonstrates tumor pushing on the dark spinal cord (arrow). (**b**) An axial T2 MR shows the spinal cord (arrow) pushed to the right by the large left posterior mediastinal mass entering into the left spinal foramen. The tumor was removed surgically with only microscopic residual. As long as biological markers are favorable, patients treated in this manner need no further therapy, with recurrences very unlikely.

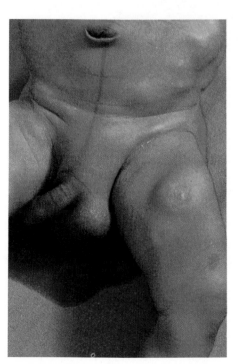

Fig. 16.16 Skin and subcutaneous metastases. Skin lesions can vary in size and are frequently smaller than seen in this infant with stage 4-S neuroblastoma.

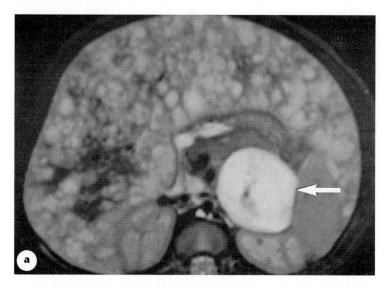

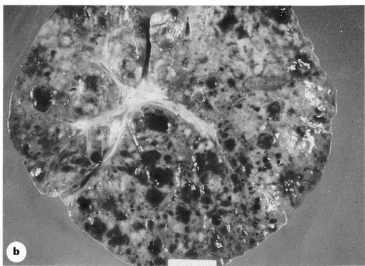

Fig. 16.17 Neuroblastoma: liver metastases. (**a**) MR scan of left adrenal primary neuroblastoma (arrow) with multiple liver metastases in a 3-month-old who was brought to the pediatrician because of increased abdominal girth. The normal liver on this T2-weighted fat-suppressed fast spin MR appears dark. A needle biopsy confirmed the diagnosis and the tumor regressed after a single dose of cyclophosphamide. (**b**) In contrast to the clinical story above, this patient had progressive enlargement of his liver despite chemotherapy and radiotherapy and eventually died of respiratory failure from mechanical compression. Autopsy specimen shows virtual replacement of the liver by metastases, many of which were hemorrhagic. The liver weighted 2374 grams.

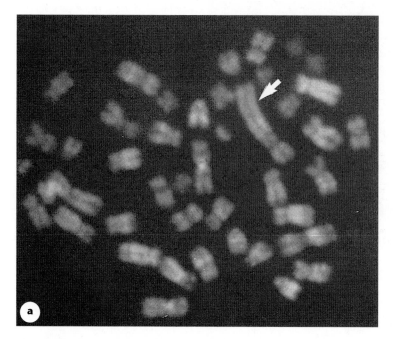

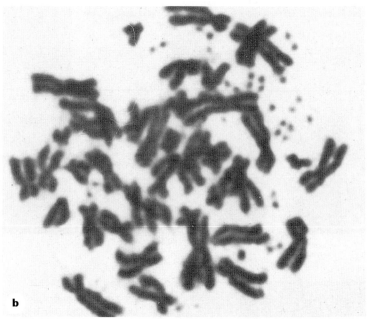

Fig. 16.18 Neuroblastoma. These chromosome spreads are from a neuroblastoma cell line with N-*myc* amplification. (**a**) On this Q-banded karyotype, there is a homogeneous staining region (HSR) on chromosome 2q (arrow). (**b**) On bright field, multiple double-minute (DM) chromosome bodies become apparent. (Courtesy of Bruch R. Korf MD, Children's Hospital, Boston, MA.)

Table 16.3 Comparison of the clinical characteristics of hepatoblastoma and hepatoma.

	Hepatoblastoma	Hepatoma
Age	0–3 years	5–18+ years
Previous liver disease	Uncommon	Common
Pain	Uncommon	Common
Jaundice	Uncommon	1/4 of cases
Elevated α-fetoprotein	2/3 of cases	1/2 of cases

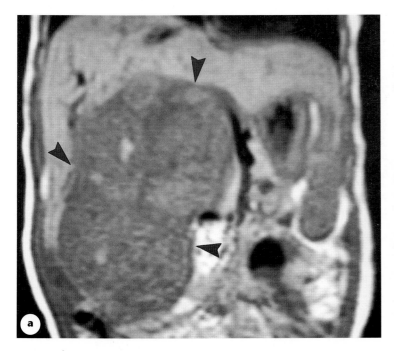

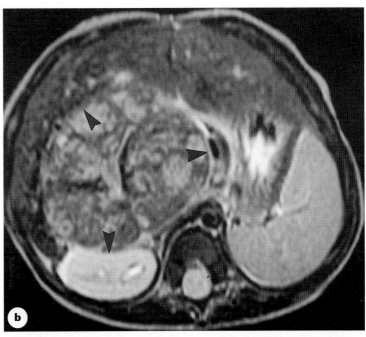

Fig. 16.19 Hepatoblastoma. This 16-month-old child presented with a rapidly enlarging abdominal mass. (**a**) T1-weighted coronal MR shows that the mass is confined to the right lobe of the liver but is contiguous with the portal vein and mesentery. (**b**) The axial T2-weighted MR demonstrates the mass extending medially to the portal vein and posteriorly to the level of the kidney. Resection of the tumor was possible after induction chemotherapy and the patient has remained well.

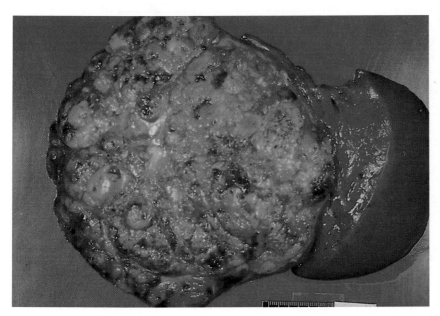

Fig. 16.20 Hepatoblastoma. Typical hepatoblastoma: a single, round, well-demarcated lobulated mass with variegated appearance and areas of necrosis and hemorrhage. Normal liver included in the resection specimen is seen at the right.

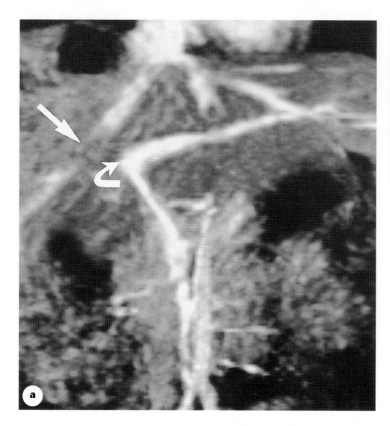

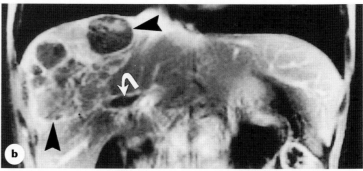

Fig. 16.21 This 9-year-old girl had a right lobe hepatoblastoma. (**a**) Coronal MRA demonstrates attenuation of the right hepatic vein (straight arrow) and interruption of the right portal vein (curved arrow). (**b**) Post-contrast T1-weighted coronal MR imaging demonstrates the mass (arrowheads) and the dark right portal vein tumor thrombus (curved arrow). MR angiography helps the surgeon by demonstrating the hepatic artery, portal vein and hepatic venous anatomy, frequently obviating the need for angiography.

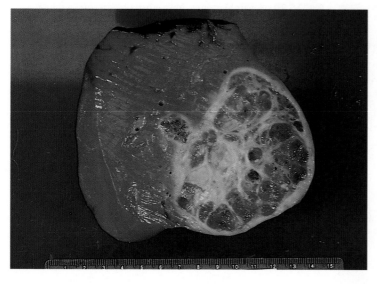

Fig. 16.22 Hepatoblastoma resected after three cycles of induction chemotherapy. The tumor is markedly reduced in size (as compared to pretreatment MR scans, not shown) and displays central scarring and necrosis along with a thick fibrous capsule. The dark, fleshy tumor seen between the central scarring and the periphery is made up of granulation tissue with hemosiderosis and scattered residual tumor cells. Normal liver is included with the specimen (on the left side).

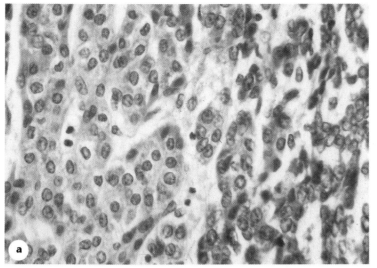

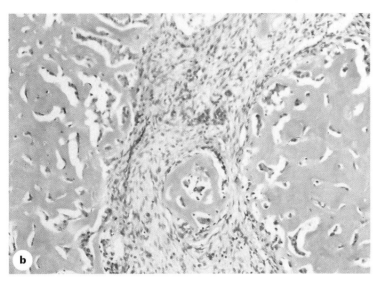

Fig. 16.23 Hepatoblastoma. (**a**) This tumor exhibits a mixture of the embryonal type (on the right) with the fetal histologic type (on the left).

(**b**) Osteoid (pinkish areas) is often observed.

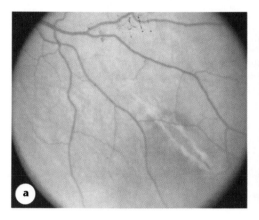

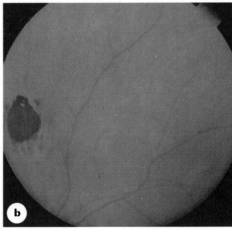

Fig. 16.24 Hepatoblastoma. Congenital hypertrophy of the retinal pigment epithelium (CHRP) is sometimes seen in patients with hepatoblastoma associated with familial polyposis coli. (**a**) The CHRP is seen as discoloration. (**b**) In another patient, the discoloration is more rounded. (Courtesy of Dr J. Garber MD, Dana-Farber Cancer Institute, Boston, MA.)

Table 16.4 IRSG presurgical staging classification

Stage	Sizes	Tumor III	Size	Node (N)	Metastasis (M)	
I	Orbit head and neck (excluding paramingeal) GU: non-bladder/non-prostate	T_1 or T_2	a or b	N_0 N_1, or b	N_x	M_o
II	Bladder/prostate, extremity, cranial, paramingeal, other (includes trunk, retroperitoneum, and so on)	T_1 or T_2	a	N_0 or N_x	M_o	
III	Bladder/prostate, extremity, cranial paramingeal, other (includes trunk, retroperitoneum, and so on)	T_1 or T_2	a	N_1	M_o	
			b	N_0, N_1, or N_x		
IV	All	T_1 or T_2	a or b	N_0 or N_1	M_1	

Tumor: T_1, confined to anatomic site of origin, (a) ≤ 5 cm in diameter in size, (b) > 5 cm in diameter in size; T_2 extension and/or fixative to surrounding tissue, (a) ≤ 5 cm in diameter in size, (b) >5 cm in diameter in size; regional nodes: N_a, regional nodes not clinically involved; N_1, regional nodes clinically involved by neoplasm; N_x clinical status of regional nodes unknown, metastasis: M_o, no distant metastasis; M_1, matastasis present. GU, genitourinary.

IRSG Postsurgical Grouping Classification	
Group 1	Localized disease, completely excersised, no microscopic residual
A	Confined to site of origin, completely resected
B	Infiltrating beyond site of origin, completely resected
Group 2	Total gross resection
A	Gross resection with evidence of micro scopic local residual
B	Regional disease with involved lymph nodes, completely resected with no microscopic residual
C	Microscopic local and/or nodal residual
Group 3	Incomplete resection or biopsy with gross residual
Group 4	Distant metastases

Fig. 16.25 IRSG post-surgical group classification.

Table 16.5 Patterns of clinical presentation in rhabdomyosarcoma

Location	Relative frequency (%)	Median age (years)	Histology
Head and neck	40	6	Embryonal > alveolar
Genitourinary	20	2–3	Embryonal
Extremity, trunk	30	12–20	Alveolar > embryonal

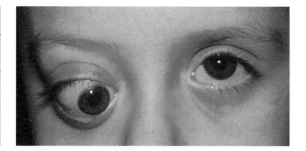

Fig. 16.26 Orbital rhabdomyosarcoma. This patient presented with unilateral proptosis of very recent onset. Often rhabdomyosarcoma develops rapidly and causes lid redness. It may be mistaken for orbital inflammation.

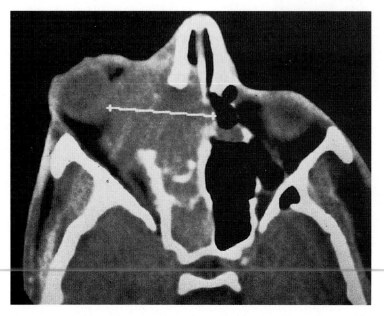

Fig. 16.27 Orbital rhabdomyosarcoma. CT scan at the level of the orbits in a patient who presented with marked unilateral proptosis shows extensive bone destruction with involvement of the ethmoid sinus.

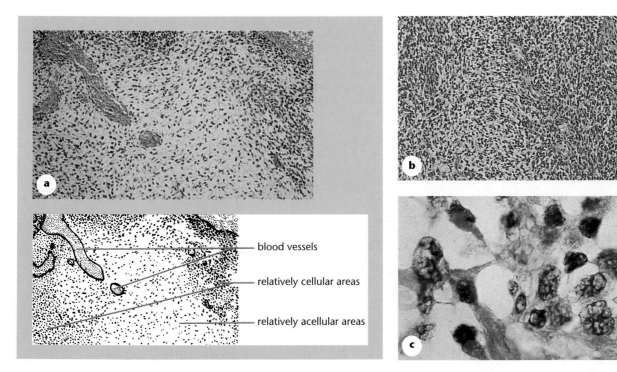

Fig. 16.28 Embryonal rhabdomyosarcoma. (**a**) Microscopy shows an embryonic cellular pattern. (**b**) Higher magnification reveals the primitive nature of the rhabdomyoblasts, which tend to cluster in groups, separated by relatively acellular areas. (**c**) Some rhabdomyoblasts exhibit characteristic cross-striations (arrow) in their cytoplasm.

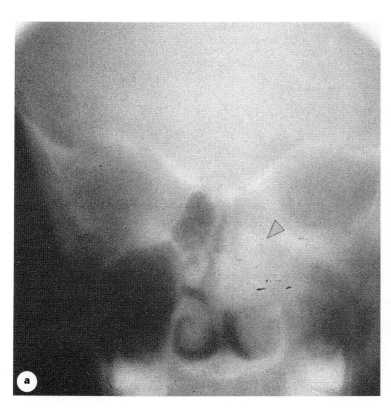

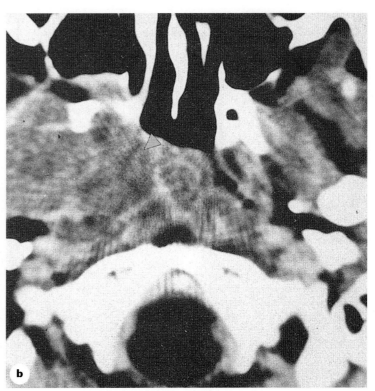

Fig. 16.29 Rhabdomyosarcoma. (**a**) Facial tomogram in a 7-year-old boy who presented with pain, swelling and inability to move the left eye laterally shows a soft tissue mass involving the left ethmoid sinus (arrow). (**b**) CT scan in a patient who presented with similar symptoms demonstrates extension of a tumor (arrow) to the base of the skull, with a significant amount of bone destruction. Such bone involvement is associated with increased risk of local recurrence.

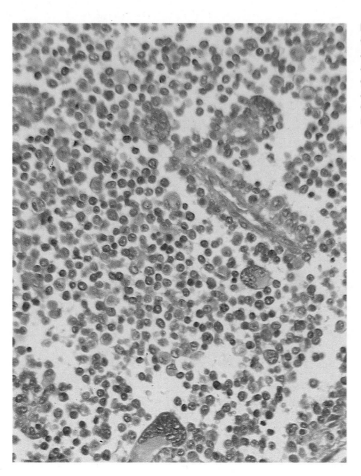

Fig. 16.30 Alveolar rhabdomyosarcoma. Characteristically, tumor cells are loosely attached to trabeculae or lie free within alveolar spaces. Occasional multinucleate giant cells are seen in this photograph and are a helpful diagnostic feature. Cross-striations are rare in this type of rhabdomyosarcoma.

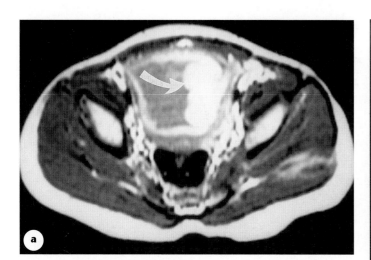

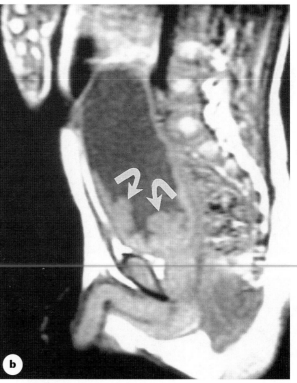

Fig. 16.31 Rhabdomyosarcoma (sarcoma botryoides). Axial (**a**) and sagittal (**b**) MR scans of a 2-year-old patient who presented with urinary obstruction. The tumor can be seen in the bladder with ball-like projections into the bladder space (arrows) as well as extension along the bladder wall. This extension usually occurs in the anatomic plane between the mucosa and the muscularis. The tumor was biopsied transurethrally during cystoscopy.

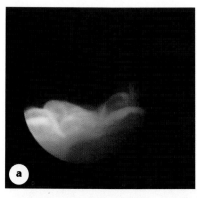

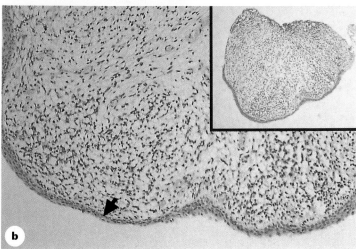

Fig. 16.32 Rhabdomyosarcoma (sarcoma botryoides). Cystoscopy (**a**) reveals the delicate, grape-like projections of tumor from the bladder wall. The pathologic section (**b**) further illustrates this process: the tumor cells push out from the bladder wall and are covered with a layer of normal mucosa (arrow). The most common site for botryoid sarcoma is the GU tract, but occasionally it presents in the gallbladder or bile duct.

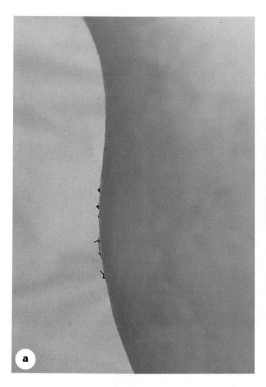

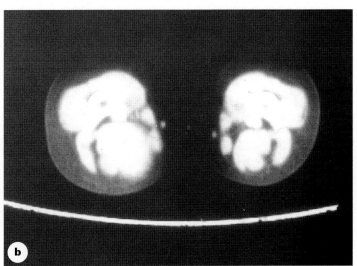

Fig. 16.33 Rhabdomyosarcoma. (**a**) A 2-year-old girl presented after her parents noticed a mass behind her right thigh, which is evident on CT scan (**b**). Most patients with extremity primary tumors are teenagers. Rhabdomyosarcomas at this location, as well as the trunk, carry a poorer prognosis than GU, orbital and head and neck tumors without extensive bone destruction. (Courtesy of Mark Gebhardt MD, Children's Hospital, Boston, MA.)

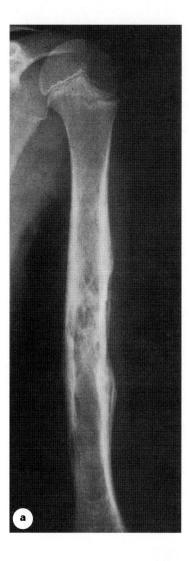

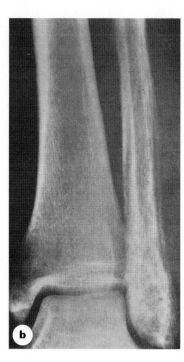

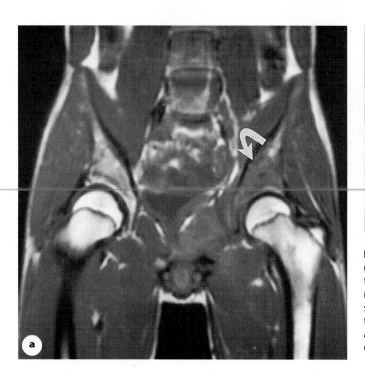

Fig. 16.34 Ewing's sarcoma/primitive neuroectodermal tumor (PNET). (**a**) The midshaft of long bones is a common site of occurrence, as illustrated here in the left humerus of a 9-year-old girl. Almost any bone in the body may be affected. (**b**) Ewing's sarcoma's classic radiographic appearance is marked by permeative bone destruction and a lamellated ('onion skinning') periosteal reaction. This 24-year-old man presented with an 8-week history of pain and swelling of his left ankle.

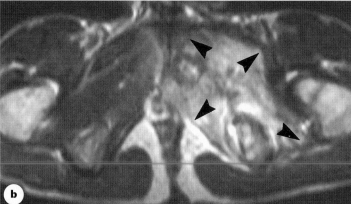

Fig. 16.35 Ewing's sarcoma/PNET. A 15-year-old developed pain in his hip. (**a**) The coronal T1-weighted MR shows dark marrow (arrow) in contrast to the bright marrow on the other side. The dark signal is due to marrow replacement with tumor. (**b**) The axial T2 MR demonstrates the typical large, soft tissue mass involving the ischium and the pubic bones as indicated by the bright signal of the tumor. Patients with pelvic primaries frequently have a long period of symptoms prior to diagnosis, since the tumor is often not evident on physical examination.

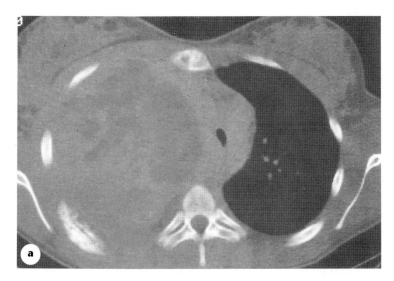

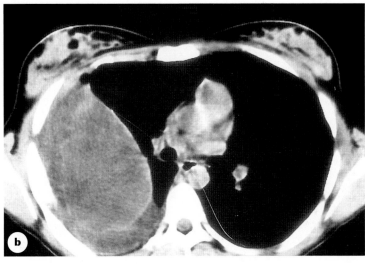

Fig. 16.36 Ewing's sarcoma/PNET (Askin tumor). A 17-year-old girl presented with weight loss and shortness of breath. (**a**) Chest CT scan reveals a massive tumor filling the right hemithorax and deviating the mediastinum to the left. Rib erosion can be seen posteriorly. (**b**) After two courses of chemotherapy, there was a dramatic response. After further shrinkage with drug therapy, the tumor was removed. The majority of the specimen showed necrosis, with only rare scattered areas of tumor remaining.

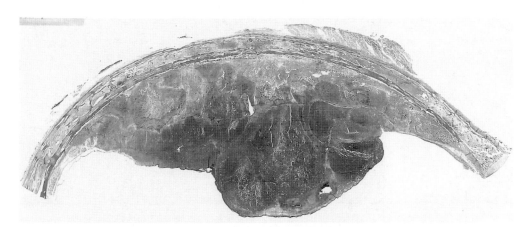

Fig. 16.37 Ewing's sarcoma/PNET. This giant histologic section shows another typical Ewing's family tumor adjacent to a rib. These lesions are commonly referred to as Askin's tumors. The bone may not be involved at all or only focally by the tumor. The tumor protrudes into the pleural cavity and may be associated with pleural fluid or pleural studding with metastases.

Fig. 16.38 PNET. (**a**) MR scan in a 12-year-old boy who presented with a mass lesion shows a soft tissue mass posterior to the spinous processes in the upper thoracic spine. Most paraspinal PNETs are deeper than this tumor, but its superficial nature allows for better appreciation of the excellent response to chemotherapy 9 weeks later (**b**).

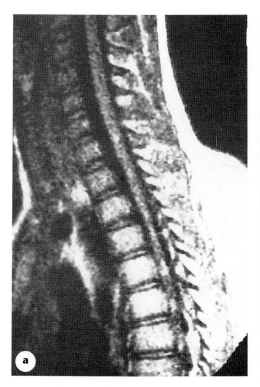

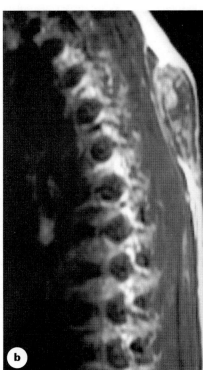

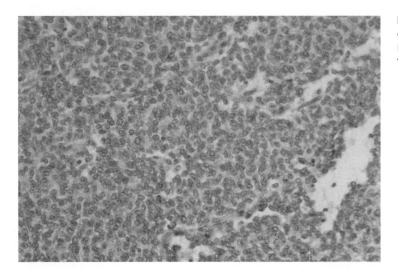

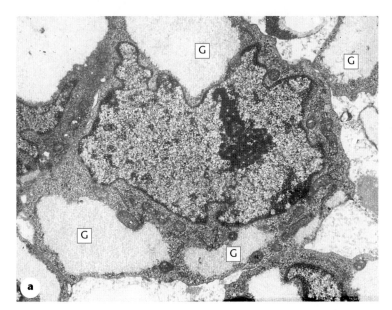

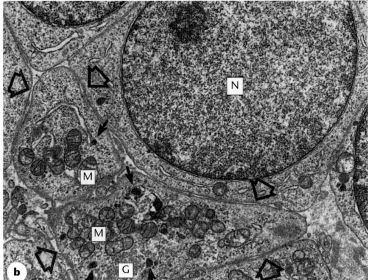

Fig. 16.39 Ewing's sarcoma/PNET. This tumor is marked by small, round blue cells. A capillary network gives a lobular pattern to the tumor. Poorly formed rosettes can be seen as in this slide. Demonstration of cytoplasmic glycogen with PAS staining (not shown) is common.

Fig. 16.40 Ewing's sarcoma/PNET. (**a**) Electron micrograph of a 'typical' Ewing's tumor shows large pools of cytoplasmic glycogen (G). (**b**) In contrast, the PNET variant tends toward neural differentiation. Neuritic processes (open arrows) contain mitochondria (m), dense-core granules (smaller arrows) and looser areas of glycogen (G). N, nucleus.

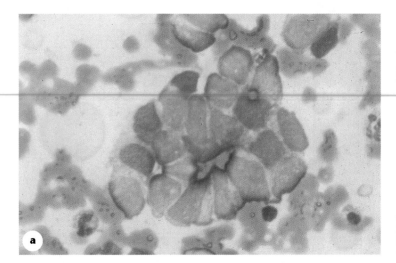

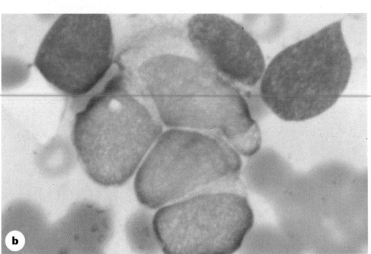

Fig. 16.41 Bone marrow metastases. (**a**) Low-power view of a bone marrow aspirate shows a clump of undifferentiated malignant cells. (**b**) Higher magnification reveals small blue cells with scanty cytoplasm and indistinct nucleoli. Unlike osteosarcoma, Ewing's sarcoma frequently spreads to bone marrow.

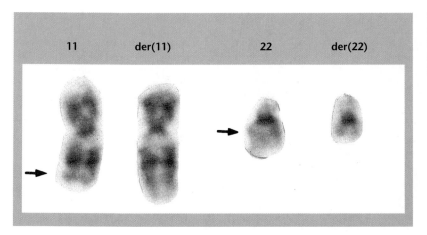

Fig. 16.42 PNET. This partial karyotype demonstrates the t(11;22) abnormally (arrows) seen in almost all cases of PNET and Ewing's sarcoma (*see also* Fig. 10.23). (Courtesy of Jonathan Fletcher MD, Dana–Farber Cancer Institute, Boston, MA.)

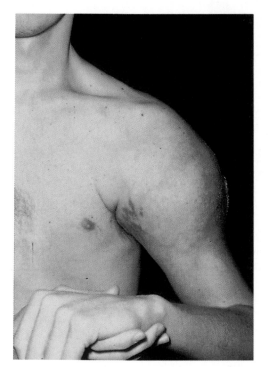

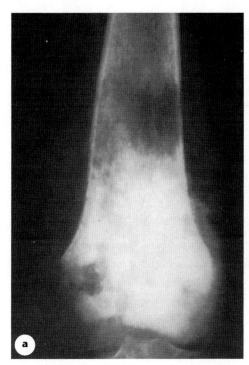

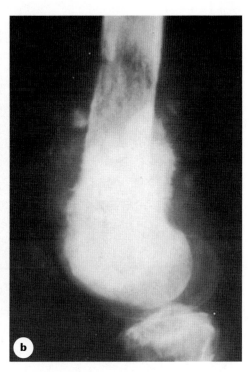

Fig. 16.43 Osteosarcoma. This 21-year-old man presented with a prominent soft tissue mass at the left proximal humerus. He first noted pain while at basic training and the mass followed a few weeks later. Proximal humoral malignancies can usually be treated with a limb-sparing operation. In this patient, however, chest wall involvement required a forequarter amputation. (Courtesy of Mark Gebhardt MD, Children's Hospital, Boston, MA.)

Fig. 16.44 Osteosarcoma. Anteroposterior (**a**) and lateral (**b**) plain films of the femur in a 19-year-old woman show a typically mixed lytic and sclerotic lesion with a periosteal reaction of the 'sunburst' type. A soft tissue mass containing tumor is quite evident, as is common with osteosarcoma. The distal femur is the most common site of occurrence.

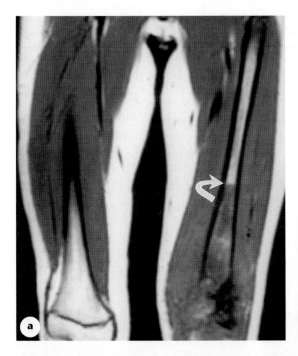
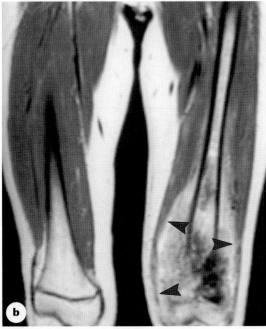

Fig. 16.45 Osteosarcoma. An 11-year-old boy presented with a mass of the distal femur. (**a**) T1-weighted coronal MRI shows the proximal extent of the tumor (curved arrow). (**b**) The gadolinium-enhanced T1 coronal MR shows the extent of the soft tissue mass (arrowheads). This patient eventually had a limb salvage operation after induction chemotherapy.

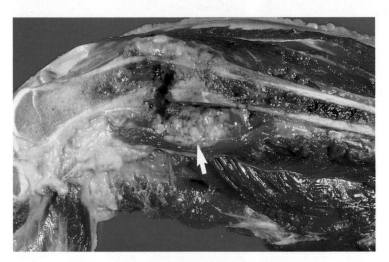

Fig. 16.46 Osteosarcoma. Sagittal section through the thigh shows a large metaphyseal mass with soft tissue extension (arrow). Note the pathologic fracture.

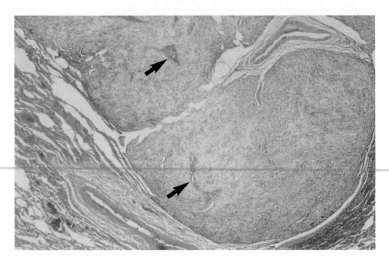

Fig. 16.47 Lung metastases. A photomicrograph of a pulmonary metastatic nodule compressing the lung parenchyma (periphery). Osteoid formation (arrows) is present within a sarcomatous stroma.

REFERENCES

Retinoblastoma

Eng C, Li FP, Abramson DH, *et al.*: Mortality from second tumors among long-term survivors of retinoblastoma. J Natl Cancer Inst 1993; 85 : 1121–1128.

Friend SH, Bernards R, Rogelj S, *et al.*: A human DNA segment with properties of the gene that predisposes to retinoblastoma and osteosarcoma. Nature 1986: 323 : 643–646.

Garber JE, Diller L: Screening children at genetic risk of cancer. Curr Opin Pediatr 1989; 5 : 712–715.

Kaste S, Jenkins J, Pratt C, *et al.*: Retinoblastoma: sonographic findings with pathologic correlation in pediatric patients. A J Roentgenol 2000; 175: 495–501.

Wetzig P: Fluorescein photography in the differential diagnosis of retinoblastoma. Am J Ophthalmol 1966; 61: 341–343.

Yandell DW, Campbell TA, Dayton SH, *et al.*: Oncogenic point mutations in the human retinoblastoma gene: their application to genetic counseling. N Engl J Med 1989; 321: 1689–1695.

Wilms' tumor

Bardeesy N, Beckwith J, Pelletier J: Clonal expansion and attenuated apoptosis in Wilms' tumors are associated with p53 gene mutations. Cancer Res 1995; 55 : 215–219.

Bonadio JF, Storer B, Norkool P, *et al.*: Anaplastic Wilms' tumor: Clinical and pathologic studies. J Clin Oncol 1985; 3 : 513–520.

Coppes MJ, Haber DA, Grundy PE: Genetic events in the development of Wilms' tumor. N Engl J Med 1994; 331 : 586–590.

D'Angio GJ, Breslow NE, Beckwith JB, *et al.*: Results of the third National Wilms' Tumor Study. Cancer 1989; 64 : 349–360.

Green DM: The treatment of children with unilateral Wilms' tumor (editorial). J Clin Oncol 1993; 1 : 1009–1010.

Tournade MF, Cam-Nougue C, Voute PA, *et al.*: Results of the sixth International Society of Pediatric Oncology Wilms' tumor trial and study: a risk-adapted therapeutic approach in Wilms' tumor. J Clin Oncol 1993; 11 : 1014–1023.

Neuroblastoma

Brodeur GM, Pritchard J, Berthold F, *et al.*: Revisions of the international criteria for neuroblastoma diagnosis, staging, and response to treatment. J Clin Oncol 1993; 11 : 1466–1477.

Castleberry R, Pritchard J, Ambros P, *et al.*: The International Neuroblastoma Risk Group (INRG): a preliminary report. Eur J Cancer 1997; 33: 2113–2116.

Look, AT, Hayes FA, Shuster JJ, *et al.*: Clinical relevance of tumor cell ploidy and n-*myc* gene amplification in childhood neuroblastoma: a Pediatric Oncology Group study. J Clin Oncol 1991; 9 : 581–591.

Nitschke R, Smith EI, Shochat S, *et al.*: Localized neuroblastoma treated by surgery: a Pediatric Oncology Group study. J Clin Oncol 1988; 6 : 1271–1279.

Philip T, Bernard JL, Zucker JM, *et al.*: High dose chemoradiotherapy with bone marrow transplantation as consolidation treatment in neuroblastoma: an unselected group of stage IV patients over 1 year of age. J Clin Oncol 1987; 5 : 266–271.

Seeger RC, Brodeur GM, Sather H, *et al.*: Association of multiple copies of the N-*myc* oncogene with rapid progression of neuroblastomas. N Engl J Med 1985; 313 : 1111–1116.

Hepatic tumors

Douglass EC, Reynolds M, Finegold M, *et al.*: Cisplatin, vincristine, and fluorouracil therapy for hepatoblastoma: a Pediatric Oncology Group study. J Clin Oncol 1993; 11 : 96–99.

Haliloglu M, Hoffer F, Gronemeyer S, *et al.*: 3D gadolinium-enhanced MRA: evaluation of hepatic vasculature in children with hepatoblastoma. J Magnet Res Imag 2000; 11: 65–68.

Ikeda H, Matsuyama S, Tanimura M: Association between hepatoblastoma and very low birth weight: a trend or a chance? J Pediatr 1997; 130: 557–560.

Lack EE, Neave C, Vawter GF: Hepatocellular carcinoma. Review of 32 cases in childhood and adolescence. Cancer 1983; 52 : 1510–1515.

Ortega JA, Krailo MD, Haas JE, *et al.*: Effective treatment of unresectable or metastatic hepatoblastoma with cisplatin and continuous infusion doxorubicin chemotherapy: a report from the Children's Cancer Study Group. J Clin Oncol 1991; 9 : 2167–2176.

Weinberg AG, Finegold NJ: Primary hepatic tumors of childhood. Hum Pathol 1983; 14 : 512–537.

Rhabdomyosarcoma

Barr FG, Chatten J, D'Cruz C, *et al.*: Molecular assays for chromosomal translocations in the diagnosis of pediatric soft tissue sarcomas. JAMA 1995; 273 : 553–557.

Maurer HM, Gehan EA, Beltangady M, *et al.*: The Intergroup Rhabdomyosarcoma Study II. Cancer 1993; 71 : 1904–1922.

Pappo AS, Shapiro DN, Crist WM, *et al.*: Biology and therapy of pediatric rhabdomyosarcoma. J Clin Oncol 1995; 13 : 2123–2139.

Pizzo PA, Triche TJ: Clinical staging in rhabdomyosarcoma: current limitations and future prospects (editorial). J Clin Oncol 1987; 5 : 8–9.

Ewing's family of tumors: Ewing's sarcoma and PNET

Delattre O, Zucman J, Melot T, *et al.*: The Ewing family of tumors – a subgroup of small round cell tumors defined by specific chimeric transcripts. N Engl Med 1994; 331 : 294–299.

Dunst J, Sauer R, Burgers JMV, *et al.*: Radiation therapy as local treatment in Ewing's sarcoma: results of the Cooperative Ewing's Sarcoma Studies CESS-81 and CESS-86. Cancer 1991; 67 : 2818–2825.

Pearlman E, Dickman PS, Askin FB, *et al.*: Ewing's sarcoma: routine diagnostic utilization of MIC2 analysis. Hum Pathol 1994; 25 : 304–307.

Shamberger RC, Tarbell NJ, Perez-Atayade AR, Grier HE: Malignant small round cell tumor (Ewings-PNET) of the chest wall in children. J Pediatr Surg 1994; 29 : 179–185.

Osteosarcoma

Goorin AM, Abelson HT, Frei E: Osteosarcoma: fifteen years later. N Engl J Med 1985; 313: 1637–1643.

Link MP, Goorin AM, Miser AW, *et al.*: The effect of adjuvant chemotherapy on relapse-free survival in patients with osteosarcoma of the extremity. N Engl J Med 1986; 314 : 1600–1606.

Look AT, Douglass EC, Meyer WH: Clinical importance of near-diploid tumor stem lines in patients with osteosarcoma of an extremity. N Engl J Med 1988; 318 : 1567–1572.

Meyers PA, Heller G, Healey JH, *et al.*: Osteogenic sarcoma with clinically detectable metastasis at initial presentation. J Clin Oncol 1993; 11 : 449–453.

17 AIDS-associated malignancies

David T. Scadden

The AIDS epidemic is now in its third decade and it is estimated that the number of people infected with the human immunodeficiency virus-1 (HIV) in the United States is 750 000, with over 36 million individuals infected worldwide. Since early in the HIV epidemic, it has been recognized that certain tumors occur with increased frequency in the setting of HIV-induced immunosuppression. These include most prominently Kaposi's sarcoma (KS), B-cell non-Hodgkin's lymphoma (NHL) and anogenital neoplasia. Less common, but also of increased frequency compared with the general population, are Hodgkin's disease and, in children, leiomyosarcomas. The advent of highly active antiretroviral therapy (HAART) has dramatically reduced the morbidity and mortality of HIV-infected individuals with access to such medications. Oncologic complications are among those markedly reduced in the era of better viral control, though the impact has not been uniform across neoplasms.

PATHOGENESIS OF AIDS-RELATED NEOPLASMS

A number of possible contributing pathophysiologic mechanisms may participate in the predisposition to neoplasms in the setting of immune deficiency, including altered immune activation, dysregulated cytokine production and inadequate control of secondary, oncogenic pathogens.

Organ transplant data indicate that the risk of tumor development increases with specific types of transplants, probably due to the intensity of immunosuppressive therapy given for specific transplanted organs (see Table 17.1). However, there are also data suggesting that immune activation may contribute to the emergence of lymphoid neoplasms. For example, there is an increased incidence in autoimmune diseases such as Sjogren's syndrome. It is therefore likely that proliferative stimuli and disordered immune regulation combine to enhance tumorigenesis.

Perturbations in the tissue cytokine milieu may provide the specific signals altering the control of cellular proliferation in tumors of immune suppression. KS serves as an example of this as KS cells, unlike normal mesenchymal cells, both secrete interleukin-6 (IL-6) and have a proliferative response to IL-6 in an autocrine fashion. Similarly, some AIDS-lymphoma cells appear to produce interleukin-10 and their growth rate is affected by it. These events may not be sufficient for tumor generation but provide the proliferative background against which transforming events may occur.

In addition, inadequate host immunologic responses to infectious agents such as EBV or human papilloma virus (HPV) may result in tumor development such as in EBV-driven lymphoproliferation seen after organ transplantation and in some AIDS-related lymphomas. The geographic clustering of KS and its association with specific sexual practices strongly supported the possibility of a secondary infectious process which has been subsequently identified as human herpesvirus-8 or Kaposi's sarcoma herpesvirus (KSHV), a member of the γ herpesvirus family. The role for immune control of KSHV and EBV in oncogenesis is now strongly supported by evidence that improved immune function with HAART dramatically reduces KSHV- and EBV-related tumors. Notably, however, data regarding the impact of HAART on HPV-related tumors are less clear and it is not yet known to what extent improved immune function will affect anogenital neoplasia. What is clear is that HIV itself does not play a direct role in tumor generation. Other than in very rare cases of T-cell lymphoma, HIV is not detectable in HIV-related malignancies. HIV provides the immunologic dysfunction permissive of tumor emergence. These tumors may be regarded as opportunistic neoplasms in much the same way as specific infections are regarded as opportunistic in the immunocompromised host.

KAPOSI'S SARCOMA

Kaposi's sarcoma is believed to arise from mesodermally derived cells, the exact nature of which remains controversial. Histologically these lesions are composed of multiple cell types, including smooth muscle, endothelial and immune cells. The histologic picture raises the unanswered question of whether this disease represents a true malignancy or is the result of dysregulated proliferation of otherwise normal cells in response to an abnormal signal. Efforts to define clonality in lesions have conflicting results, showing that clonal disease may evolve, but polyclonality is common. The abnormal drive for cell proliferation may be due to products of KSHV itself such as a constitutively active G-protein coupled receptor the virus encodes. In addition, the HIV gene product, *tat*, may induce enhanced proliferation, possibly accounting for the extraordinary predilection for KS seen in HIV-infected individuals above that of other immunosuppressed populations. The epidemiology of KS is outlined in Figures 17.1 and 17.2.

KS lesions occur clinically in the skin, on mucosal surfaces and in lymph nodes and involve solid organs, most commonly the lung and gastrointestinal tract. Cutaneous manifestations vary from erythematous, macular lesions to raised, nodular masses with a violaceous hue. Large plaque-like lesions may develop when clusters of tumors coalesce and central necrosis can occur. KS tends to appear at multiple sites concurrently, with no ordered pattern of spread. An important differential diagnosis is bacillary angiomatosis, which is an infectious disease occurring in HIV patients caused by *Bartonella* organisms. Also, cutaneous *Pneumocystis carinii* infection has been reported to cause an erythematous lesion resembling KS. Thus biopsy of clinically suspected KS lesions is recommended at the time of first clinical presentation.

Mucosal involvement by KS may occur in the oral cavity, conjunctiva or more rarely the urethral meatus and may result in local discomfort. Cutaneous lesions, however, are mostly of cosmetic significance and their successful treatment can overcome a major source of distress in affected patients. Approximately one-half of patients with mucocutaneous disease will also have KS involving other organs. While skin disease usually accompanies organ involvement, up to 15% of patients have been reported to have lymph node, GI or lung KS without skin manifestations.

Pulmonary KS may involve the large airways, the interstitium, alveoli or pleural surfaces and the clinical features vary accordingly. Patients may complain of dyspnea, cough, hemoptysis or wheezing, but the disease is often asymptomatic. When parenchymal involvement is extensive, it may be life threatening, prompting most clinicians to treat aggressively with chemotherapy those patients in whom infiltrates on chest X-ray are thought to be due to KS. GI tract lesions are generally asymptomatic but may result in non-specific symptoms such as abdominal pain and bloating. These lesions may be the cause of minor chronic blood loss, but massive hemorrhage is uncommon.

Finally, KS can involve lymph nodes and local lymphatics, causing marked local edema. This is exacerbated by the increased permeability of the vascular component of KS and by a permeability factor elaborated by KS cells, vascular endothelial growth factor (VEGF). Edema is commonly seen in the groin, distal lower extremities or head and neck regions and is a major cause of morbidity. It is the most common cause of symptoms from KS and is generally regarded by us as an indication to proceed with a more aggressive treatment approach. A system for clinically staging KS is outlined in Table 17.2.

NON-HODGKIN'S LYMPHOMA

The increased incidence of NHL in AIDS patients was first noted in 1984 and became recognized as an AIDS-defining illness in 1987. The estimated incidence of NHL in patients ranges from 1.6% to 2.0% per year with patients from all HIV risk groups being susceptible to the disease. It is likely that HIV lymphoma is at least partially responsible for the 60% increase in NHL that has occurred in the US since 1976.

The pathogenesis of AIDS-lymphoma is related to underlying immune dysfunction, with possible participation of co-infecting organisms such as EBV or the effects of cytokines acting in an abnormal fashion. There is a clear link between EBV and CNS lymphoma in the HIV population, but association with the virus in systemic AIDS-lymphoma is less clear. Large cell or immunoblastic lymphomas are associated with EBV in up to 75% of cases and in virtually all CNS lymphomas, while small non-cleaved cell or Burkitt-like lymphomas are EBV associated in only 20–35%. The pattern of EBV expression differs from that in lymphomas following transplant. In systemic AIDS lymphomas a unique combination of Epstein–Barr nuclear antigen (EBNA)-1 and latent membrane protein (LMP)-1 expression occurs. In post-transplant patients and primary CNS AIDS lymphomas, EBNA-2–5 are expressed along with LMP-1 and -2. Transplant-related neoplasms may regress upon withdrawal of administered immunosuppressive agents or occasionally with antiviral therapy. However, this is not the case in AIDS where tumor regression is rare even in the face of improved immune function with HAART.

A number of genetic abnormalities have been found in AIDS-NHL. Rearrangements of the c-*myc* proto-oncogene located on chromosome 8 with the immunoglobulin genes situated on chromosomes 14 and 2 are the commonest mutations noted, with a frequency of 23–79%. The rearrangement occurs in the mature B-cell in which immunoglobulin gene rearrangement has already occurred. The resultant juxtaposition of the c-*myc* and immunoglobulin genes may

play a central role in the transformation of cells bearing this molecular translocation. Other oncogene mutations that occur less frequently than that involving c-*myc* include abnormalities of the *p53* tumor suppressor gene and the ras oncogene.

Histologically, AIDS-lymphomas are B-cell intermediate or high-grade tumors demonstrating very aggressive clinical behavior. Rarely, T-cell malignancies such as large granular lymphoproliferative disease, Sézary syndrome or angiocentric immunoblastic lymphadenopathy are encountered in HIV-infected patients. In some cases, these rare T-cell malignancies have been demonstrated to harbor HIV, some of which have integrated into the host genome resulting in a transforming mutation.

The clinical features of AIDS-NHL are similar to those of aggressive lymphomas in general. Of note, however, is the high proportion of patients with 'B' symptoms, i.e. weight loss, fevers and night sweats. Patients presenting with such symptoms should have a thorough microbiologic evaluation to exclude bacterial, viral, fungal or parasitic disease. Advanced-stage disease and extranodal sites of involvement are the rule in AIDS-lymphoma (*see* Fig. 17.3). Sites of disease may vary with histologic types; for example, large cell tumors have a predilection for the GI tract and CNS while small non-cleaved (Burkitt or Burkitt-like) tumors often involve the bone marrow.

Prognosis has been shown to be closely linked to the status of the immunodeficiency (as indicated by CD4 count and prior AIDS diagnosis) as well as tumor-related factors. The international prognostic index has not been extensively evaluated in AIDS-related lymphoma, but limited data suggest that it will be useful. However, the status of HIV disease itself must always be kept in mind, as prognosis and tolerance of therapy are different for patients with advanced AIDS failing antiretrovirals compared with those tolerating and benefiting from HAART.

Primary CNS lymphoma is an important subgroup of HIV-associated lymphoma and comprises 15–20% of all AIDS-NHL. It tends to occur in patients with more advanced immunosuppression; one study demonstrated a mean CD4 count of 30 cells/mm^3 in primary CNS lymphoma vs 190 cells/mm^3 in patients with systemic NHL. Primary CNS lymphoma in AIDS resembles transplant lymphoma in that it is of immunoblastic histology and is virtually always associated with the EBV genome (*see* Table 17.3). This is in contrast to systemic HIV-lymphoma, which differs from lymphoma developing in patients who are immunocompromised for other reasons (*see* Table 17.4). This subset of HIV-associated lymphomas has substantially declined in the era of HAART. The improved immune function associated with more effective control of HIV likely accounts for the decrease in patients with this devastating complication. Clinical presentation is with neurologic symptoms which may be as vague as subtle personality changes with a CNS mass lesion found by radiographic imaging studies. In AIDS patients, lymphoma needs to be distinguished from toxoplasma or other infectious brain abscess and progressive multifocal leukoencephalopathy. Certain radiologic criteria are useful in differentiating lymphoma from toxoplasma lesions: NHL is typically located centrally, is often larger than 2 cm and may cross the midline, while converse features may suggest toxoplasmosis. Brain biopsy is required to establish a definitive diagnosis, but the presence of EBV by cerebrospinal fluid PCR strongly supports a lymphoma diagnosis and has a sensitivity and specificity of greater than 90% in patients with a negative toxoplasma titre who have been on trimethoprim-sulfa prophylaxis. For those in whom ambiguity remains, a therapeutic trial of anti-toxoplasma therapy may be useful as a majority of patients with toxoplasma infection will respond within 2 weeks.

Certain aspects of the management of systemic AIDS-lymphoma require special consideration. First, the CNS should be examined carefully with radiologic scanning and cytologic analysis of the cerebrospinal fluid (CSF) due to the high incidence of CNS involvement by these lymphomas. Many centers administer intrathecal chemotherapy to prevent CNS relapse even if there is no evidence of disease in the CSF initially. A recent study suggests that the presence of EBV in the primary tumor is highly associated with CNS involvement and may be useful in discriminating those patients who most benefit from prophylactic therapy to the CNS. Patients with B symptoms must be evaluated to exclude coincident HIV-related infections which can cause symptoms such as fever and weight loss and which would require a different treatment approach. In general, patients should receive prophylaxis for *Pneumocystis carinii* infection while undergoing chemotherapy. During treatment of lymphoma in the HIV population, the physician should be particularly wary of the myelotoxic effects of chemotherapy as these may be compounded by the concomitant administration of drugs for *Pneumocystis carinii* prophylaxis (trimethoprim-sulfamethoxazole) as well as by antiretroviral agents (zidovudine). Granulocyte colony-stimulating factor (G-CSF) and granulocyte macrophage colony stimulating factor (GM-CSF) have been useful in mitigating neutropenia in this setting.

Treatment of systemic disease is usually with standard combination chemotherapy regimens such as CHOP, which have yielded response rates of 50–70% with some patients achieving a durable long-term remission. Lower dose regimens have been tested in comparison to full-dose regimens with comparable results; however, these studies were conducted prior to the availability of HAART and the low-dose regimens should probably be reserved for those patients with advanced AIDS who have failed antiretroviral therapy. Chemotherapy regimens using continuous infusion schedules have been very encouraging and, if confirmed in larger studies, may herald a new approach to these patients. Trials assessing the benefit of combined monoclonal antibody therapy plus chemotherapy are in progress. For those individuals failing initial therapy, a standard salvage regimen has not been defined. Ongoing studies are testing the use of stem cell transplantation in this disease though participation in studies at centers with particular expertise in this patient population is recommended.

Treatment of CNS lymphoma is generally limited to radiation therapy and corticosteroids although high-dose methotrexate has also been useful. Combination chemotherapy and radiation therapy appears to add little beyond toxicity. The overall prognosis in this group of patients is grim, with survival estimated to be 2–5 months limited approximately equally by recurrent lymphoma and other complications of AIDS.

HODGKIN'S DISEASE

Hodgkin's disease occurs more frequently in AIDS patients than in the general population, but of a magnitude less pronounced than NHL (an approximately fivefold increase compared with a 60-fold increase for NHL). The subtypes of disease are also different in the context of HIV infection with the mixed cellularity histologic subtype seen more commonly. Presentation is usually with advanced stage disease – 82% of cases having stage III or IV disease at diagnosis. There is a propensity for extranodal and bone marrow involvement with 67% and 48% respectively in one series. Treatment consists of standard Hodgkin's disease approaches based on stage with durable remissions well documented. As with the care of any malignancy in HIV disease the vigor with which a curative strategy is pursued should be tempered by the status of the HIV infection itself. Individuals with end-stage AIDS who have failed all available antiretroviral therapy may be better approached with a palliative intent. Chemotherapy regimens such as ABVD may require additional supportive measures and attention must be paid to the prevention and treatment of opportunistic infections.

SQUAMOUS EPITHELIAL LESIONS

Anal intraepithelial neoplasia and invasive squamous cell cancer are increased among men who have sex with men. The additional risk imposed by HIV infection is substantial for dysplasia, though the impact on frank invasive cancer is more ambiguous. Similarly, dysplasia of the uterine cervix is increased in HIV-infected women, though a substantial increase in invasive cervical cancer has not been detected in most studies. Whether more lengthy follow-up of patients on HAART will reveal the emergence of an increased frequency of squamous cell cancer is not known, but certainly of concern. Anogenital squamous cell neoplasia in the setting of HIV disease is highly linked to human papilloma virus (HPV) infection with known oncogenic serotypes. The ability to intervene to eradicate HPV is extremely limited at this time. Therefore, therapeutic strategies aimed at this disease are focused on discerning whether cancer is present and, if so, undertaking definitive therapy. For women, the guidelines for treating cervical dysplasia and cancer outside the context of HIV disease are those generally applied. Additional vigilance in screening and following women with HIV infection for the presence of high-grade dysplasia, recurrent dysplasia or frank cancer is warranted. For anal and perianal dysplasia, the therapeutic options are less clear and therefore guidelines for treatment not well established and screening quite controversial. At present, patients with dysplasia on the anal verge may benefit from topical therapy with agents such as imiquimod and lesions in the anal canal from local therapies with cryo- or laser surgery. For patients with invasive anal cancer, the combination of chemotherapy and radiation therapy is recommended and can result in long-term elimination of the disease.

Occurring in the Mediterranean basin – generally elderly males often with immunologic abnormalities

Occurring in Central Africa – male predominance, antedated the HIV epidemic

Post-transplant on immunosuppressive drugs

HIV-related – 20,000-fold increased incidence over the general population

Fig. 17.1 Epidemiology of Kaposi's sarcoma.

Table 17.1 Incidence of post-transplant lymphoproliferative disorders based on data using historic immunosuppression regimens. Incidence figures would be expected to be lower using current protocols.

Transplant type	Incidence (%)
Renal	1.0
Heart	1.8
Liver	2.2
Heart and lung	5.0
Bone marrow (BM)	<1.0
T cell-depleted BM	12.0
Mismatched, T cell-depleted BM	24.0

Predominantly in homosexual/bisexual risk group for HIV

Incidence in HIV-positive homosexual males is 15-20% (decreased from 48% in 1981 pre-HAART*; much reduced (<5% on HAART)

Associated with infection by human herpesvirus 8 (HHV-8), also know as Kaposi's sarcoma herpesvirus (KSHV)

*HAART, highly active antiretroviral therapy

Fig. 17.2 HIV-associated Kaposi's sarcoma.

Table 17.2 Staging system (TIS) for HIV-associated Kaposi's sarcoma.

	Good risk (all of the following)	Poor risk (any of the following)
Tumor (T)	Confined to skin and/or lymph nodes and/or minimal oral disease	Tumor-associated edema or ulceration Extensive KS Gastrointestinal disease Other visceral involvement.
Immune system (I)	CD4 > 200 cells/μl	CD4 < 200 cells/μL
Systemic Illness (S)	No opportunistic infections or thrush (candida) No 'B' symptoms Karnofsky score > 70%	History of or current opportunistic infection or thrush 'B' symptoms Karnofsky score < 70% Other HIV-related illness (CMV, PCP, MAI, PML)

CMV, cytomegalovirus; PCP, *Pneumocystis carinii*; PML, progressive multifocal leukoencephalopathy; MAI; *Mycobacterium ovium-introcellulare*

Histology

Small noncleaved cell (Burkitt-like)	(36%)
Immunoblastic	(21%)
Diffuse large cell	(24%)
Other type	(9%)

Stage at presentation

I, II	(27%)
III, IV	(73%)

Extranodal sites

CNS	(23%)
Bone marrow	(23%)
GI Tract	(21%)
Liver	(18%)

Fig. 17.3 HIV-associated non-Hodgkin's lymphoma.

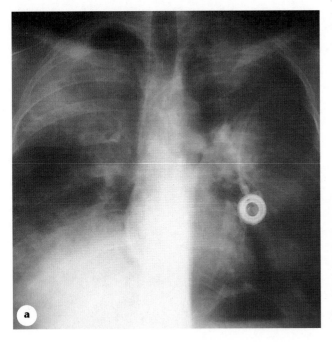

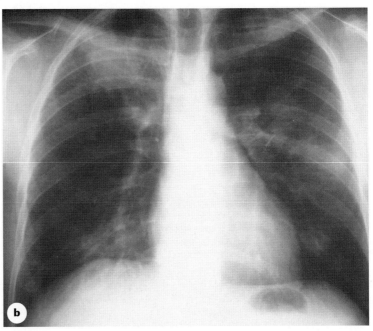

Fig. 17.4 Pulmonary Kaposi's sarcoma (KS). (**a**) A 28-year-old patient with known HIV infection developed progressive shortness of breath, cough and hemoptysis. Evaluation for an infectious etiology as the basis for the multiple infiltrates was negative. Bronchoscopy revealed multiple endobronchial KS lesions and a gallium-67 citrate scan was negative (characteristic of KS, but not infection). Treatment with chemotherapy initially resulted in resolution of his respiratory symptoms and improvement of his chest X-ray. (**b**) However, 6 months later new infections interrupted his KS therapy. He developed progressive respiratory compromise, worsening of the KS infiltrates and new pleural effusions.

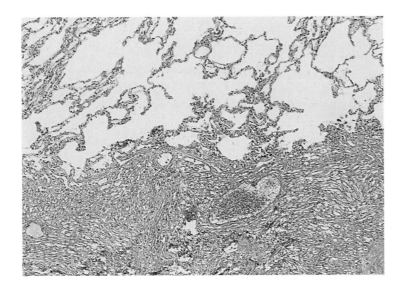

Fig. 17.5 Pulmonary Kaposi's sarcoma. A 27-year-old graduate student with a history of asthma presented with progressive dyspnea on exertion unresponsive to antiasthma medications and a declining DLCO. Chest X-ray revealed patchy areas of consolidation (not shown). Thoracoscopic biopsy revealed KS adjacent to normal lung parenchyma. Low-power microscopic view shows infiltration of the lung by a spindle cell neoplasm with large and small thin-walled vascular spaces. With ongoing chemotherapy the patient became oxygen independent with no respiratory symptoms 1 year following diagnosis. He had no mucocutaneous KS when he initially presented, a situation that may occur in up to 20% of patients with pulmonary KS. (Courtesy of Dr Bradford Sherburne.)

Table 17.3 Primary CNS and systemic HIV lymphoma. (Adapted from Levine, 1996)

	Primary CNS	Systemic
CD4 (cells/µl)	~30	~189
Prior AIDS	~73%	~37%
Immunoblastic histology	~100%	18–43%
EBV genome detected	~100%	38–68%
Median survival	2–5 months	4–7 months

Table 17.4 Features of lymphoma in immunosuppressed patients. SNCC, small non-cleaved cell (Burkitt-like).

Feature	Organ transplantation patients	AIDS patients
EBV GENOME	–100%	38–68%
SNCC histology	~1%	36%
myc translocation	not reported	30–80%

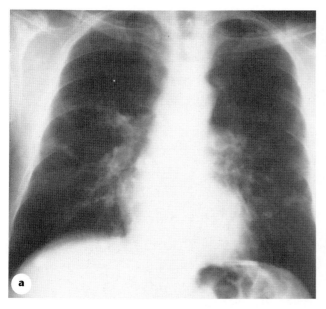

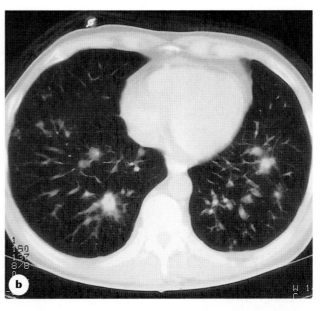

Fig. 17.6 Pulmonary Kaposi's sarcoma. A 41-year-old man previously diagnosed with cutaneous KS developed persistent cough without fever. Chest X-ray revealed hilar fullness and parenchymal nodules (**a**) more clearly defined on chest CT scan (**b**). This radiographic appearance is common for pulmonary KS.

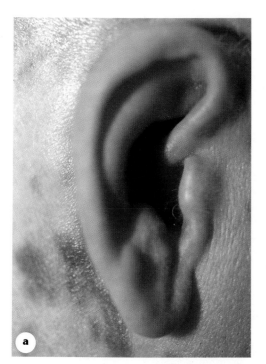

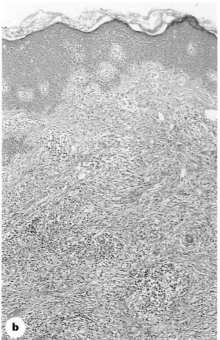

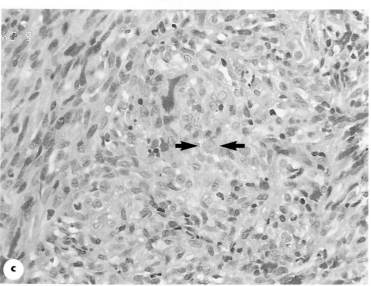

Fig. 17.7 Cutaneous Kaposi's sarcoma. (**a**) Typical appearance of cutaneous KS with irregularly shaped, macular papular lesions of erythematous or violaceous hue. There is often a surrounding halo of pigment representing the breakdown of heme pigments from red cells that diapedese into KS lesions. (**b**) Skin punch biopsy from an erythematous macule reveals a dermal infiltrate of spindle cells forming vascular arrays expanding the reticular dermis (× 40). This is a characteristic appearance of KS in the skin. (**c**) A higher-magnification view (× 100) of the biopsy specimen in (**b**) reveals spindle cell vascular channels with enlarged 'boxcar nuclei' in parallel bundles arranged haphazardly. These are interspersed between scattered mononuclear inflammatory cell infiltrates. In the center there are eosinophilic cytoplasmic droplets characteristic of KS (arrows). (Courtesy of Dr Steven Tahan.)

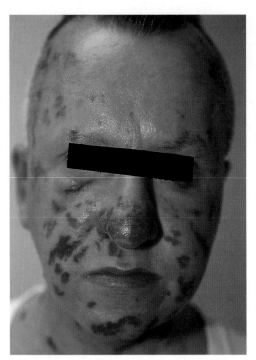

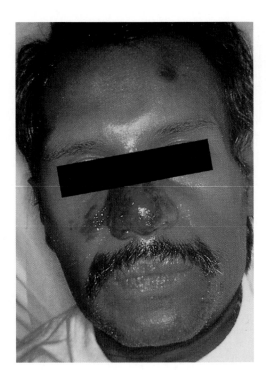

Fig. 17.8 Cutaneous Kaposi's sarcoma. The marked disfigurement evident in this photograph demonstrates why patients with only cutaneous involvement may seek aggressive therapy. This 32-year-old clerk also has evidence of early periorbital edema.

Fig. 17.9 Cutaneous Kaposi's sarcoma. Facial KS often has a predilection for the nose. In this 26-year-old male this resulted in marked edema of the nose and eventual sloughing of the overlying skin. The latter is a rare complication.

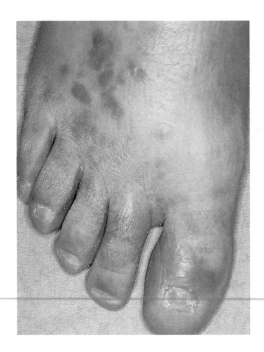

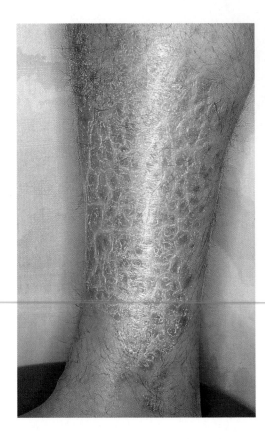

Fig. 17.10 Cutaneous Kaposi's sarcoma. Involvement of the skin can often result in local edema. In this patient, painful swelling of the first two digits occurred from cutaneous involvement.

Fig. 17.11 Cutaneous Kaposi's sarcoma. Extensive KS can become consolidated and can result in marked local edema. This is particularly true in the lower extremity – as evident in this photograph – often resulting in joint stiffness and discomfort limiting mobility.

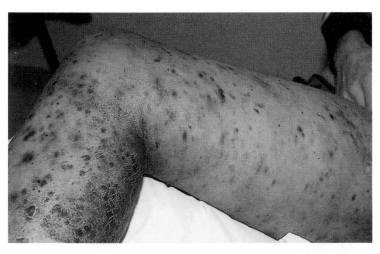

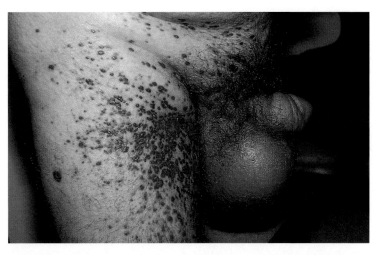

Fig. 17.12 Cutaneous Kaposi's sarcoma. Massive edema from presumed lymph node involvement can accompany local skin involvement. This 28-year-old male developed complete immobility of his right lower extremity that confined him to bed despite aggressive treatment.

Fig. 17.13 Cutaneous Kaposi's sarcoma. Edema of the lower extremities, peripubic area, genitalia and face is common in advanced KS. This can often result in extreme discomfort and immobility. This patient had complete resolution of genital and peripubic edema with systemic chemotherapy. Remaining woody edema of the upper thigh did not compromise the mobility of his leg function and he was able to continue his career for 9 months after beginning chemotherapy.

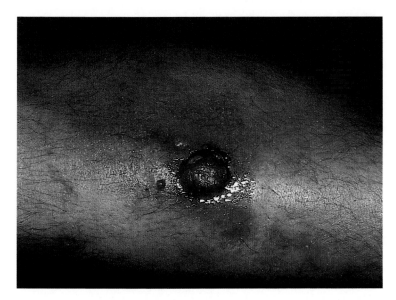

Fig. 17.14 Cutaneous Kaposi's sarcoma. Extensive KS can occasionally ulcerate as in this 54-year-old woman. The ulcer occurred in the setting of extensive local edema and radiation therapy. The resulting ulcer and surrounding cellulitis slowly responded to antibiotics and fastidious wound care.

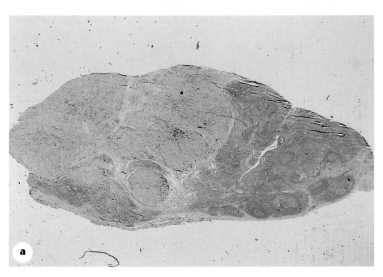

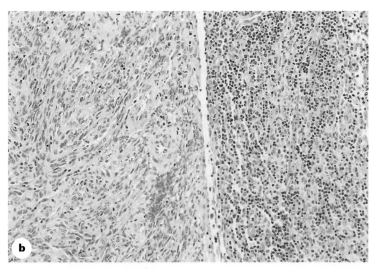

Fig. 17.15 Cutaneous Kaposi's sarcoma: lymphadenopathy. A 23-year-old patient, seropositive for HIV and previously diagnosed with KS of the extremities and hard palate, developed unilateral inguinal adenopathy and woody edema of the thigh. (**a**) A lymph node biopsy revealed Kaposi's sarcoma disrupting the normal architecture of the node (× 2.5). (**b**) Higher power shows lymphoid tissue on right with reactive changes (increase in macrophages, small lymphocytes and endothelial cells and venules) with sharp transition to Kaposi's infiltrate consisting of spindle cells and frequent extravasated red blood cells (×50). No infectious organisms or lymphoma were noted. The patient improved on systemic chemotherapy but did not have resolution of the edema and died of an opportunistic infection 6 months later. (Courtesy of Dr Bradford Sherburne.)

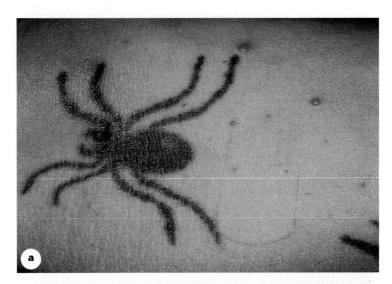

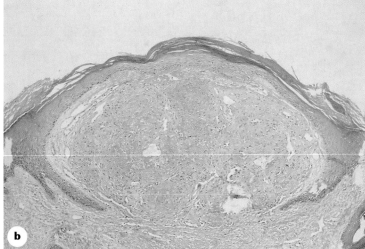

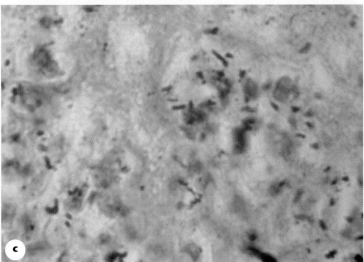

Fig. 17.16 Cutaneous lesions: bacillary angiomatosis. An important differential diagnosis in pigmented skin lesions in HIV-infected patients is bacillary angiomatosis. (**a**) Seen here on the tattooed forearm of a 26-year-old male, these lesions may be mistaken for KS and have very different implications for therapy. (**b**) A characteristic collar of epidermis around a dermal papule is seen (× 40) on skin punch biopsy of one of the lesions shown in (**a**) This appearance is classic for bacillary angiomatosis. (**c**) Warthin–Starry silver stain reveals organisms consistent with *Bartonella*, confirming the diagnosis of bacillary angiomatosis. (**a**: Courtesy of Dr Richard Johnson; **b, c**: Courtesy of Dr Steven Tahan.)

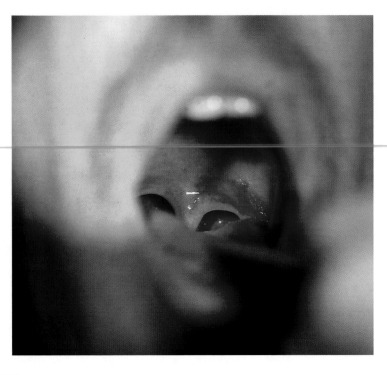

Fig. 17.17 Mucosal Kaposi's sarcoma. Typical appearance of oral KS visualized here on the soft palate of a 44-year-old man. Note the erythematous, patchy, raised lesions.

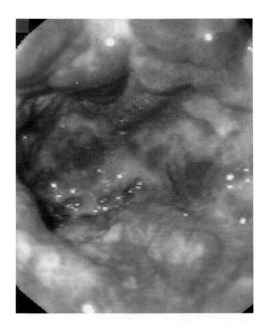

Fig. 17.18 Mucosal Kaposi's sarcoma. Mucosal involvement by KS is common. Note the red, violaceous, raised colonic nodules. It is often noted as an asymptomatic finding on either bronchoscopy or GI endoscopy. The colonoscopic findings depicted above were thought to be a potentially contributory factor, but unlikely to be the primary cause, of intractable, watery diarrhea. (Courtesy of Dr Harry Anastopoulos.)

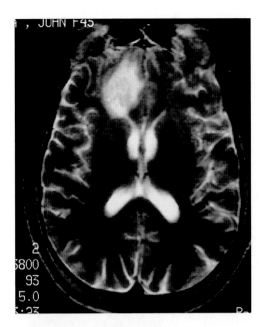

Fig. 17.19 Central nervous system lesions: cytomegalovirus. A 20-year-old male with a history of *Pneumocystis carinii* pneumonia (PCP) and CMV retinitis developed headache, lethargy and irritability. MRI revealed a space-occupying lesion in the frontal lobe which enhanced with gadolinium and on T2-weighted image. He transiently responded to therapy, but relapsed and died of intractable seizures 3 months later.

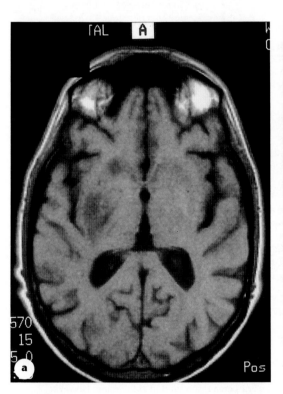

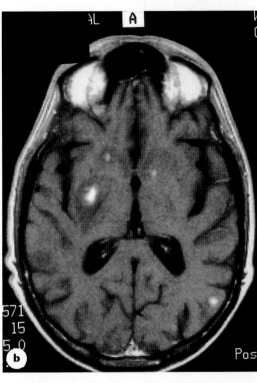

Fig. 17.20 Central nervous system lesion: toxoplasmosis. A 26-year-old female with multiple prior opportunistic infections developed left-sided motor and sensory deficits. MR scan revealed multiple focal defects on T1-weighted imaging (**a**) which enhanced with gadolinium (**b**). The patient failed to respond to empiric antitoxoplasma therapy, but on stereotactic biopsy had histologically confirmed toxoplasma abscess to which she rapidly succumbed.

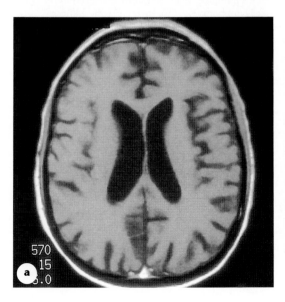

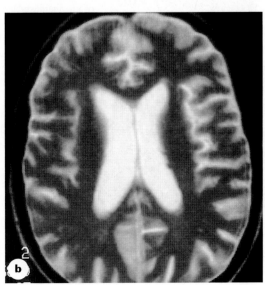

Fig. 17.21 Central nervous system lesion: progressive multifocal leukoencephalopathy. A 44-year-old man who had been HIV seropositive for 10 years had three episodes of PCP. He developed profound wasting, recurrent fevers, generalized weakness and ataxia. MRI revealed a low-signal intensity T1 (**a**), high-signal intensity T2-weighted image lesion (**b**) which did not enhance or show mass effect which was consistent with localized demyelination. The presumptive diagnosis was PML. The patient had progressive neurologic deterioration and generalized wasting and died from pneumonia 4 weeks later.

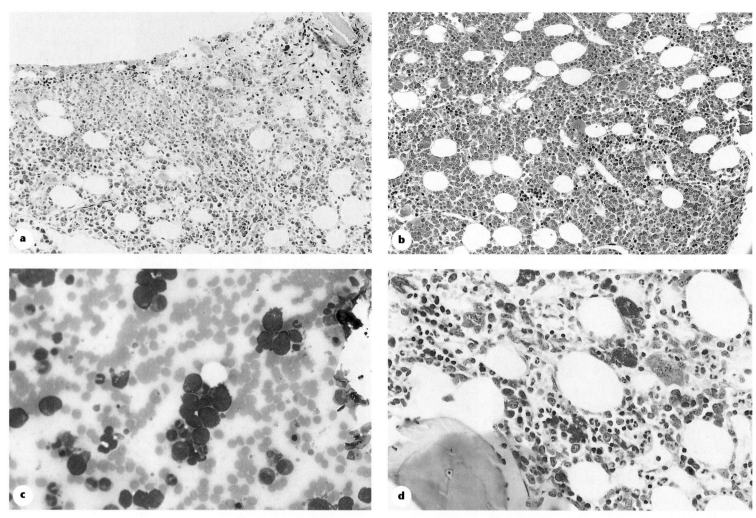

Fig. 17.22 Bone marrow findings in HIV disease. Bone marrow morphology of patients with HIV disease is often abnormal. Typically cellularity will be normal or increased, mild dysplastic changes will be noted, often accompanied by increased plasma cells, eosinophils and reticulin. Atypical lymphoid aggregates are often noted (**a**). These are to be distinguished from the infiltrating involvement by lymphoma seen in approximately 23% of patients with AIDS-related lymphoma (**b**). The small non-cleaved cell lymphoma seen in (**b**) was further evident in the accompanying bone marrow aspirate (**c**). Whenever evaluating patients with cytopenia and fever in AIDS, it is particularly important to exclude lymphoma or infiltrating infectious diseases such as those caused by mycobacteria and fungi. Abundant acid-fast organisms are noted in bone marrow (**d**) from a patient presenting with fever and cytopenia, splenomegaly and retroperitoneal adenopathy. (Courtesy of Dr Bradford Sherburne.)

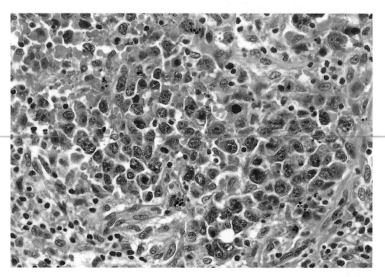

Fig. 17.23 AIDS-associated lymphomas. A 54-year-old male developed idiopathic thrombocytopenic purpura (ITP) and was found to be HIV seropositive. His thrombocytopenia responded to zidovudine. However, 2 years later he developed a scalp nodule which on biopsy revealed high-grade anaplastic large B-cell lymphoma (× 100). He is currently without evidence of disease in his second remission 12 months after diagnosis. (Courtesy of Dr Bradford Sherburne.)

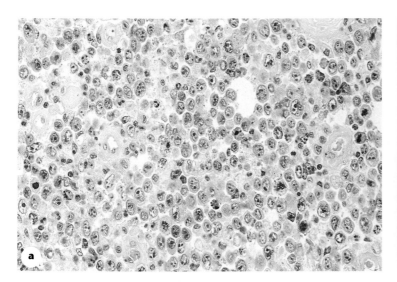

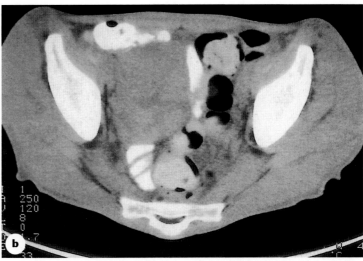

Fig. 17.24 AIDS-associated lymphomas. A 41-year-old male known to be HIV seropositive presented with fever, hematuria, hepatosplenomegaly and inguinal adenopathy. Cystoscopic and inguinal lymph node biopsy revealed diffuse large B-cell lymphoma with immunoblastic histology (**a**) (× 100). The patient failed to respond to chemotherapy and developed hepatosplenomegaly and a lower abdominal mass (**b**). On autopsy, he was found to have a large pelvic tumor mass as well as extensive lymphomatous involvement of the right ventricle of the heart, liver, spleen and bladder. (**a**: Courtesy of Dr Bradford Sherburne.)

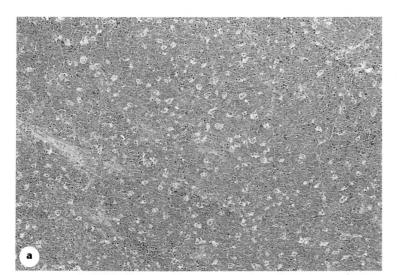

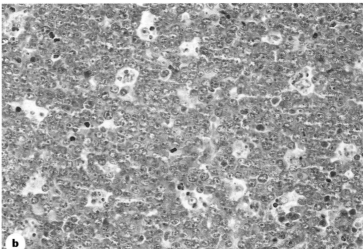

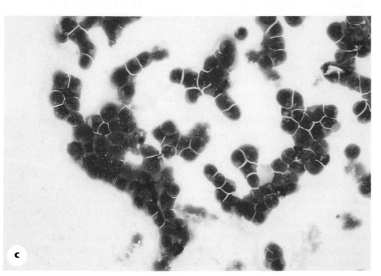

Fig. 17.25 AIDS-associated lymphomas. (**a, b**) A 26-year-old male noted a swelling in the left axilla. He was otherwise well and had no prior knowledge of HIV infection. A lymph node biopsy revealed a small non-cleaved cell lymphoma (**a**: × 25; **b**: × 100) and a serologic test for HIV was positive. Note the 'starry-sky' appearance of the lymph node due to the presence of light-staining benign histiocytes among a diffuse population of Burkitt-like undifferentiated lymphoma cells. He initially responded to chemotherapy. However, he developed perioral numbness and radicular back pain 6 months after his original diagnosis. He was found to have CSF involvement with relapsed lymphoma that was refractory to therapy (**c**). (**a,b**: Courtesy of Dr Bradford Sherburne.)

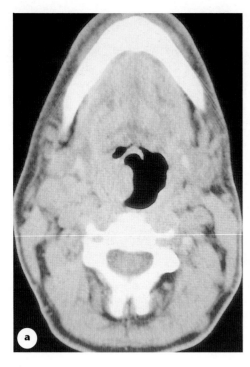

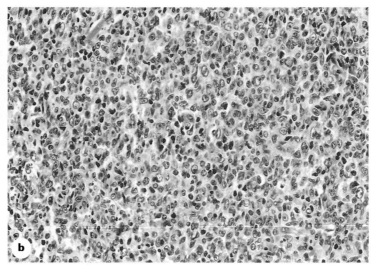

Fig. 17.26 AIDS-associated lymphomas. A 38-year-old male with a remote history of IV drug use presented with persistent hoarseness and dysphagia. The patient was found to have extensive involvement of the tonsil, piriform fossa, cervical nodes and associated soft tissue (**a**). Excisional biopsy of the tonsil revealed diffuse large cell lymphoma (**b**, × 100). He received chemotherapy and is disease free with an excellent performance status and CD4 count of 350 cells/mm³ 18 months after diagnosis. (**b**: Courtesy of Dr Bradford Sherburne.)

REFERENCES

Epidemiology

Besson C, Goubar A, Gabarre J, *et al.*: Changes in AIDS-related lymphoma since the era of highly active antiretroviral therapy. Blood 2001; 98(8): 2339-2344.

International Collaboration on HIV and Cancer: Highly active antiretroviral therapy and incidence of cancer in human immunodeficiency virus-infected adults. J Natl Cancer Inst 2000; 92: 1823-1830.

Kaposi's sarcoma

Chang Y, Cesarman E, Pessin MS, *et al.*: Identification of herpesvirus-like DNA sequences in AIDS-associated Kaposi's sarcoma. Science 1994; 266: 1865–1869.

Gill P, Tulpule A, Espina B, *et al.*: Paclitaxel is safe and effective in the treatment of advanced AIDS-related Kaposi's sarcoma. J Clin Oncol 1999; 17: 1876–1883.

Gill PS, Wernz J, Scadden DT, *et al.*: Randomized phase III trial of liposomal daunorubicin versus doxorubicin, bleomycin, and vincristine in AIDS-related Kaposi's sarcoma. J Clin Oncol 1996; 14: 2353–2364.

Karcher DS, Alkan S: Human herpesvirus-8-associated body cavity-based lymphoma in human immunodeficiency virus-infected patients: a unique B-cell neoplasm. Hum Pathol 1997; 28: 801–805.

Martin JN, Ganem DE, Osmond DH, Page-Shafer KA, Macrae D, Kedes DH: Sexual transmission and the natural history of human herpesvirus 8 infection. N Engl J Med 1998; 338: 948–954.

Northfelt DW, Dezube BJ, Thommes JA, *et al.*: Efficacy of pegylated-liposomal doxorubicin in the treatment of AIDS-related Kaposi's sarcoma after failure after of standard chemotherapy. J Clin Oncol 1997; 15: 653–659.

Sgadari C, Barillari G, Toschi E, *et al.*: HIV protease inhibitors are potent anti-angiogenic molecules and promote regression of Kaposi sarcoma. Nature Med 2002; 8(3): 225-232.

Whitby D, Boshoff C: Kaposi's sarcoma herpesvirus as a new paradigm for virus-induced oncogenesis. Curr Opin Oncol 1998; 10: 405–412.

Non-Hodgkin's lymphoma

Antinori A, Ammassari A, De Luca A, *et al.*: Diagnosis of AIDS-related focal brain lesions: a decision-making analysis based on clinical and neuroradiologic characteristics combined with polymerase chain reaction assays in CSF. Neurology 1997; 48: 687–694.

Cingolani A, Gastaldi R, Fassone L, *et al.*: Epstein–Barr virus infection is predictive of CNS involvement in systemic AIDS-related non-Hodgkin's lymphomas. J Clin Oncol 2000; 18: 3325–3330.

Jacomet C, Girard PM, Lebrette MG, Farese VL, Monfort L, Rozenbaum W: Intravenous methotrexate for primary central nervous system non-Hodgkin's lymphoma in AIDS [see comments]. *Aids* 1997; 11: 1725–1730.

Kaplan LD, Straus DJ, Testa MA, *et al.*: Low-dose compared with standard-dose m-BACOD chemotherapy for non Hodgkin's lymphoma associated with human immunodeficiency virus infection. N Engl J Med 1997; 336: 1641–1648.

Kirk O, Pederson C, Cozzi-Lepri A, *et al.*: Non-Hodgkin lymphoma in HIV-infected patients in the era of highly active antiretroviral therapy. Blood 2001; 98(12): 3406-3412.

Little RF, Butierrez M, Jaffe ES, *et al.*: HIV-associated non-Hodgkin's lymphoma: incidence, presentation, and prognosis. J Am Med Assoc 2001; 285(14):1880-1885.

Rabkin CS, Yang Q, Goedert JJ, Nguyen G, Mitsuya H, Sei S: Chemokine and chemokine receptor gene variants and risk of non-Hodgkin's lymphoma in human immunodeficiency virus-1-infected individuals. Blood 1999; 93: 1838–1842.

Ratner L, Lee J, Shengui T, *et al.*: Chemotheryapy for HIV-associated non-Hodgkin's lymphoma in combination with highly active antiretroviral therapy. J Clin Oncol 2001; 19: 2171-2178.

Straus DJ, Huang J, Testa MA, Levine AM, Kaplan LD: Prognostic factors in the treatment of human immunodeficiency virus associated non-Hodgkin's lymphoma: analysis of AIDS Clinical Trials Group protocol 142 – low-dose versus standard-dose m-BACOD plus granulocyte-macrophage colony-stimulating factor. National Institute of Allergy and Infectious Diseases. J Clin Oncol 1998; 16: 3601–3606.

Hodgkin's disease

Levine AM: HIV-associated Hodgkin's disease. Biologic and clinical aspects. Hematol Oncol Clin North Am 1996; 10: 1135–1148.

Re A, Casari S, Cattaneo C, *et al.*: Hodgkin disease developing in patients infected by human immunodeficiency virus results in clinical features and a prognosis similar to those in patients with human immunodeficiency virus-related non-Hodgkin lymphoma. Cancer 2001; 92(11): 2739-2745.

Anogenital neoplasm

Frisch M, Biggar RJ, Goedert JJ: Human papillomavirus-associated cancers in patients with human immunodeficiency virus infection and acquired immunodeficiency syndrome. J Natl Cancer Inst 2000; 92(18) 1500-1510.

Palefsky JM, Holly EA, Ralston ML, Jay N: Prevalence and risk factors for human papillomavirus infection of the anal canal in human immunodeficiency virus (HIV)-positive and HIV-negative homosexual men. J Infect Dis 1998; 177: 361–736.

Peddada AV, Smith DE, Rao AR, Frost DB, Kagan AR: Chemotherapy and low-dose radiotherapy in the treatment of HIV-infected patients with carcinoma of the anal canal. Int J Radiat Oncol Biol Phys 1997; 37: 1101–1105.

Sun XW, Kuhn L, Ellerbrock TV, Chiasson MA, Bush TJ, Wright TC Jr: Human papillomavirus infection in women infected with the human immunodeficiency virus [see comments]. N Engl J Med 1997; 337: 1343–1349.

Systemic and mucocutaneous reactions to chemotherapy

Joseph P. Eder, Arthur T. Skarin

18

INTRODUCTION

Cancer chemotherapy is a major component of cancer therapy, along with surgery and radiation. Cancer chemotherapy agents differ from most drugs in that they are intentionally cytotoxic to human cells. This aspect of cancer chemotherapeutic agents produces a narrow therapeutic index (desired vs undesired) for most, but not all, agents in this class. The target of cancer chemotherapeutic agents is the proliferating cancer cell. While many normal tissues are non-proliferating, others are and toxicity of this class tends to overlap proliferating tissues preferentially – hematopoietic, gastrointestinal mucosa and skin. In addition, each agent often has specific organ toxicity related to its chemical class or unique mechanism of action.

The major groups of cancer chemotherapeutic agents are the direct-acting alkylating agents, the indirect-acting anthracyclines and topoisomerase inhibitors, the antimetabolites, the tubulin-binding agents, hormones and a class of miscellaneous agents. Despite the disparate nature of this broad class of agents, some generalizations about the effects of chemotherapy are still possible.

ACUTE HYPERSENSITIVITY REACTIONS

Acute hypersensitivity can occur with any drug. However, several cancer chemotherapeutic agents are derived from hydrophobic plant chemicals and must be solubilized with agents with a marked propensity for causing acute hypersensitivity reactions, especially histamine-mediated anaphylactic reactions, such as the Cremophor used with paclitaxel. Docetaxel has a lower incidence of this complication.

The incidence of severe hypersensitivity reactions with paclitaxel may be up to 25% without ancillary measures. With antihistamine H1 and H2 blockade with corticosteroids, the incidence falls to 2–3%. Hypersensitivity reactions occur in up to 40% of patients receiving single agent 1-asparaginase but only 20% when administered in combination therapy with glucocorticoids and 6-mercaptopurine, perhaps as a result of immunosuppression. The hypersensitivity usually occurs after several doses and in successive cycles. The reaction may be only urticaria but may be severe with laryngospasm or, rarely, serum sickness. Fatal reactions occur <1% of the time. Changing the source of enzyme is the appropriate initial step. Two other proteins in clinical use, tostuzimab and traztuzumab, have a similar incidence of hypersensitivity reactions.

Certain drugs such as etoposide are associated with a greater incidence of reactions but most are not true hypersensitivity reactions. The Tween diluant in the clinical etoposide formulation produces hypotension, rash and back pain. The platinum compounds, carboplatin and cisplatin, are associated with hypersensitivity reactions, particularly on subsequent cycles. Liposomal encapsulated anthracyclines are associated with a much increased incidence of hypersensitivity compared with the parent drugs.

ALOPECIA

Many antineoplastic drugs can produce marked hair loss. This includes not only scalp hair but also facial, axillary, pubic and all body hair. The germinating hair follicle has an approximately 24-hour doubling time. Cancer chemotherapy agents preferentially affect actively growing (anagen) hairs. The interruption of mitosis produces a structurally weakened hair prone to fracture easily from minimal trauma such as brushing. Since 80–90% of scalp hairs are in anagen phase, the degree of hair loss can be substantial. Hair loss, while often emotionally difficult for patients, is reversible, although hair may regrow more curly and of a slightly different color.

STOMATITIS/MUCOSITIS

The oral complications of cancer chemotherapy are many and frequently severe. The disruption of the protective mucosal barrier serves as a portal of entry for pathogens which, especially when combined with chemotherapy – induced neutropenia, predisposes to local infection and systemic sepsis. Once established, these infections may be difficult to eradicate in immunocompromised patients. The most common infectious organisms are *Candida albicans*, herpes simplex virus, β-hemolytic streptococci, staphylococci, opportunistic Gram-negative bacteria and mouth anaerobes.

Several agents of the antimetabolite class of cancer chemotherapeutic agents, especially those that target pyrimidine biosynthesis such as methotrexate, 5-fluorouracil and cytosine arabinoside, and the anthracycline agents, such as doxorubicin and daunorubicin, are particularly toxic to the mucosal epithelium. These agents have a marked capacity to produce more severe injury in irradiated tissues, even if the radiation is temporally remote. These agents produce marked ulceration and erosion of the mucosa. These lesions occur initially on those mucosal surfaces that abrade the teeth and gums, such as the sides of the tongue, the vermillion border of the lower lip and the buccal mucosa. More advanced mucosal injury may occur on the hard and soft palate and the posterior oropharynx. These ulcerations cannot often be distinguished from those caused by infectious organisms. Appropriate tests must be performed to exclude viral, fungal and bacterial causes or superinfection.

In addition to the risk of infection, the resultant pain makes patients unable to maintain adequate nutrition and hydration. This may compromise the capacity to complete a course of chemotherapy and require prolonged administration of parenteral fluids and even parenteral nutrition.

DERMATITIS, SKIN RASHES AND HYPERPIGMENTATION

Superficial manifestations of cancer chemotherapy agents is noted frequently by patients, although much less often is it considered significant by clinicians. The cosmetic changes may be disturbing to patients without requiring discontinuation of therapy.

Of the direct-acting alkylating agents, busulfan has been associated with a wide variety of specific and non-specific cutaneous changes. Diffuse hyperpigmentation has been noted, which resolves with discontinuation of therapy. Systemic mechlorethamine (nitrogen mustard) has no cutaneous toxicity. However, when applied topically for cutaneous T-cell lymphomas, telangiectasias, hyperpigmentation and allergic contact dermatitis may occur. The development of more effective, safer alternative agents has rendered busulfan and mechlorethamine to essentially historical interest only or narrow indications (busulfan in allogeneic bone marrow transplant for hematologic malignancies). Cyclophosphamide, ifosfamide and melphalan produce hyperpigmentation of nails, teeth, gingiva and skin.

The antimetabolites methotrexate and 5-fluorouracil are frequently associated with cutaneous reactions. In contrast, the purine antimetabolites 6-mercaptopurine, 6-thioguanine, cladribine, fludarabine and pentostatin are devoid of cutaneous toxicity. Methotrexate, a folate antagonist, may cause reactivation of ultraviolet burns when given in close proximity to previous sun exposure. This is not prevented by leucovorin, a reduced folate that prevents the myelosuppression and stomatitis of high doses of methotrexate. Methotrexate should be given more than a week after a significant solar burn. It may cause stomatitis and cutaneous ulcerations at high dose, despite the use of leucovorin. Extensive epidermal necrolysis may occur and be fatal. Multiple areas of vesiculation and erosion over pressure areas have been noticed.

5-fluorouracil (5-FU) is an antimetabolite with steric properties similar to uracil. Like methotrexate, 5-FU produces increased sensitivity to ultraviolet-induced toxic reactions in large number of patients, over 35% in one study. Enhanced sunburn erythema and increased posterythema hyperpigmentation characterize these reactions. A hyperpigmentation reaction over the veins in which the drug is administered may occur. This is likely hyperpigmentation secondary to chemical phlebitis due to chemotherapeutic agents in the superficial venous system. Nail and generalized skin hyperpigmentation have been reported with 5-FU. Occasionally, acute inflammation of existing actinic keratosis is seen in patients receiving 5-FU. This differs from a drug reaction in that it occurs in discrete inflamed regions only in sun-exposed areas, not in a generalized distribution. The end result is usually the disappearance of the actinic keratosis as a result of an inflammatory infiltration into the atypical epidermis and resultant removal of atypical cells.

When 5-FU is given by intravenous continuous infusion, the most common dose-limiting toxicity is erythromalagia, the so-called 'hand–foot' syndrome. The hands and feet become red, edematous and often painful. The skin often peels afterward. The nails become dry and brittle and develop linear cracks. This may occur at doses less than those that produce the hand–foot syndrome. A similar reaction occurs with 5-FU or 5-FU prodrugs administered orally on a daily schedule. Capecitabine, an oral prodrug that is eventually converted to 5-FU intracellularly, produces erythromalagia as its most common toxicity. Interestingly, oral 5-FU does not produce this syndrome when combined with enyluracil, an irreversible inhibitor of dihydropyrimidine dehydrogenase, the major enzyme in 5-FU catabolism.

High doses of cytosine arabinoside may produce ocular toxicity through an ulcerating keratoconjunctivitis. This may be prevented by the prophylactic administration of steroid eyedrops. Excessive lacrimation may be noted with 5-FU therapy due to lacrimal duct stenosis. This is corrected by surgical dilatation of the duct.

The indirect anticancer drugs may produce superficial cutaneous toxicity. The anthracyclines doxorubicin, daunorubicin, epirubicin and idarubicin produce complete alopecia. Radiation recall reactions are frequent, even when the two modalities are separated by years.

Skin, nail and mucous membrane hyperpigmentation may be striking; these may be localized or general. Hyperpigmentation of the hands, feet and face may occur in patients of African descent. Liposomal anthracyclines, such as Doxil (doxorubicin) and Daunosome (daunomycin), may produce a severe erythromalagia with palmar and plantar erythema and desquamation similar to 5-FU. Actinomycin D produces a characteristic skin eruption in many patients. Beginning 3–5 days after drug administration, patients develop facial erythema followed by papules, pustules and plugged follicles similar to the open comedones of acne. This eruption is benign, self-limited and not a reason to stop therapy. A similar acneform skin rash occurs in patients taking the new oral epidermal growth factor receptor inhibitors such as Iressa (ZD-1839) and Tarceva (OSI-774). In most patients the rash is mild and may regress with continued treatment. When severe, the skin lesions will rapidly regress with discontinuation of the drug.

Bleomycin is actually a mixture of peptides isolated from *Streptomyces verticuillus*. Its most common toxic effects involve the lungs and skin because of high concentrations in these organs due to the deficiency of the catabolic enzyme bleomycin hydrolase in these tissues. Cutaneous toxicity occurs in the majority of patients treated with bleomycin doses in excess of 200 mg. Bleomycin causes a morbilliform eruption 30 minutes to 3 hours after administration in approximately 10% of patients. It most likely represents a transient hypersensitivity response (it may be accompanied by fever). Linear or 'flagellate' hyperpigmentation may occur on the trunk. This may likewise represent postinflammatory hyperpigmentation. Bleomycin may cause a scleroderma-like eruption of the skin. Infiltrative plaques, nodules and linear bands of the hands have been described. Pathologic findings include dermal sclerosis and appendage entrapment similar to that seen in scleroderma. These changes are reversible when the drug is stopped.

Etoposide has relatively few cutaneous manifestations at standard doses (<600 mg/m^2). At higher doses (1800–4200 mg/m^2), a generalized pruritic, erythematous, maculopapular rash occurs in approximately 25% of patients. The most severe toxicity occurs at the highest doses. In these patients, an intense, well-defined palmar erythema develops. Affected areas become edematous, red and painful. Bullous formation and desquamation follow. The severity of the reaction is related to dose. A short course (3–5) days of corticosteroids controls the symptoms.

SKIN ULCERATION AND EXTRAVASATION

Vesicant reactions from extravasated cancer chemotherapeutic agents are one of the most debilitating complications seen with cancer therapy. The anthracyclines, especially doxorubicin, are particularly noted for an intense inflammatory chemical cellulitis caused by subcutaneous extravasation. This results in ulceration and necrosis of affected tissue. No local measures have proven unequivocally helpful once the accident has occurred. Doxorubicin should be stopped immediately but the i.v. left in place. Dilution of doxorubicin with sodium bicarbonate and the local installation of steroids prior to catheter withdrawal are standard measures but their efficacy is uncertain. Rest and warm compresses are recommended. If healing does not proceed well, excision of the affected area and surgical grafting are recommended to avoid excess morbidity. Other agents with vesicant properties include the vinca alkaloids (vincristine, vinblastine, vinorelbine) and actinomycin. General recommendations for the administration of vesicant drugs includes the use of veins as far away from the hands and joints as possible and that the i.v. be able to infuse at a rapid rate and have a good blood return.

The use of venous access devices is accepted as appropriate in this situation unless contraindicated on specific clinical grounds.

Generalized skin ulceration is an infrequent albeit dramatic occurrence. Mucocutaneous ulcerations are frequently noted with bleomycin. These begin as edema and erythema over pressure points such as elbows, knees and fingertips and in intertrigenous areas such as the groin and axillae. These areas then proceed to shallow ulcerations. These ulcerations may also occur in the oral cavity. Biopsy shows epidermal degeneration and necrosis with dermal edema. Total epidermal necrosis can even be found, without any dermal changes. This suggests that the epidermal toxicity is the primary event.

NAIL CHANGES

Banding of the nails is the appearance of linear horizontal depressions in the nails that occur as a result of growth interruptions in the nail germinal cell layer by a cytostatic effect from the administration of cancer chemotherapy agents. These occur in other disease settings and are called Beau's lines. The direct–acting alkylating agents cyclophosphamide, ifosfamide and melphalan may also produce hyperpigmentation of nails. The nails may exhibit linear or transverse banding or hyperpigmentation. These changes begin proximally and progress distally and clear, proximally to distally, when the agents are discontinued. Similar effects are seen with the indirect-acting anthracyclines, such as doxorubicin, and bleomycin. The anthracyclines may cause hyperpigmentation of the hyponychia (the soft layer of skin beneath the nail), especially in dark-skinned persons.

Onycholysis is separation of the nail plate from the nail bed. Anthracyclines, anthracenediones and taxanes are the drugs most frequently associated with onycholysis. The combination of these agents is most frequently reported with onycholysis. Most of the reports are associated with docetaxel, either administered weekly or every 3 weeks. These changes occur after hyperpigmentation of the hyponychia, often with hyperkeratosis and splinter hemorrhages. Ultraviolet light may be a facilitating factor. Onycholysis can occur within weeks or months of the initiation of therapy.

RADIATION RECALL

Radiation recall dermatitis is a cutaneous toxicity that develops in patients with prior exposure to therapeutic doses of radiation and subsequent treatment with a cancer chemotherapeutic agent. These reactions occur in the previously irradiated field and not elsewhere. A previous cutaneous reaction at the time of irradiation is not a prerequisite. The onset of symptoms is days to weeks after drug treatment and can occur any time after radiation, even years later. Cutaneous manifestations include erythema with maculopapular eruptions, vesiculation and desquamation. The intensity of the cutaneous response can vary from a mild rash to skin necrosis. Radiation recall reactions in other organs can produce gastrointestinal mucosal inflammation (stomatitis, esophagitis, enteritis, proctitis), pneumonitis and myocarditis.

An extensive number of anticancer agents have been implicated in radiation recall reactions. The anthracyclines (doxorubicin as an example), bleomycin, dactinomycin, etoposide, the taxanes, vinca alkaloids and antimetabolites (hydroxy-carbamide, fluorouracil, methotrexate, gemcitabine) are the most commonly implicated in cutaneous toxicity.

Methotrexate and dactinomycin are reported to cause radiation enhancement in the central nervous system (CNS). The antimetabolites, doxorubicin, dactinomycin and bleomycin enhance gastrointestinal toxicity from radiation. Cyclophosphamide, taxanes, hydroxy-carbamide, doxorubicin, dactinomycin, gemcitabine, cytosine arabinoside and, most importantly, bleomycin exacerbate pulmonary radiation toxicity. Optic toxicity is increased by treatment with fluorouracil and cytosine arabinoside. Radiation lowers the dose of doxorubicin that produces cardiomyopathy.

ORGAN TOXICITY
Cardiac toxicity

Cardiotoxicity is a well-recognized consequence of anthracycline use, especially doxorubicin because of its wide spectrum of antineoplastic therapy. This peculiar and potentially lethal problem can be classified as acute or chronic. The acute toxicity is usually asymptomatic arrhythmias, including heart block. Acute myopericarditis occurs at low total doses in an idiosyncratic fashion or at high single doses >110–120 mg/m^2. Fever, pericarditis, and congestive heart failure (CHF) are the clinical manifestations. Chronic cardiomyopathy is characterized by progressive myofibrillar damage with each dose, dilatation of sarcoplasmic reticulum, loss of myofibrils and myocardial necrosis/fibrosis.

A doxorubicin total dose <550 mg/m^2 has 1–10% of CHF (daunorubicin 900–1000 mg/m^2), a 40% incidence at 800 mg/m^2 of doxorubicin, and the incidence of CHF approaches 100% at 1 g/m^2. Cardiac function is tested using non-invasive techniques to measure the resting and exercise ejection fraction, including radionuclide ventriculograms and echocardiograms, or invasively by cardiac biopsy. Factors that increase the risk of developing CHF include pre-existing heart disease, hypertension and cardiac XRT. Concomitant dosing with trastuzamab (Herceptin) increases the cardiac toxicity of doxorubicin. Cardiac toxicity is a function of *peak* dose level, so continuous infusions or weekly dosing decrease the risk. Desrazoxane (ICRF-187), an iron chelator, decreases cardiotoxicity and is approved for use.

Biochemical mechanisms implicated include calcium-mediated damage to the sarcoplasmic reticulum (SR), which increases calcium ion (Ca^{++}) release with increased Ca^{++} uptake in mitochondria in preference to ATP. Lipid peroxidations of the SR, which decrease high Ca^{++} binding sites, and lipid peroxidation due to drug $^\bullet$Fe^{3+} complexes with hydroxyl (OH) radical generation may contribute to cardiotoxicity. The heart has no catalase and anthracyclines decrease glutathione peroxidase activity, which increases the sensitivity of the myocardium to oxidative damage.

Idarubicin and epirubicin have less cardiotoxicity but are still capable of causing cardiotoxicity. High-dose cyclophosphamide, at doses >60 mg/kg as used in bone marrow transplantation, can cause a hemorrhagic cardiomyopathy. Paclitaxel produces clinically insignificant atrial arrhythmias. Agents which can produce arterial smooth muscle spasm may produce ischemic myocardial infarction in the absence of fixed coronary vascular disease. These agents include 5-FU, vincristine and vinblastine.

Pulmonary toxicity

Bleomycin produces pulmonary toxicity which is the major problem with subacute or chronic interstitial pneumonitis complicated by late-stage fibrosis. The incidence is 3–5% with doses <450 u/m^2, in patients over 70, with emphysema and after high single doses (>25 u/m^2). The incidence rises to 10% at doses >450 mg/m^2, but can occur at cumulative doses <100 mg. Pulmonary injury can occur during high FiO$_2$ and volume overload during surgery for many years after exposure.

Toxicity results from free radicals produced by an intercalated Fe(II)–bleomycin–O$_2$ complex between DNA strands. Intercalation of drug into DNA is the first step, then Fe(II) is oxidized and O_2 is reduced to oxygen ($^{\bullet}O_2^-$) or hydroxyl radicals $^{\bullet}OH$. DNA cleavage occurs after the activated bleomycin complex is assembled. Strand breakage absolutely requires O_2, which is converted to O_2^- and $^{\bullet}OH$, and peroxidation products of DNA (and protein) are formed. Free radical scavengers and superoxide dismutase (SODM) inhibit DNA breakage. Bleomycin is hydrolyzed by bleomycin hydrolase, a cysteine present in normal and malignant cells but decreased in lung and skin.

Busulfan, mitomycin C and carmustine are direct-acting alkylating agents that can cause chronic interstitial pneumonitis and fibrosing alveolitis. This chronic fibrosis produces the clinical picture of progressive, often fatal, restrictive lung disease. The symptoms occur insidiously, often after prolonged therapy. The chronic use of busulfan for the treatment of chronic myelogenous leukemia is now a historical footnote but carmustine remains the mainstay of treatment for glioblastoma and anaplastic astrocytomas. Cyclophosphamide has been implicated in chronic pulmonary toxicity but rarely as a single agent, more often after radiation.

The antimetabolite methotrexate may produce an acute eosinophilic pneumonitis, which represents an allergic reaction. Cytosine arabinoside and gemcitabine (2,2'-difluoro-deoxycytosine) may also cause an acute pneumonitis, which may be fatal if unrecognized. In these circumstances, withdrawal of the offending agent, supportive care and corticosteroids may prevent a fatal outcome.

Hepatotoxicity

The liver is a frequent organ for toxicity with cancer chemotherapeutic agents. Centrilobular hepatocyte injury is the frequent histologic finding, elevated transaminases the biochemical manifestation. Antimetabolite drugs such as cytosine arabinoside, methotrexate, hydroxy-carbamide and 6-mercaptopurine are all associated with hepatic injury. 6-mercaptopurine produces a cholestatic picture, with an elevated alkaline phosphatase and bilirubin. L-asparaginase and carmustine cause hepatotoxicity as well. The injury reverses with discontinuation of the drug. Chronic methotrexate administration, such as in the treatment of autoimmune diseases, is associated with irreversible fibrosis and cirrhosis.

Hepatic vascular injury is another type of injury to the liver associated with cancer chemotherapeutic agents. Hepatic veno-occlusive (VOD) disease may occur in up to 20% of patients receiving high-dose chemotherapy in conjunction with bone marrow transplantation, with a mortality up to 50%. Jaundice, ascites and hepatomegaly are the full manifestations of VOD but right upper quadrant pain and weight gain occur more frequently. Obliteration of the central hepatic venules and resulting pressure necrosis of hepatocytes is seen at autopsy. Many regimens and many individual drugs have been implicated. With busulfan, adjustment of the plasma concentration-time profile may reduce the risk. Dacarbazine, a monofunctional alkylating agent, may produce an eosinophilic centrilobular injury with hepatic vein thromboses.

Gastrointestinal toxicity

Chemotherapy-induced diarrhea has been described with several drugs including the fluoropyrimidines (particularly 5-FU), irinotecan, methotrexate and cisplatin. However, it is the dose-limiting and major toxicity of regimens containing a fluoropyrimidine and/or irinotecan. Both 5-FU and irinotecan cause acute damage to the intestinal mucosa, leading to loss of epithelium. 5-FU causes a mitotic arrest of crypt cells, leading to an increase in the ratio of immature secretory crypt cells to mature villous enterocytes. The increased volume of fluid that leaves the small bowel exceeds the absorptive capacity of the colon, leading to clinically significant diarrhea.

In patients treated with irinotecan, early-onset diarrhea, which occurs during or within several hours of drug infusion in 45–50% of patients, is cholinergically mediated. This effect is thought to be due to structural similarity with acetylcholine. In contrast, late irinotecan-associated diarrhea is not cholinergically mediated. The pathophysiology of late diarrhea appears to be multifactorial with contributions from dysmotility and secretory factors as well as a direct toxic effect of the drug on the intestinal mucosa.

Irinotecan produces mucosal changes associated with apoptosis, such as epithelial vacuolization, and goblet cell hyperplasia, suggestive of mucin hypersecretion. These changes appear to be related to the accumulation of the active metabolite of irinotecan, SN-38, in the intestinal mucosa. SN-38 is glucuronidated in the liver and is then excreted in the bile. The conjugated metabolite SN-38G does not appear to cause diarrhea. However, SN-38G can be deconjugated in the intestines by β-glucuronidase present in intestinal bacteria. A direct correlation has been noted between mucosal damage and either low glucuronidation rates or increased intestinal β-glucuronidase activity. Severe toxicity has been described following irinotecan therapy in patients with Gilbert's syndrome, who have defective hepatic glucuronidation. Experimental studies have shown that inhibition of intestinal β-glucuronidase activity with antibiotics protects against mucosal injury and ameliorates the diarrhea.

Neurotoxicity

Neurotoxicity from cancer chemotherapeutic agents is an increasingly recognized consequence of cancer treatment. The toxicities observed may affect the brain and spinal cord (CNS), peripheral nerves (PNS) or the supporting neurologic tissues such as the meninges. Neurotoxicity from cancer therapeutic drugs must be distinguished from the effects of space-occupying metastatic lesions, toxic metabolic effects from disorders of blood chemistry, adjunctive drugs (such as opiate narcotics) and paraneoplastic syndromes. Toxicity may be acute, subacute or chronic, reversible or irreversible.

The direct-acting alkylating agents ifosfamide and carmustine cause somnolence, confusion and coma at high doses. The toxicity of ifosfamide is secondary to accumulation of a metabolite, chlorethyl aldehyde, in cerebrospinal fluid. Renal dysfunction may cause CNS toxicity at low doses when acidosis results in increased chlorethyl aldehyde levels.

Damage from the antimetabolite methotrexate occurs in three forms and is worse when given intrathecally with radiation. Chemical arachnoiditis, characterized by headache, fever and nuchal rigidity, is the most common and most acute toxicity. This may be due to additives in the diluent (benzoic acid in sterile water). Subacute toxicity is delayed 2–3 weeks after administration and is characterized by extremity motor paralysis, cranial nerve palsy seizures and coma. This is due to prolonged exposure to high doses of methotrexate. Chronic demyelinating encephalitis produces dementia and spasticity. There is cortical thinning with enlarged ventricles and cerebral calcifications. Types 2 and 3 may be increased after irradiation especially if concomitant systemic therapy with high (or intermediate) doses is used.

Cytosine arabinoside, when given at high doses, produces cerebral and cerebellar dysfunction due to Purkinje cell necrosis and damage. At standard doses, leukoencephalopathy occurs rarely. When given intrathecally, cytosine arabinoside can produce transverse myelitis with resulting paralysis. 5-FU may produce acute cerebellar toxicity due to inhibition of the aconintase, an enzyme in the cerebellar Krebs cycle. The purine adenine deaminase inhibitors, pentostatin and fludarabine, may produce several types of neurotoxicity. Pentostatin produces somnolence and coma at high doses. Fludarabine may causes delayed-onset coma or cortical blindness at high doses, peripheral neuropathy at low doses. Peripheral neuropathy is a frequent toxicity encountered with many cancer chemotherapeutic agents of many classes. Cisplatin and oxaliplatin, the vinca alkaloids and the taxanes all produce peripheral neuropathy in a cumulative dose-dependent manner.

Nephrotoxicity

One of the most serious side-effects of chemotherapeutic agents is nephrotoxicity. Any part of the kidney structure, (e.g. the glomerulus, the tubules, the interstitium or the renal microvasculature) could be vulnerable to damage. The clinical manifestations of nephrotoxicity can range from an asymptomatic elevation of serum creatinine to acute renal failure requiring dialysis. Intravascular volume depletion secondary to ascites, edema or external losses, concomitant use of nephrotoxic drugs, urinary tract obstruction secondary to the underlying malignancy, tumor infiltration of the kidney and intrinsic renal disease can potentiate renal dysfunction in the cancer patient.

Platinum compounds are the agents most associated with renal toxicity. Cisplatin is one of the most commonly used and effective chemotherapeutic agents available and also the best studied antineoplastic nephrotoxic drug. It is a potent tubular toxin, particularly in a low chloride environment, such as the interior of cells. Cell death results via apoptosis or necrosis as in DNA-damaged cells enter the cell cycle. Approximately 25–35% of patients will develop a mild and partially reversible decline in renal function after the first course of therapy. The incidence and severity of renal failure increase with subsequent courses, eventually becoming in part irreversible. As a result, discontinuing therapy is generally indicated in those patients who develop a progressive rise in the plasma creatinine concentration. In addition to this rise, potentially irreversible hypomagnesemia due to urinary magnesium wasting may occur in over one-half of cases.

There is suggestive evidence that the nephrotoxicity of cisplatin can be diminished by vigorous hydration and perhaps by giving the drug in a hypertonic solution. A high chloride concentration may minimize both the formation of the highly reactive platinum compounds described above and the uptake of cisplatin by the renal tubular cells. Amifostine, an organic thiophosphate, appears to diminish cisplatin-induced toxicity by donating a protective thiol group, an effect that is highly selective for normal, but not malignant, tissue. Discontinuation of platinum therapy once the plasma creatinine concentration begins to rise should prevent progressive renal failure.

Carboplatin has been synthesized as a non-nephrotoxic platinum analog. But even though it is less nephrotoxic, it is not free of potential renal injury. Hypomagnesemia appears to be the most common manifestation of nephrotoxicity. Other, less common renal side-effects include recurrent salt wasting. No significant clinical nephrotoxicity due to oxaliplatin has yet been reported. Limited data have shown no exacerbation of pre-existing mild renal impairment. Studies of oxaliplatin in patients with progressive degrees of renal failure are in progress.

Cyclophosphamide may produce significant side-effects involving the urinary bladder (hemorrhagic cystitis). The primary renal effect of this agent is hyponatremia, which is due to impairment of the ability of the kidney to excrete water. The mechanism appears to be due to a direct effect of cyclophosphamide on the distal tubule and not to increased levels of antidiuretic hormone. Hyponatremia usually occurs acutely and resolves upon discontinuation of the drug (approximately 24 hours). It is recommended that isotonic saline be infused prior to cyclophosphamide administration, in order to ameliorate this effect.

Ifosfamide nephrotoxicity has a primary renal effect to produce tubular renal toxicity. The damage produced by ifosfamide is concentrated in the proximal renal tubule and a Fanconi syndrome has been observed after therapy. Other clinical syndromes that have been associated with ifosfamide include nephrogenic diabetes insipidus, renal tubular acidosis and rickets. Pre-existing renal disease is an important risk factor for ifosfamide nephrotoxicity.

Carmustine, lomustine and semustine are lipid-soluble nitrosureas which have been used against brain tumors. The exact mechanism of nephrotoxicity, however, is incompletely understood. High doses of semustine in children and adults have been associated with progressive renal dysfunction to marked renal insufficiency 3–5 years after therapy. The characteristic histologic changes include glomerular sclerosis without immune deposits and interstitial fibrosis. The incidence of nephrotoxicity was reported at 26% in patients with malignant melanoma treated with methyl CCNU in the adjuvant setting. Nephrotoxicity has been reported in 65–75% of patients treated with streptozotocin for prolonged periods of time. Proteinuria is often the first sign of renal damage. This is followed by signs of proximal tubular damage, such as phosphaturia, glycosuria, aminoaciduria, uricosuria and bicarbonaturia. Renal toxicity lasts approximately 2–3 weeks after discontinuing the drug.

The most common form of nephrotoxicity associated with mitomycin C is hemolytic uremic syndrome. It has been reported in patients who were treated with total doses of mitomycin C in excess of 60 mg/m². The renal damage caused by this antineoplastic agent appears to be direct endothelial damage. The incidence of this syndrome ranges from 4% to 6% of patients who receive this drug alone or in combination.

Low or standard doses of methotrexate are usually not associated with renal toxicity, unless patients have underlying renal dysfunction. High doses (1–15 g/m²) are associated with a 47% incidence of renal toxicity, accompanied by methotrexate crystals in the urine. The mechanism for methotrexate-induced nephrotoxicity is explained in part by its limited solubility at an acid pH, which leads to intratubular precipitation. Patients who are volume depleted and excrete an acidic urine are at higher risk for nephrotoxicity. With aggressive hydration and urine alkalinization, the incidence of renal failure with high doses of methotrexate can be decreased. The clinical picture of methotrexate-induced renal failure is that of a non-oliguric renal failure. Preventive measures when using high doses of methotrexate include aggressive intravenous hydration with saline and urine alkalinization with sodium bicarbonate to maintain a urine pH around 7.0. If renal failure develops, methotrexate levels will increase and the risk for systemic toxicity will also be enhanced. In addition to supportive measures, patients should be started on folinic acid rescue, until levels of methotrexate fall below 0.5 uM.

LATE COMPLICATIONS OF CANCER CHEMOTHERAPY

As cancer therapy has become increasingly effective and more patients live longer, late complications have become apparent separate from the direct toxic effects on organ system function described above. Gonadal dysfunction is one. In males, the primary lesion is depletion of germinal epithelium of seminiferous tubules with marked decrease in testicular volume, oligo- or azoospermia and infertility. There is an increase in follicle-stimulating hormone (FSH) and occasionally in luteinizing hormone (LH). No change is seen in serum testosterone. Alkylating agents (and irradiation) are the most damaging and toxicity is dose related. About 80% of males with Hodgkin's disease treated with MOPP are oligo-azoospermic. About half recover in up to 4 years. Procarbazine is a major offender. Anthracyclines also cause azoospermia in a dose-related fashion. In females, the primary lesion is ovarian fibrosis and follicle destruction. Amenorrhea ensues with increase in FSH and LH and a decrease in estradiol leading to vaginal atrophy and endometrial hypoplasia. Onset and duration are dose and age related. Alkylating agents (and irradiation) again are the worst offenders.

In children, the prepubertal effects may be less profound and reversible in males, though the pubertal effects may be more severe with often irreversible azoospermia, decreased testosterone and increased FSH and LH. Less is known about females, but young girls appear quite resistant to alkylating agents.

No more tragic toxicity is seen with cancer chemotherapeutic agents than the induction of a second, treatment-related cancer in a patient cured of one cancer. Of the wide variety of environmental and chemical agents causing cancer, there is one common thread in their mode of action–interaction with DNA. Clinical studies detailing this consequence of therapy have many problems, including the inherent bias of reporting index cases, the retrospective nature of many reports, the lack of reliable information on drug dosage, total amount of drug given and duration of therapy and the underlying incidence of second malignancy. The direct-acting alkylating agents are most often implicated and chronic, low-dose administration is a greater risk factor. Acute non-lymphocytic leukemia or myelodysplasia is the best described. The indirect-acting topoisomerase II agents produce a specific 11q23 translocation.

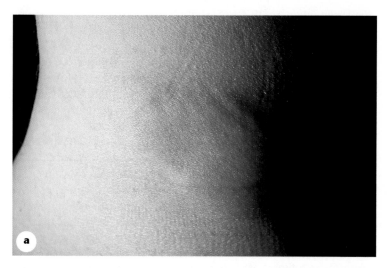

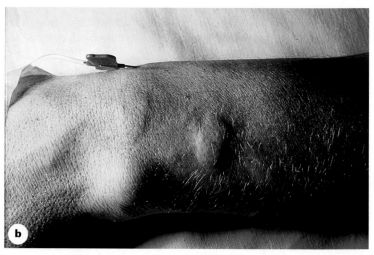

Fig. 18.1 Acute hypersensitivity reactions. (**a**) Urticaria, with giant localized hives, occurred in a 40-year-old man within a few minutes of receiving intravenous 5-fluorouracil and (**b**) in the lower arm of a 50-year-old man after receiving adriamycin. The urticaria was self-limited in both patients.

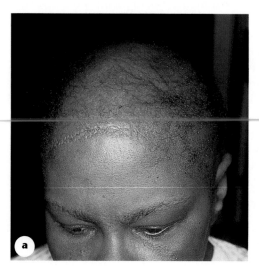

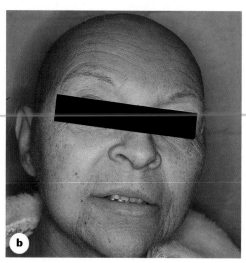

Fig. 18.2 Alopecia. (**a**) Near-total alopecia in a 38-year-old woman receiving cyclophosphamide and adriamycin. Note loss of eyebrow and eyelid hair. (**b**) Total alopecia developed in this 64-year-old woman due to chemotherapy and cranial irradiation for brain metastases. The duration of alopecia after both treatment modalities may be many months or even permanent in some patients. In this woman, the scalp edema and erythema are related to an allergic cutaneous reaction from diphenylhydantonin.

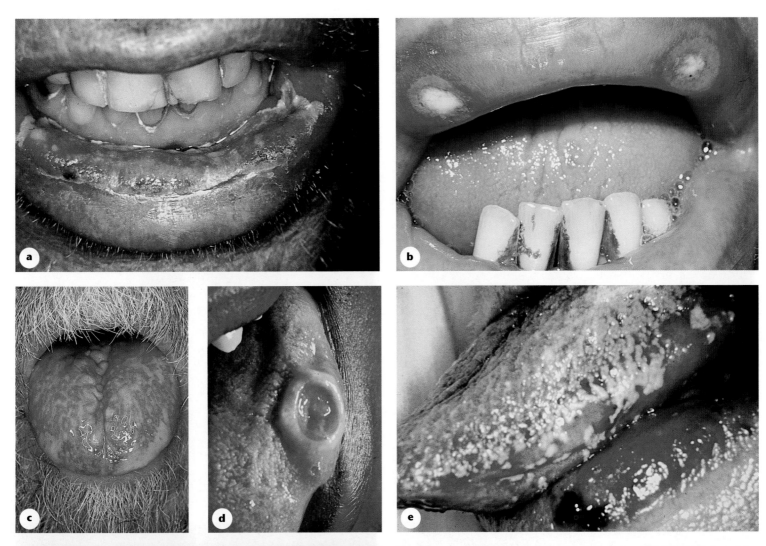

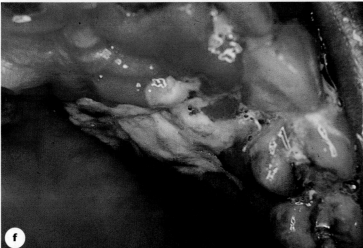

Fig. 18.3 Stomatitis and mucositis. (**a**) Marked stomatitis in a patient receiving methotrexate. (**b**) Aphthous stomatitis related to severe granulocytopenia after chemotherapy. The ulcers may be due to herpes simplex or other infection. (**c**) Mucositis in a patient receiving combination chemotherapy for head and neck cancer. (**d**) Marked ulcer of the tongue in a 32-year-old man receiving induction chemotherapy for acute leukemia. (**e**) Mucositis of the tongue due to monilia infection (thrush) in a patient receiving corticosteroids for brain metastases. (**f**) Marked oral mucositis due to mixed infection in a patient receiving chemotherapy for acute leukemia.

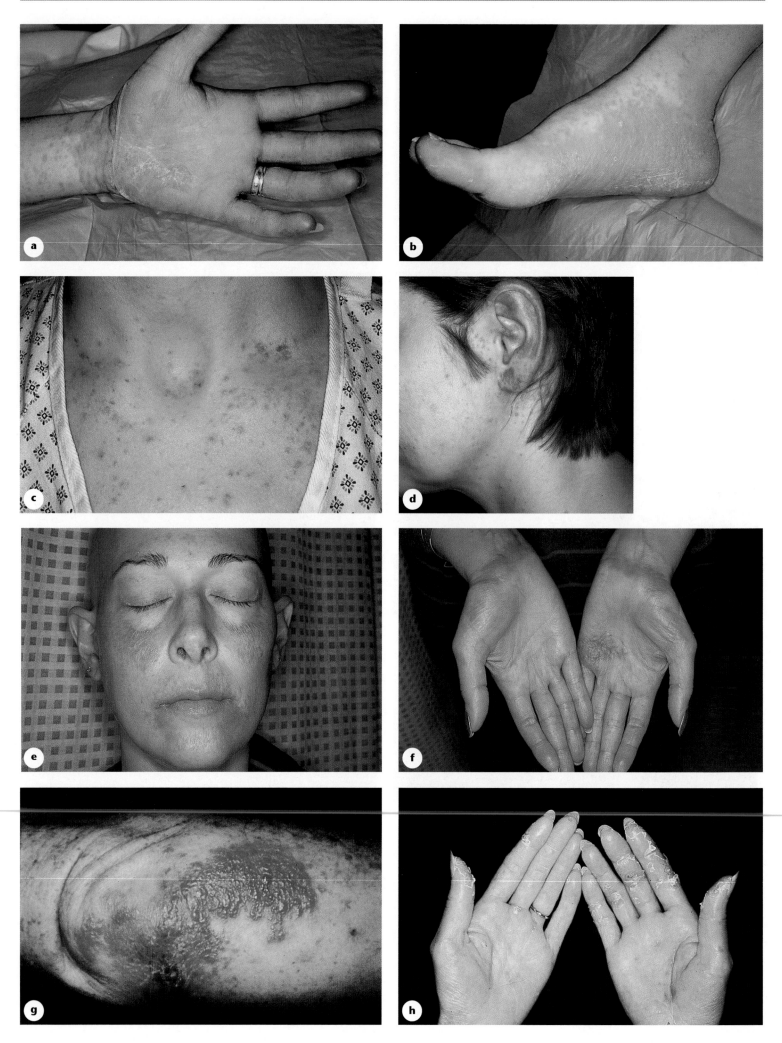

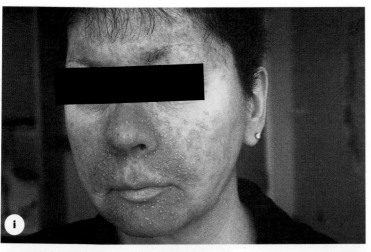

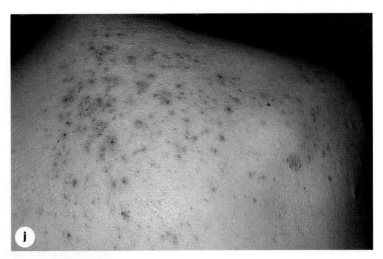

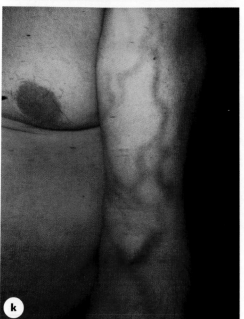

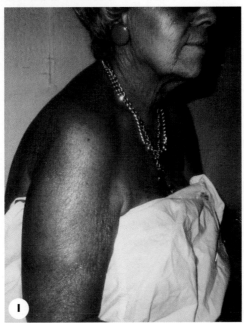

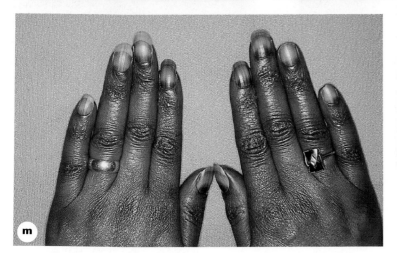

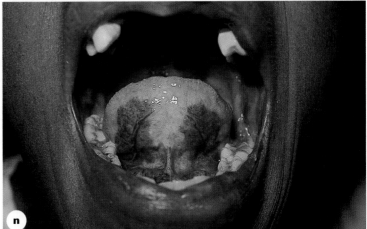

Fig. 18.4 (**a,b**) Dermatitis, skin rashes and hyperpigmentation: hand–foot syndrome related to 5-fluorouracil chemotherapy in metastatic colon cancer. Note the erythema, edema, rash and early skin desquamation. Severe pain is associated with this toxic reaction. (**c,d**) Skin reaction to Ara-C. Note erythematous macular rash on chest and diffuse erythema and edema of ears in this 22-year-old woman receiving Ara-C for acute leukemia. (**e,f**) Skin reaction to docetaxel. Note periorbital and malar flush along with erythema and edema of palms in this patient. (**g,h**) Cutaneous reactions to bleomycin include raised, erythematous and pruritic lesions around pressure points, especially the elbows (**g**), also desquamation of skin (**h**). (**i,j**) Acne-form skin lesions occur in patients on ZD-1839 (Iressa), especially on the face (**i**), chest and back (**j**). These rashes may regress when the drug is temporarily withheld or the dose is lowered. Similar skin reactions occur after actinomycin-D and corticosteroids. (**k**) Hyperpigmentation of the skin along veins occurs after use of many chemotherapeutic agents, including navelbine, actinomycin-D and 5-fluorouracil infusion, as in this patient. In many cases, the veins become sclerotic due to thrombophlebitis. (**l–n**) Hyperpigmentation of the skin occurs after 5-fluorouracil (**l**), adriamycin (**m**) and other drugs, while increased pigment in the mucous membranes (**n**) and nails (**m**) is mainly related to adriamycin. (Also see Fig. 18.6b).

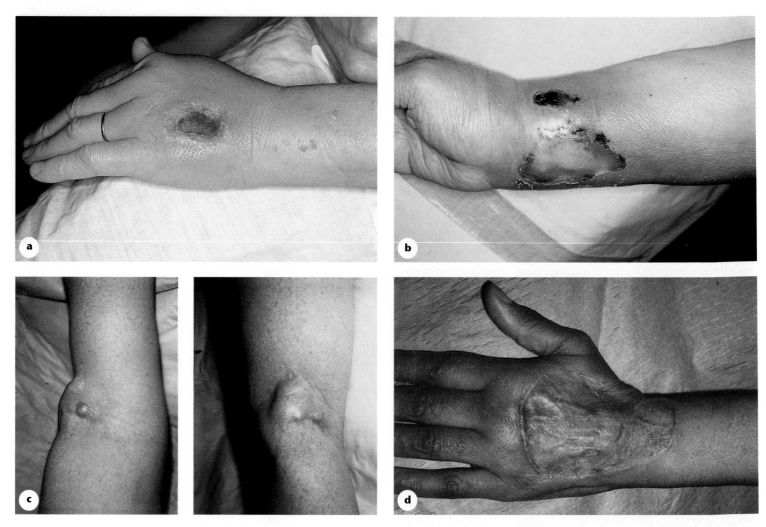

Fig. 18.5 (**a–d**) Extravasation of drugs and skin ulcers occurs with vesicant drugs including adriamycin (**a,b** acute changes, **c** chronic healed scarring), mitomycin-C (**d**), actinomycin-D, vincristine and navelbine. Immediate medical attention is necessary and sometimes skin grafts are required (see text).

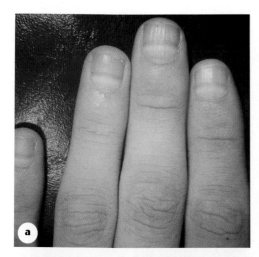

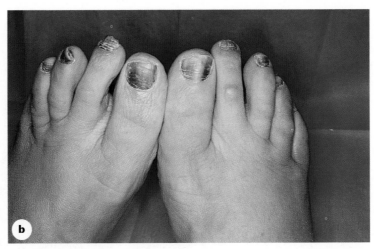

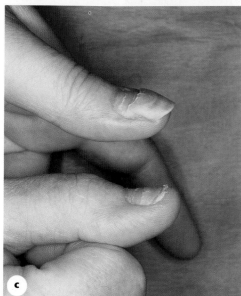

Fig. 18.6 Nail changes are often seen after prolonged chemotherapy. (**a**) Banding of the nails results from growth interruptions in the nail germinal cell layer by the cytostatic effect of chemotherapy. These white bands (called Mee's lines) will grow outward eventually. Beau's lines are transverse grooves across the nail plate due to temporary nail matrix malfunction, seen with chemotherapy or associated with other illnesses (acute coronary or severe febrile episodes). Nail hyperpigmentation occurs occasionally after prolonged use of adriamycin (**b**) especially in people with dark skin. Onycholysis or separation of the nail from its bed is associated with use of adriamycin (**c**), cyclophosphamide and the taxanes. (Also see Fig. 8.82).

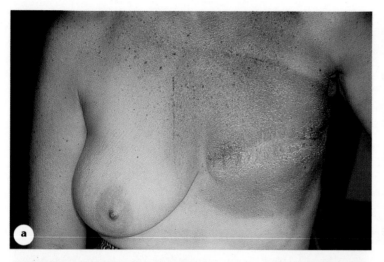

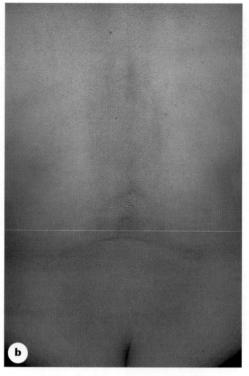

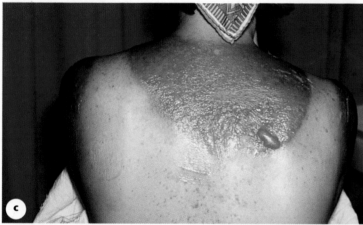

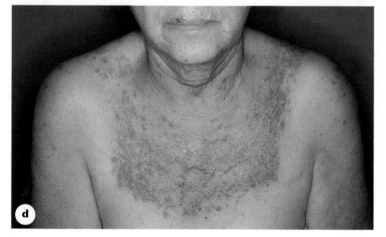

Fig. 18.7 Radiation recall dermatitis may occur in a radiotherapy treatment field after systemic chemotherapy, with development of hyperemia and then hyperpigmentation in the healing phase (**a**). The patient in (**a**) received adjuvant alkeran 1 month after postoperative radiation to the chest wall. (**b**) This patient had radiation therapy to the lower spine for bone metastases from breast cancer and developed recall dermatitis 6 months later, when gemcitabine was administered. (**c**) Chemotherapy can also sensitize the skin to adverse reactions to solar radiation. This young woman developed severe dermatitis in a sun-exposed area while taking methotrexate. (**d**) This patient also developed acute dermatitis in a sun-exposed area while receiving 5-fluorouracil. See text for discussion of radiation recall in organs such as the heart, lung and esophagus.

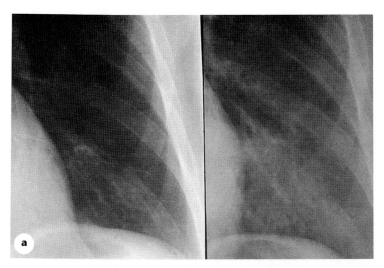

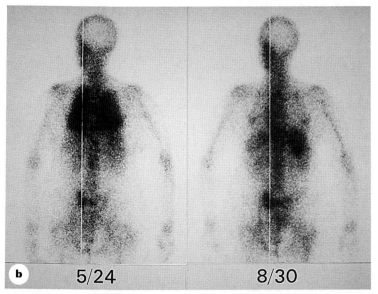

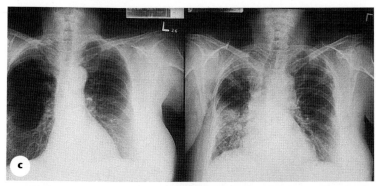

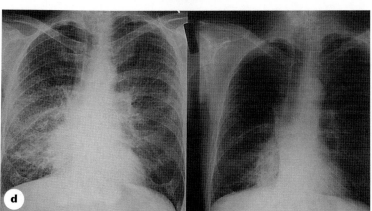

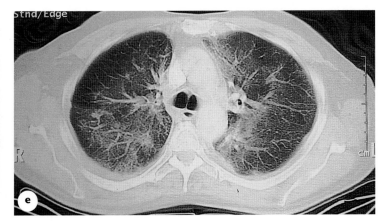

Fig. 18.8 Organ toxicity. Non-mucocutaneous toxicity of chemotherapeutic agents is covered in the text. The lung may be affected by several agents including bleomycin. (**a**) The earliest radiographic changes are linear infiltrates in the lower lung fields. (**b**) Gallium-67 uptake is quite striking but is reversible, as this serial study demonstrates. (**c**) While usually dose related, progressive changes may occur resulting in fibrosis and pulmonary insufficiency. Other drugs such as alkylating agents and high-dose methotrexate (**d**) may result in diffuse infiltrates, which were reversible 4 months later. (**e**) In this patient several courses of gemcitabine resulted in acute dyspnea and decreased oxygen saturation. Evaluation with lung biopsy and other studies showed no evidence of infection, pulmonary emboli or other diagnosable disease. Use of prednisone led to rapid improvement and regression of the interstitial infiltrates.

REFERENCES

Adrian RM, Hood, AF, Skarin AT. Mucocutaneous reactions to antineoplastic agents. CA J Clin 1980; 30 : 143–157.

Attar EC, Ervin T, Janicek M, Deykin A, Godleski J: Acute interstitial pneumonitis related to gemcitabine. J Clin Oncol 2000; 18 : 697–698.

Burstein H: Radiation recall dermatitis from gemcitabine. J Clin Oncol 2000; 18 : 693–694.

Chabner BA, Longo DL: Cancer Chemotherapy and Biotherapy, 2nd edn. Lippincott–Raven, Philadelphia, 1996.

DeVita VT Jr, Hellman S, Rosenberg SA: Cancer: Principles and Practice of Oncology, 4th edn. Lippincott, Philadelphia, 1993.

Darnell J, Lodish H, Baltimore D: Molecular Cell Biology, 3rd edn. W.H. Freeman, New York, 1995.

Eder, JP: Neoplasms. In: Page CP, Curtis MJ, Sutter MC, Walker MJA, Hoffman BB, eds: Integrated Pharmacology. Mosby–Times Mirror International, London, 1997 : 501–522.

Hussain S, Anderson DN, Salvatti ME, Adamson B, McManus M, Braverman AS: Onycholysis as a complication of systemic chemotherapy. Cancer 2000; 88 : 2367–2371.

Perry MD: The Chemotherapy Source Book. Williams and Wilkins, Baltimore, 1992.

Skeel RT: Handbook of Cancer Chemotherapy. Little, Brown, Boston, 1991.

Sonis ST, Fey EG. Oral complications of cancer therapy. Oncology 16: 680–691, 2002.

Index